ANNUAL REVIEW OF NUTRITION

ANNUAL REVIEW OF NUTRITION

VOLUME 2, 1982

WILLIAM J. DARBY, *Editor*
Nutrition Foundation

HARRY P. BROQUIST, *Associate Editor*
Vanderbilt University

ROBERT E. OLSON, *Associate Editor*
St. Louis University

ANNUAL REVIEWS INC.   4139 EL CAMINO WAY,   PALO ALTO, CALIFORNIA 94306 USA

ANNUAL REVIEWS INC.
Palo Alto, California, USA

International Standard Serial Number: 0199-9885
International Standard Book Number: 0-8243-2802-7

Annual Reviews Inc. and the Editors of its publications assume no responsibility for the statements expressed by the contributors to this *Review*.

PREFACE

In planning the second volume of the *Annual Review of Nutrition* the Editorial Committee has adhered to the intention that guided selection of topics for the initial volume—to display the wide scope of the subject through "critical, authoritative surveys of the original literature describing the current developments in the science of nutrition." As the complexity and breadth of nutrition cannot be explored fully in a single volume, we plan to concentrate on the major aspects of the field in turn, cycling at multi-year intervals to reassess topics reviewed in the past. Matters of immediate interest, or in which rapid advance is currently taking place, will be reviewed promptly.

Since the production process at Annual Reviews does not enable us to co-position related chapters within each volume, our dual Table of Contents displays both the usual sequence of chapters by page number, and related chapters grouped by category of interest. For the convenience of the reader, the categorical Table of Contents for the current volume also lists the chapters of Volume 1.

The continued excitement of discovery in the science of nutrition is evident to the reader of these reviews. Equally clear is the satisfying evidence of the vast improvement in health care, preventive medicine, and therapy that is occurring through assimilation into practice of the basic scientific understanding generated by research—experimental, observational, chemical, and genetic, whether in vivo, in vitro, clinical, or epidemiologic.

The opening chapter of this second volume is timely because its publication coincides with that of several recent accounts of the long evolution of the understanding of pellagra. Dr. William Bean's essay brings the reader a series of fascinating personal reflections concerning the elucidation of this clinical syndrome. It is written by a scholar who was associated with two prolific centers of study (Birmingham and Cincinnati) from which came notes, papers, and observations that contributed to definition of the role(s) of B-vitamins in clinical nutrition. Dr. Bean's recollections of and reflections on human experimentation provide much ethical wisdom for today's investigator of newly recognized syndromes of nutritional origin. Readers who enjoy perusing this essay will also want to reread Dr. Bean's 1952

Presidential Address to the American Society of Clinical Nutrition (The Clinician Interrogates Nutrition. *Am. J. Clin. Nutr.* 13:263-74), including its text of the Pellagra Song.

The Editors are grateful both to the authors who have so generously contributed to this second volume and to the staff of Annual Reviews Inc. for their painstaking efforts throughout the planning and production of Volume 2.

William J. Darby
Harry P. Broquist
Robert E. Olson

Annual Review of Nutrition
Volume 2, 1982

CONTENTS

CONTENTS OF VOLUMES 1 AND 2 ARRANGED BY CATEGORY

RELATED ARTICLES IN OTHER *ANNUAL REVIEWS*

From the *Annual Review of Physiology*, Volume 44 (1982):

   Energetics and Mechanics of Terrestrial Locomotion, C. R. Taylor and N. C. Heglund

From the *Annual Review of Public Health*, Volume 3 (1982):

   Reproductive Toxicity of Environmental Agents, K. S. Rao and B. A. Schwetz

   Epidemiological Approaches to Cancer Etiology, J. F. Fraument, Jr.

   Drinking Water and Cancer: Review of Recent Epidemiological Findings and Assessment of Risks, K. S. Crump and H. A. Guess

   Water and Wastewater Quality Control and the Public Health, B. B. Berger

   Health Consequences of Wastewater Reuse, H. J. Ongerth and J. E. Ongerth

From the *Annual Review of Medicine*, Volume 33 (1982):

   Major Drug Interactions: Effect of Liver Disease, Alcohol, and Malnutrition, A. M. Hoyumpa, Jr. and S. Schenker

   Thirst and Its Disorders, B. Andersson and M. Rundgren

   Effects of Alcohol on Hepatic Transport of Proteins, E. Baraona and C. S. Lieber

   The Effects of Alcohol on Folate Metabolism, R. S. Hillman and S. E. Steinberg

   Clinical Removal of Iron, R. Propper and D. Nathan

   Clinical Disorders of Hyperkalemia, R. A. DeFronzo, M. Bia, and D. Smith

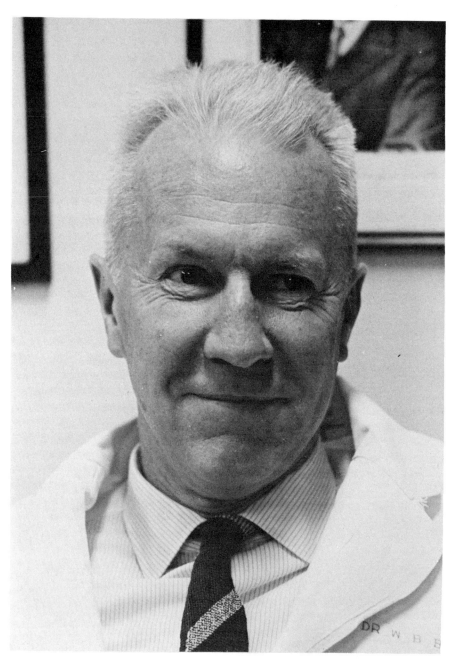

Ann. Rev. Nutr. 1982. 2:1-20

PERSONAL REFLECTIONS ON CLINICAL INVESTIGATIONS

William B. Bean[1]

Department of Internal Medicine, University of Iowa, Iowa City, IA 52240

Introduction

I was fortunate to participate in one of the explosive phases of clinical nutrition more than 40 years ago, just before World War II began. At that time water-soluble vitamin B was becoming the vitamin-B complex, budding off many separate new vitamins. These were being discovered by students of animal nutrition and biochemistry, and by those interested in the nutritional growth requirements of such lowly organisms as bacteria, yeasts, and fungi.

As an undergraduate medical student at the University of Virginia, I saw pellagra. We were told about malnutrition and Goldberger's work. I saw one pellagra patient on the Osler Service at Johns Hopkins in 1935–1936. The next year, when I went to the Thorndike Laboratory, Soma Weiss and Robert Wilkins were in the midst of their exciting studies demonstrating that vitamin B_1, thiamin, quieted the alarming and precarious hyperdynamic state of the circulation in beri-beri, then so prevalent among the alcoholic gentry who crowded into the Boston City Hospital.

In 1937 I went to work in Marion Blankenhorn's Department of Medicine in Cincinnati. It was an exciting place to be. Gene Stead, Gene Ferris, Johnson McGuire, Leon Schiff, Lee Foshay, and others there were stimulating young investigators and teachers. Tom Spies had done excellent clinical studies on pellagra at the Lakeside Hospital in Cleveland and the Cincinnati General Hospital. Near the end of my year as a senior medical resident an

---

[1]William B. Bean, medical scholar—physician, clinical investigator, editor, teacher, writer, and medical philosopher—was intimately involved in clinical nutrition research during the exciting era of discoveries of the 1930s–1950s. His reflections on clinical research in and knowledge of nutrition during that period of more direct, relatively uncomplicated, less restrictive investigations provide much wisdom for consideration by investigative-minded physicians today.

1

0199-9885/82/0715-0001$.02.00

opportunity arose to work as a Fellow in nutrition. I had no special competence in the field of human nutrition but had helped Soma Weiss and Bob
Wilkins in some of their clinical experiments. A good friend of Blankenhorn, Dr. James McLester of Birmingham, Alabama, still skeptical of the
ideas introduced by Goldberger, welcomed Tom Spies to Birmingham to see
if he could get the same good results in treating desperately ill pellagrins
there that he had obtained in Ohio. The mobility of the staff, which shifted
to Birmingham for the spring and summer months and then returned to
Cincinnati for the fall and winter months, was remarkable. Richard and Sue
Vilter and I had the main clinical and laboratory responsibilities. In the
considerable outpouring of papers from the nutrition clinic, Spies's name
led all the rest. Charles Aring, Cincinnati neurologist, essayist, and scholar,
made prominent contributions to the thiamin and beri-beri studies. Many
physicians, biochemists, nurses, dentists, and others from various medical
schools in the country were eager participants. In addition to A. B. Chinn
and Blankenhorn, the following co-workers are listed alphabetically: W. F.
Ashe, A. E. Axelrod, W. Beckh, C. E. Bills, Hugh Butt, C. Cogswell, Clark
Cooper, Zola K. Cooper, G. Delfs, R. Eakin, Conrad Elvehjem, Joe P.
Evans, E. Gross, Morton Hamburger, Harold E. Himwich, M. P. Hudson,
T. H. Jukes, Walter F. Lever, J. B. McLester, A. W. Mann, V. Minnick,
Carl V. Moore, Robert A. Moore, Gordon R. Morey, Milton Rosenbaum,
J. M. Ruegsegger, E. E. Snell, S. R. Stanbury, R. E. Stone, E. P. Swain,
Emory D. Warner, R. J. Williams. After I had left Carl Vilter and Wally
Frommeyer were important contributors.

A Note on the History of Pellagra

Three recently published books (25a, 27a, 40a) afford detailed accounts of
the history of pellagra. These and the earlier compilation of selected reprints
of Joseph Goldberger and an evaluation of his classical studies of the
disease, *Goldberger on Pellagra* by Milton Terris (62a), make it redundant
to detail here an account of the evolution of understanding of this fascinating deficiency syndrome. Rather, I recall here but a few especially poignant
personal recollections pertinent to my own early involvement with clinical
evidence concerning pellagra.

For more than two hundred years the nature of pellagra had been a
subject of great debate and confusion (32). Many drugs had been tested on
severely ill pellagrins brought into a hospital, put to bed, and given fluids
and good nursing care. For a brief time many experienced clinical improvement. Spies had shown that this might occur even while they were eating
a pellagra-producing diet or given nothing but salt solution and dextrose.
Such a program, however, could not be continued long or the patients
would suddenly get sicker and might die if the elements missing from the
diet were not restored in ample quantities.

Perhaps the first controlled study in human nutrition after Lind's observation on scurvy was Cerri's study of pellagra carried out in Milan, Italy in 1795 and 1796 (32). Cerri was convinced that a diet made up largely of corn and corn products somehow explained the very high incidence of pellagra among the country folk. He selected ten of them, who for two years moved to town and ate the diet common to those in the city. On this regimen no signs of pellagra developed, while in the peasant controls in the country the incidence remained high. The following year the subjects were allowed to revert to their polenta (corn meal) diet, and pellagra returned as usual. One, however, was so much impressed that he got work in the city and never had pellagra again. These observations have been largely neglected by those who have written on pellagra.

A good example of the pre-Goldberger confusion is found in a 1912 book entitled *Report of the Pellagra Commission of the State of Illinois* (40). It describes the distressing outbreak of pellagra in Illinois mental hospitals from 1909–1911. Of the 258 patients with pellagra in Peoria, 128 died. In Kankakee, with fewer patients, 40% died, and about a third died at the Elgin State Hospital [subsequently the site of a long series of remarkable studies by Horwitt et al, in which deficiencies of niacin, thiamine, riboflavin, or tocopherol were induced by feeding diets deficient in the nutrients. These studies were made in collaboration between the Food and Nutrition Board of the National Research Council and the Elgin State Hospital over a 23-year period (33a)]. At that time all the Commission could think of were infections. Study of fecal bacteria occupied 105 pages of the special report, which then proceeded to complement fixation tests, cutaneous tests with corn extracts in pellagrins, and a learned discourse on black flies and buffalo gnats, including beautiful drawings of the various larval phases of the Simulium in Illinois. An essay on the protozoan infections was followed by dietary studies from the hospital concerned only with the food as issued, not the food as eaten. A corn-free diet was compared with a mainly-corn diet without definite conclusions. The experiment is a good example of how not to do a study comparing one food with another. In the summary the authors wrote that "the lack of definite information regarding the food requirements and metabolism in the class of subjects experimented upon has made it difficult to interpret the results obtained in these studies." A rather wistful comment added that "the experimental work here reported is in itself brief and is not extensive enough to allow any broad interpretation."

Joseph Goldberger Solves the Problem

The spectacular prevalence of pellagra in the Southern states seemed related to poverty. Of course, infection was known to follow poverty fairly closely. In 1914, Joseph Goldberger of the US Public Health Service, the old Marine Hospital Service, was sent to Georgia to see if the peculiar epidemiology of pellagra indicated an infection. The seasonal peak of pellagra occurred in the late spring and early summer, some two or three months before the peak intensity of sunshine and heat. In cotton towns the disease clustered among the homes of workers who lived in poor quarters, often along the banks of streams or rivers subjected to flooding, and largely without plumbing. Goldberger's work in solving certain epidemics of insect-borne skin disorders made him a logical person to find some kind of infecting organism. In the South, Goldberger was under the triple jeopardy of being a Yankee, a Federal Government worker, and a Jew. His assignment seemed to add Northern insult to Southern injury, though eventually some southerners accepted the surprising results of his heroic experiments.

Goldberger not only tormented himself as an experimental subject, he also used his wife as a subject in hair-raising ingestions or injections of horrible samples of the effluvia of very ill victims of pellagra. While this ranks high as an example of heroic autoexperimentation and of a wife's devotion, it failed to reveal any infecting organism. Indeed, Goldberger was well aware of the fact that nurses, attendants, and physicians almost never got pellagra in asylums, hospitals, or prisons. Thus having found no infection, he turned to study of diet. After he learned what the people who developed pellagra customarily ate, he obtained convict volunteers as subjects, promised them early reprieve, and fed them the same food as customarily eaten by those developing pellagra. After many months the prisoners developed pellagra, which cleared up on a good diet. Goldberger found, in particular, that inexpensive brewer's yeast was a good biological food for treatment or prevention. He suspected that an amino acid deficiency, particularly that of tryptophane, was important—a suggestion made by Sandwith as early as 1913 (29–31, 41a).

Nicotinic Acid: The New Era

In 1937, Elvehjem, Woolley, and their associates (27) found that canine black tongue, which Goldberger had identified as a good experimental model of human pellagra, was relieved dramatically by nicotinic acid. It was most interesting to see the spectacular and sometimes astonishing efforts to establish priority of publication in nailing nicotinic acid to the clinical mast. In New Orleans, Durham, Augusta, Birmingham, and Cincinnati there was a great scurrying around to find out what nicotinic acid might do for sick pellagrins.

The name nicotinic acid for this derivative of nicotine was rather frightening (48–52), and the term niacin was coined to avoid any implication of a toxic material. A dramatic and alarming, but fortunately innocuous, event occurred when Spies and his associates each took a quantity of nicotinic acid by mouth. Soon, to their astonishment, they developed a blotchy erythema of the face and upper body. Some experienced a pounding headache and a little nausea. No doubt anxiety was a part of the reaction, which fortunately soon passed without damage.

Later on I studied whether nicotinic acid and related compounds that did not produce flushing were effective in the prevention and treatment of pellagra. Several, indeed, had this property. In order to study the great variety of compounds to determine what specifically caused the flushing, it was necessary to measure skin temperature in fasting subjects. Since many compounds had to be prepared and were available in small quantities, the tests involved the intravenous injection of 20 mg of the experimental compounds, each of which I had previously tested on myself. Subjects lay flat on their backs, lightly clad, in a constant-temperature room at 20°C. This produced a steady state of vasoconstriction so that vasodilation could be measured readily. Skin temperatures were read off a galvanometer. The specific molecules that produced flushing were those of nicotinic acid and its various salts. Pellagra could be treated effectively with nicotinamide, which did not produce the unpleasant flush (3).

The Self as Subject

As illustrated by this experience, autoexperimentation was usually the beginning of clinical research in nutrition. I have done hundreds of such experiments with no apparent ill effects. A near miss occurred, however, when I was a busy nutrition Fellow with many clinical and teaching responsibilities. For nearly two weeks I took a pellagra-producing diet and lost ten pounds in ten days, mostly from an inability to eat enough of the cornbread, hominy, fat back, and molasses to supply calories. I was exhausted and unable to do my work, so I stopped the test, which was not expected to produce results for months. This experience made me acutely aware of the other side of the patient-physician interaction. Therefore, in testing various compounds for effects on malnourished persons we ate or injected them into ourselves before giving them to patients. Later, extensive experiments of many kinds were done in the Army with the medical officers undergoing practically all of the test routines before or while our soldier subjects were tested.

The Inertia and Momentum of Clinical Signs of Malnutrition

Food provides material for constructing the fabric of the body and for the energy for the multitude of functions that constitute cell life. After growth is complete, repair and renewal require energy, as do the daily metabolic functions of the body.

Malnutrition begins when supplies are low. For water-soluble vitamins this occurs more rapidly than with fat-soluble vitamins, some of which are retained with great tenacity. A deficiency at the biochemical level begins to interfere with various functions, causing pathophysiological changes. The organic lesions of niacin deficiency are at first microscopic but become grossly visible as clinical hallmarks of disease of gut, skin, and nervous system. Stomatitis and diarrhea occur. The initial changes in the skin of the malnourished look like a second degree burn, a mild scald, or a severe sunburn. The skin becomes pigmented, desquamates, and sometimes regenerates with the cracking of crazy-pavement epithelium. In localization, regional forces are important. A skin lesion may be progressing in one place while it is healing and regenerating in another. Individual variation in susceptibility is also significant.

It was logical to suppose that nicotinic acid played its role through its function in respiratory enzyme systems. For this reason it was important to find chemical methods to obtain information about the blood level of such enzymes. In 1939, Richard and Sue Vilter published with Tom Spies a microbiological method for determining the level of codehydrogenase (cozymase) in the blood and urine of pellagrins and normal persons (64, 65, 67). The assay of the enzymes was a logical approach to classification and measurement, but later clinical study provided most of the key information on nicotinic acid deficiency. Levels of these pyridine compounds were low in people with pellagra, but also in many persons with diabetes, leukemia, Roentgen sickness, and pneumococcal pneumonia (9, 64, 65). Sometimes the levels were decreased in other infections, in various fevers, and after extreme physical exercise.

It was a puzzling problem to Spies and others that while eating the pellagra-producing diets, pellagrins who are hospitalized might have their lesions improve or even disappear. It began to be obvious that the upset balance between demand and supply could be rectified temporarily by reducing the need as well as by normalizing or increasing the intake. Any agent given at this time that had no specific effect might be credited for the therapeutic improvement that followed.

Biosynthesis, which is important in ruminants, is much less significant in human beings since the colon, where most bacterial action occurs, is too far down the alimentary canal for very effective absorption.

Indirect effects of test substances must also be remembered in therapeutic testing. For instance, if nicotinic acid is given to someone with pellagra and beri-beri while the individual remains on a poor diet, digestion and absorption may improve enough so that thiamin is absorbed in quantities adequate to correct the thiamin deficiency and thus relieves the beri-beri (16).

Deficiencies may take months or years to produce clinical changes. It is not surprising that restoring the missing vitamins and providing a balanced diet do not always produce rapid effects. This is particularly true in lesions involving the nervous system. When a nerve cell is killed, no treatment can repair the damage. However, in many patients with the peripheral neuropathies of beri-beri, slow improvement occurs over a period of months of carefully continued treatment (16).

Because of the diversified metabolic missions of various cells, specific deficiencies may interfere with certain functions of cells before others. The study of nutrition is full of surprises. Krehl, Elvehjem, and colleagues (34) found that the essential amino acid, tryptophane, can be converted into niacin and thus can prevent or cure pellagra. This was a unique example of the conversion of an essential amino acid into an essential vitamin. On the other hand, an abundance of niacin does not take the place of tryptophane in human nutrition, so it is a one way street. It is of note that Goldberger suggested tryptophane deficiency as a contributory mechanism in the development of pellagra (31).

Vitamins undoubtedly may serve as placebos. The confidence engendered by coming to a famous nutrition clinic well-known for benefiting many persons may assist in generating great subjective improvement. Where most manifestations are subjective, the interpretation of improvement must be made in the light of this significant point. Hospitals have lost some of their terror and famous clinics have achieved famous cures. Faith has helped ailing humanity, as at Lourdes. Psychosomatic factors must be investigated, controlled, and evaluated, particularly where manifestations contain so much that is subjective (16).

My observations on pellagra led me to believe that a major source of the arguments and disagreements among observers resulted from significant variation in the quality of corn in different southern regions—i.e. from the amount of nicotinic acid and perhaps of tryptophane in the diet. Certainly when we learned about tryptophane a number of mysteries were cleared up. Diets with more nicotinic acid were sometimes associated with more pellagra, rather than the other way around. Later studies of bound niacin further clarified concepts.

It is still a matter of conjecture why mechanical defects such as intestinal shunts may be followed now by pellagra, now by beri-beri, now by macrocytic or microcytic anemia, or by apparently reasonable health in what seem to be precisely comparable circumstances (4, 6). (See the review by Young & Blass in this volume.)

Unilateral and Experimental Lesions Produced Without Sunlight

Goldberger, who made so many capital observations on pellagra, observed that atypical lesions may readily occur.

It may be stated as the rule, that if the back of one hand, or one foot, one elbow, one knee, one side of the neck, one cheek, or the lid of one eye is affected then the corresponding part of the other side of the body is assumed to become similarly affected and affected to almost exactly the same degree. This rule, however, is not without many exceptions. It must not be hastily assumed, therefore, that the possibility of pellagra is necessarily excluded because the back of the head or of one foot or of one side of the neck alone seems to be involved or is involved to so slight an extent to be almost nothing in comparison with the other side.

Stannus, in his classic review of the theories of the cause of pellagra (62), observed that "the facts in regard to the distribution of the exanthem in pellagra may be stated in reality quite simply, though they appear to have escaped the observations of most pellagrologists. The exanthem tends to appear in those areas of the skin which in any particular individual have *undergone certain changes* as the result of the action *in the past* of traumata of various kinds including solar radiation, exposure to cold, friction, pressure, irritants, etc." This is also true of skin lesions in many other diseases.

I made a careful study in 1940 and 1941 of a series of patients who had asymmetric or unilateral lesions as well as bilaterally symmetrical ones (8). Five cases of asymmetric lesions were observed in persons with varicose veins that were more severe on one side than the other. Trauma, pressure, and irritation were found to be the cause in five other cases. Infection was responsible in two, paralysis was found in one, and no cause could be found in two. Asymmetrical lesions on the elbow occurred only in patients confined to bed who, if right-handed, rested on the left elbow. A one-sided lesion was associated with asymmetrical varicose veins in patients who were ambulatory. In none of the patients we observed was sunlight a provoking cause, although Plunkett (39) noticed that a one-sided exposure to sunlight or wind damaged the skin and gave rise to asymmetrical localization.

In the middle 1930s Spies had demonstrated that glossitis was a much more sensitive gauge of the clinical stage of pellagra than the skin; skin lesions might clear up while patients were eating a pellagra-producing diet. Such a diet might ultimately lead to skin lesions in persons not exposed to sun. Dermatitis in the pudendal region had been known for a long time. There was thus much argument about the specificity of sunlight in the disease. For this reason, early in 1941 I undertook to determine whether by reducing the blood flow to the skin and increasing its metabolism by the use of a heating pad the localization of skin lesions could be encouraged. This had to be done during the prodromal stage of the disease, perhaps months and certainly weeks before the clinical manifestations were expected. For one or two hours a day for a period of more than two weeks, I put a cuff on my arm, set the pressure well over the level of systolic blood pressure, and wrapped an electric heating pad around. After several days' testing the skin developed the so-called fire stains, or *erythema ab igne,* the reticulated, mottled, pigmented network seen in those who have used a hot water bottle or an electric heating pad for a long time or have sat long in front of an open fire or a hot water radiator. No other manifestation occurred, and after a few weeks my arm resumed its normal appearance. I concluded that the method was probably safe to use in persons whose history led us to believe they would develop an annual relapse in pellagra. We used the tourniquet method of producing ischemia in several persons before encountering an example of neuropathy. This mishap occurred in a malnourished man in his early 30s who had had annual attacks of pellagra for several years. I used the method of heat and ischemia that I had used on myself, but only for 15 minutes. To my surprise and consternation, this produced a neuropathy that included both paralysis of the muscles and a loss of the sensations of touch and pain. Fortunately, the condition cleared up in a few hours. This led me to use simple sandbags to weight the electric heat pad. The weight of the sandbags in place 30 minutes was sufficient without heat to cause reactive hyperemia, indicating effective oxygen deprivation. No further neuropathy occurred, and we used the method in a study of thiamin metabolism and beri-beri. An effective variation of the method was to have the patient lie supine on a firm examining table. The weight of the leg induced ischemia on the back of the calf. In two of five persons with latent pellagra, the induction of ischemia plus heat produced changes in the skin that resulted in a unilateral lesion during a clinical relapse of the disorder in which bilateral dermatitis developed in other parts.

Secondary Pellagra

My studies of diarrheal diseases that give rise to pellagra got me interested in going over the records of all patients with pellagra in the modern period at Lakeside Hospital in Cleveland and at the Cincinnati General Hospital (6). This review was supplemented by an intensive literature search which I had been conducting for years on the history and current understanding of pellagra. Strictly secondary pellagra can be established only when a person on a fixed diet develops pellagra following the development of a disease and gets rid of the pellagra when the disease is reduced or cured. To be sure, the diet is likely to be marginal, but not in itself sufficient to produce the disease. The current state of medicine and science has generally determined current thoughts about pellagra. When first described, its cause was thought to be a toxin or poison on corn, analogous to ergot on rye (32a). In the last third of the 19th century infection dominated thoughts of etiology and convinced many that pellagra was an infection. Sambon incriminated the buffalo gnat. For sixty years the belief that pellagra was an infection prevented progress.

Clearly any disease can dispose to the development of pellagra by disorganizing a person's relationship to his environment. Disorders of the body politic give rise to war and famine, upheavals in personality lead to food fads, dietary cults, and addiction to alcohol; other disabling upsets, including insanity, are important in the background upon which pellagra develops. Even epilepsy, hemiplegia, and parkinsonism may have pellagra engrafted upon them.

It is not easy to separate symptoms of pellagra from those of the diseases of the alimentary canal upon which it may be engrafted. We must consider intestinal hypermotility, decreased enzymatic digestion, inadequate absorption, abnormal bacterial flora, destruction or utilization of vitamins by bacteria, inactivation or binding by various constituents, liver damage and such abnormalities of function as nausea, vomiting, loss of appetite, infection and fever. Thus the alimentary canal from one end to the other can influence nutrition—e.g. damaged teeth or their absence, disease in the gullet, trouble in the stomach including cancer, ulcer, inflammation, syphilis, and a host of diseases of the remaining alimentary canal: parasitism, obstruction, granulomas, tuberculosis, ulcerative colitis, Crohn's disease, shunts, operations, strictures, and functional disorders of the alimentary canal. All such conditions cause conditioned malnutrition. Liver disease, operations, anesthesia, infection, and fever are all important. Women need more nutrients during pregnancy, lactation, and childbirth in order to produce the fetus and placenta and to supply milk later. In addition, a mother is likely to sacrifice her own food in order to feed her child. Hypertension, congestive heart failure, and radiation sickness have had meager systematic study but may have special mechanisms of reducing the pyridine coenzymes. Drugs, chemicals, hemorrhage, and a vast miscellany of nonspecific disorders may also condition occasional instances. It has not been possible to study in isolation a genetic liability to pellagra, mainly because people inherit not only their genes but also, to a surprising degree, their environments. During the period of the Birmingham studies among a large Negro population, blacks provided only 9% of all pellagra patients whereas in Ohio pellagra was two or three times as common in blacks as in whites. It has been my impression that in the old South blacks usually had white friends or a white family who were genuinely concerned with their well-being and saw to it that they got food.

Pellagra in Ohio Hospitals in 1941 and 1949

I did two studies (5, 15) of pellagra in Ohio Hospitals, in Cleveland and Cincinnati (1942) and the other in Cincinnati (1949), where pellagra had been under intensive study for nearly 15 years and underestimation of its frequency, therefore, was unlikely when we studied the effectiveness of new remedies. During the depression in Cleveland and Cincinnati the disease was prevalent, constituting one or two percent of the admissions to the medical services. The figure doubled if readmissions were counted. Despite emphasis on early signs of deficiency, the 1949 study disclosed a spectacular decrease in the frequency beginning between 1939 and 1940. In 1939, 44 pellagrins were admitted to the Cincinnati General Hospital. In 1940 there were three, and by 1946–1947 none. Changes in the vitamin content of white flour began in 1942, two years after pellagra experienced its sharp decline. Vitamin tablets were not used by the Cincinnati patients. The improvement of the economy with retooling for World War II must have improved the diet of many persons who during the depression rarely had food adequate in quality or quantity.

The Birmingham Scene

The social milieu of Birmingham, its southern culture and graces, made it a pleasant place to work. The many visitors to the Spies clinic were entertained as guests at the Mountainbrook Country Club—not only scientists and nutritionists but also publicists, those in pharmaceutical and manufacturing firms, and a number of private persons who were generous and sometimes lavish contributors to the work of Tom Spies and the nutrition clinic. It was my good fortune to more or less fall into the responsibility of looking out for visitors, meeting them at trains and planes and otherwise spending time with them. In this way I had the uncommon and pleasant experience of getting to know Paul DeKruif (26), John Steinbeck, and others who spent weeks or months there gathering information. De Kruif, the gifted author of *Hunger Fighters,* wrote many popular articles about the colorful Dr. Spies and his nutrition clinic. (I do not think Steinbeck ever used his experience in a book.) Joseph Goldberger's widow, who belonged to a prominent New Orleans family, was a charming guest enormously interested in anything having to do with pellagra, nutrition in the South and, naturally, her husband. From the back numbers of the *Southern Medical Journal* I compiled into one volume all the pellagra articles by Goldberger I could find; this volume, supplemented with his papers in the US Public Health Reports, made a nearly complete file of Goldberger's published studies. Mrs. Goldberger was astonished that we knew so much about her husband, that our admiration of him was so great, and that his contributions had been every bit as valuable as she believed. Despite a steady inflow of bourbon whiskey, DeKruif was a vivid and entertaining conversationalist; and once one had penetrated the protective cover of the very shy Steinbeck, whose face was disfigured with acne scars, he, too, was delightful, perceptive, and extremely warm and gentle as well as profoundly intelligent. Just as knowing history gives us a clearer view of reality, so knowing individuals gives us special insights into their creative works and achievements.

In the spring of 1940, Tom Spies told me that I was to present a paper at the New York meeting of the American Medical Association (AMA) and discuss a hundred patients with diarrheal diseases who had developed pellagra (4). I had been in the clinic only a couple of months and could not find any satisfactory records. It was clear to me that we needed to devise accurate, quantitative clinic records and that I would have to find some way of straightening out the strange fascination with round numbers that seemed to exist in the clinic. The only records available had been those kept by the excellent nurses and social workers in the clinic, so I designed a record that became the standard nutritional form in the clinic and is displayed in Spies's paper in the 1943 handbook (38).

I was interested in a variety of clinical observations by that time on fingernails, skin mottling, the triple response, and vascular spiders. These, therefore, were included on the form. The nutrition clinic in Birmingham was the focus of such enormous interest that visitors from all over the country, indeed from many parts of the world, were coming and going. Each was given a copy of the nutrition form, and I became inadvertently responsible for a rather casual assumption that anything found in a pellagra clinic must have something to do with pellagra. Some of the visitors even wrote learned articles about vascular spiders and such things as signs of pellagra. It took a long time to get this heresy removed.

Urinary Pigments in Pellagra

One of the interesting misinterpretations of the early studies was in the Beckh, Ellinger & Spies (BES) tests for pigments in the urine of pellagrins (25). In Spies's article, "The Principles of Diet and the Treatment of Disease" in the 1943 American Medical Association Handbook of Nutrition, he stated that the BES Test for porphyrins in the urine was of "considerable clinical use in detecting small quantities of abnormal pigments" in persons with subclinical and clinical deficiency states. While it is perfectly true that the BES Test will be positive in people who excrete much corproporphyrins and other porphyrins, Cecil Watson and his colleagues (69) in Minneapolis demonstrated that in most malnourished persons the main pigment was indole acetic acid or its chromogen, again a tryptophane-related compound.

In 1940 I presented a paper on the subject before the American Society for Clinical Investigation, but by this time it was recognized that the test was not in any sense diagnostic of porphyrin. My paper may have increased interest in the matter, since I discussed the notion of photosensitivity and pellagrous dermatitis. At this time it was not clear that exposure to sunlight was unnecessary to the production of the pellagraderm.

Adenylic Acid

Many studies were done with adenylic acid from yeast and muscle in malnourished patients (55). We reported improvement of ulcers in the mouths of several patients following daily intravenous administration of 50 mg of adenylic acid. Because the adenylic acid produced disagreeable symptoms we did not recommend its use clinically. Such lesions generally healed promptly in pellagrins after administration of nicotinic acid and an improved diet. Often ulcers were swarming with Vincent's organisms and this condition also cleared up. Neither diet nor adenylic acid administration was effective in treating the ordinary aphthous ulcer or canker sore, a lesion that produces discomfort out of proportion to its usual small size.

Roentgen Sickness

In 1944 Bean, Spies & R. W. Vilter (9) published a series of studies on irradiation sickness—the nausea, vomiting, headache, cramps, diarrhea, and general feeling of illness that may follow therapeutic irradiation. We found that persons on a diet very poor in B-complex vitamins developed Roentgen sickness that could be prevented or ameliorated by giving supplements of nicotinic acid or thiamin a few days before irradiation. Well-fed persons had no untoward reaction to 400 roentgen units administered from a distance of 27 cm.

Glossitis

In the effort to compare the speed with which various compounds, diets, or procedures brought about the healing of glossitis, Vance and I published a table in the *Journal of Clinical Nutrition* in 1953 (18) indicating the rapidity with which glossitis underwent characteristic improvement (Table 1).

Ration Testing For Military Use

My introduction to ration testing in the Army in 1942 was to follow Ancel Keys in the California desert and study the acceptibility of the K-ration. He had written a favorable report. We found that one could track a light tank batallion on maneuvers by following a trail of discarded K-rations. In

Table 1 Speed with which various compounds, diets, or procedures bring about the healing of glossitis

Agent	Time for effect
Cozymase	few minutes to several hours
Nicotinic acid	few hours to days
Tryptophane	few hours to days
ACTH + diet	one to three days
Rest in bed	one to three days
Crude liver extract	one to five days
Yeast	three to fifteen days
Diet alone	three to thirty days

the winter of 1942–1943 it became obvious to everyone that the US battle rations were not good. In North Africa our military debut was anything but a success. In order to get into each day's ration and preferably each item a proportion of the daily vitamin requirement while staying within the space and weight allowances it was necessary to make the ration biscuits with yeast, liver extract, and soybean flour. They had a very high satiety value, soon became rancid, and thus were not eaten. Then serious difficulties arose. The Surgeon General ordered me to write a critique of Army Emergency Rations. I emphasized two disregarded facts (7): (a) A ration is no good if it is not eaten. All the vitamin king's horses and all the procuring king's men cannot feed an Army if the soldier will not eat the food provided. Soldiers are people and eat things they are familiar with. (b) Variety encourages eating. I emphasized that a ration had to be palatable; it must "fill the belly," and be usable in extremes of heat and cold. The fare should consist of common foods, bland and not heavily seasoned. I was directed to design a ration and, using a thousand soldiers, test it against the various rations already procured (11). I obtained from the large food stores a list of the 20 most popular meal items purchased by the American housewife. From the list I selected foods that could be procured readily and developed a ration in which there was no repetition of major item for nine meals. Such meals as chicken stew and ham with lima beans were most popular.

I was then put in charge of a ration test in the Pike National Forest. Our subjects were the 201st Infantry Regiment, whose officers had seen combat in a 20-month stay in the Aleutians and were serious about discipline and training. Expert consultants included John B. Youmans, Virgil P. Sydenstricker, Frederick J. Stare, W. Henry Sebrell, Julian Ruffin, R. H. Kampmire, W. F. Freedman, and M. Corlette. We organized a complicated experiment involving 10 physical fitness tests, 30 biochemical tests, and a complete nutritional examination, recording 200 items on every soldier. By means of a questionnaire each ration item was rated at each meal. The regiment's six companies, separated from each other so there was no opportunity to exchange food, underwent a rigorous training program. Daily records of ration evaluation, biochemical tests, the fitness scores and evaluations by the officers were transferred to IBM cards and sent to the Corps Area Headquarters in Omaha, Nebraska, from which we got reports twice a week. We compared rations as issued, one ration per day of varying calorie content (some being 20% greater than others), with rations issued so that each man received the same number of calories per day. Rapid data processing enabled us to complete a book nearly 250 pages long for distribution 3 months after the test. We found no vitamin deficiencies. The sun and the semiarid weather chaffed the soldiers' lips, and trauma to their gums from chewing K-ration biscuits at first caused concern. The biochemical tests revealed no abnormalities; physical fitness improved; muscle mass increased. The thin soldiers gained weight, those of average weight added muscle and lost fat, and the heavy ones lost a great deal more fat than they gained in muscle mass. Every tenth soldier, the total coming to about 100, was examined independently on four occasions by at least three different clinicians. After careful instructions and agreement on the criteria for diagnosis, we published a detailed account of the subjective factors in these clinical examinations in nutrition which had accounted for some of the polemics of the past. These are important in all clinical judgments. Since then, diagnostic variability has been demonstrated in measurement of blood pressure, interpretation of X-rays, and numerous other clinical matters. Extremes present no problem of observer differences, but borderline manifestations—potentially so important in finding trouble early—are difficult. On our Army ration evaluation team, each observer had a pattern of diagnostic habits. The less experienced tended to overdiagnose and the more experienced found no significant lesions.

The surprising outcome of this study was that military authorities in Washington procured the new and improved C-ration, shipped millions of dollars worth to the Pacific, and sent me with three colleagues to test various old and new rations in ten different places in the Pacific, including observations made on Iwo Jima and Luzon on soldiers immediately out of combat (12–14). The most spectacular results we saw were in the 38th Infantry Division in Luzon, who had been fighting the Japanese for four and a half months, subsisting on the improved C-ration. The soldiers, though low on praise, were still eating the food. They had the best physical fitness record of any group we tested and exhibited no clinical or biochemical abnormalities.

The rations had been designed without much sophisticated metabolic theory but with practical common sense. Here was a unique example of the recognition of a clinical Army problem, a diagnosis, a proposal for change in the form of preventive therapy, a test under conditions of training but not combat, a procurement of the ration, and a final study right out of combat. The food did indeed work in the circumstances for which it was designed.

The development of large-scale rations tests and the improvement of Army emergency rations were a natural outgrowth of the work I had done in the field of nutrition in association with Spies, the Vilters, and many others. Several important lessons came from these studies. The most important, but little recognized, was that the acceptability of a ration is essential for its use. It is better to have an imperfect ration that is eaten than a theoretically perfect one that is not eaten or is eaten only in unbalanced fractions.

Tropical Nutrition

Our ration study group (R. E. Johnson, C. R. Henderson, L. M. Richardson, and myself) in the US Army and that of R. M. Kark and associates in the Canadian Army used identical reagents and methods to demonstrate that there was no form of deterioration peculiar to the tropics (33). Isolation, boredom, homesickness, and abuse of alcohol were just as prevalent in various parts of the United States as they were in tropical regions. Such deterioration as occurred was not related to any peculiar tropical requirement for food or supplements.

The Canadian study of Kark and associates in Southeast Asia demonstrated that animal protein, riboflavin, and ascorbic acid levels were definitely lower in East Indian natives and Japanese prisoners than in US troops. Racial and religious dietary preferences resulted in lower values for hemoglobin, serum proteins, serum and urine ascorbic acid, and urinary riboflavin in Indian soldiers than in Americans; but interestingly enough, no classical disease of nutritional deficiency was found. Japanese prisoners were seriously malnourished, and many had vitamin deficiency diseases. A regiment of Gurkhas with the highest fitness record and almost no physical signs of deterioation or malfunction had much lower values of serum protein and urinary riboflavin than US troops. Food habits, customs, and adaptation must explain this.

Establishment of a Metabolism Unit in Iowa

After extensive clinical research on nutrition and human work and climate physiology in World War II, I established a metabolism unit at Iowa City, where P. C. Jeans had done such splendid work in pediatric nutrition. Kate Daum's section dealt with the biochemistry of nutrition, to which was added my own interest in B-complex vitamin deficiencies and the use of vitamin antagonists (16–22, 24, 35, 63). We published extensively on pantothenic acid deficiency and later on combinations of pantothenic and pyridoxine deficiency. We were trying hard to see whether vitamin antagonists would produce vitamin deficiencies that might be important in reducing antigen-antibody reactions and, thus, play a useful role in organ transplant. We did, indeed, find that many antibody reactions were diminished or prevented by the combination of pantothenic acid and pyridoxine deficiency. The catch was that this deficiency also prevented normal wound healing, perhaps partly owing to local infections. Thus the idea had to be discarded because of interfering complications.

Moral and Ethical Problems in Human Experimentation

I discussed Walter Reed and human experiments in the Garrison Lecture (24). Nearly thirty years before that I had presented my concern with moral responsibilities in clinical research in the Presidential Address of the Central Society for Clinical Research in November, 1951 (17a). This has recently been updated in the December 1981 issue of the *Journal of Laboratory and Clinical Medicine* (17b). Though I saw no examples of disregard for the patients' safety and well-being in studies in Birmingham or Cincinnati, this owed more to the backgrounds and training of those involved than to any formal evaluation or obtaining of written consent. During World War II we had done all manner of experiments on physical fitness, adaptation to extremes of heat and cold, and water and salt requirements; we had done extensive ration tests involving a great variety of clinical, biochemical, and performance evaluations without formally obtaining consent, though the procedures had been explained to the subjects in detail. Though an occasional soldier departed without leave, in general the morale was splendid and the rate of AWOL was much smaller in our experimental subjects than in the units from which they were drawn. We agreed with the English investigator, L. J. Witts, who believed that if one does any investigation on oneself first then it is permissible to do it on others after genuine efforts to explain it to the subjects and after obtaining informed consent. No set of formal and codified rules or laws will be satisfactory in all cases, particularly if the experimenters do not have high ethical standards.

Despite the fact that we tested on ourselves the drugs we used and the compounds that had been effective in animal experiments, we made no systematic efforts to get what we now call informed consent, nor was there any document for the patients to sign. The only signed releases I saw were those that physicians and patients signed for photographs or moving pictures for education and promotion. The subject usually was paid, as token payment, a dollar and signed without any question. There was exhibited a further very important, but scarcely studied influence of faith and belief at the nutrition clinic in Birmingham, Alabama, where the famous Dr. Spies had created an effect resembling, but by no means as evident as that at Lourdes. This similarly exists in some centers today, centers of legitimate as well as pseudoscientific nutrition fame.

From the moral and ethical point of view, the fact that we had tested new compounds or diets on ourselves, orally or by injection, made us feel, in those informal days of confidence and trust, that we had done what was required to safeguard our subjects. I believe that most if not all of our studies would have been approved by the array of committees set up today to monitor moral and ethical guides in experiments on volunteers. I am unaware of any harm that resulted from our studies. A great deal of good resulted.

Literature Cited

1. Aring, C. D., Bean, W. B., Roseman, E., Rosenbaum, M., Spies, T. D. 1941. The peripheral nerves in cases of nutritional deficiency. *Arch. Neurol. Psychol.* 48:772–87
2. Bean, W. B., Vilter, R. W., Spies, T. D. 1939. The effect of Roentgen-ray on the blood codehydrogenase I and II. *Ann. Intern. Med.* 13:783–86
3. Bean, W. B., Spies, T. D. 1940. A study of the effects of nicotinic acid and related pyridine and pyrazine compounds on the temperature of the skin of human beings. *Am. Heart J.* 20(1):62–78
4. Bean, W. B., Spies, T. D. 1940. Vitamin deficiencies in diarrheal states. *J. Am. Med. Assoc.* 115:1078–81
5. Bean, W. B., Spies, T. D., Blankenhorn, M. A. 1942. The incidence of pellagra in Ohio hospitals, *J. Am. Med. Assoc.* 118:1176–79
6. Bean, W. B., Spies, T. D., Blankenhorn, M. A. 1944. Secondary pellagra. *Medicine* 23:1–77
7. Bean, W. B. 1944. A critique of army rations: acceptability and dietary requirements. *Armored Med. Res. Lab. Rep.*
8. Bean, W. B., Spies, T. D., Vilter, R. W. 1944. Asymmetric cutaneous lesions in pellagra. *Arch. Derm. Syph.* 49:335–45
9. Bean, W. B., Spies, T. D., Vilter, R. W. 1944. A note on irradiation sickness. *Am. J. Med. Sci.* 208:46–54
10. Bean, W. B. 1944. Remarks on the incidence, manifestations and treatment of nutritional deficiency diseases. *Nebr. State Med. J.* 29 (8):241–44
11. Bean, W. B., Youmans, J. B., Nelson, N., Bell, D. M., Richardson, L. M. Jr., French, C. E., Henderson, C. R., Johnson, R. E. 1944. Final report on tests of the acceptability and adequacy of U.S. Army C, K, 10-in-1 and Canadian Army mess tin ration. *Armored Med. Res. Lab. Rep.*
12. Bean, W. B., Johnson, R. E., Henderson, C. R., Richardson, L. M. 1946. Nutrition survey in Pacific theater of operations. *Bull. U. S. Army Med. Dept.* V:697–705
13. Bean, W. B. 1948. Field testing of army rations. *J. Appl. Physiol.* 1:448–57
14. Bean, W. B. 1948. An analysis of subjectivity in the clinical examination in nutrition. *J. Appl. Physiol.* 1:458–68
15. Bean, W. B., Vilter, R. W., Blankenhorn, M. A. 1949. Incidence of pellagra. *J. Am. Med. Assoc.* 140:872–73
16. Bean, W. B. 1950. Control in research in human nutrition. *Nutr. Rev.* 8:97–99
17. Bean, W. B., Franklin, M., Daum, K. 1951. A note on trytophane and pellagrous glossitis. *J. Lab. Clin. Med.* 38:167–72
17a. Bean, W. B. 1952. A testament of duty: some strictures on moral responsibility in clinical research. *J. Lab. Clin. Med.* 39:3–9
17b. Bean, W. B. 1981. "A testament of duty" revisited. *J. Lab. Clin. Med.* 98(6):795–99
18. Bean, W. B., Vance, M. 1953. Some aspects of the tongue in pellagrous glossitis. *J. Clin. Nutr.* 1:267–74
19. Bean, W. B., Hodges, R. E., 1954. Pantothenic acid deficiency induced in human subjects. *Proc. Soc. Exp. Biol. Med.* 86:693–98
20. Bean, W. B., Hodges, R. E., Daum, K. 1955. Pantothenic acid deficiency induced in human subjects. *J. Clin. Invest.* 34:1073–84
21. Bean, W. B. 1955. Research: prelude and first movement. *Circ. Res.* 3:317–19
22. Bean, W. B. 1955. Vitaminia, polypharmacy and witchcraft. *Am. Med. Assoc. Arch. Intern. Med.* 96:137–41
23. Bean, W. B. 1963. Presidential address: the clinician interrogates nutrition. *Am. J. Clin. Nutr.* 13:263–74
24. Bean, W. B. 1977. Walter Reed and the ordeal of human experiments. *Bull. Hist. Med.* 51:75–92
25. Beckh, W., Ellinger, P., Spies, T. D. 1937. Porphyrinuria in pellagra. *Q. J. Med. New Ser.* VI:305–19
25a. Carpenter, K. J. 1981. *Pellagra.* Stroudsburg, PA: Hutchinson Ross. 391 pp.
26. de Kruif, P. 1940. Famine fighters. *Readers Digest* Dec., 1940, pp. 11–16
27. Elvehjem, C. A., Madden, R. J., Strong, F. M., Woolley, D. W. 1939. Relation of nicotinic acid and nicotinic acid amide to canine black tongue. *J. Am. Chem. Soc.* 59:1767
27a. Etheridge, E. W. 1972. *The Butterfly Caste: A Social History of Pellagra in the South.* Westport, CT: Greenwood. 278 pp.
28. Frommeyer, W. B. Jr., Spies, T. D., Vilter, C. F., English, A. 1946. Further observations on the antianemic properties of 5-methyl uracil. *J. Lab. Clin. Med.* 31:643–49
29. Goldberger, J. 1916. The transmissibility of pellagra. *Pub. Health Rep.* 31:3159–73
30. Goldberger, J., Wheeler, G. A. 1920. Experimental pellagra in white male convicts. *Arch. Int. Med.* 25:451–71

31. Goldberger, J., Tanner, W. F. 1922. Amino-acid deficiency probably the primary etiological factor in pellagra. *Publ. Health Rep.* 37:462–86

32. Harris, H. F. 1919. *Pellagra.* NY: MacMillan

32a. Hirsch, A. 1855. *Handbook of Geographical and Historical Pathology.* Tranl. from 2nd German ed. by C. Creighton, M. D., vol. 2, Ch. 6. London: New Sydenham Soc.

33. Kark, R. M., Aiton, H. F., Pease, E. D., Bean, W. B., Henderson, C. R., Johnson, R. E., Richardson, L. M. 1947. Tropical deterioration and nutrition. *Medicine.* 26:1–40

33a. King, C. G. 1976. *A Good Idea: The History of The Nutrition Foundation.* NY: Nutr. Fnd. pp. 210–41

34. Krehl, W. A., Tepley, L. J., Savma, P. S., Elvehjem, C. A. 1945. Growth retarding effect of corn in nicotinic acid-low rations and its counteraction by tryptophane. *Science* 101:489

35. Lubin, R., Daum, K. A., Bean, W. B. 1956. Studies of pantothenic acid metabolism. *Am. J. Clin. Nutr.* 4:420–33

36. Moore, C. V., Vilter, R., Minnich, V., Spies, T. D. 1944. Nutritional macrocytic anemia in patients with pellagra or deficiency of the vitamin B complex. *J. Lab. Clin. Med.* 29:1226–55

37. Moore, R. A., Spies, T. D., Copper, Z. K. 1942. Histopathology of the skin in pellagra. *Arch. Derm. Syph.* 46:100–11

38. Handbook of Nutrition. A symposium prepared under the auspices of the Council of Foods and Nutrition of the American Medical Association. 1943. Chicago: American Medical Association. 586 pp.

39. Plumbett, O. R. L. L. 1939. Observations and clinical notes on some cases of pellagra seen in cypress. *J. R. Army M. Corps.* 72:317

40. Report of the Pellagra Commission of the State of Illinois. November, 1911. Published in Springfield, Illinois, Illinois State Journal Co., State Printers, in 1912. 250 pages.

40a. Roe, D. A. 1973. *A Plague of Corn: The Social History of Pellagra.* Ithaca, NY: Cornell Univ. Press. 217 pp.

41. Ruegsegger, J. M., Hamburger, M. Jr., Turk, A. S., Spies, T. D., Blankenhorn, M. A. 1941. The use of 2-sulfanilamidopyrazine in pneumococcal pneumonia. A preliminary report. *Am. J. Med. Sci.* 202:432–35

41a. Sandwith, F. M. 1913. Is pellagra a disease due to a deficiency of nutrition? *Trans. Soc. Trop. Med. Hyg.* 6:143

42. Spies, T. D. 1932. Pellagra: etiology, response to a deficient diet. *South. Med. Surg.* 44:128–36

43. Spies, T. D. 1932. Pellagra: improvement while taking so-called "pellagra-producing" diet. *Am. J. Med. Sci.* 184:837–46

44. Spies, T. D. 1933. Skin lesions of pellagra. An experimental study. *Arch. Intern. Med.* 52:945–47

45. Spies, T. D. 1935. Relationship of pellagrous dermatitis to sunlight. *Arch. Intern. Med.* 56:920–26

46. Spies, T. D. 1935. The treatment of pellagra. *J. Am. Med. Assoc.* 104:1377–80

47. Spies, T. D., Chinn, B., McLester, J. B. 1937. Treatment of endemic pellagra. *South. Med. J.* 30:18–22

48. Spies, T. D. 1938. The response of pellagrins to nicotinic acid. *The Lancet* 1:252–59

49. Spies, T. D., Aring, C. D. 1938. Effect of vitamin B_1 on the peripheral neuritis of pellagra. *J. Am. Med. Assoc.* 110:1081–1084

50. Spies, T. D., Aring, C. D., Gelperin, J., Bean, W. B. 1938. The mental symptoms of pellagra: their relief with nicotinic acid. *Am. J. Med. Sci.* 196:461–75

51. Spies, T. D., Bean, W. B., Stone, R. E. 1938. The treatment of subclinical and classic pellagra; use of nicotinic acid, nicotinic acid amide and sodium nicotinate, with special reference to the vasodilator action and the effect on mental symptoms. *J. Am. Med. Assoc.* 111:584–90

52. Spies, T. D., Cooper, C., Blankenhorn, M. A. 1938. The use of nicotinic acid in the treatment of pellagra. *J. Am. Med. Assoc.* 110:622–27

53. Spies, T. D., Bean, W. B., Ashe, W. F. 1939. A note on the use of vitamin B_6 in human nutrition. *J. Am. Med. Assoc.* 112:2414–15

54. Spies, T. D., Bean, W. B., Vilter, R. W., Huff, N. E. 1940. Endemic riboflavin deficiency in infants and children. *Am. J. Med. Sci.* 220:697–701

55. Spies, T. D., Bean, W. B., Vilter, R. W. 1940. Adenylic acid in human nutrition. *Ann. Intern. Med.* 13:1616–18

56. Spies, T. D., Ladisch, R. K., Bean, W. B. 1940. Vitamin B_6 (pyridoxin) deficiency in human beings. Further studies, with special emphasis on the urinary excretion of pyridoxin. *J. Am. Med. Assoc.* 115:839–40

57. Spies, T. D., Butt, H. R. 1942. Vitamins and avitaminoses. In *Diseases of Metabolism*, ed. G. G. Duncan, pp. 366–502. Philadelphia: Saunders

58. Spies, T. D., Bradley, J., Rosenbaum, M., Knott, J. R. 1943. Emotional disturbances in persons with pellagra, beriberi and associated deficiency states. *Res. Publ. Assn. Nerv. Ment. Dis.* 22: 122–40

59. Spies, T. D., Cogswell, R. C., Vilter, C. 1944. Detection and treatment of severe atypical deficiency disease. *J. Am. Med. Assoc.* 126:752–58

60. Spies, T. D., Vilter, C. F., Koch, M. B., Caldwell, M. H. 1945. Observations on the anti-anemic properties of synthetic folic acid. *South. Med. J.* 38:707–9

61. Spies, T. D., Frommeyer, W. B. Jr., Vilter, C. F., English, A. 1946. Anti-anemic properties of thymine. *Blood* 1:185–88

62. Stannus, H. S. 1937. Pellagra, theories of causation. *Trop. Dis. Bull.* 34:183

62a. Terris, M. 1964. *Goldberger on Pellagra.* Baton Rouge, LA: Louisiana State Univ. Press. 395 pp.

63. Thornton, G. H. M., Bean, W. B., Hodges, R. E. 1955. The effect of pantothenic acid deficiency on gastric secretion and motility. *J. Clin. Invest.* 34:1085–91

64. Vilter, R. W., Vilter, S. P., Spies, T. D. 1939. Relationship between nicotinic acid and a codehydrogenase (cozymase) in blood of pellagrins and normal persons. *J. Am. Med. Assoc.* 112:420–22

65. Vilter, R. W., Bean, W. B., Ruegsegger, J. M., Spies, T. D. 1940. The role of coenzymes I and II in blood of persons with pneumococcal pneumonia. *J. Lab. Clin. Med.* 25:897–99

66. Vilter, R. W., Mueller, J. F., Bean, W. B. 1949. The therapeutic effect of tryptophane in human pellagra. *J. Lab. Clin. Med.* 34:409–13

67. Vilter, S. P., Spies, T. D., Mathews, A. P. 1938. A method for the determination of nicotinic acid, nicotinamide, and possibly other pyridine-line substances in human urine. *J. Biol. Chem.* 125: 85–98

68. Warner, E. D., Spies, T. D., Owen, C. A. 1941. Hypoprothrombinemia and vitamin K in nutritional deficiency states. *South. Med. J.* 34:161–63

69. Watson, C. J. 1939. Further observations on red pigments of pellagra urines. *Proc. Soc. Exp. Biol. Med.* 41:591–95

Ann. Rev. Nutr. 1982. 2:21–50

LIVER DISEASE
AND PROTEIN NEEDS

Esteban Mezey

Department of Medicine of the Baltimore City Hospitals and The Johns
Hopkins University School of Medicine, Baltimore, Maryland 21224

CONTENTS

0199-9885/82/0715-0021$02.00

INTRODUCTION

The liver plays a central role in the metabolism of nutrients. Protein deficiency, often associated with liver disease, may be caused by decreased intake, decreased absorption, abnormalities in metabolism, or increased requirements for protein. Deficiencies of other nutrients in patients with liver disease, such as of carbohydrates and vitamins, also adversely affect the metabolism of protein. Abnormalities in the metabolism of protein in liver disease play a role in the pathogenesis of many of the clinical complications of liver disease.

DIETARY INTAKE AND NUTRITIONAL STATUS IN PATIENTS WITH LIVER DISEASE

Poor dietary intake is probably the principal cause of protein deficiency in liver disease. Decreased dietary intake is caused by symptoms of anorexia and nausea in association with liver disease, often compounded by minimal appeal of the special diets, restricted in salt and protein, that are prescribed for the patient. In alcoholic patients, additional causes of inadequate food intake are epigastric discomfort caused by gastritis, the high caloric value of alcohol, limited finances, a disorganized family and social life, and therefore a disrupted meal schedule.

Dietary histories are generally unreliable, especially in alcoholic patients. Nevertheless, a history of grossly substandard diets was obtained in 73% of 124 alcoholic patients with cirrhosis and hepatic failure (132), and in 64% of 172 alcoholic patients with various types of liver disease (79). In another study (113) poor dietary intake, defined as less than one meal per day for a period of 10 days before admission to the hospital, was found in 68% of 56 alcoholic patients with hepatomegaly caused by fatty infiltration of the liver.

The dietary intake of the alcoholic patient consists mostly of carbohydrate with inadequate amounts of protein and vitamins (132). During drinking sprees food intake is negligible, being often no more than a bowl of soup and a pretzel. In a study by Patek et al (133) a mean daily caloric intake in alcoholic patients with cirrhosis was in the range of 3200–3500, with alcohol contributing 51–58% of the calories, while protein intake was 50 g/day and contributed only 6% of the calories. Alcoholics without cirrhosis had a 13% higher intake of calories and protein than found in those with cirrhosis. In another group of alcoholics with cirrhosis the mean intake of protein was 56 g/day (136). In a study in France, alcoholics with cirrhosis had a mean caloric consumption of 3435 with alcohol contributing 31% of the calories; protein intake however was 81 g/day (only slightly lower than that of 89 g/day of a control population) and contributed 13% of the calories. Total protein intake is only slightly influenced by the protein content of the alcoholic beverages ingested (134). Distilled spirits such as gin, rum, whiskey, and vodka contain no protein, while the protein content of one American beer (alcohol content, 3.6 w/v) and of one liter of wine (alcohol content, 9.9 w/v) are 1.1 g and 1.0 g, respectively (24).

A history of weight loss is obtained in most alcoholic patients with (132) and without cirrhosis (113), and almost invariably weight is gained following abstinence and reinstatement of a normal diet. A mean weight gain of 3.1 kg was found over a 3 week period in one study of 56 alcoholic patients after admission to the hospital (113). In a study by Leevy et al (2) circulating levels of water-soluble vitamins were frequently found deficient in alcoholic patients. Folic acid is the vitamin most commonly found deficient, low serum levels occuring in 30% of those with normal liver, 40% with fatty liver, and 47% with cirrhosis (79). Low serum levels of thiamine, riboflavin, nicotinic acid, and pyridoxine were found in 23% of patients with cirrhosis, whereas 20% had low levels of vitamin B_{12}, panthotenic acid, or biotin. Clinical stigmata of vitamin B deficiency were regularly associated with low serum vitamin levels. The serum albumin is usually normal in chronic alcoholics with no or mild hepatomegaly due to fatty infiltration (115) but was found decreased in 87% of patients with symptomatic fatty liver (75) and in 90% of patients with cirrhosis and hepatic failure (132). Lean body mass estimated from measurement of total body potassium using ^{40}K and whole body counting was found to be decreased in alcoholic cirrhosis (142); by contrast, skeletal mass determined by measurements of total body calcium using total body neutron activation analysis, and by bone mineral content of the radius using the photon absorption technique, was not decreased. Consequently, patients with alcoholic cirrhosis have a decrease in the ratio of lean body mass to skeletal mass.

Nonalcoholic patients with cirrhosis have also been documented to have decreased dietary intake. In a study of 39 patients a history of decreased caloric intake and dietary intake was found in 44 and 20% of the patients, respectively (120). The protein intake in 10 patients (26%) was below 55 g/day, but in all cases it was above the minimum of 0.85 g/kg body weight. In addition 18% of the patients were underweight by a mean of 9.3 kg below ideal weight. The fat-soluble vitamins were the principal vitamins found deficient. The plasma levels of vitamins A and E were low in 42 and 38% of the patients, respectively. In contrast to the alcoholic patients, deficiencies in the water-soluble vitamins (thiamine, riboflavin, and nicotinic acid) were found only once, each in a different patient. However, leukocyte ascorbic acid levels and serum folate were decreased in 35 and 17% of patients, respectively, whereas serum vitamin B_{12} was decreased in three patients.

DIGESTION AND ABSORPTION

Patients with liver disease often have abnormalities of digestion and absorption of nutrients that may contribute to protein deficiency. The disturbances in digestion and absorption may be related principally to alcoholism or may be associated with cirrhosis alone.

Alcoholism

Alcoholics with minimal hepatomegaly owing to fatty infiltration or no demonstrable liver disease frequently have abnormalities in intestinal absorption and pancreatic dysfunction after heavy alcohol ingestion. The substances that have been shown to be malabsorbed are: D-xylose, thiamine, folic acid, and fat (111). An increase in the fecal excretion of nitrogen (> 2.75 g/24 hr) was found in 52% of alcoholic patients in one study (141). Radiological studies of the small bowel are normal and jejunal biopsies reveal no abnormalities of the mucosa when examined by light microscopy; but ultrastructural changes have been described in the jejunal mucosa of patients fed ethanol with an adequate diet (149). Pancreatic function assessed by means of the secretin stimulation test in one study was abnormal in 44% of 32 patients tested. Frequent abnormalities of pancreatic secretion in these patients are decreased outputs of bicarbonate, amylase, lipase, and chymotrypsin, but normal or increased volume output and normal trypsin output (114). Steatorrhea correlates best with a low lipase output (114). The abnormalities of intestinal absorption and pancreatic function are reversible to normal in most patients after abstinence from alcohol and ingestion of an adequate diet.

Both a direct toxic effect of ethanol and malnutrition have been considered as causes of the absorption and pancreatic abnormalities. The acute administration of large doses of ethanol (0.8 g per kg of body weight, or more) in man has been shown to inhibit intestinal absorption of thiamine and folic acid in a few patients, and of D-xylose in all patients studied (111). The chronic administration of ethanol in man together with an adequate dietary intake has resulted in a decrease in vitamin B_{12} absorption in all of the patients studied (84), a decrease in folate absorption in only a few (42), but no changes in D-xylose absorption (111).

In support of the role of malnutrition as a factor in malabsorption and pancreatic dysfunction is the demonstration of the recovery to normal of D-xylose and folic acid absorption, the disappearance of steatorrhea (111), and the return to normal of exocrine pancreatic function (114) in patients after institution of a normal diet despite continuation of ethanol feeding in doses averaging 250 g per day (equivalent to 24 ounces of 86 proof whiskey per day). Exocrine pancreatic function in malnourished alcoholics ingesting

250 g of ethanol per day was shown to be dependent on the protein content of the diet. It remained abnormal as long as the patients were maintained on a low protein (25 g) 1800 calorie diet, but returned promptly to normal after institution of a normal protein (100 g) 2600 calorie diet. Furthermore readministration of the low protein diet resulted in decreased outputs of amylase and chymotrypsin (114).

Most likely, both alcohol and nutritional factors in combination are the cause of the malabsorption and pancreatic dysfunction. This is suggested by studies showing that, although neither the administration of ethanol nor the feeding of a folate-deficient diet alone resulted in malabsorption of folic acid and D-xylose, the combination of both did produce malabsorption of these substances (42). Also, chronic administration of ethanol decreased the pancreatic content of enzymes in rats fed a low protein diet, while increasing them in rats fed a high protein and high lipid diet (155).

Effects of Ethanol on Amino Acid Absorption

Ethanol has been shown to inhibit small intestinal transport of amino acids. In man the direct addition of ethanol to intestinal perfusates in a concentration of 2% was found to inhibit the intestinal uptake of L-methionine (57). In the rat intragastric administration of ethanol in a dose of 2.5 g/kg body weight together with the amino acid resulted in 50% inhibition of the absorption of L-phenylalanine, but did not modify the absorption of D-phenylalanine, an amino acid that is not actively absorbed (56). In everted sacs of small intestine 3% ethanol inhibited the transport of L-phenylalanine, L-leucine, glycine, L-alanine, L-methionine, and L-valine (16). L-alanine flux across the rabbit jejunal mucosa in Ussing Chambers was partially depressed by 3% ethanol and completely suppressed by 5.4% ethanol (72). Ethanol at these concentrations also decreased transport of sodium and 3-o-methylglucose, and decreased electrical potential difference and short circuit current. The effect of ethanol in inhibiting transport was found when added to the mucosal or to both the mucosal and serosal sides, but not when added to the serosal side alone, indicating that its effect was on active transport and not on permeability nor due to damage of the cellular membrane. The inhibitory effect of ethanol on amino acid transport is probably due to its inhibitory effect on the activity of intestinal basolateral membrane Na^+-K^+ ATPase (52). Besides its effect on inhibition of active transport, ethanol also causes an increase in intestinal permeability demonstrated by increases in serosal to mucosal flux of sodium, 3-o-methylglucose, and L-alanine (72). The increase in permeability is more marked at higher concentrations of ethanol, which are also known to result in erosions of the gastric and intestinal mucosa (8).

Cirrhosis

Steatorrhea is the most common manifestation of malabsorption in patients with cirrhosis. It occurs in about 50% of patients with cirrhosis whether or not they are alcoholic, and in the latter patients it persists even after several weeks of abstinence from alcohol. The steatorrhea is usually mild, not exceeding 10 g/day; however in 10% of cases it exceeds 30 g/day (85). The most common cause of steatorrhea in cirrhosis is decreased synthesis and biliary excretion of bile salts, resulting in decreased intestinal bile salt concentration for the formation of micelles (4). D-xylose malabsorption has been found in some (7, 36) but not in other (29, 176) studies of cirrhotic patients. The digestion and absorption of protein in patients with cirrhosis appear to be normal. Stool nitrogen excretion was not increased above normal at protein intakes as high as 100 g/day in one study (38). An increased gastrointestinal loss of albumin has been found in some patients with cirrhosis. In one study, there were positive correlations between protein loss into the intestine and the severity of the liver disease, the depression of the serum albumin, and the elevation of portal pressure (54). The increased losses of albumin into the gastrointestinal tract are probably the result of increased lymph flow and lymph pressure with resulting decreased drainage of lymph from the intestine caused by postsinusoidal obstruction to portal blood flow. Radiology of the small intestine has demonstrated thickening of the mucosal folds (7), which is more common in patients with hypoalbuminemia and probably is secondary to edema. Histological examination of the intestine in one study revealed edema, inflammation, and fibrosis of the villi, and dilation of the crypts of Lieberkühn (2); however, most recent studies have revealed little or no change in jejunal histology (101, 173).

Neomycin used in the treatment of hepatic encephalopathy, because it alters the intestinal flora that produce ammonia, may be a cause of malabsorption and steatorrhea. Changes produced by neomycin that may be responsible for the malabsorption and steatorrhea are: direct toxicity to the mucosal cell of the intestine, inhibition of intraluminal hydrolysis of long chain triglycerides, and precipitation of bile salts and fatty acids (178).

Intestinal Bacterial Overgrowth

An increase in small intestinal flora and an alteration in its composition have been found in patients with cirrhosis. Martini et al (102) found an increased total coliform count in the duodenum, jejunum, and ileum in one half of the patients studied; in addition, *Streptococcus fecalis* was present in the jejunum of 25% patients with cirrhosis but in none of the normal subjects examined. Examination of the feces revealed a higher incidence of atypical coliform bacteria such as *Escherichia freundii* in patients with cirrhosis. Lal et al (74) reported an increase in urea-splitting bacteria, predominately *Klebsiella* and *Proteus* strains, in the small and large bowel of 88% of patients with cirrhosis. Contamination of the small bowel with these organisms was found in 5% of the patients. Some of the *Klebsiella* organisms were resistant to the action of neomycin. Intestinal bacterial overgrowth can have a deleterious effect on nitrogen metabolism (62). It can contribute to catabolism of ingested protein, increased loss of endogenous protein, and diminished absorption of protein. In addition it can alter the composition of amino acids and nitrogen breakdown products that are available for absorption (177). Rats with blind loops and bacterial overgrowth have decreased gain in body weight, steatorrhea, increased urinary excretion of bacterial degradation products from ingested protein, and increase in fecal nitrogen excretion (117, 127). In man bacterial overgrowth due to a blind loop was associated with decreased plasma concentration of essential amino acids, decreased synthesis of albumin and fibrinogen with an increased synthesis of urea (65); these data suggest that intestinal bacteria deaminate large quantities of protein with the formation of ammonia which is then available for incorporation into urea.

PROTEIN REQUIREMENTS AND PROTEIN METABOLISM

Nitrogen Balance

The protein requirements of most patients with liver disease for maintenance of nitrogen balance are not different from those of normal individuals. In one study most of the patients with cirrhosis were in nitrogen equilibrium or in positive balance at protein intakes of 35–50 g/day (38, 39), which is in the range of the minimal requirement for normal adults. In patients with decompensated cirrhosis, manifested by the presence of ascites, an intake up to 75 g of protein a day may be necessary to maintain nitrogen balance, indicating an increased requirement of protein. With improvement in the clinical condition of these patients, and maintenance on the same protein intake, there was a decrease in the urinary nitrogen excretion, suggesting a defect in utilization of dietary protein in the presence of active disease and a more efficient utilization with improvement. Catabolism of endogenous protein does not account for the increased urinary excretion of nitrogen, since administration of a diet low in protein (4.3–13.0 g per day) but adequate in carboyhdrate reduced urinary nitrogen excretion to minimal levels (< 4.6 g/ day) (38). Ingestion of 400 g of glucose a day in this study provided sufficient calories to prevent utilization of significant quantities of nitrogen. Also in another study the normal ability to conserve nitrogen was demonstrated in cirrhotics placed on an even lower protein (2 g) diet for 8–10 days. On the other hand, an excessive degree of positive nitrogen balance was observed in these patients upon institution of a high protein diet (120 g/day) after a period of 8–10 days on the low protein diet. This excessive degree of nitrogen balance was associated with a subnormal urinary excretion of urea and no gain in body weight, suggesting that it was caused by a decrease in the synthesis of urea (151). Although estimates of total body nitrogen balance do not seem to be altered significantly in cirrhosis, there are profound alterations in the distribution of nitrogen between the liver and other organs, and in intermediary nitrogen metabolism. An increased demand for protein after liver injury drains nitrogen from other organs, leading to deficiencies in those other organs. Increases in plasma glucagon and an increase in the glucagon to insulin ratio results in increased gluconeogenesis with release of amino acids from muscle (168). The altered distribution of amino acids may contribute to the muscle wasting commonly observed in patients with cirrhosis (39).

Chronic ethanol feeding results in increased urinary excretion of nitrogen in rats (140) and in man (90). The increased excretion of nitrogen in man was associated with a negative nitrogen balance and weight loss. Possible causes for these findings are effects of ethanol in decreasing protein synthesis or in enhancing protein catabolism. Recent studies in rats show that chronic ethanol feeding decreases whole body protein synthesis and that this is due to reduced efficiency in recycling nitrogen for protein synthesis. An accompanying decrease in protein catabolism was not enough to maintain growth of the animals at levels similar to controls (17). Chronic ethanol feeding increases urea synthesis in liver slices of rats (58), while ethanol in concentrations of 50 and 100 mM decreases urea synthesis in isolated rat hepatocytes (123). Relatively low concentrations of ethanol and acetaldehyde inhibit protein synthesis by isolated muscle and liver mitochondria (150), and acetaldehyde depresses microsomal protein synthesis in the heart (157).

Amino Acids

Changes in the plasma concentrations of amino acids and increases in the urinary excretion of some amino acids are found in acute and chronic liver disease, but are most prominent during massive hepatic necrosis and in association with hepatic encephalopathy. Experimentally, in the dog, more than 85% of the liver must be removed before disturbances in amino acid patterns become apparent (97). The normal breakdown of tissue proteins results in a release of amino acids into the blood stream. These amino acids are continuously deaminated to serve as sources of energy. The catabolism of many of the amino acids occurs in the liver, whereas essential branched chain amino acids such as valine, leucine, and isoleucine, and many of the nonessential amino acids, are preferentially taken up by extrahepatic tissues (118). In chronic liver disease there is a tendency for an increase in plasma concentrations of the amino acids normally removed by the liver, and a fall in the amino acids principally taken up by extrahepatic tissues. Therefore, the most common amino acid pattern observed in chronic liver disease consists of rises in the aromatic amino acids, tyrosine and phenylalanine, and glutamic acid, methionine, and sometimes cystine, and a fall in the branched chain amino acids, valine, leucine, and isoleucine (55, 126, 180, 186, 190). Increases in plasma tryptophan have been found only in cirrhotic patients with encephalopathy (50).

Increases in the circulating levels of both insulin and glucagon (100, 162) found in cirrhosis may be partly responsible for the changes in plasma amino acids observed. Elevated levels of insulin, by stimulating increased peripheral uptake of branched chain amino acids (138), contributes to their low levels in the circulation (162). On the other hand, elevated levels of glucagon stimulate gluconeogenesis and the release of amino acids from muscle, with a resulting accumulation of the aromatic amino acids which the diseased liver fails to metabolize. The principal cause of the high insulin levels found in cirrhosis appears to be insulin hypersecretion in association with insulin resistance. This is suggested by findings of inappropriately high plasma insulin levels in response to glucose administered either orally or intravenously (9, 20), increased insulin response even when glucose tolerance is normal (110, 158), and a diminished response of glucose to injected insulin (21). Decreased degradation of insulin does not appear to be a factor because rates of disappearance of injected insulin were found to be normal (21). Elevated levels of free fatty acids (9), fasting growth hormone (22), and glucagon (100, 162) as well as hepatic damage may be causes of insulin resistance. Glucagon levels are particularly high after portacaval shunting (162). Hyperammonemia may be a stimulus for increased secretion of glucagon, since plasma levels of glucagon correlated with elevated levels of blood ammonia (152), and administration of ammonia salts to normal dogs resulted in hypergluconemia (171).

The increase in the plasma levels of aromatic amino acids in liver disease as mentioned previously is due to a combination of increased release of amino acids from muscle and a decrease in their metabolism. In a recent study, Heberer et al (44) showed a decrease in the elimination of intravenously administered L-phenylalanine, associated with a decreased formation of tyrosine in patients with cirrhosis and acute hepatitis, but not in those with alcoholic hepatitis. The activity of hepatic phenylalanine hydroxylase was decreased in patients with cirrhosis and acute alcoholic hepatitis. The total phenylalanine hydroxylase activity in patients with cirrhosis was estimated to be 20% of the normal value, suggesting that reduced enzyme activity was the principal cause of the decreased metabolism of this amino acid. In another study (59) the elimination of L-phenylalanine from the plasma was normal in patients with cirrhosis, but the total body clearance was decreased, owing to a decrease in the volume of the central compartment of distribution. This compartment corresponds to highly perfused organs, such as the liver, that rapidly equilibrate with plasma. The elimination of tyrosine, the metabolic product of phenylalanine, had been shown to be decreased in cirrhosis (83). A decrease in the elimination of orally administered methionine has also been demonstrated in cirrhosis (51); the simultaneous decrease in urine sulfate excretion suggested that the retarded elimination of methionine is due to a block in the transsulfuration pathway. The increases in plasma free tryptophan may be the result of decreased binding of tryptophan to plasma albumin due to a decreased concentration of albumin and a raised concentration of free fatty acids that compete for binding to albumin (109).

Ethanol feeding for two or four weeks to alcoholic volunteers resulted in increases in plasma α-amino-n-butyric acid and the branched chain amino acid isoleucine (160). Studies in rats and baboons demonstrated that the increased concentration of plasma α-amino-n-butyric acid was caused by an increased hepatic production and release into the circulation of this amino acid following chronic ethanol ingestion (161). It is postulated that the increased production of α-amino-n-butyric acid may be due to increased catabolism of threonine, serine, and methionine to α-ketobutyrate, which is then transaminated to α-amino-n-butyric acid. In another study, chronic ethanol feeding in rats resulted in increases in plasma and muscle, but not in the hepatic concentration of α-amino-n-butyric acid (169), while the concentration of leucine was increased in plasma, muscle, and liver. Most of these amino acid changes were prevented by the addition of pyruvate, dihydroacetone, and riboflavin to the diet. Alanine concentration in plasma and liver, but not in muscle, is decreased by chronic ethanol feeding. The decrease in alanine is observed despite the fact that ethanol inhibits its conversion to glucose by gluconeogenesis; rather the alanine is converted to lactate via pyruvate (71). Ethanol (80–100 mM) inhibits basal and insulin-stimulated uptake of the nonmetabolizable amino acid, α-amino-isobutyric acid, by rat hepatocytes in culture (143). The inhibition of insulin-stimulated transport was greater than that of basal transport, suggesting an effect on the "A" system of amino acid transport in the liver (18). The "A" system of transport, which is Na^+-dependent and requires energy, serves mainly for short-chain amino acids such as alanine, glycine, and serine. The effect of ethanol was not inhibited by pyrazole, suggesting that it is a direct physical effect of ethanol on the cell membrane. A number of recent studies have demonstrated that ethanol in vitro increases membrane fluidity; by contrast, chronic ethanol administration increases resistance to the fluidizing effect of ethanol (175). These changes appear to be caused by alterations in the composition of membrane phospholipids (182).

Urea Synthesis

The normal liver disposes of the nitrogen in amino acids by transamination with formation of glutamic acid. In addition, ammonia produced in various tissues can be removed by amination of glutamic acid with the formation of glutamine. The nitrogen is then released in the liver as ammonia and enters the urea cycle with the eventual formation of urea (Figure 1). In patients with liver disease there is a decrease in the synthesis of urea with the resultant accumulation of ammonia. Maximal rates of urea synthesis have been shown to be decreased in patients with cirrhosis to values ranging from 10–90% of normal. In a study of 34 cirrhotic patients, mean maximal rate of urea synthesis was 27 mg of urea N/hr/kg of body weight, as compared with a rate of 65 mg of urea N/hr/kg of body weight in normal subjects (152). The depressed maximum rate of urea synthesis correlated strongly with elevated fasting venous ammonia, impaired ammonia tolerance, elevations in plasma glutamine and glycine, and a prior history of hepatic encephalopathy (1). The increase in plasma glutamine is most likely the result of a reaction of excess ammonia with α-ketoglutarate; however, the mechanism for the hyperglycinemia is unknown. Maximum rate of urea synthesis showed no correlation with serum levels of albumin, bilirubin, and glutamic oxaloacetic transaminase, or with prothrombin time or hemoglobin concentration (1, 152). A decrease in the ability to synthesize urea could be detected earlier in the natural history of cirrhosis than hyperammonemia, hyperaminoacidemia, and hepatic encephalopathy. A further decrease in the maximal rate of urea synthesis occurs after venous shunts for the therapy of bleeding esophageal varixes, and this decrease is more marked after total portacaval shunts, which divert blood flow from the liver, than after selective splenorenal shunts, which only decompress the varixes (40). The greater decrease in maximal rate of urea synthesis after portacaval shunt is associated with a higher incidence of hepatic encephalopathy. Decreases in urea synthesis have also been demonstrated in perfused livers of rats made cirrhotic with a diet deficient in choline and protein (66) or with the administration of carbon tetrachloride (135).

Factors that may be responsible for the decreased urea synthesis in liver disease are: decreases in the enzymes or substrates of the Krebs-Henseleit urea cycle, a reduced hepatic blood flow, and a smaller functional hepatic

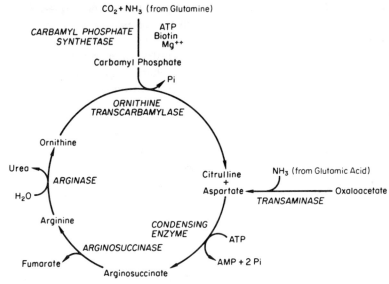

Figure 1 Reactions involved in the utilization of ammonia and formation of urea. Reproduced from (111a).

mass. The activities of all five enzymes that catalyze the steps of the urea cycle—i.e. of carbamyl phosphate synthetase, ornithine carbamyltransferase, arginosuccinate synthetase, arginosuccinate lyase, and arginase—are decreased in cirrhosis (68, 94). The most likely limiting enzymes in the urea cycle on the basis of tissue enzyme levels are carbamyl phosphate synthetase and arginosuccinate synthetase (68, 159). The decreases in the activities of these enzymes in cirrhosis were of the order of 60% for carbamyl phosphate synthetase and 37% for arginosuccinate synthetase (154). Patients with chronic active hepatitis had decreases in all the five enzymes similar to those found in cirrhosis (154), while patients with alcoholic hepatitis only had decreases in the activities of carbamyl phosphate synthetase and arginase, but not in the other three enzymes (95). No changes in enzyme activity were demonstrated in patients with fatty liver. However, substrate availability rather than enzyme activity may be rate-limiting for the urea cycle under physiologic conditions. A direct relationship exists between dietary protein intake and urea synthesis (156). Feeding of a low protein diet results in a greater decrease in urea synthesis by the perfused rat liver than the associated decrease in the activity of ornithine carbamyltransferase, while the addition of ornithine and acetylglutamate to the perfusate enhances the rate of urea synthesis (154). Similarly, urea synthesis in the perfused liver which had been made cirrhotic by carbon tetrachloride was found to exceed the decrease in the activity of the arginine synthetase system (66). Alterations in portal blood flow due to portal hypertension and the presence of spontaneous venous collaterals or surgically constructed portal-systemic shunts also contribute to decreases in urea synthesis and the disposition of ammonia (40, 185). The diversion of portal blood flow causes hepatocellular atrophy and a decrease in the enzyme activities of the urea cycle in experimental animals (99); furthermore, the shunting of portal blood to the systemic circulation not only reduces the ammonia immediately available for extraction by the liver, but also reduces the concentrations of amino acids necessary for maximal activity of the urea cycle. Finally, a direct correlation between decreased liver mass produced by partial hepatectomy and urea synthesis was demonstrated in rats (12).

The administration of corticosteroids to patients with cirrhosis and chronic active hepatitis results in an increase in urea synthesis (64). In patients with chronic active hepatitis, corticosteroid-induced histological and laboratory remission of the disease is associated with a return to normal of the activities of the urea cycle enzymes (93). By contrast, corticosteroid administration did not improve depressed activities of the enzymes of the urea cycle in patients with alcoholic hepatitis.

HEPATIC ENCEPHALOPATHY

The abnormalities of nitrogen metabolism, amino acid metabolism, and urea formation found in chronic liver disease are important in the pathogenesis of hepatic encephalopathy.

Nitrogenous Breakdown Products

Nitrogenous breakdown products produced by the action of bacteria in the large intestine have ready access to the systemic circulation and brain in patients with a diseased liver and portal-systemic collaterals. Of these nitrogenous products ammonia is the best studied and is the principal potential substance in the pathogenesis of hepatic encephalopathy. Elevations of ammonia are common in patients with encephalopathy, and decreases in levels after treatment often correlate with improvement of the encephalopathy, whereas administration of ammonia or substances that give rise to it often precipitates encephalopathy; however, the correlation is far from perfect, and in fact about 10% of patients with encephalopathy have normal arterial levels (174). Of course, it is likely that blood ammonia does not reflect brain ammonia concentration. Mercaptans, which are derived from bacterial metabolism of methionine, can produce coma in animals and have synergistic properties when administered with ammonia and fatty acids (188). Changes in the blood concentration of methanethiol (methyl mercaptan) were found to correlate with changes in the severity of encephalopathy in man (106).

Amino Acid Imbalance

A number of recent studies have suggested that changes in plasma and, hence, brain amino acids may be important in the pathogenesis of hepatic encephalopathy by their production of changes in central neurotransmitters (28, 31, 187). Fischer et al found a correlation between the degree of hepatic encephalopathy and the molar ratio of the branched chain amino acids, valine, leucine, and isoleucine, to the aromatic amino acids, phenylalanine and tyrosine, in dogs (33) and man (34). The normal value for the ratio is approximately 3.0, and in severe hepatic encephalopathy the value drops to 1.0. In other studies, an excellent correlation was found between elevation of plasma free tyrptophan, or the ratio between free tryptophan to branched chain amino acids, and the grade and evolution of hepatic encephalopathy (15, 98). These amino acids compete for entry across the blood-brain barrier (128); hence, a decrease in the plasma concentrations of branched chain amino acids would result in an increased entry and brain concentration of the aromatic amino acids, which are the precursors of central neurotrans- mitters. Indeed an increased transport of the neutral amino acids trypto- phan, phenylalanine, tyrosine, and leucine from plasma into brain was demonstrated in rats after portacaval anastomosis (60). Elevated ammonia levels may contribute to the entry of these amino acids into the brain due to the increased formation of glutamine in the brain. The increased efflux of glutamine from the brain stimulates influx of other neutral amino acids by a mechanism of exchange using the neutral amino acid carrier system (61). Decreases in the brain concentration of the normal neurotransmitter norepinephrine (23) and increases in the false neurotransmitters (β-hydrox- ylated phenylethylamines and octopamine) were demonstrated in experi- mental hepatic encephalopathy (32). In patients, elevations of serum phenylethanolamine (14) and serum octopamine (96) were found to corre- late with the degree of hepatic encephalopathy. The hypothesis has been challenged, however, by the observation that the intraventricular infusion of octopamine, resulting in very high brain concentrations of octopamine and a reduction in brain norepinephrine and dopamine, failed to result in hepatic encephalopathy in rats (189). Of course, dopamine may not act alone and may not be the principal false neurotransmitter responsible for hepatic encephalopathy. Also in one study a significant decrease in the molar ratio of valine, leucine, and isoleucine to phenylalanine and tyrosine was found in severe liver disease irrespective of the presence or absence of encephalopathy (121).

Therapy of Hepatic Encephalopathy

Present therapy of hepatic encephalopathy results in the development of a negative nitrogen balance because it is largely based on decreasing the production of ammonia and other nitrogenous breakdown products in the intestine by limiting protein intake. Additional measures that decrease ammonia production are the administration either of antibiotics such as neomycin, which decreases the flora of ammonia-producing organisms, or of lactulose, which traps nitrogen and increases its fecal loss (184). Efforts have been made recently to treat hepatic encephalopathy while maintaining an adequate nitrogen balance. This has been attempted by the administration of special mixtures of amino acids to normalize plasma amino acids or by the administraiton of keto analogs of amino acids to offset both hyperammonemia and protein deficiency. Parenteral administration of mixtures of amino acids, high in branched chain but low in aromatic amino acids, has resulted in normalization of plasma amino acids and improvement in hepatic encephalopathy in some patients (34). In rats studied after portacaval shunt, administration of the same mixture of amino acids, resulting in normalization of most of the plasma and brain amino acids, was shown to be associated with a positive nitrogen balance (144). Improvement of hepatic encephalopathy in man has also been reported after the intravenous infusion of the single branched chain amino acid valine (70) or leucine (27). Administration of the keto analogs of the essential amino acids, valine, leucine, isoleucine, methionine, and phenylalanine, resulted in an increase in the plasma concentrations of the amino acids corresponding to the infused analogs, and an increase to normal of the ratio of essential to nonessential plasma amino acids. There was a delayed but only slight decrease in blood ammonia. Clinical improvement as assessed by mental and psychological studies was obtained in 8 of the 11 patients studied (92). More recently the administration of ornithine salts of branched chain ketoacids by nasogastric tube was found to be more effective than that of branched chain amino acids in improving encephalopathy (47). In both cases there was an improvement in nitrogen balance equal to the nitrogen content of the medication. The administration of ornithine α-ketoglutarate was not effective in improving the encephalopathy. L-Dopa has been used in the therapy of hepatic encephalopathy with the idea that it may replenish the normal neurotransmitters dopamine and norepinephrine and displace the false neurotransmitters that accumulate. Although a few patients have awakened from hepatic coma after the administration of L-Dopa, no efficacy was demonstrated in the one controlled trial that has been done (116). In chronic hepatic encephalopathy a change from animal-protein to a vege-

table-protein diet has been found to result in improvement of the encephalopathy in association with decreased arterial ammonia levels (41). The
exact mechanism whereby vegetable-protein is better tolerated than animal-
protein is unknown. However, vegetable-protein contains smaller amounts
of ammonia, methionine, and aromatic amino acids and also results in
alterations of small intestinal and colonic bacteria flora. The beneficial
effects of a vegetable-protein and lactulose on hepatic encephalopathy were
additive.

PROTEIN SYNTHESIS

Proteins synthesized by the liver are frequently decreased in patients with
liver disease. This is manifested clinically by decreases in circulating proteins such as albumin, clotting factors, ceruloplasmin, transferrin, and retinol-binding protein.

Albumin

Albumin is normally the most abundant of the serum proteins synthesized
in the liver. The synthesis of albumin is normal in most cases of viral
hepatitis and only decreased in severe cases (105). In patients with cirrhosis,
hypoalbuminemia, and ascites, albumin synthesis although depressed in
some cases is more often normal or elevated (147). The exchangeable pool
of albumin is often normal, or greater than normal, owing to expansion of
the plasma volume and leakage of albumin into the ascitic fluid, whereas
the catabolic rate of albumin is frequently decreased (10, 43, 147). A very
important factor affecting albumin synthesis in liver disease is nutrition.
Protein deficient diets can result in decreases in albumin synthesis and
albumin levels of more than 50%, and this effect is readily reversed by the
administration of either protein or amino acids (69, 165, 183). Both an
adequate supply of total amino acids and an availability of individual amino
acids are important for albumin synthesis. Tryptophan, which is the least
abundant amino acid in the hepatic intracellular amino acid pool, is often
rate-limiting in albumin synthesis (146, 164). Animals fed tryptophan-
deficient amino acid diets have disaggregation of polysomes and depressed
hepatic protein synthesis, which reverts to normal following tryptophan
administration (146, 164). Acute exposure of the liver to ethanol either by
the oral route or in the perfused liver inhibits albumin synthesis, which,
however, can be prevented by the simultaneous addition of a mixture of
amino acids (148). Chronic ethanol administration, on the other hand, was
reported to increase the synthesis of albumin but inhibit its export into the
circulation (5). The decrease in the export of albumin coincided with decreases in polymerized tubulin and the number of visible microtubules

(137). These decreases were also demonstrated in vitro by incubation of hepatocytes with either ethanol (50 mM) or acetaldehyde (mean concentration of 234 μM). Acetaldehyde may be responsible for the observed effects since pyrazole, an inhibitor of alcohol dehydrogenase, blocked the effect of ethanol on microtubules in isolated hepatocytes (104). In addition disulfiram, an inhibitor of aldehyde dehydrogenase, exaggerated the in vivo effect of ethanol on either microtubules or polymerized tubulin (6), and acetaldehyde has been shown to compete with colchicine binding to liver tubulin (37). In another study, however, no change in albumin synthesis was found after chronic administration of ethanol to rabbits (145). Also, ethanol in vitro in a concentration of 50 mM had no effect on the polymerization of purified bovine neurotubulin, while acetaldehyde produced only slight inhibition at a concentration of 1 mM, which is much higher than micromolar concentrations found after ethanol ingestion (63). Furthermore, ethanol in concentrations of 50 and 100 mM did not inhibit the release of prelabelled total export proteins and albumin from isolated hepatocytes (122).

Increases in the gastrointestinal loss of albumin, mentioned in a previous section, can also contribute to hypoalbuminemia in some patients with cirrhosis (32).

Clotting Factors

The clotting factors most likely to be decreased in parenchymal liver disease are factors II, VII, IX, and X. Fibrinogen and factor V are reduced only in severe liver disease. In one study, 85% of patients with liver disease had at least one abnormal clotting test and 15% had abnormal bleeding (25). Decreases in clotting factors can be caused by decreased synthesis or increased utilization. Decreased synthesis is the principal cause of decreases in clotting factors in liver disease. Vitamin K controls the synthesis of prothrombin (factor II) and also of factors VII, IX, and X. Deficiency of this vitamin, owing to decreased intake or to decreased absorption, is a cause for the decrease of the above clotting factors, with resultant prolongations of the one-stage prothrombin time (affected by factors II, V, VII, and X) and of the partial thromboplastin time (affected by factors II, V, VIII, IX, and X). Vitamin K deficiency is readily corrected by the parenteral administration of aqueous preparations of vitamin K. The administration of 15 mg of Aquamephyton® will result in a return of vitamin K-dependent clotting factors (assessed by the determination of the prothrombin time) to normal within 48 hr of its administration in patients with vitamin K deficiency. However, patients with severe acute liver disease or advanced chronic liver disease there often is a parenchymal defect in the synthesis of clotting factors not correctable with vitamin K. In these cases, measurements of the prothrombin time after vitamin K repletion are useful clinically in the assessment of the severity and prognosis of the liver disease. Clotting factors may also be decreased because of increased utilization due to disseminated intravascular coagulation and excessive fibrinolysis, which occur on occasion in various types of liver disease (139).

VITAMIN DEFICIENCIES AND PROTEIN METABOLISM

Vitamin deficiencies that are found commonly in patients with liver disease contribute to abnormalities of protein metabolism and cell replication. Deficient dietary intake is the principal cause of the vitamin deficiencies. In addition malabsorption, decreased storage, defects in their metabolism to their active forms, and increased requirements of some of the vitamins after liver injury also contribute significantly to vitamin deficiencies in liver disease.

Thiamine

Red blood cell transketolase activity is dependent on thiamine pyrophosphate and, therefore, subject to the ability of the liver to phosphorylate thiamine. Administration of thiamine to thiamine-deficient alcoholic patients with cirrhosis and peripheral neuropathy resulted in an increase in blood thiamine levels, but no significant change in red blood cell transketolase activity and no effect on peripheral neuropathy (30). In vitro addition of thiamine pyrophosphate to red cell hemolysates resulted in increases in enzyme activity of the hemolysates from thiamine deficient patients with liver disease, but not in those with cirrhosis. These studies suggest that alcoholic patients without liver disease have a defect in the conversion of thiamine to thiamine pyrophosphate (the active form of the vitamin). Patients with liver disease in addition may have poor utilization of the active form of the vitamin. The Wernicke-Korsakoff syndrome probably occurs only in individuals who have a genetically determined abnormal transketolase enzyme with a low affinity for its coenzyme thiamine pyrophosphate (11).

Folic Acid

The metabolic conversion of absorbed folic acid (pteroylglutamic acid) to 5-methyltetrahydrofolic acid, which is the principal circulating form of folate, occurs in the liver. 5-methyltetrahydrofolic acid is also the folate coenzyme that serves as a donor of methyl units for the conversion of deoxyuridylate to methyl deoxyuridylate (thymidylate), which is necessary for the synthesis of DNA. Folate is stored in the liver predominantly as reduced polyglutamate forms (163). Ethanol has been shown to suppress the hematological response of anemic, folate-deficient patients to folic acid (172). Also, the acute administration of ethanol results in a fall in serum folate levels in alcoholic patients and normal subjects, suggesting that ethanol interferes with the formation or release of 5-methyltetrahydrofolic acid (131). Recent studies in the rat show that ethanol inhibits folate excretion into the bile by shunting pteroylglutamic acid, returning via the enterohepatic circulation to the liver for reduction and methylation, into a hepatic pentaglutamate storage pool. The resulting decrease in folate in the enterohepatic cycle probably explains the fall in serum folate after the acute administration of ethanol (49). In one study, the induction of moderate alcoholic hepatitis with alcohol despite a normal diet was associated with a low serum folate level and decreased in vitro hepatic DNA synthesis, which could be corrected to normal by the administration of extra folate despite continuation of alcohol intake (77, 80).

Vitamin B_6

The biologically active form of vitamin B_6 compounds is the coenzyme pyridoxal-5'-phosphate (PLP). The liver is the principal site of PLP formation (88). Decreases in plasma PLP have been demonstrated in alcoholic patients with (73, 119) and without liver dysfunction (89). The decreases in PLP are not due to a decrease in its formation but rather the result of an acceleration of its degradation. Acetaldehyde acts by displacing PLP from its binding protein, thereby making it susceptible to hydrolysis by membrane-bound alkaline phosphatase (89). In patients with cirrhosis an increased clearance of PLP after its intravenous administration and an increased excretion of 4-pyridoxic acid after the oral administration of either pyridoxine or PLP (119) also suggests that increased degradation of PLP is the principal cause of low plasma PLP in these patients. However, the mechanism for the increased degradation of PLP in cirrhosis remains unknown. The aminotransferases require PLP as a cofactor. Pyridoxine deficiency in rats results in a greater decrease in the liver and serum glutamate pyruvic transaminase (SGPT) than in the liver and serum glutamate oxalacetic transaminase (SGOT) (87). Also, lower levels of GPT were found in patients with alcoholic liver disease as compared with normal individuals and those with viral hepatitis (103), suggesting that low levels of SGPT in alcoholic hepatitis are due to decreased hepatic concentration available for release into the circulation.

Vitamin A

Vitamin A is transported in the plasma by a retinol binding-prealbumin complex. In patients with acute and chronic liver disease, the complex is decreased in association with decreases in plasma vitamin A. These studies suggest that the decrease in plasma vitamin A in patients with liver disease may be attributable in part to a decrease in its release from the liver because of decreased synthesis of the retinol-binding protein and prealbumin necessary for its transport (166). This is supported by the finding of an increased percentage of unbound retinyl esters to total vitamin A in the fasting serum of cirrhotics with abnormal dark adaptation (153). In a few cirrhotic patients with low serum vitamin A and low zinc concentrations, and impaired dark adaptation with poor or no response to vitamin A administration, the administration of zinc sulfate resulted in improved or normal dark adaptation (124). Decreased plasma retinol-binding protein (167) or decreased retinal alcohol dehydrogenase activity (53), both of which have been demonstrated in zinc-deficient rats, may account for the association between zinc deficiency and impaired dark adaptation.

Vitamin D

Vitamin D is metabolized to 25-hydroxyvitamin D in the liver, and this metabolite is converted in the kidney to 1, 25-hydroxyvitamin D, which is the most active form of vitamin D. An increased incidence of osteoporosis has been described in chronic liver disease in association with low serum 25-hydroxyvitamin D levels (19, 46, 179). Therapy of patients with large doses of vitamin D corrects serum 25-hydrovitamin D levels to normal, but fails to prevent the progression of the osteoporosis, suggesting that factors other than the hepatic conversion of vitamin D to 25-hydroxyvitamin D plays a role in the development of bone disease (86). Ethanol administration in chickens decreased renal 25-hydroxyvitamin D-l-α-hydroxylase, which catalyzes the formation of 1,25-hydroxyvitamin D, while it increased the activity of 25-hydroxyvitamin D-24-hydroxylase, which catalyzes the formation of 24,25-hydroxyvitamin D, probably an inactive metabolite (67).

HEPATIC REGENERATION

An increased requirement for protein and vitamins for use in tissue regeneration occurs after liver injury. In addition, alcohol increases nutritional requirements and has adverse effects on hepatic regeneration. Partial hepatectomy has been the principal model for the study of mechanisms of hepatic regeneration and the factors that influence it.

Liver mass is restored with extraordinary rapidity following partial hepatectomy in experimental animals and in man. In the rat following partial hepatectomy, DNA synthesis increases after a lag of 12 hr, reaching a maximum at 20 hr followed 6–8 hr later by mitosis (13). An increase in protein synthesis is detectable at about 12 hr and reaches a peak at 36 hr. The increase in protein synthesis is accompanied by an increase in free amino acid pools, which in the case of some amino acids such as lysine appears to be due to a decrease in their catabolism (48). The residual lobe after partial hepatectomy in rats doubles in size in two days and the liver is almost back to normal weight in seven days (13). Administration of a protein-free diet results in a delay in DNA synthesis and protein accumulation in partially hepatectomized rats, which is readily eliminated by the administration of casein hydrolysate, but not by glucose or incomplete amino acid mixtures (108). The early increase in hepatic protein after partial hepatectomy is more the result of a cessation of protein breakdown than due to an increase in protein synthesis, and the decrease in degradation is less in animals protein-depleted prior to hepatectomy (3). The administration of ammonia in the form of ammonium acetate inhibited the incorporation of ^{3}H-thymidine into hepatic DNA after partial hepatectomy (26). In carbon tetrachloride-induced hepatic injury there are decreases in liver folate during the first 24 hr owing to release of folate in the serum, followed by further decreases during maximum regeneration 48 hr after the administration of carbon tetrachloride. This is accompanied by a reduction in DNA synthesis, which is corrected by folate administration (78). In rats with thiocetamide-induced cirrhosis the incorporation of ^{3}H-thymidine into hepatic DNA was only slightly delayed as compared to controls, and the final level of incorporation was similar (170).

Acute and chronic ethanol administration were found to depress ^{3}H-thymidine incorporation into DNA, mitotic activity, and protein synthesis of the regenerating rat liver after partial hepatectomy (35, 181). Yet despite these effects, ethanol had no effect on total DNA and the restoration of liver mass (35, 129), suggesting that ethanol does not influence the overall ability of the liver to regenerate. Total hepatic protein was increased in ethanol-fed animals before and after hepatectomy as compared with controls (129). Increases in enzymes of short half-life such as ornithine decarboxylase and tyrosine aminotransferase (137), which occur in the regenerating liver after partial hepatectomy, were more pronounced in animals ingesting ethanol. The increase in these enzymes appeared to be caused by a decrease in their degradation. Accumulation of these enzymes and other proteins as a result of decreased degradation may contribute to the observed increase in total hepatic protein caused by ethanol in normal and regenerating liver.

In man a 65–90% hepatectomy for tumor or abscess results in a fall in serum albumin and clotting factors during the first week following operation to dangerously low levels (107, 130). The development of both of these deficiencies needs to be anticipated and prevented by the administration of parenteral albumin and plasma during the immediate post-operative period (107). Both liver function and mass return to normal in six weeks to six months following partial hepatic resection (107, 130).

The treatment of alcoholic liver disease has consisted of abstinence from alcohol, bed rest, and intake of a diet of normal or high protein content, provided there is no evidence of encephalopathy. Fatty liver and alcoholic hepatitis produced by chronic administration of ethanol while on a normal diet is associated with low serum levels of folate, thiamine, riboflavin, vitamin B_6, and nicotinic acid (81). About 20% of the patients with alcoholic hepatitis have negligible in vitro hepatic DNA synthesis, which is restored to normal by administration of vitamins found deficient (76, 78). In a recent study, administration of 70–80 g of parenteral amino acids a day of either 7% Aminosyn® or 8.5% Travasol® for four weeks in patients with alcoholic hepatitis resulted in greater clinical and laboratory improvement and less mortality than found in a control group (125). The administration of prednisolone was shown to increase survival in a subgroup of severely ill patients manifested by encephalopathy in one study (45), and this effect was associated with an increased caloric intake, suggesting that this was a factor in the decreased mortality. However, in another study by the same group prednisolone was again demonstrated to increase survivial in patients with alcoholic hepatitis and encephalopathy as compared to those receiving oral or intravenous nutrient supplements of at least 1600 calories a day, leading to the conclusion that the effect of prednisolone was not related to total caloric intake (82). The administration of prednisolone results in a more prompt decrease in serum bilirubin and prothrombin time, and increases serum albumin (91). The effect of corticosteroids in decreasing mortality in severely ill patients with alcoholic hepatitis was confirmed by another group of investigators (91); however, it was found of no benefit in other studies in which all patients with alcoholic hepatitis were grouped together regardless of the severity of the disease (112).

SUMMARY

Protein deficiency is often associated with liver disease. The principal cause of protein deficiency is decreased dietary intake. Deficiencies in digestion and absorption that are common in alcoholics contribute to protein deficiency in alcoholic liver disease. The protein requirements in most patients with compensated chronic liver disease are not different from normal, but increase during episodes of hepatocellular deterioration. An increased demand for protein after liver injury drains nitrogen from other organs such as muscle. Aromatic amino acids released from muscle in increased amounts accumulate in the circulation of patients with chronic liver disease because of their decreased hepatic metabolism. By contrast branched chain amino acids decrease in the circulation because of their preferential uptake by extrahepatic tissues. Decreases in urea synthesis in liver disease result in the accumulation of ammonia. The causes of the decrease in urea synthesis include decreases in the enzymes and substrates of the urea cycle, alterations in portal blood flow, and a decrease in total hepatic mass. The resulting increase in ammonia in association with an increased accumulation and entry of aromatic amino acids into the brain are important factors in the pathogenesis of hepatic encephalopathy. Circulating proteins synthetized by the liver, such as albumin and clotting factors, are frequently decreased in chronic liver disease. Vitamin deficiencies that are common in liver disease contribute to abnormalities of protein metabolsim. Hepatic regeneration following hepatic resection or injury is adversely affected by protein and vitamin deficiencies and by alcohol ingestion.

ACKNOWLEDGMENTS

The support of the United States Public Health Service, grant AA00626, and the United States Brewers Inc. is gratefully acknowledged.

Literature Cited

1. Ansley, J. D., Isaacs, J. W., Rikkers, L. F., Kutner, M. H., Nordlinger, B. M., Rudman, D. 1978. Quantitative tests of nitrogen metabolism in cirrhosis: Relation to other manifestations of liver disease. *Gastroenterology* 75:570–79
2. Astaldi, G., Strosseli, E. 1960. Peroral biopsy of the intestinal mucosa in hepatic cirrhosis. *Am. J. Dig. Dis.* 5:603–12
3. Augustine, S. A., Swick, R. W. 1980. Turnover of total proteins and ornithine aminotransferase during liver regeneration in rats. *Am. J. Physiol.* 238:E46–E52
4. Badley, B. W. D., Murphy, G. M., Bouchier, I. A. D., Sherlock, S. 1970. Diminished micellar phase lipid in patients with chronic nonalcoholic liver disease and steatorrhea. *Gastroenterology* 58:781–89
5. Baraona, E., Leo, M. A., Borowsky, S. A., Lieber, C. S. 1977. Pathogenesis of alcohol-induced accumulation of protein in the liver. *J. Clin. Invest.* 60:546–54
6. Baraona, E., Matsuda, Y., Pikkarainen, P., Finkleman, F., Lieber, C. S. 1979. Exaggeration of the ethanol-induced decrease in liver microtubules after chronic ethanol consumption: role of acetaldehyde. *Gastroenterology* 76:1274 (Abstr.)
7. Baraona, E., Orrego, H., Fernandez, O., Amenabar, E., Maldonado, E., Tag, F., Salinas, A. 1962. Absorptive function of

the small intestine in liver cirrhosis. *Am. J. Dig. Dis.* 7:318–30
8. Baraona, E., Pirola, R. C., Lieber, C. S. 1974. Small intestinal damage and changes in cell population produced by ethanol ingestion in the rat. *Gastroenterology* 66:226–34
9. Berkowitz, D. 1969. Glucose tolerance, free fatty acid and serum insulin responses in patients with cirrhosis. *Am. J. Dig. Dis.* 14:691–99
10. Bianchi, R., Mariani, G., Pilo, A., Toni, M. G. 1974. Serum albumin turnover in liver cirrhosis. *J. Nucl. Biol. Med.* 18:20–29
11. Blass, J. P., Gibson, G. E. 1977. Abnormality of a thiamine-requiring enzyme in patients with Wernicke-Korsakoff Syndrome. *N. Engl. J. Med.* 297:1367–70
12. Brewer, T. G., Dunn, M. A., Berry, W. R., Harmon, J. W. 1980. Urea synthesis reflects hepatic mass in rats. *Gastroenterology* 79:1007 (Abstr.)
13. Bucher, N. L. R. 1967. Experimental aspects of hepatic regeneration. *N. Engl. J. Med.* 277:686–96, 738–46
14. Cangiano, C., Rossi-Fanelli, A., Bozzi, A., Calcaterra, V., Cascino, A., Capocaccia, L. 1978. Plasma phenylethalonamine in hepatic encephalopathy. *Eur. J. Clin. Invest.* 8:183–84
15. Cascino, A., Cangiano, C., Calcaterra, V., Rossi-Fanelli, A., Capocaccia, L. 1978. Plasma amino acid imbalance in

patients with liver disease. *Am. J. Dig. Dis.* 23:591–98

16. Chang, T., Lewis, J., Glazko, A. J. 1967. Effect of ethanol and other alcohols on the transport of amino acids and glucose by everted sacs of rat small intestine. *Biochim. Biophys. Acta* 135:1000–7

17. Chapman, S., Ward, L. C., Cooksley, W. G. 1979. Effect of ethanol on dietary protein concentration on whole body protein synthesis rates in rats. *Nutr. Rep. Int.* 20:329–34

18. Christensen, H. N. 1975. *Biological Transport,* p. 178. London: W. A. Benjamin, Inc. 514 pp. 2nd ed.

19. Collesson, L., Grilliat, J. P., Mathieu, J., Laurent, J. 1965. L'osteose rarefiante dans les cirrhoses de foie. *Presse. Med.* 73:2571–74

20. Collins, J. R., Crofford, O. B. 1969. Glucose tolerance and insulin resistance in patients with liver disease. *Arch. Intern. Med.* 124:142–48

21. Collins, J. R., Lacy, W. W., Stiel, J. N., Crofford, O. B. 1970. Glucose intolerance and insulin resistance in patients with liver disease. II. A study of etiologic factors and evaluation of insulin actions. *Arch. Intern. Med.* 127:608–14

22. Conn, H. O., Daughaday, W. H. 1970. Cirrhosis and diabetes. V. Serum human growth hormone levels in Laennec's cirrhosis. *J. Lab. Clin. Med.* 76:678–88

23. Dodsworth, J. M., James, J. H., Cummings, M. C., Fischer, J. E. 1974. Depletion of brain norepinephrine in acute hepatic coma. *Surgery* 75:811–20

24. Darby, W. J. 1979. The nutrient contributions of fermented beverages. In *Fermented Food Beverages in Nutrition,* ed. C. F. Gastineau, W. J. Darby, T. B. Turner, pp. 61–79. NY: Academic. 537 pp.

25. Deutsch, E. 1965. Blood coagulation changes in liver disease. In *Progress in Liver Diseases,* ed. H. Popper, F. Schaffner, 2:69–83. NY: Grune & Stratton. 554 pp.

26. Ellis, W. R., Chu, P. K., Murray-Lyon, I. M. 1979. The influence of ammonia and octanoic acid on liver regeneration in the rat. *Clin. Sci.* 56:95–97

27. Eriksson, S., Hagenfeldt, L., Wahren, J. 1981. A comparison of the effects of intravenous infusion of individual branched-chain amino acid levels in man. *Clin. Sci.* 60:95–100

28. Faraj, B. A., Bowen, P. A., Isaacs, J. W., Rudman, D. 1976. Hypertyra-minemia in cirrhotic patients. *N. Engl. J. Med.* 294:1360–64

29. Fast, B. B., Wolfe, S. J., Stormont, J. M., Davidson, C. S. 1959. Fat absorption in alcoholics with cirrhosis. *Gastroenterology* 37:321–24

30. Fennelly, J., Frank, O., Baker, H., Leevy, C. M. 1967. Red blood cell transketolase activity in malnourished alcoholics with cirrhosis. *Am. J. Clin. Nutr.* 20:946–49

31. Fernstrom, J. D., Wurtman, R. J. 1972. Brain serotonin content: physiological regulation by plasma neutral amino acids. *Science* 178:414–16

32. Fischer, J. E., Baldessarini, R. J. 1971. False neurotransmitters and hepatic failure. *Lancet* 2:75–79

33. Fisher, J. E., Funovics, J. M., Aguirre, A., James, J. H., Keane, J. M., Wesdorp, R. I. C., Yoshimura, N., Westman, T. 1975. The role of plasma amino acids in hepatic encephalopathy. *Surgery* 78:276–90

34. Fischer, J. E., Rosen, H. M., Ebeid, A. M., James, J. H., Keane, J. M., Soeters, P. B. 1976. The effect of normalization of plasma amino acids on hepatic encephalopathy in man. *Surgery* 80:77–91

35. Frank, W. O., Rayyes, A. N., Washington, A., Holt, P. R. 1979. Effect of acute ethanol administration upon hepatic regeneration. *J. Lab. Clin. Med.* 93:402–13

36. Friedman, A. I., McEwan, G. 1963. Small bowel absorption in portal cirrhosis with ascites. *Am. J. Gastroenterol.* 39:114–22

37. Gabriel, L., Bonelli, G., Dianzani, M. U. 1977. Inhibition of colchicine binding to rat liver tubulin by aldehydes and by linolenic acid hydroperoxide. *Chem. Biol. Interact.* 19:101–9

38. Gabuzda, G. J. Jr., Davidson, C. S. 1954. Protein metabolism in patients with cirrhosis of the liver. *Ann. NY Acad. Sci.* 57:776–85

39. Gabuzda, G. J., Shear, L. 1970. Metabolism of dietary protein in hepatic cirrhosis. Nutritional and clinical considerations. *Am. J. Clin. Nutr.* 23:479–87

40. Galambos, J. T., Warren, W. D., Rudman, D., Smith, R. B. III, Salam, A. A. 1976. Selective and total shunts in the treatment of bleeding varices. A randomized controlled trial. *N. Engl. J. Med.* 295:1089–95

41. Greenberger, N. J., Carley, J., Schenker, S., Bettinger, I., Stamnes, C., Beyer, P. 1977. Effect of vegetable and animal protein diets in chronic hepatic

encephalopathy. *Am. J. Dig. Dis.* 22: 845–55

42. Halsted, C. H., Robles, E. A., Mezey, E. 1973. Intestinal malabsorption in folate-deficient alcoholics. *Gastroenterology* 64:526–32

43. Hasch, E., Jarnum, S., Tygstrup, N. 1967. Albumin synthesis rate as a measure of liver function in patients with cirrhosis. *Acta Med. Scand.* 182:83–92

44. Heberer, M., Talke, H., Maier, K. P., Gerok, W. 1980. Metabolism of phenylalanine in liver diseases. *Klin. Wochenschr.* 58:1189–96

45. Helman, R. A., Temko, M. H., Nye, S. W., Fallon, H. J. 1971. Alcoholic hepatitis. Natural history and evaluation of prednisolone therapy. *Ann. Intern. Med.* 74:311–21

46. Hepner, G. W., Roginsky, M., Moo, H. F. 1976. Abnormal vitamin D metabolism in patients with cirrhosis. *Am. J. Dig. Dis.* 21:527–32

47. Herlong, H. F., Maddrey, W. C., Walser, M. 1980. The use of ornithine salts of branched-chain ketoacids in portal-systemic encephalopathy. *Ann. Intern. Med.* 93:545–50

48. Higashino, K., Lieberman, I. 1965. Lysine catabolism by liver after partial hepatectomy. *Biochim. Biophys. Acta* 111:346–48

49. Hillman, R. S., McGuffin, R., Campell, C. 1977. Alcohol interference with the folate enterohepatic cycle. *Trans. Assoc. Am. Physns.* 90:145–56

50. Hirayama, C. 1971. Tryptophan metabolism in liver disease. *Clin. Chim. Acta* 32:191–97

51. Horowitz, J., Rypins, E., Henderson, M., Chipponi, J., Rudman, D. 1981. Impairment of transsulfuration pathway in cirrhosis. *Clin. Res.* 29:510A (Abstr.)

52. Hoyumpa, A. M. Jr., Nichols, S. G., Wilson, F. A., Schenker, S. 1977. Effect of ethanol on intestinal (Na,K)ATPase and intestinal thiamine transport in rats. *J. Lab. Clin. Med.* 90:1086–95

53. Huber, A. M., Gershoff, S. N. 1975. Effects of zinc deficiency on the oxidation of retinol and ethanol in rats. *J. Nutr.* 105:1486–90

54. Iber, F. L. 1966. Protein loss into the gastrointestinal tract in cirrhosis of the liver. *Am. J. Clin. Nutr.* 19:219–22

55. Iber, F. L., Rosen, H., Levenson, S. M., Chalmers, T. C. 1957. The plasma amino acids in patients with liver failure. *J. Lab. Clin. Med.* 50:417–25

56. Israel, Y., Salazar, I., Rosenmann, E. 1968. Inhibitory effects of alcohol on intestinal amino acid transport *in vivo* and *in vitro*. *J. Nutr.* 96:499–504

57. Israel, Y., Valenzuela, J. E., Salazar, I., Ugarte, G. 1969. Alcohol and amino acid transport in the human small intestine. *J. Nutr.* 98:222–24

58. Israel, Y., Videla, L., MacDonald, A., Bernstein, J. 1973. Metabolic alterations produced in the liver by chronic ethanol administration. Comparison between the effects produced by ethanol and by thyroid hormones. *Biochem. J.* 134:523–29

59. Jagenburg, R., Olsson, R., Regardh, C. G., Rodjer, S. 1977. Kinetics of intravenous administered L-phenylalanine in patients with cirrhosis of the liver. *Clin. Chim. Acta* 78:453–63

60. James, J. H., Escourrou, J., Fischer, J. E. 1978. Blood-brain neutral amino acid transport activity is increased after portacaval anastomosis. *Science* 200:1395–97

61. James, J. H., Ziparo, V., Jeppsson, B., Fischer, J. E. 1979. Hyperammonemia, plasma aminoacid imbalance, and blood-brain aminoacid transport: A unified theory of portal-systemic encephalopathy. *Lancet* 2:772–75

62. Jeejeebhoy, K. N. 1964. Endogenous protein loss into the bowel as a cause of hypoalbuminemia. In *The Role of the Gastrointestinal Tract in Protein Metabolism*, ed. H. N. Munro, pp. 357–83. Philadelphia: F. A. Davis. 402 pp.

63. Jennett, R. B., Tuma, D. J., Sorrell, M. F. 1980. Effect of ethanol and its metabolites on microtubule formation. *Pharmacology* 21:263–68

64. Jones, E. A., Cain, G. D., Dickinson, G. 1972. Corticosteroid-induced changes in urea metabolism in patients with hepatocellular disease. *Gastroenterology* 62:612–17

65. Jones, E. A., Craigie, A., Tavill, A. S., Franglen, G., Rosenoer, V. M. 1968. Protein metabolism in the intestinal stagnant loop syndrome. *Gut* 9: 466–69

66. Kekomäki, M., Schwartz, A. L., Pentikäinen, P. 1970. Rate of urea synthesis in normal and cirrhotic rat liver with reference to the arginine synthetase system. *Scand. J. Gastroent.* 5:375–80

67. Kent, J. C., Devlin, R. D., Gutteridge, D. H., Retallack, R. W. 1979. Effect of alcohol on renal vitamin D metabolism in chickens. *Biochem. Biophys. Res. Commun.* 89:155–61

68. Khantra, B. S., Smith, R. B. III, Millikan, W. J., Sewell, C. W., Warren, W. D., Rudman, D. 1974. Activities of Krebs-Henseleit enzymes in normal and

cirrhotic human liver. *J. Lab. Clin. Med.* 84:708–15

69. Kirsch, R., Frith, L., Black, E., Hoffenberg, R. 1968. Regulation of albumin synthesis and catabolism by alteration of dietary protein. *Nature* 217:578–79

70. Kleinberger, G., Ferenci, P., Gassner, A., Lochs, H., Pall, H., Pichler, M. 1977. Behandlung des Coma hepaticum durch vollständige parenterale Ernährung und L-Valin. *Schweiz. Med. Wochenschr.* 107:1639

71. Kreisberg, R. A., Siegal, A. M., Owen, W. C. 1972. Alamine and gluconeogenesis in man: Effect of ethanol. *J. Clin. Endocrinol. Metab.* 34:876–83

72. Kuo, Y. J., Shanbour, L. L. 1978. Effects of ethanol on sodium, 3-0-methylglucose, and L-alanine transport in the jejunum. *Dig. Dis.* 23:51–56

73. Labadarios, D., Rossouw, J. E., McConnell, J. B., Davis, M., Williams, R. 1977. Vitamin B$_6$ deficiency in chronic liver disease—evidence for increased degradation of pyridoxal 5'-phosphate. *Gut* 18:23–27

74. Lal, D., Gorbach, S. L., Levitan, R. 1972. Intestinal microflora in patients with alcoholic cirrhosis: Urea-splitting bacteria and neomycin resistance. *Gastroenterology* 62:275–79

75. Leevy, C. H. 1962. Fatty liver: A study of 270 patients with biopsy-proven fatty liver and a review of the literature. *Medicine* 41:249–78

76. Leevy, C. M. 1966. Abnormalities of hepatic DNA synthesis in man. *Medicine* 45:423–33

77. Leevy, C. M. 1967. Clinical diagnosis, evaluation and treatment of liver disease in alcoholics. *Fed. Proc.* 26:1474–81

78. Leevy, C. M. 1967. Observations on hepatic regeneration in man *Adv. Intern. Med.* 13:97–126

79. Leevy, C. M., Baker, H., ten Hove, W., Frank, O., Cherrick, G. R. 1965. B-complex vitamins in liver disease of the alcoholic. *Am. J. Clin. Nutr.* 16:339–46

80. Leevy, C. M., Thompson, A., Baker, H. 1970. Vitamins and liver injury. *Am. J. Clin. Nutr.* 23:493–98

81. Leevy, C. M., Valdellon, E., Smith, F. 1971. Nutritional factors in alcoholism and its complications. In *Biological Basis of Alcoholism,* ed. Y. Israel, J. Mardones, pp. 365–82. NY: Wiley. 453 pp.

82. Lesesne, H. R., Bozymski, E. M., Fallon, H. J. 1978. Treatment of alcoholic hepatitis with encephalopathy. Comparison of prednisolone with caloric supplements. *Gastroenterology* 74:169–73

83. Levine, R. J., Conn, R. J. 1967. Tyrosine metabolism in patients with liver disease. *J. Clin. Invest.* 46:2012–20

84. Lindenbaum, J., Lieber, C. S. 1969. Alcohol-induced malabsorption of vitamin B$_{12}$ in man. *Nature* 224:806

85. Linscheer, W. G. 1970. Malabsorption in cirrhosis. *Am. J. Clin. Nutr.* 23:488–92

86. Long, R. G., Skinner, R. K., Sherlock, S., Wills, M. R. 1977. 25-Hydroxylation of vitamin D in primary biliary cirrhosis. *Lancet* 1:720–21

87. Ludwig, S., Kaplowitz, N. 1980. Effect of pyridoxine deficiency on serum and liver transaminases in experimental liver injury in the rat. *Gastroenterology* 79:545–49

88. Lumeng, L., Brashear, R. E., Li, T. K. 1974. Pyridoxal 5'-phosphate in plasma: source, protein-binding, and cellular transport. *J. Lab. Clin. Med.* 84:334–43

89. Lumeng, L., Li, T. K. 1974. Vitamin B$_6$ metabolism in chronic alcohol abuse. Pyridoxal phosphate levels in plasma and the effects of acetaldehyde on pyridoxal phosphate synthesis and degradation of human erythrocytes. *J. Clin. Invest.* 53:693–704

90. MacDonald, J. T., Margen, S. 1976. Wine versus ethanol in human nutrition. I. Nitrogen and calorie balance. *Am. J. Clin. Nutr.* 29:1093–103

91. Maddrey, W. C., Boitnott, J. K., Bedine, M. S., Weber, F. L. Jr., Mezey, E., White, R. I. Jr. 1978. Corticosteroid therapy in alcoholic hepatitis. *Gastroenterology* 75:193–99

92. Maddrey, W. C., Weber, F. L. Jr., Coulter, A. W., Chura, C. M., Chapanis, N. P., Walser, M. 1976. Effects of keto analogues of essential amino acids in portal-systemic encephalopathy. *Gastroenterology* 71:190–95

93. Maier, K. P., Talke, H., Heimsoeth, H., Gerok, W. 1978. Influence of steroids on urea-cycle enzymes in chronic human liver disease. *Klin. Wochenschr.* 56:291–95

94. Maier, K. P., Talke, H., Gerok, W. 1979. Activities of urea-cycle enzymes in chronic liver disease. *Klin. Wochenschr.* 57:661–65

95. Maier, K. P., Volk, B., Hoppe-Seyler, G., Gerok, W. 1974. Urea-cycle enzymes in normal liver and in patients with alcoholic hepatitis. *Eur. J. Clin. Invest.* 4:193–95

96. Manghani, K. K., Lunzer, M. R., Billing, B. H., Sherlock, S. 1975. Urinary and serum octopamine in patients with portal-systemic encephalopathy. *Lancet* 2:943–46
97. Mann, F. C. 1927. The effects of complete and of partial removal of the liver. *Medicine* 6:419–511
98. Marchesini, G., Zoli, M., Dondi, C., Cecchini, L., Angiolini, A., Bianchi, F. B., Pisi, E. 1980. Prevalence of subclinical hepatic encephalopathy in cirrhotics and relationship to plasma amino acid imbalance. *Dig. Dis. Sci.* 25:763–68
99. Marchioro, T. L., Porter, K. A., Brown, B. I., Otte, J. B., Starzl, T. E. 1967. The effect of partial portacaval transposition on the canine liver. *Surgery* 61:723–32
100. Marco, J., Diego, J., Villanueva, L., Diaz-Fierros, M., Valverde, I., Segovia, J. M. 1973. Elevated plasma glucagon levels in cirrhosis of the liver. *N. Eng. J. Med.* 289:1107–11
101. Marin, G. A., Clark, M. L., Senior, J. R. 1969. Studies of malabsorption occuring in patients with Laennec's cirrhosis. *Gastroenterology* 56:727–36
102. Martini, G. A., Phear, E. A., Ruebner, B., Sherlock, S. 1956. The bacterial content of the small intestine in normal and cirrhotic subjects: relation to methionine toxicity. *Clin. Sci.* 16:35–51
103. Matloff, D. S., Selinger, M. J., Kaplan, M. M. 1980. Hepatic transaminase activity in alcoholic liver disease. *Gastroenterology* 78:1389–92
104. Matsuda, Y., Baraona, E., Salaspuro, M., Lieber, C. S. 1979. Effects of ethanol on liver microtubules and golgi apparatus. *Lab. Invest.* 41:455–63
105. Mayer, G., Shomerus, H. 1975. Synthesis rates of albumin and fibrinogen during and after acute hepatitis. *Digestion* 13:261–71
106. McClain, C. J., Zieve, L., Doizaki, W. M., Gilberstadt, S., Onstad, G. R. 1980. Blood methanethiol in alcoholic liver disease with and without hepatic encephalopathy. *Gut* 21:318–23
107. McDermott, W. V. Jr., Greenberger, N. J., Isselbacher, K. J., Weber, A. L. 1963. Major hepatic resection: diagnostic techniques and metabolic problems. *Surgery* 54:56–66
108. McGowan, J., Atryzek, V., Fausto, N. 1979. Effects of protein-deprivation on the regeneration of rat liver after partial hepatectomy. *Biochem. J.* 180:25–35
109. McMenamy, R. H., Oncley, J. L. 1958. The specific binding of L-trypophan to serum albumin. *J. Biol. Chem.* 233:1436–47

110. Megyensi, C., Samols, E., Marks, V. 1967. Glucose intolerance and diabetes in chronic liver disease. *Lancet* 2: 1051–55
111. Mezey, E. 1975. Intestinal function in chronic alcoholism. *Ann. NY Acad. Sci.* 252:215–27
111a. Mezey, E. 1979. Nutritional effects of hepatic failure. In *Nutrition: Metabolic and Clinical Applications*, ed. R. E. Hodges, pp. 141–68. NY: Plenum
112. Mezey, E. 1982. Alcoholic liver disease. In *Progress in Liver Diseases*, ed. H. Popper, F. Schaffner, 7. New York: Grune & Stratton. In press
113. Mezey, E., Faillace, L. A. 1971. Metabolic impairment and recovery time in acute ethanol intoxication. *J. Nerv. Ment. Dis.* 153:445–52
114. Mezey, E., Potter, J. J. 1976. Changes in exocrine pancreatic function produced by altered protein intake in drinking alcoholics. *Johns Hopkins Med. J.* 138: 7–12
115. Mezey, E., Tobon, F. 1971. Rates of ethanol clearance and activities of the ethanol-oxidizing enzymes in chronic alcoholic patients. *Gastroenterology* 61: 707–15
116. Michel, H., Salere, M., Granier, P., Cauvet, G., Bali, J. P., Pons, F., Bellet-Herman, H. 1980. Treatment of cirrhotic hepatic encephalopathy with L-dopa. A controlled trial. *Gastroenterology* 79:207–11
117. Miller, B., Mitchison, R., Tabaqchali, S., Neale, G. 1971. The effects of excessive bacterial proliferation on protein metabolism in rats with self-filling jejunal sacs. *Eur. J. Clin. Invest.* 2:23–31
118. Miller, L. L. 1962. The role of the liver and the non-hepatic tissues in the regulation of free amino acid levels in the blood. In *Amino Acid Pools, Distribution: Formation & Function of Free Amino Acids*, ed. J. T. Holden, pp. 708–21. Amsterdam: Elsevier. 815 pp.
119. Mitchell, D., Wagner, C., Stone, W. J., Wilkinson, J. R., Schenker, S. 1976. Abnormal regulation of plasma pyridoxal 5'-phosphate in patients with liver disease. *Gastroenterology* 71:1043–49
120. Morgan, A. G., Kelleher, J., Walker, B. E., Losowsky, M. S. 1976. Nutrition in cryptogenic cirrhosis and chronic aggressive hepatitis. *Gut* 17:113–18
121. Morgan, M. Y., Milsom, J. P., Sherlock, S. 1978. Plasma ratio of valine, leucine and isoleucine to phenylalanine and tyrosine in liver disease. *Gut* 19:1068–73

122. Mørland, J., Rothschild, M. A., Oratz, M., Mongelli, J., Donor, D., Schreiber, S. S. 1979. The lack of effect of ethanol on protein export in isolated rat hepatocytes. *Gastroenterology* 77:A29 (Abstr.)

123. Mørland, J., Rothschild, M. A., Oratz, M., Mongelli, J., Donor, D., Schreiber, S. S. 1981. Protein secretion in suspension of isolated rat hepatocytes: No influence of acute ethanol administration. *Gastroenterology* 80:159–65

124. Morrison, S. A., Russell, R. M., Carney, E. A., Oaks, E. V. 1978. Zinc deficiency: A cause of abnormal dark adaptation in cirrhotics. *Am. J. Clin. Nutr.* 31:176–81

125. Nasrallah, S. M., Galambos, J. T. 1980. Aminoacid therapy of alcoholic hepatitis. *Lancet* 2:1276–77

126. Ning, M., Lowenstein, L. M., Davidson, C. S. 1967. Serum amino acid concentrations in alcoholic hepatitis. *J. Lab. Clin. Med.* 70:554–62

127. Nygaard, K. 1968. Nutrition and absorption after resections and by-pass-operations on the small intestine in rats. *Acta Chir. Scand.* 134:63–77

128. Oldendorf, W. H. 1971. Brain uptake of radiolabelled amino acids, amines and hexoses after arterial injection. *Am. J. Physiol.* 221:1629–39

129. Orrego, H., Crossley, I. R., Saldivia, V., Medline, A., Varghese, G., Israel, Y. 1981. Long-term ethanol administration and short-and long-term liver regeneration after partial hepatectomy. *J. Lab. Clin. Med.* 97:221–30

130. Pack, G. T., Mollander, D. W. 1960. Metabolism before and after hepatic lobectomy for cancer. *Arch. Surg.* 80: 685–92

131. Paine, C. J., Eichner, E. R., Dickson, V. 1973. Concordance of radioassay and microbiologic assay in the study of the ethanol-induced fall in serum folate level. *Am. J. Med. Sci.* 266:135–38

132. Patek, A. J. Jr., Post, J., Ratnoff, O. D., Mankin, H., Hillman, R. W. 1948. Dietary treatment of cirrhosis of the liver. *J. Am. Med. Assoc.* 138:543–49

133. Patek, A. J. Jr., Toth, I. G., Saunders, M. G., Castro, G. A. M., Engel, J. J. 1975. Alcohol and dietary factors in cirrhosis. An epidemiological study of 304 alcoholic patients. *Arch. Intern. Med.* 135:1053–57

134. Pequignot, G., Tuyns, A. J. 1980. Compared toxicity of ethanol on various organs. In *Alcohol and the Gastrointestinal Tract*, ed. C. Stock, H. Sarles, pp. 17–32. Paris: INSERM. 540 pp.

135. Perez, G. O., Rietenberg, B., Owens, B., Parker, T., Obaya, H., Schiff, E. R. 1979. Urea synthesis by perfused rat liver. Studies of CCl₄-induced cirrhosis. *Biochem. Pharmacol.* 28:485–88

136. Pitchumoni, C. S., Sonnenshein, M., Candido, F. M., Panchacharam, P., Cooperman, J. M. 1980. Nutrition in the pathogenesis of alcoholic pancreatitis. *Am. J. Clin. Nutr.* 33:631–36

137. Pösö, H., Pösö, A. R. 1980. Stabilization of tyrosine aminotransferase and ornithine decarboxylase in regenerating liver by ethanol treatment. *FEBS Lett.* 113:211–14

138. Pozefsky, T. J., Felig, P., Tobin, J. D., Soeldner, J. S., Cahill, G. F. Jr. 1969. Amino acid balance across tissues of the forearm in post-absorptive man: effects of insulin at two dose levels. *J. Clin. Invest.* 48:2273–82

139. Roberts, H. R., Cederbaum, A. I. 1972. The liver and blood coagulation: physiology and pathology. *Gastroenterology* 63:297–320

140. Rodrigo, C., Antezana, C., Baraona, E. 1971. Fat and nitrogen balances in rats with alcohol-induced fatty liver. *J. Nutr.* 101:1307–10

141. Roggin, G. M., Iber, F. L., Kater, R. M. H., Tobon, F. 1969. Malabsorption in the chronic alcoholic. *Johns Hopkins Med. J.* 125:321–30

142. Roginsky, M. S., Zanzi, I., Cohn, S. H. 1976. Skeletal and lean body mass in alcoholics with and without cirrhosis. *Calcif. Tiss. Res* 21:(Suppl.) 386–91

143. Rosa, J., Rubin, E. 1980. Effects of ethanol on amino acid uptake by rat liver cells. *Lab. Invest.* 43:366–72

144. Rosen, H. M., Soeters, P. B., James, J. H., Hodgman, J., Fischer, J. E. 1978. Influences of exogenous intake and nitrogen balance on plasma and brain aromatic amino acid concentrations. *Metabolism* 27:393–404

145. Rothschild, M. A., Oratz, M., Schreiber, S. S. 1979. Albumin synthesis studied in livers from rabbits chronically exposed to ETOH. *Gastroenterology* 77:A35 (Abstr.)

146. Rothschild, M. A., Oratz, M., Mongelli, J., Fishman, L., Schreiber, S. S. 1969. Amino acid regulation of albumin synthesis. *J. Nutr.* 98:395–403

147. Rothschild, M. A., Oratz, M., Zimon, D., Schreiber, S. S., Weiner, I., van Caneghem, A. 1969. Albumin synthesis in cirrhotic subjects with ascites studied with carbonate-¹⁴C. *J. Clin. Invest.* 48:344–50

148. Rothschild, M. A., Oratz, M., Schreiber, S. S. 1974. Alcohol, amino acids, and albumin synthesis. *Gastroenterology* 67:1200–13

149. Rubin, E., Ryback, B. J., Lindenbaum, J., Gerson, C. D., Walker, G., Lieber, C. S. 1972. Ultrastructural changes in the small intestine induced by ethanol. *Gastroenterology* 63:801–14

150. Rubin, E., Beattie, D. S., Lieber, C. S. 1970. Effects of ethanol on the biogenesis of mitochondrial functions. *Lab. Invest.* 23:620–27

151. Rudman, D., Akgun, S., Galambos, J. T., McKinney, A. S., Cullen, A. B., Gerron, G. G., Howard, C. H. 1970. Observations on the nitrogen metabolism of patients with portal cirrhosis. *Am. J. Clin. Nutr.* 23:1203–11

152. Rudman, D., DiFulco, T. J., Galambos, J. T., Smith, R. B. III, Salam, A. A., Warren, W. D. 1973. Maximal rates of excretion and synthesis of urea in normal and cirrhotic subjects. *J. Clin. Invest.* 52:2241–49

153. Russell, R. M., Morrison, S. A., Smith, F. R., Oaks, E. V., Carney, E. A. 1978. Vitamin A reversal of abnormal dark adaptation in cirrhosis. Study of effects on the plasma retinol transport system. *Ann. Intern. Med.* 88:622–26

154. Saheki, T., Tsuda, M., Tanaka, T., Katunuma, N. 1975. Analysis of regulatory factors for urea synthesis by isolated perfused liver. II. Comparison of urea synthesis in livers of rats subjected to different dietary conditions. *J. Biochem.* 77:671–78

155. Sarles, H., Figarella, C., Clemente, F. 1971. The interaction of ethanol, dietary lipid and proteins on the pancreas. *Digestion* 4:13–22

156. Schimke, R. T. 1962. Adaptive characteristics of urea cycle enzymes in the rat. *J. Biol. Chem.* 237:459–68

157. Schreiber, S. S., Oratz, M., Rothschild, M. A., Reff, F., Evans, C. 1974. Alcoholic cardiomyopathy. II. Inhibition of cardiac microsomal protein synthesis by acetaldehyde. *J. Mol. Cell Cardiol.* 6:207–13

158. Sestoft, L., Rehfeld, J. F. 1970. Insulin and glucagon metabolism in liver cirrhosis and in liver failure. *Scand. J. Gastroenterol.* 7:133–36 (Suppl.)

159. Shambaugh, G. E. III. 1977. Urea biosynthesis. 1. The urea cycle and relationships to the citric acid cycle. *Am. J. Clin. Nutr.* 30:2083–87

160. Shaw, S., Lieber, C. S. 1978. Plasma amino acid abnormalities in the alcoholic. Respective role of alcohol, nutri-

tion and liver injury. *Gastroenterology* 74:677–82

161. Shaw, S., Lieber, C. S. 1980. Increased hepatic production of alpha-amino-n-butyric acid after chronic alcohol consumption in rats and baboons. *Gastroenterology* 78:108–13

162. Sherwin, R., Joshi, P., Hendler, R., Felig, P., Conn, H. O. 1974. Hyperglucagonemia in Laennec's cirrhosis. The role of portal-systemic shunting. *N. Engl. J. Med.* 290:239–42

163. Shin, Y. S., Williams, M. A., Stokstad, E. L. R. 1972. Identification of folic acid compounds in rat liver. *Biochem. Biophys. Res. Commun.* 47:35–43

164. Sidransky, H., Sarma, D. S. R., Bongiorno, M., Verney, E. 1968. Effect of dietary tryptophan on hepatic polyribosomes and protein synthesis in fasted mice. *J. Biol. Chem.* 243:1123–32

165. Skillman, J. J., Rosenoer, V. M., Smith, P. C., Fang, M. S. 1976. Improved albumin synthesis in post-operative patients by amino acid infusion. *N. Engl. J. Med.* 295:1037–40

166. Smith, F. R., Goodman, D. S. 1971. The effects of diseases of the liver, thyroid, and kidneys on the transport of vitamin A in human plasma. *J. Clin. Invest.* 50:2426–36

167. Smith, J. E., Brown, E. D., Smith, J. C. Jr. 1974. The effect of zinc deficiency on the metabolism of retinol-binding protein in the rat. *J. Lab. Clin. Med.* 84:692–97

168. Soeters, P. B., Fisher, J. E. 1976. Insulin, glucagon amino acid imbalance and hepatic encephalopathy. *Lancet* 2:880–82

169. Stanko, R. T., Morse, E. L., Adibi, S. A. 1979. Prevention of effects of ethanol on amino acid concentrations in plasma and tissues by hepatic lipotropic factors. *Gastroenterology* 76:132–38

170. Stocker, E., Wullstein, H. K. 1975. Capacity of liver regeneration after partial hepatectomy in cirrhotic and CCl_4 intoxicated old rats. In *Liver Regeneration after Experimental Injury*, ed. R. Lesch, W. Reutter, pp. 66–74. NY: Stratton Int. Med. Book Corp. 249 pp.

171. Strombeck, D. R., Rogers, Q., Stern, J. S. 1978. Effects of intravenous ammonia infusion on plasma levels of amino acids glucagon and insulin in dogs. *Gastroenterology* 74:1165 (Abstr.)

172. Sullivan, L. W., Herbert, V. 1964. Suppression of hematopoiesis by ethanol. *J. Clin. Invest.* 43:2048–62

173. Summerskill, W. H. J., Moertel, C. G. 1962. Malabsorption syndrome asso-

ciated with anicteric liver disease. *Gastroenterology* 42:380–92

174. Summerskill, W. H. J., Wolfe, S. J., Davidson, C. S. 1957. The metabolism of ammonia and α-keto-acids in liver disease and hepatic coma. *J. Clin. Invest.* 36:361–72

175. Sun, A. Y. 1979. Biochemical and biophysical approaches in the study of ethanol-membrane interaction. In *Biochemistry and Pharmacology of Ethanol,* ed. E. Majchrowicz, E. P. Noble, 2:81–100. NY/London: Plenum. 600 pp.

176. Sun, D. C., Albacete, R. A., Chen, J. K. 1967. Malabsorption studies in cirrhosis of the liver. *Arch. Intern. Med.* 119:567–72

177. Tabaqchali, S. 1970. The pathophysiological role of small intestinal bacterial flora. *Scand. J. Gastroenterol.* 6:(Suppl.)139–63

178. Thompson, G. R., Barrowman, J., Gutierrez, L., Dowling, R. H. 1971. Actions of neomycin on the intraluminal phase of lipid absorption. *J. Clin. Invest.* 50:319–23

179. Wagonfeld, J. B., Nemchausky, B. A., Bolt, M., Horst, J. V., Boyer, J. L., Rosenberg, I. H. 1976. Comparison of vitamin D and 25-hydroxyvitamin D in the therapy of primary biliary cirrhosis. *Lancet* 2:391–93

180. Walshe, J. M., Senior, B. 1955. Disturbances of cystine metabolism in liver disease. *J. Clin. Invest.* 34:302–10

181. Wands, J. R., Carter, E. A., Bucher, N. L. R., Isselbacher, K. J. 1979. Inhibition of hepatic regeneration in rats by acute and chronic ethanol intoxication. *Gastroenterology* 77:528–31

182. Waring, A. J., Rottenberg, H., Ohnishi, T., Rubin, E. 1981. Membranes and phospholipids of liver mitochondria from chronic alcoholic rats are resistant to membrane disordering by alcohol. *Proc. Natl. Acad. Sci. USA* 78:2582–86

183. Waterlow, J. C. 1968. Observations on the mechanism of adaptation to low protein intakes. *Lancet* 2:1091–97

184. Weber, F. L. Jr. 1979. The effect of lactulose on urea metabolism and nitrogen excretion in cirrhotic patients. *Gastroenterology* 77:518–23

185. White, L. P., Phear, E. A., Summerskill, W. H. J., Sherlock, S. 1955. Ammonium tolerance in liver disease: observations based on catherization of the hepatic veins. *J. Clin. Invest.* 34:158–68

186. Wu, C., Bollman, J. L., Butt, H. R. 1955. Changes in free amino acids in the plasma during hepatic coma. *J. Clin. Invest.* 34:845–49

187. Wurtman, R. J., Larin, F., Mostafapour, S., Fernstrom, J. D. 1974. Brain catechol synthesis: Control by brain tyrosine concentration. *Science* 185: 183–84

188. Zieve, L., Doizaki, W. M., Zieve, F. J. 1974. Synergism between mercaptans and ammonia or fatty acids in the production of coma: a possible role for mercaptans in the pathogenesis of hepatic coma. *J. Lab. Clin. Med.* 83:16–28

189. Zieve, L., Olsen, R. L. 1977. Can hepatic coma be caused by a reduction of brain noradrenalin or dopamine? *Gut* 18:688–91

190. Zinneman, H. H., Seal, U. S., Doe, R. P. 1969. Plasma and urinary amino acids in Laennec's cirrhosis. *Am. J. Dig. Dis.* 14:118–26

Ann. Rev. Nutr. 1982. 2:51–71

THE RELATIONS OF ALCOHOL AND THE CARDIOVASCULAR SYSTEM

Arthur L. Klatsky

Cardiovascular Division, Department of Medicine, Kaiser-Permanente Medical Center, Oakland, California.

CONTENTS

INTRODUCTION

Much has been learned about relations between alcohol and heart disease during more than a century of interest by investigators and clinicians. However, the clinical, epidemiologic, and physiologic evidence cannot yet be integrated into definitive concepts. Past attempts to generalize have impeded progress in understanding this subject. However, some apparent paradoxes disappear when we consider the following premises.

51

0199-9885/82/0715-0051$02.00

1. The apparent roles of alcohol in various cardiovascular disorders are disparate. For example, the relation of alcohol to cardiomyopathy, hypertension, and the various manifestations of coronary disease has features unique to each condition.

2. The relation of alcohol to a specific cardiovascular disorder is likely to vary with the amount used.

3. Alcohol most often plays an indirect or partial role in specific cardiovascular disorders. It is best to think of alcohol as a conditioning factor or risk factor in these conditions. Although alcohol is statistically associated with some cardiovascular disorders, a cause-and-effect relation has yet to be proved between alcohol and any cardiovascular condition.

HISTORICAL REVIEW

Because there have been intellectual digressions, the history of alcohol and heart disease is worth reviewing. Some of the great clinicians and pathologists of the 19th and early 20th centuries perceived an association between the regular use of large amounts of alcohol and nonspecific heart disease. Thus in 1861 Friedreich (45) described heart enlargement associated with alcoholism, and in 1873 Walsche (155) used the term "patchy cirrhosis of the heart." The "*Münchener Bierherz*" was considered a common condition in the Bavarian capital in the late 19th century. Böllinger (17) described the entity as a nonspecific dilatation and thickening of the heart chambers and also mentioned estimates of an average annual per capita beer consumption of 432 liters in Munich (compared with 82 liters elsewhere in Germany). In 1893 Graham Steell (149) reported a series of 25 cases of alcohol-induced heart disease and stated, "Not only do I recognize alcoholism as one of the causes of muscle failure of the heart but I find it a comparatively common one." James MacKenzie (87) made similar observations in 1902 and may have been the first to use the term "alcoholic heart disease."

An epidemic of heart muscle disease due to contamination of beer by arsenic occurred in 1900 in England (53, 120, 126–128, 150). After this epidemic, Steell (150) adopted the view that the "heart condition" due to use of substantial amounts of alcohol was largely the result of arsenic. From 1900 to the late 1920s, there was general doubt that alcohol had a substantial, direct role in heart muscle disease, although Vaquez (154) strongly believed in such a relation.

From the late 1920s to about 1950, the entity "beriberi heart disease" became the dominant theme in the medical literature concerning the effects of alcohol on the heart. The general interest then rapidly turned back in the 1950s to possible direct effects of alcohol on the heart muscle, separate from or in addition to deficiency states. The terms "alcoholic heart disease" and "alcoholic cardiomyopathy" have been increasingly used, and the existence of such an entity has become more accepted than ever before.

Since William Heberden's classical description in 1786 of angina pectoris (59), some have felt that alcohol might be beneficial in coronary disease. Heberden described subjective benefit for angina, but there is evidence (19, 132) that the subjective benefit is the result entirely of dulled perception of the discomfort. Since 1970, largely through epidemiologic studies, considerable interest has arisen in possible relations of chronic alcohol use to both hypertension and coronary atherosclerotic disease. Evidence is increasing that hypertension is more prevalent among heavy drinkers and that coronary disease is more prevalent among abstainers.

EFFECTS OF ALCOHOL ON CARDIOVASCULAR FUNCTION, BIOCHEMISTRY, AND STRUCTURE

Knowledge of the cardiovascular effects of alcohol, especially with respect to the effects of chronic alcohol use, is incomplete. Most experimental work on animals and humans has concerned the effects of acutely administered alcohol. In many instances, the results of such investigations cannot be applied directly to the relations of alcohol and chronic disorders.

Heart Rate, Blood Pressure, and Blood Vessel Tone

It has long been known that in healthy humans alcohol doses of 30–75 ml (equivalent to 2–5 ordinary drinks) produce slightly increased heart rate, blood pressure (systolic more than diastolic), and cardiac output (34, 55, 67, 123). How much these changes are direct effects of alcohol on the circulation and how much they represent indirect nervous system regulation is unclear. Overall peripheral vascular resistance changes little; blood vessels in the skin dilate (producing the familiar facial flush), but blood vessels in skeletal muscles and internal organs constrict (41). It has also long been known (34) that doses of alcohol sufficient to produce severe intoxication also produce hypotension, bradycardia, and, ultimately, death from cardiac standstill. Nervous system reflexes are believed to predominate in these effects.

There are suggestions of possible links between alcohol and several abnormal physiologic processes in humans that have been implicated in experimental or clinical hypertension. These tentative links include increases in renin and aldosterone (85) as well as elevation in cortisone-like hormones to produce a state resembling Cushing's syndrome (111, 112, 145).

Effects on Heart Pumping Action

GENERAL SUMMARY   The effects of alcohol on heart muscle have been explored in numerous studies of normal and diseased humans, intact animals, and isolated animal heart muscle preparations. The results vary according to dose, route, duration, and frequency of administration, parameters measured, and pathologic state of subjects. Most studies indicate that alcohol in sufficient doses decreases myocardial contractility. The dose required for this effect in humans may be lower if there is clinical evidence of heart muscle disease or if the subject has ingested substantial amounts of alcohol for a long time.

ACUTE STUDIES   Depressed contractility has been convincingly demonstrated in isolated heart muscle fibers exposed to alcohol (47, 146). Other studies provide evidence of depressed heart muscle contraction in anesthetized dogs (93, 116, 156, 157) and in conscious dogs (62) at blood alcohol levels of 100 mg/100 ml. Discharge of the adrenal glands and sympathetic nervous system as a compensatory mechanism has also been demonstrated (165), although other investigators (65) could not confirm this.

In normal humans, depressed contraction of the left ventricle has been found at blood alcohol levels of 75–250 mg/100 ml (93, 97). These levels could represent very mild to severe intoxication. Similar findings have been demonstrated with various indirect methods such as systolic time interval (2) and echocardiographic measurements (31, 90) at blood levels of 75–138 mg/100 ml. This decreased force of contraction was not always associated with decreased cardiac output (2, 31), leading to the suggestion that a direct myocardial depressant effect of alcohol brought compensatory mechanisms into play to preserve overall circulatory integrity. Poor correlation of the observed effects with doses of alcohol within the ranges studied (31, 67) also can be interpreted as evidence for the development of compensatory mechanisms. Still more evidence of physiologic compensation is provided by studies of near-maximal cardiac exercise performance that showed little effect of blood alcohol levels of 85–200 mg/100 ml in normal humans (16, 123).

The acute depressant effects of alcohol on heart muscle contraction may be more pronounced and may occur with smaller alcohol doses in persons with preexisting heart disease not related to drinking. A study of patients with coronary artery disease (29) led to the conclusion that "three or four whiskeys" profoundly depressed heart muscle. Similar results have been reported with doses of 60 ml of alcohol (equivalent to five 12-ounce cans of beer or 5 ounces of 80-proof whiskey) administered to volunteers with various types of heart disease (50, 51). Analogous evidence is provided by a study of anesthetized dogs to which a standard nonpenetrating blow was given to the chest (83). Prior administration of alcohol greatly increased the mortality of the blow and decreased the performance of the traumatized heart.

CHRONIC STUDIES   Deleterious effects on heart function have been shown in well-nourished mice fed large amounts of alcohol for only 7–10 weeks (20). A study of rats that received 25% of their calorie intake as alcohol showed a decrease in force of heart muscle contraction (88), but no abnormality was seen (86) in the same species given 15% of their food intake as alcohol. One study of dogs fed about one third of their calorie intake as alcohol (100) showed no functional cardiovascular abnormalities after several months, but another study (115) of dogs fed a like proportion of their calories as alcohol showed definite impairment of heart function after 18 months. Thus dose and duration of chronic alcohol use are both important in production of functional cardiac abnormalities in animals. No experiment has yet produced frank congestive failure in well-nourished animals.

There is much evidence that humans with a long history of substantial alcohol intake and without clinical evidence of heart disease often have abnormal myocardial function. This phenomenon, which is considered by many to represent preclinical heart muscle disease, has been demonstrated by physiologic studies (52, 84, 117) as well as by indirect noninvasive tests (89, 147, 166). Men may be more susceptible than women to these effects (166). A recent report (7) suggests that the functional abnormality in humans may represent primarily decreased left ventricular compliance.

Coronary Circulation

The substantial body of data showing that ethanol adversely affects heart muscle function is not paralleled by similar consistency in known effects of alcohol on the blood supply to the heart muscle (the coronary circulation). In fact, some of the experiments showing acute impairment of heart muscle contractile force (93, 117) in humans and dogs showed concomitant increase in coronary blood flow. Ganz (46) also found evidence suggesting increased coronary blood flow from acute exposure to alcohol. Nevertheless, there are experiments that suggest decreased coronary blood flow (116, 156) or no effect (138, 160). Studies of humans with coronary disease who were monitored by electrocardiograph while exercising suggest no benefit or possible worsening of impaired coronary blood flow (99, 132). It should be kept in mind that responses of normal coronary vessels to pharmacologic agents may differ from responses of diseased vessels, which have limited capacity to dilate. A recent study in dogs (44) suggests that alcohol increases blood flow in nonischemic myocardium but that, in acute experimental ischemia, there is an unfavorable redistribution of myocardial blood flow.

Alcohol Versus Acetaldehyde

The physiologic response to acetaldehyde, the first metabolite of alcohol, has been the subject of some investigation. In dogs, a pressor effect and an increased coronary blood flow have been demonstrated (91), but this effect was the result of secondary catechol release. In another dog experiment (44), ethanol and acetaldehyde (at levels produced by alcohol metabolism) had opposite effects upon cardiac function; alcohol depressed myocardial performance, but acetaldehyde improved cardiac performance secondary to peripheral vasodilation. Both substances appeared to increase coronary flow in this study.

Myocardial Biochemistry

Because there is no apparent metabolism of alcohol in heart muscle cells, the mechanism of possible myocardial injury in heart muscle cells presumably differs from the situation in the liver (65). Mitochondrial oxidation of fatty acids represents the major source of myocardial cell energy. In isolated heart muscle cells, alcohol inhibits fatty acid oxidation (86). In humans, blood alcohol levels of 100–200 mg/100 ml can cause leakage of mitochondrial enzymes (116, 117, 159). Furthermore, chronic alcohol administration in animals appears to reduce cardiac mitochondrial capacity to oxidize a number of other substrates (100). Chronic alcohol feeding in dogs reduces the activity of intramitochondrial isocitrate dehydrogenase and also reduces calcium binding to sarcoplasmic reticulum (119, 129, 135). An analogous effect upon skeletal muscle has been shown in human volunteers with short-term experiments (130). Because myocardial contraction requires calcium release by sarcoplasmic reticulum, this biochemical effect is likely to have functional correlates. Reduced protein synthesis (139) and altered phospholipid composition of cardiac cell membranes (114) have also been demonstrated. Additional acute effects of alcohol upon cardiac muscle cells include the inhibition of Na-K ATPase activity (164) and direct influence upon contractile proteins (109).

Effects on Heart Muscle Structure

Enlarged scarred hearts were described as early as 1861 (45) among some chronic heavy users of alcohol. A number of modern descriptions are available (3, 4, 21, 136). Grossly, the hearts show hypertrophy, dilatation, fibrosis, and mural thrombus formation. Under the optical microscope, there is variation in muscle fiber size; cellular swelling, vacuolization, fatty droplet infiltration, and focal scarring or inflammation. These abnormalities have been observed in very heavy drinkers with no clinical heart disease evident during life (136). The coronary vessels have generally been unobstructed, but there has been a report of fibrosis in small coronary branches (39).

Electron microscopy shows evidence of damage in various ultrastructural components including mitochondria, myofibrils, intercalated discs, and the sarcoplasmic reticulum (4, 19, 21, 94). Histochemical studies show an increased accumulation of fat droplets and a decrease in oxidative enzymes. None of the gross, optical microscopic, electron microscopic, or histochemical findings are specific enough to distinguish heart muscle disease in users of large amounts of alcohol from cardiomyopathy in other persons.

Animal experiments have shown production of similar ultrastructural abnormalities with chronic feeding of large amounts of alcohol (20, 115, 141). The accumulation of Alcian blue-staining material (presumably glycoproteins) may correlate with the increased functional stiffness of the myocardium (115). The animal experiments, in which all essential nutrients were supplied, given evidence that alcohol toxicity to the heart muscle is not related to associated nutritional deficiency. However, neither gross cardiac dilatation nor congestive heart failure has yet been produced in animal experiments.

ALCOHOL AND SPECIFIC CARDIOVASCULAR DISEASES

Alcoholic Cardiomyopathy

Much of the evidence described above clearly suggests a direct myocardial toxic effect by alcohol or one of its metabolites. The existence of at least one chronic disorder due to this direct, toxic effect is widely accepted by clinical cardiologists and is usually called alcoholic cardiomyopathy, or alcoholic heart disease. The circumstantial evidence for the existence of this condition is substantial, although some (142) question it.

EVIDENCE FOR ALCOHOLIC CARDIOMYOPATHY   The condition has often been reported by excellent clinicians and pathologists of the past two centuries. The reports represent various types of practices and populations (3, 4, 17, 18, 21, 37, 38, 56, 87, 106, 143, 149, 154).

Further evidence is the fact that long-standing use of substantial amounts of alcohol has been found in a large proportion of patients with unexplained heart disease (3, 56, 134, 143). Alexander (3) made an attempt at control. He reported that 80% of patients hospitalized at the Minneapolis Veterans Administration Hospital for primary myocardial disease were defined as heavy drinkers compared with 28% of patients with other diagnoses admitted to the same medical service. This difference, although impressive, apparently represented a hospital population with a large proportion of substantial alcohol users. On the other hand, the proportion of alcohol users in some series of cardiomyopathy patients has been much lower; Goodwin (49) stated that "alcohol is certainly not the cause of congestive cardiomyopathy in the majority of patients."

Other evidence consists of a few well-documented case reports. Congestive heart failure developed in one well-nourished patient during a 4-month period when he ingested 12–16 ounces (390–518 ml) of Scotch whiskey daily; the clinical abnormality subsided after he ceased drinking (117). Other such cases have been reported (140); many must have been seen and not reported.

An important study (32) documented more frequent regression of clinical abnormality in cardiomyopathy patients who abstained compared with those who continued to drink.

Other indirect evidence is the documented existence of both acute and chronic peripheral skeletal muscle damage related to alcohol use (105, 129). Data concerning an association with cardiomyopathy are sparse, but a case has been reported (107). Affected skeletal muscles have shown microscopic evidence of inflammation, intercellular edema, and ultrastructural abnormalities of the mitochondria and myofibrils. These abnormalities are similar to the cardiac abnormalities seen in cardiomyopathy (105, 129).

Another example of circumstantial evidence is the observation of heart rhythm disturbances in relation to drinking (35). This phenomenon has been given the colorful name "holiday heart syndrome" (36). More serious arrhythmias are believed to be related to acute alcohol use (144). A recent case has been reported of an alcoholic patient in whom ventricular tachycardia could be provoked only after alcohol ingestion (54).

Perhaps the strongest circumstantial evidence for alcoholic cardiomyopathy are facts already cited in detail: (a) autopsy studies showing abnormalities in large proportions of alcoholics with no clinical evidence of heart disease; (b) acute and chronic interference with heart function and metabolism by alcohol; and (c) structural abnormalities in human and animal heart muscle cells related to alcohol ingestion.

CLINICAL FEATURES   Early signs or symptoms are nonspecific electrocardiographic (ECG) changes and rhythm disturbances, often minor. The holiday heart syndrome (36) following spree drinking has already been mentioned. Nonspecific ST-T variations on the electrocardiogram, as well as arrhythmias, occur among some nonspree drinkers and regress when drinking is reduced or stopped. Evans (37) described T-wave configurations that he considered relatively specific for early alcoholic heart disease, but others (10, 101, 108) have not often observed these "characteristic" ECG findings. The prevalence of such early nonspecific evidence of cardiac susceptibility to alcohol is unknown. The likelihood of progression to chronic myocardial disease is also unknown and probably low. However, it seems reasonable to suppose that these persons represent a high-risk group, and there is evidence that reversibility is maximal at early stages of alcoholic heart disease.

The late clinical picture, a chronic congestive cardiomyopathy, is described in several excellent reports (3, 18, 21, 102, 106, 134). Congestive heart failure, chronic rhythm disturbances, conduction abnormalities on the ECG, and a high incidence of embolic complications are characteristic. Although the development is usually insidious, a number of patients seem to have an acute onset of severe heart failure and do not come to medical attention before the late stage has been reached. Even at this point, some patients show partial regression, but many progress inexorably despite abstinence from alcohol and optimal medical therapy. Except for the relation to alcohol use, this clinical picture cannot be distinguished from chronic congestive cardiomyopathy of any cause.

DIAGNOSIS AND TREATMENT   The diagnosis of alcoholic cardiomyopathy is always presumptive, since there are no specific symptoms, signs, tests, or pathologic findings. A high clinical index of suspicion and skillful interpretation of nonspecific evidence are necessary. Basically, the two necessary diagnostic features are a compatible drinking history and the exclusion of other causes of heart disease. Little is known about the minimum amount and duration of alcohol use that may lead to cardiomyopathy, but it is generally believed that very heavy drinking over many years is necessary. One investigator (78) has suggested as a criterion for diagnosis of alcoholic cardiomyopathy a drinking habit equal to or greater than 125 ml of ethanol daily for 10 years or longer. Even among very heavy drinkers, the prevalence is probably low, distinctly lower than the prevalence of liver damage. The exclusion of other types of heart disease is necessary for reasonable certainty of diagnosis, but there is no logical reason that a person might not have both alcoholic heart disease and another type of heart disease. Existence of another type of heart disease might actually predispose to heart muscle damage by alcohol.

Abstinence from alcohol is the mainstay of treatment. Rest, digitalis, diuretics, antiarrhythmic drugs, and other measures appropriate to the individual's clinical picture should be employed. With abstinence, the recovery rate is good in early disease. Even with advanced disease, a marked degree of recovery is possible (32, 113, 140), although there is a high death rate from congestive heart failure, sudden death due to arrhythmias, and embolism.

RISK FACTORS AND COFACTORS   Aside from the possible greater susceptibility of men (166), little is known about the reasons for individual susceptibility to alcohol's toxic effects on the heart. It seems fairly certain that alcohol itself is the major toxin, but a role for other constituents of wine, beer, or certain types of distilled spirits may exist.

The concept of synergistic toxicity to the heart by alcohol and other cofactors is supported by two well-documented historical episodes. The first was a major epidemic at the turn of the century in and near Manchester, England, due to accidental contamination of beer by arsenic (53, 120, 126–128). This episode caused a major intellectual digression in the development of the concept of alcoholic heart disease. The second occurred 65 years later in several locations in North America and in Belgium and was due to the use of cobalt as a foaming agent in beer (5, 6, 71, 92, 95, 151). In both epidemics, there was an abrupt, severe illness characterized principally by acute heart muscle failure in chronic drinkers of large amounts of beer. Those who recovered appeared able to resume their beer-drinking habit without apparent harm. The amounts of cobalt and arsenic alone were insufficient to account for the heart damage. Although no biochemical mechanisms were established, these events strongly suggest synergistic toxicity (the enhancement of the effect of one substance by the presence of another chemical).

The parallels between the arsenic and cobalt beer episodes make it likely that other metals and chemicals can act synergistically with alcohol to produce cardiomyopathy. Thus it seems reasonable that multiple factors may be involved in many instances of cardiomyopathy. Possibilities include iron, copper, and drugs with heart-damaging properties (emetine, adriamycin, and tricyclic antidepressants are a few). Furthermore, it is known that myocarditis occurs with many viral illnesses, and the possibility exists that residual heart damage acts as a cofactor in other heart muscle diseases. In fact, a synergistic link between almost any type of heart muscle impairment and alcohol is a reasonable hypothesis. A similar role of vitamin or nutritional deficiencies (e.g., selenium) may exist.

Cardiovascular Beriberi

For several decades, the concept of cardiovascular beriberi dominated thinking about the relation of alcohol to heart disease. Although the condition was well known previously, the classic detailed description by Aalsmeer & Wenckebach (1) clearly defined a clinical picture of heart failure with high cardiac output. Beriberi in persons in the Orient who subsisted on polished rice was caused by thiamine (vitamin B_1) deficiency. Because some patients in Western countries had a similar clinical picture and responded well to thiamine, it was assumed (70) that most heart failure in heavy drinkers was caused by associated nutritional deficiencies. In the 1960s (12) and 1970s (79), high-output cardiovascular beriberi was studied by modern physiologic techniques in a few cases. These patients showed some of the highest cardiac outputs at rest ever measured. The major cardiovascular physiologic consequence of thiamine deficiency in most appeared to be dilatation of peripheral small blood vessels with the creation, in effect, of a large arteriovenous shunt. Some responded remarkably rapidly (hours to days) to thiamine, with apparent complete recovery. The clinical observations of Aalsmeer & Wenckebach were confirmed.

In Western countries, the cases presumed to represent vitamin-deficiency-induced heart failure all used large amounts of alcohol (70). It gradually became apparent that only a minority fit the rice beriberi picture. Many, if not most, had good nutritional state, responded poorly if at all to thiamine administration, and had low-output heart failure with predominant left ventricular failure (in contrast to the right ventricular failure so evident in Oriental beriberi) (158). A widely held view was that in long-standing thiamine deficiency, chronic myocardial damage occurred that no longer responded to thiamine (14, 15). One reported patient (124) demonstrated two syndromes in sequence. He first had a high-cardiac-output state that responded to thiamine, then somewhat later developed low cardiac heart failure that was unresponsive to thiamine. This was interpreted as representing beriberi followed by alcoholic cardiomyopathy.

It became the prevalent view (66) that chronic thiamine deficiency as a cause of congestive cardiomyopathy has been poorly documented but that thiamine deficiency may be a conditioning factor in some cases. Thiamine deficiency is probably, at most, a contributory factor in the "atypical" cases of beriberi. Blacket & Palmer (12) stated it well: "It [beriberi] responds completely to thiamine but merges imperceptibly into another disease called alcoholic cardiomyopathy, which does not respond to thiamine."

Alcohol and Hypertension

Strong epidemiologic evidence exists that regular use of large amounts of alcohol is associated with a substantially higher prevalence of hypertension. On the other hand, persons who use small amounts of alcohol, up to the amounts contained in one or two drinks daily, seem to fare slightly better than nondrinkers with regard to blood pressure measurements. This possible environmental link to a common serious condition is of both theoretical and practical importance.

The reports (11, 27, 30, 33, 68, 89, 96, 110, 111) of an alcohol-blood pressure link represent varied populations. By far the largest study (77) used data gathered at checkup examinations given at the Kaiser-Permanente Medical Care Program in Northern California. These data showed a statistically strong association between blood pressure and known drinking habits of 83,947 men and women of three races. After cross-classification, this relation proved to be independent of smoking, coffee use, salt use, blood group, educational attainment, and adiposity (height/weight index).

The difference in mean blood pressure in the Kaiser-Permanente study translated into a doubled prevalence of hypertension (defined as blood pressure of 160–95 mm Hg or higher) in white men and women who took six or more drinks daily compared with nondrinkers or users of two or fewer drinks daily. The doubled prevalence among the white heavier drinkers was quite similar to the findings in other studies (30, 68) in which the methods of classifying data allowed comparison.

In view of agreement among various studies, some type of association between alcohol use and blood pressure is established. However, various types of indirect association have not been ruled out. These include (*a*) psychosocial stress as an underlying factor, (*b*) a common hereditary predilection both for use of alcohol and hypertension, (*c*) other environmental factors such as dietary habits, and (*d*) alcohol withdrawal, which is associated with higher pressures in some heavier drinkers.

The blood pressure elevations among heavier drinkers, whether direct or indirect, could be a temporary effect that disappears, at least in part, with reduced drinking. The study of Du Pont employees (30) supports this possibility. On the other hand, there was a residual increase in hypertension prevalence in presumably abstinent alcoholics among the Du Pont workers. A physiologic mechanism is not established. The effects of acutely administered alcohol on blood pressure do not provide a ready explanation. Evidence is limited about pathophysiologic actions of chronic substantial drinking that could account for blood pressure elevations. In view of the uncertainty about the nature of the alcohol–blood pressure association and the absence of a proven mechanism, a causal relation has not been proved.

Alcohol and Coronary Atherosclerotic Disease

In coronary atherosclerosis, the factors involved in the production of the underlying occlusive process are not identical to those that immediately provoke symptoms or clinical events. Furthermore, present knowledge suggests that the role of alcohol should be considered separately for each of the three major clinical expressions of the condition: angina pectoris, acute myocardial infarction, and sudden death.

ANGINA PECTORIS Heberden's classic description of angina (59) included the statement that "wine and spiritous liquors afford considerable relief." Over the ensuing two centuries, it was widely presumed (82, 161) that alcohol was a coronary vasodilatator. However, studies of exercise performance ability using electrocardiographic evidence of ischemia have shown either no benefit (132) or, with doses of 65–320 ml of alcohol, decreased exercise performance ability (99). However, in contrast to the effects of other types of ingested foodstuffs, the *perception* of ischemic discomfort with exercise—anginal distress—did not occur sooner when alcohol was given.

Attempts to study coronary blood flow in relation to acutely administered alcohol have yielded conflicting findings (46, 93, 117, 138, 157, 160). Furthermore, the acute blood pressure and heart rate effects of doses of 30–75 ml of alcohol (34, 55, 67, 123) may affect the occurrence of myocardial ischemia, independent of any possible action of alcohol on the coronary circulation itself. Thus an ambiguous relation exists between alcohol ingestion and angina pectoris due to coronary atherosclerotic disease. Subjective benefit is probably not related to concurrent improvement in myocardial oxygen supply but presumably is the result of anesthetic or tranquilizing effects of alcohol.

MYOCARDIAL INFARCTION AND CORONARY DISEASE MORTALITY The relation of alcohol consumption to myocardial infarction and death from coronary disease has aroused much recent interest and some controversy. Some of the earlier population studies (26, 104) showed no association between alcohol use and major coronary events. The data were not apparently controlled for cigarette smoking, a well-established predictor of coronary events and a strong correlate of alcohol use (72, 74, 76, 137). The Framingham Heart Study reported data (153) showing a slight but statistically insignificant inverse relation (drinkers at less risk) between use of 30 or more ounces of alcohol per month and myocardial infarction, even without apparent control for smoking.

In a population study well controlled for smoking and other established coronary risk factors (43), there was a statistically significant inverse relation of alcohol use and heart attack among members of the Northern California Kaiser-Permanente Medical Care Program (73). A slightly inverse, but not statistically significant, relation between drinking and sudden cardiac death (42) was also found in the Kaiser-Permanente study. The inverse drinking-coronary relation was slightly progressive up to users of six or more drinks per day, although the largest difference in coronary risk was the difference between nondrinkers and users of two or fewer drinks daily.

In a study of Japanese men in Honolulu, a statistically significant inverse relation was found between drinking and both myocardial infarction and coronary mortality (13, 167).

A report from the Boston Collaborative Drug Surveillance Program (148) showed a slight inverse relation between alcohol use and nonfatal myocardial infarction. Another recent study in Boston (60) showed an inverse relation between alcohol use and death from coronary disease. In a later report (61), the relation was shown independently for users of beer, wine, or distilled spirits. A second study from the Kaiser-Permanente Medical Care Program (72, 75) showed a significantly lower hospitalization incidence and mortality for coronary disease among drinkers than among nondrinkers.

On the other hand, a number of studies (23, 30, 33, 137, 163) among problem drinkers or alcoholics have presented data showing a higher risk of myocardial infarction or coronary death among these persons. Among these studies, several (30, 33, 137) are comparisons between groups not controlled for important coronary risk factors, including smoking. Only one, a study of Swedish Temperance Board Registrants (163), showed a statistically significant increased risk of both nonfatal myocardial infarction and coronary death with control for smoking and other coronary risk factors.

Thus, most of the population studies suggest that drinkers suffer fewer major coronary events, whereas the studies of alcoholics show the opposite. It is possible that large amounts of alcohol have effects in coronary disease quite different from those of smaller amounts, but other explanations for this discrepancy are more likely. There are two possible explanations for a spurious association in the population studies. First, former drinkers, a subset of the nondrinkers in several of the studies, may be at especially high coronary risk. Second, there may be indirect association through ethnic factors, psychological traits, or other unknown risk factors. Explanations for a possible spurious association between very heavy drinking and coronary events include: (a) An indirect relation of very heavy drinking and coronary events through established coronary risk factors (e.g. hypertension and smoking) is almost certain. (b) An indirect relation may exist through other possible risk factors, such as psychosocial stress, which could be related to both heavy drinking and heart attack. (c) A possible erroneous diagnosis of coronary disease among alcoholics who die of other cardiac conditions, such as alcoholic cardiomyopathy, may also be made.

In the first half of this century, there were a number of reports (22, 64, 81, 103, 162) of an apparent inverse relation between chronic substantial alcohol use and atherosclerotic disease, including coronary disease, diagnosed at autopsy. However, this was dismissed by some (103, 131) as a statistical artifact because the premature deaths of many alcoholic persons might preclude the development of atherosclerotic vascular disease. Recent work by Barboriak and colleagues (8, 9) showed that, among 900 patients examined by coronary arteriography, drinkers had significantly less atherosclerotic occlusion than nondrinkers, although the drinkers smoked more. Recent experimental data (28) concerning monkeys fed 36% of their calorie intake as alcohol indicate that alcohol at this level apparently reduces the development of experimental coronary atherosclerosis.

POSSIBLE EXPLANATIONS FOR THE INVERSE ALCOHOL-CORONARY DISEASE RELATION   The emergence of a plausible mechanism for a protective effect of alcohol in coronary disease increases the possibility that such an effect exists. The mechanism is based on the observation that alcohol raises high-density lipoprotein (HDL) cholesterol levels in blood (25, 63, 80, 122). Elevated HDL is inversely related to coronary atherosclerotic disease (24, 48, 121) and may have a protective role by aiding in removal of cholesterol from the body or by retarding the formation of atherosclerotic plaques. The effect of alcohol in raising HDL levels is generally proportional to the amount regularly taken (63). Alcohol-induced HDL elevations decrease in days to weeks when drinking is stopped (63, 80). There is evidence that the site of action of alcohol's influence on HDL is the liver; some integrity of liver function is needed, as evidenced by the fact that some persons with acute, severe alcohol hepatotoxicity have very low HDL levels (80, 133). At ordinary levels of alcohol use, it has been suggested (152) that alcohol facilitates HDL production by facilitating influx of triglyceride-carrying lipoproteins to the liver cells.

Alcohol may also protect against major coronary events by a mechanism other than prevention of atherosclerotic occlusion. Although this has not been studied extensively, evidence for such an action has been reported (57). Such protection might be mediated by inhibition of platelet aggregation (58).

Alcohol and Other Cardiovascular Diseases

STROKE   A positive relation between drinking and stroke incidence has been reported (13, 24, 69, 72). The relation is stronger for hemorrhagic than for thrombotic stroke (13, 72) and is felt to be not entirely explained by the association of both drinking and stroke with hypertension. A bleeding tendency due to alcohol has been implicated (13) as a possible additional explanation.

AORTIC AND PERIPHERAL VESSEL ATHEROSCLEROSIS   There is little epidemiologic evidence to suggest a relation to alcohol use (72).

NONCORONARY ATHEROSCLEROTIC DISEASE   An unusual form of angina pectoris, known as Prinzmetal variant angina, is widely believed to be related in some patients to reversible spasm of large coronary vessels (125). Although alcohol has been reported to be one of the pharmacologic agents that can induce this phenomenon (40), the association has not been widely observed.

Regan (118) reported a number of cases of myocardial infarction among alcoholics with no evidence of atherosclerotic or thrombotic occlusion. He postulated a mechanism of external constriction of coronary vessels by scarring due to alcoholic cardiomyopathy. Myocardial infarction without atherosclerosis is a poorly understood event that also occurs occasionally in nonalcoholics (125).

OTHER CONDITIONS   Substantial alcohol use has been reported to be associated with a higher incidence of venous conditions (72) such as phlebitis and varicose veins. Heavy maternal drinking is associated with congenital anomalies of the heart (septal defects and patent ductus arteriosus) in offspring (98).

Table 1 summarizes the disparate relations of alcohol use and cardiovascular conditions. A recent report on hospitalization incidence in a large number of persons with various alcohol habits (72) demonstrated this disparity in a single cohort. The heaviest drinkers fared worst because of a higher risk of hypertension, stroke, congestive failure, arrhythmias, venous conditions, and cardiomyopathy. Moderate drinkers (two or fewer drinks per day) fared best with respect to overall incidence of hospitalization for cardiovascular causes. Nondrinkers fared substantially worse than the moderate drinkers, primarily because of a higher incidence of coronary heart disease. Hospitalizations for coronary events showed a pattern distinctly different from that for any other cardiovascular condition, with nondrinkers at significantly greater risk.

PUBLIC HEALTH ASPECTS OF ALCOHOL AND CARDIOVASCULAR DISEASES

The American public, aware of advances in knowledge in the alcohol-cardiovascular area, expects sound advice based on current knowledge, although it is probably easier to counsel individual patients than to formulate general pronouncements. Most health professionals would probably agree on a few basic facts: (a) There is substantial evidence that use of large amounts of alcohol carries heavy medical and social risks. The medical risks include cardiovascular and noncardiovascular disorders. (b) The threshold dose for possible harmful effects of alcohol is not known and probably varies from person to person. (c) Many persons should not drink at all—those

Table 1   Disparate relations of alcohol and cardiovascular conditions

	Apparent relation to use of alcohol	
	Small amounts	Large amounts
Beriberi	None	None (cause is thiamine deficiency)
Alcoholic cardiomyopathy	None	Direct myocardial toxicity in susceptible persons
Arsenic (As) beer drinkers' disease	None	Synergistic myocardial toxicity of As, alcohol
Cobalt (Co) beer drinkers' disease	None	Synergistic myocardial toxicity of Co, alcohol
Hypertension	None or slightly inverse (less hypertension)	Direct (more hypertension)
Atherosclerotic coronary	Inverse (less disease)	Conflicting evidence
Stroke	?	Direct (stronger for hemorrhagic than thrombotic stroke)
Venous conditions	None	Direct

with a history of a drinking problem or at special risk of a drinking problem, those with certain medical illnesses, and those with idiosyncratic reactions to alcohol.

The majority of US adults use alcohol in amounts that could be defined as moderate (76). These persons can be reassured that their drinking habit carries no known detrimental cardiovascular effects and may in fact place them in the most favorable risk category for overall cardiovascular disease incidence. With respect to alcohol use in relation to specific conditions, the following guidelines seem reasonable to the author.

1. Persons with chronic congestive heart failure or major arrhythmia problems should be extremely cautious about use of alcohol (no more than one drink per occasion).

2. Up to two drinks a day seems safe for hypertensive patients or persons at special risk of hypertension. Three or more drinks a day (35 ml or more of alcohol) probably increases the risk of hypertension.

3. Drinking before exercise is dangerous to patients with angina pectoris. Drinking before exercise is probably unwise for all persons.

4. Although a protective effect has not been proved, the evidence is mounting that use of alcohol is associated with a slower rate of development of coronary atherosclerotic occlusion and a lower incidence of myocardial infarction. There is more epidemiologic evidence for this possible benefit at low to moderate levels of drinking (up to 30 ml of alcohol per day). At higher levels of drinking, the possible protection from coronary disease may be attenuated and, in any case, is outweighed by other cardiovascular risks.

68   KLATSKY

Literature Cited

1. Aalsmeer, W. C., Wenckebach, K. F. 1929. *Wien. Arch. Inn. Med.* 16:193–272
2. Ahmed, S. S., Levinson, G. E., Regan, T. J. 1973. *Circulation* 48:378–85
3. Alexander, C. S. 1966. *Am. J. Med.* 41:213–28
4. Alexander, C. S. 1966. *Am. J. Med.* 41:229–34
5. Alexander, C. S. 1968. *J. Lab. Clin. Med.* 72:850 (Abstr.)
6. Alexander, C. S. 1969. *Ann. Intern. Med.* 70:411–13
7. Askanas, A., Udoshi, M., Sadjadi, S. A. 1980. *Am. Heart J.* 99:9–16
8. Barboriak, J. J., Anderson, A. J., Rimm, A. A. 1979. *Alcohol. Clin. Exp. Res.* 3:29–32
9. Barboriak, J. J., Rimm, A. A., Anderson, A. J., Schmidhoffer, M., Tristani, F. E. 1977. *Br. Heart J.* 39:289–93
10. Bashour, T. T., Fahdul, H., Cheng, T. O. 1975. *Chest* 68:24–27
11. Beevers, D. G. 1977. *Lancet* 2:114–15
12. Blacket, R. B., Palmer, A. J. 1960. *Br. Heart J.* 22:483–501
13. Blackwelder, W. C., Yano, K., Rhoads, G. G., Kagan, A., Gordon, T., Palesch, Y. 1980. *Am. J. Med.* 68:164–69
14. Blankenhorn, M. A. 1945. *Ann. Intern. Med.* 23:398–404
15. Blankenhorn, M. A., Vilter, C. F., Scheinker, I. M., Austin, R. S. 1946. *J. Am. Med. Assoc.* 131:717–27
16. Blomqvist, G., Saltin, B., Mitchell, J. H. 1970. *Circulation* 42:463–70
17. Böllinger, O. 1884. *Dtsch. Med. Wochenschr. (Stuttgart)* 10:180
19. Bulloch, R. T., Pearce, M. B., Murphy, M. L., Jenkins, B. J., Davis, J. L. 1972. *Am. J. Cardiol.* 29:15–25
20. Burch, G. E., Colcolough, H. L., Harb, J. M., Tsui, C. Y. 1971. *Am. J. Cardiol.* 27:522–28
21. Burch, G. E., Phillips, J. H. Jr., Ferrans, V. J. 1966. *Am. J. Med. Sci.* 252:89–104
22. Cabot, R. C. 1904. *J. Am. Med. Assoc.* 43:774–75
23. California State Department of Public Health, Division of Alcoholic Rehabilitation. 1961. *Alcoholism and California, Publication No. 6.* Berkeley: Calif. State Dept. Publ. Health, Div. Alcohol. Rehab.
24. Castelli, W. 1980. Presented at 20th Ann. Conf. Cardiovasc. Epidemiol., San Diego, 1980
25. Castelli, W. P., Gordon, T., Hjortland, M. C., Kagan, A., Doyle, J. T., Hames,

C. G., Zukel, W. J. 1977. *Lancet* 2:153–55
26. Chapman, J. M., Massey, F. J. Jr., Coulson, A., Sayre, J. 1974. *Final Report to National Institute on Alcohol Abuse and Alcoholism* Rockville, Md: Natl. Inst. Alcohol Abuse and Alcoholism
27. Clark, V. A., Chapman, J. M., Coulson, A. H. 1967. *J. Chron. Dis.* 20:571–81
28. Clarkson, T. 1981. Presented at 20th Ann. Conf. Cardiovasc. Epidemiol., San Diego, 1980
29. Conway, N. 1968. *Br. Heart J.* 30:638–44
30. D'Alonzo, C. A., Pell, S. 1968. *J. Occup. Med.* 10:344–50
31. Delgado, C. E., Fortuin, N. J., Ross, R. S. 1975. *Circulation* 51:535–40
32. Demakis, J. G., Proskey, A., Rahimtoola, S. H., Jamil, M., Sutton, G. C., Rosen, K. M., Gunnar, R. M., Tobin, J. R. Jr. 1974. *Ann. Intern. Med.* 80:293–97
33. Dyer, A. R., Stamler, J., Paul, O., Berkson, D. M., Lepper, M. H., McKean, H., Shekelle, R. B., Lindberg, H. A., Garside, D. 1977. *Circulation* 56:1067–74
34. Eliaser, M., Giansiracusa, F. J. 1956. *Calif. Med.* 84:234–36
35. Ettinger, P. O., Wu, C. F., De La Cruz, C. Jr., Weisse, A. B., Regan, T. J. 1976. *Am. J. Cardiol.* 37:134 (Abstr.)
36. Ettinger, P. O., Wu, C. F., De La Cruz, C. Jr., Weisse, A. B., Ahmed, S. S., Regan, T. J. 1978. *Am. Heart J.* 95:555–62
37. Evans, W. 1959. *Br. Heart J.* 21:445–56
38. Evans, W. 1961. *Am. Heart J.* 61:556–67
39. Factor, S. M. 1976. *Am. Heart J.* 92:561–75
40. Fernandez, D., Rosenthal, J. E., Cohen, L. S., Hammond, G., Wolfson, S. 1973. *Am. J. Cardiol.* 32:238–39
41. Fewings, J. D., Hanna, M. J., Walsh, J. A., Whelan, R. F. 1966. *Br. J. Pharmacol. Chemother.* 27:93–106
42. Friedman, G. D., Klatsky, A. L., Siegelaub, A. B. 1975. *Circulation* 51/52: (Suppl. 3) 164–69
43. Friedman, G. D., Klatsky, A. L., Siegelaub, A. B., McCarthy, N. 1974. *Am. J. Epidemiol.* 99:101–16
44. Friedman, H. S., Matsuzaki, S., Choe, S., Fernando, H. A., Celis, A., Zaman, Q., Lieber, C. S. 1976. *Cardiovasc. Res.* 13:477–86
45. Friedreich, N. 1861. *Die Krankheiten des Herzens.* Erlangen: Ferdinand Enke
46. Ganz, V. 1963. *Am. Heart J.* 66:494–97

47. Gimeno, A. L., Gimeno, M. F., Webb, J. L. 1962. *Am. J. Physiol.* 203:194–96
48. Goldbourt, U., Medalie, J. H. 1977. *CVD Epidemiol. Newsl.* 22:23
49. Goodwin, J. F. 1972. *Mod. Concepts Cardiovasc. Dis.* 41:41–46
50. Gould, L., Zahir, M., DeMartino, A., Gomprecht, R. F. 1971. *J. Am. Med. Assoc.* 218:1799–802
51. Gould, L., Zahir, M., DeMartino, A., Gomprecht, R. F., Jaynal, F. 1972. *Q. J. Stud. Alcohol* 33:714–21
52. Gould, L., Zahir, M., Mahmood, S., Di Lieto, M. 1969. *Ann. Intern. Med.* 71:543–53
53. Gowers, W. R. 1901. *Lancet* 1:98–100
54. Greenspon, A. J., Stang, J. M., Lewis, R. P., Schaal, S. F. 1979. *N. Engl. J. Med.* 301:1049–50
55. Grollman, A. 1930. *J. Pharmacol. Exp. Ther.* 39:313–27
56. Hamby, R. I. 1970. *Medicine (Baltimore)* 49:55–78
57. Hartz, A. J., Anderson, A. J., Barboriak, P. N., Barboriak, J. J., Hoffman, R. G. 1979. *Circulation* 60: (Suppl. 2) 68 (Abstr.)
58. Haut, M. J., Cowan, D. H. 1974. *Am. J. Med.* 56:22–23
59. Heberden, W. 1786. *Med. Trans. R. Coll. Physicians (London)* 2:59–67
60. Hennekens, C. H., Rosner, B., Cole, D. S. 1978. *Am. J. Epidemiol.* 107:196–200
61. Hennekens, C. H., Willett, W., Rosner, B., Cole, D. S., Mayrent, S. L. 1979. *J. Am. Med. Assoc.* 242:1973–74
62. Horwitz, L. D., Atkins, J. M. 1974. *Circulation* 49:124–28
63. Hulley, S. 1981. *Circulation* 64:(Suppl. 3) 57–63
64. Hultgen, J. F. 1910. *J. Am. Med. Assoc.* 55:279–81
65. Isselbacher, K. J. 1977. *N. Engl. J. Med.* 296:612–16
66. Jones, R. H. 1959. *Circulation* 19: 275–81
67. Juchems, R., Klobe, R. 1969. *Am. Heart J.* 78:133–35
68. Kannel, W. B., Sorlie, P. 1974. In *Hypertension in Framingham: Epidemiology and Control of Hypertension,* ed. O. Paul, pp. 553–92. NY: Stratton Intercontinental Medical Book
69. Katsuki, S. 1971. *J. Jpn. Soc. Intern. Med.* 60:3–17
70. Keefer, C. S. 1930. *Arch. Intern. Med.* 45:1–22
71. Kesteloot, H., Roelandt, J., Willems, J., Claes, J. H., Joossens, J. V. 1968. *Circulation* 37:854–64
72. Klatsky, A. L., Friedman, G. D., Siegelaub, A. B. 1981. *Circulation* 64:(Suppl. 3) 32–41
73. Klatsky, A. L., Friedman, G. D., Siegelaub, A. B. 1974. *Ann. Intern. Med.* 81:294–301
74. Klatsky, A. L., Friedman, G. D., Siegelaub, A. B. 1979. In *Metabolic Effects of Alcohol,* ed. B. Avogaro, G. Marchetti, C. R. Sirtori, E. Tremoli, Amsterdam: Elsevier/North Holland
75. Klatsky, A. L., Friedman, G. D., Siegelaub, A. B. 1981. *Ann. Intern. Med.* 95:139–45
76. Klatsky, A. L., Friedman, G. D., Siegelaub, A. B., Gérard, M. J. 1977. *Am. J. Epidemiol.* 105:311–23
77. Klatsky, A. L., Friedman, G. D., Siegelaub, A. B., Gérard, M. J. 1977. *N. Engl. J. Med.* 296:1194–200
78. Koide, T., Ozeki, K. 1974. *Jpn. Heart J.* 15:337–48
79. Kozam, R. L., Esguerra, O. E., Smith, J. J. 1972. *Am. J. Cardiol.* 30:418–22
80. La Porte, R., Valvo-Gerard, L., Kuller, L., Dai, W., Bates, M., Cresenta, J., Williams, K., Palkrn, D. 1981. *Circulation* 64:(Suppl. 3) 67–72
81. Leary, T. 1931. *N. Engl. J. Med.* 205:231–42
82. Levine, S. A. 1951. *Clinical Heart Disease.* Philadelphia: W. B. Saunders. 4th ed.
83. Liedtke, A. J., DeMuth, W. E. 1975. *Am. J. Cardiol.* 35:243–50
84. Limas, C. J., Guiha, N. H., Lekagul, O., Cohn, J. N. 1974. *Circulation* 49: 755–60
85. Linkola, J. 1979. *N. Engl. J. Med.* 300:680 (Letter)
86. Lochner, A., Cowley, R., Brink, A. J. 1969. *Am. Heart J.* 78:770–80
87. MacKenzie, J. 1902. *The Study of the Pulse.* Edinburgh: Y. J. Pentland. p. 237
88. Maines, J. E., Aldinger, E. E. 1967. *Am. Heart J.* 73:55–63
89. Mathews, J. D. 1976. *Clin. Sci. Mol. Med.* 51:(Suppl. 3) 661s–63s
90. Matthews, E. C. Jr., Gardin, J. M., Henry, W. L., Del Negro, A. A., Fletcher, R. D., Snow, J. A., Epstein, S. E. 1981. *Am. J. Cardiol.* 47:570–78
91. McCloy, R. B., Prancan, A. V., Nakano, J. 1974. *Cardiovasc. Res.* 8: 216–26
92. McDermott, P. H., Delaney, R. L., Egan, J. D., Sullivan, J. F. 1966. *J. Am. Med. Assoc.* 198:163–66
93. Mendoza, L. C., Hellberg, K., Rickart, A., Tillich, G., Bing, R. J. 1971. *J. Clin. Pharmacol.* 11:165–76

94. Mitchell, J. H., Cohen, L. S. 1970. *Mod. Concepts Cardiovasc. Dis.* 39:109–13
95. Morin, Y., Daniel, P. 1967. *Can. Med. Assoc. J.* 97:926–28
96. Myrhed, M. 1974. *Acta Med. Scand., Suppl.* 567:40–46
97. Newman, W. H., Valicenti, J. F. Jr. 1971. *Am. Heart J.* 81:61–68
98. Noonan, J. A. 1978. *Am. J. Cardiol.* 37:160 (Abstr.)
99. Orlando, J., Aronow, W. S., Cassidy, J., Prakash, R. 1976. *Ann. Intern. Med.* 84:652–55
100. Pachinger, O. M., Tillmanns, H., Mao, J. C., Fauvel, J.–M., Bing, R. J. 1973. *J. Clin. Invest.* 52:2690–96
101. Pader, E. 1973. *Q. J. Stud. Alcohol* 34:774–85
102. Parker, B. M. 1974. *J. Am. Med. Assoc.* 228:741–42
103. Parrish, H. M., Eberly, A. L. Jr. 1961. *J. Indiana Med. Assoc.* 54:341–47
104. Paul, O., Lepper, M. H., Phelan, W. H., Dupertuis, G. W., MacMillan, A., McKean, H., Park, H. 1963. *Circulation* 28:20–36
105. Perkoff, G. T., Dioso, M. M., Bleisch, V., Klinkerfuss, G. 1967. *Ann. Intern. Med.* 67:481–92
106. Pintar, K., Wolanskyj, B. M., Gubbay, E. R. 1965. *Can. Med. Assoc. J.* 93:103–7
107. Prasad, P., Tabatznik, B., Kotler, M. N. 1974. *Johns Hopkins Med. J.* 134:226–32
108. Priest, R. G., Binns, J. K., Kitchin, A. H. 1966. *Br. Med. J.* 1:1453–55
109. Puskin, S., Rubin, E. 1975. *Science* 188:1319–22
110. Ramsay, L. E. 1977. *Lancet* 2:111–14
111. Ramsay, L. E. 1979. *Pract. Cardiol.* 5:27–32
112. Rees, L. H., Besser, G. M., Jeffcoate, W. J., Goldie, D. J., Marks, V. 1977. *Lancet* 1:726–28
113. Reeves, W. C., Nanda, N. C., Gramiak, R. 1978. *Am. Heart J.* 95:578–83
114. Reitz, R. C., Helsabeck, E., Mason, D. P. 1973. *Lipids* 8:80–84
115. Regan, T. J., Khan, M. I., Ettinger, P. O., Haider, B., Lyons, M. M., Oldewurtel, H. A. 1974. *J. Clin. Invest.* 54:740–52
116. Regan, T. J., Koroxenidis, G., Moschos, C. B., Oldewurtel, H. A., Lehan, P. H., Hellems, H. K. 1966. *J. Clin. Invest.* 45:270–80
117. Regan, T. J., Levinson, G. E., Oldewurtel, H. A., Frank, M. J., Weisse, A. B., Moschos, C. B. 1969. *J. Clin. Invest.* 48:397–407
118. Regan, T. J., Wu, C. F., Weisse, A. B., Moschos, C. B., Ahmed, S. S., Lyons, M. M. 1975. *Circulation* 51:453–61
119. Retig, J. N., Kirchberger, M. A., Rubin, E., Katz, A. M. 1977. *Biochem. Pharmacol.* 26:393–96
120. Reynolds, E. S. 1901. *Lancet* 1:166–70
121. Rhoads, G. G., Gulbrandsen, C. L., Kagan, A. 1976. *N. Engl. J. Med.* 294:293–98
122. Rhoads, G. G., Kagan, A., Yano, K. 1976. *Circulation* 54:(Suppl. 2) II–53 (Abstr.)
123. Riff, D. P., Jain, A. C., Doyle, J. T. 1969. *Am. Heart J.* 78:592–97
124. Robin, E., Goldschlager, N. 1976. *Am. Heart J.* 80:103–8
125. Rosenblatt, A., Selzer, A. 1977. *Circulation* 55:578–80
126. Royal Commission Appointed to Inquire into Arsenical Poisoning from the Consumption of Beer and other Articles of Food or Drink. 1903. *Final Report*. Part I. London: Wyman and Sons
127. Royal Commission on Arsenical Poisoning. 1901. *Lancet* 2:218
128. Royal Commission on Arsenical Poisoning. 1910. *Lancet* 1:672–73
129. Rubin, E. 1979. *N. Engl. J. Med.* 301:28–33
130. Rubin, E. 1981. Alcohol: Toxic or tonic? *Cardiovasc. Rev. Rep.* 2:23–27
131. Ruebner, B. H., Miyai, K., Abbey, H. 1961. *Lancet* 2:1435–36
132. Russek, H. I., Naegele, C. F., Regan, F. D. 1950. *J. Am. Med. Assoc.* 143:355–57
133. Sabesin, S. 1981. *Circulation* 64:(Suppl. 3)72–84
134. Sanders, V. 1963. *Arch. Intern. Med.* 112:661–76
135. Sarma, J. S. M., Ikeda, S., Fischer, R., Maruyama, Y., Weishaar, R., Bing, R. J. 1976. *J. Mol. Cell. Cardiol.* 8:951–72
136. Schenk, E. A., Cohen, J. 1970. *Pathol. Microbiol.* 35:96–104
137. Schmidt, W., de Lint, J. 1972. *Q. J. Stud. Alcohol* 33:171–85
138. Schmitthenner, J. E., Hafkenschiel, J. H., Forte, I., Williams, A. J., Riegel, C. 1958. *Circulation* 18:778 (Abstr.)
139. Schreiber, S. S., Briden, K., Oratz, M., Rothschild, M. A. 1973. *J. Clin. Invest.* 51:2820–26
140. Schwartz, L., Sample, K. A., Wigle, E. D. 1975. *Am. J. Cardiol.* 36:963–66
141. Segel, L. D., Rendig, S. V., Choquet, Y., Chacko, K., Amsterdam, E. A., Mason, D. T. 1975. *Cardiovasc. Res.* 9:649–63
142. Sereny, G., Mehta, B., Sethna, D. 1978. *Drug Alcohol Depend.* 3:331–43

143. Shugoll, G. I., Bowen, P. J., Moore, J. P., Lenkin, M. L. 1972. *Arch. Intern. Med.* 129:67–72
144. Singer, K., Lundberg, W. B. 1972. *Ann. Intern. Med.* 77:247–48
145. Smals, A., Kloppenborg, P. 1977. *Lancet* 1:1369 (Letter)
146. Spann, J. F. Jr., Mason, D. T., Beiser, G. D., Gold, H. K. 1968. *Clin. Res.* 16:249 (Abstr.)
147. Spodick, D. H., Pigott, V. H., Chirife, R. 1972. *N. Engl. J. Med.* 287:677–80
148. Stason, W. B., Neff, R. K., Miettinen, O. S., Jick, H. 1976. *Am. J. Epidemiol.* 104:603–8
149. Steell, G. 1893. *Med. Chron. Manchester* 18:1–22
150. Steell, G. 1906. *Textbook on Diseases of the Heart.* Philadelphia: Blakiston. p. 79
151. Sullivan, J. F., George, R., Bluvas, R., Egan, J. D. 1969. *Ann. Intern. Med.* 70:177–282
152. Tall, A. R., Small, D. M. 1978. *N. Engl. J. Med.* 299:1232–36
153. US National Heart Institute. 1966. *U.S. Publ. Health Serv. Publ. No. 1515.* Washington DC: USGPO
154. Vaquez, H. 1921. *Maladies du Coeur.* Paris: Bailliere et Fils. p. 308
155. Walsche, W. H. 1873. *Disease of the Heart and Great Vessels.* London: Smith, Elder. 4th ed.
156. Webb, W. R., Degerli, I. U. 1965. *J. Am. Med. Assoc.* 191:1055–58
157. Webb, W. R., Degerli, I. U., Cook, W. A., Unal, M. O. 1966. *Ann. Surg.* 163:811–17
158. Weiss, S., Wilkins, R. W. 1937. *Ann. Intern. Med.* 11:104–48
159. Wendt, V. E., Ajluni, R., Bruce, T. A., Prasad, A. S., Bing, R. J. 1966. *Am. J. Cardiol.* 17:804–12
160. Wendt, V. E., Stock, T. B., Hayden, R. O., Bruce, T. A., Gudbjarnason, S., Bing, R. J. 1962. *Med. Clin. North. Am.* 46:1445–69
161. White, P. D. 1931. *Heart Disease.* NY: Macmillan. p. 436
162. Wilens, S. L. 1947. *J. Am. Med. Assoc.* 135:1136–39
163. Wilhelmsen, L., Wedel, H., Tibblin, G. 1973. *Circulation* 48:950–58
164. Williams, E. S., Li, T. K. 1977. *J. Mol. Cell. Cardiol.* 9:1003–11
165. Wong, M. 1973. *Am. Heart J.* 86:508–15
166. Wu, C. F. Sudhakar, M., Jaferi, G., Ahmed, S. S., Regan, T. J. 1976. *Am. Heart J.* 91:281–86
167. Yano, K., Rhoads, G. G., Kagan, A. 1977. *N. Engl. J. Med.* 297:405–9

Ann. Rev. Nutr. 1982. 2:73–89

REGULATION OF WATER INTAKE

B. Andersson, L. G. Leksell, and M. Rundgren

Department of Physiology, College of Veterinary Medicine, Swedish University of Agricultural Sciences, S-750 07 Uppsala, and Department of Physiology, Karolinska Institutet, S- 104 01 Stockholm, Sweden

CONTENTS

INTRODUCTION

Supplied with unlimited fresh water, humans and apparently most mammals satisfy their need for water by anticipatory, habitual, or prandial drinking not motivated by true thirst (23). Nevertheless, an efficient thirst mechanism and appropriate regulation of the liberation of water-retaining antidiuretic hormone (ADH, vasopressin) are indispensable for optimal water balance, the maintenance of which has high homeostatic priority.

73

0199-9885/82/0715-0073$02.00

Thus during severe dehydration the craving for water becomes tormenting and constitutes one of the most urgent of human needs (79). Normally, all derangements of fluid balance that elicit thirst also induce hypersecretion of ADH from the neurohypophysis (although the reverse is sometimes not the case). This implies that water intake and ADH secretion are predominantly regulated by similarly functioning enteroreceptors, which have a lower stimulus threshold for initiating ADH liberation than for eliciting the urge to drink. Hence, research on the regulation of ADH secretion is relevant to the etiology of thirst, and studies on thirst may contribute to our understanding of ADH release. Here we review the regulation of both water intake and ADH secretion, citing current evidence for (*a*) the contribution of cerebral sensory mechanisms to the control of water balance, and (*b*) the role played by the brain as coordinator of relevant afferent signals. We discuss controversies in the area and briefly review certain clinical manifestations of disturbed cerebral regulation of water intake.

DEVIATIONS FROM FLUID BALANCE ELICITING THIRST AND ADH RELEASE

Osmotic Regulation

The deviations from fluid balance that most efficaciously elicit thirst and hypersecretion of ADH are (*a*) deficit of water without corresponding loss of Na (hypovolemic hypernatremia, Figure 1 D), and (*b*) osmotic shift of water from the cells to the extracellular fluid (ECF) induced by excessive Na intake (hypervolemic hypernatremia, Figure 1 A). The latter condition does not involve any net loss of water, but characteristics common to both conditions are cellular dehydration, hyperosmolality of the body fluids, and elevated extracellular Na concentration. Of these three factors, cellular dehydration is generally considered to constitute the crucial thirst and ADH stimulus. Such regulation is designated osmotic in the light of Verney's (75) fundamental investigations, which imply that ADH release is negatively correlated to the cell volume of hypothalamic osmoreceptors. Whether the sensory mechanism disclosed by Verney in fact consists of osmoreceptors, or elements more specifically sensitive to Na (5), has recently been debated (see the section below on Sensors of Osmotic Regulation). Be that as it may, more than 90% of the osmolality of the interstitial fluid and the blood plasma is created by Na and its associated anions. These particles also exert the effective (cell-dehydrating) tonicity of the ECF since Na is continuously extruded from the cells in exchange for K by active, enzymatic cation transport. In reality, therefore, the osmotic regulation of water intake and ADH release serves as a protector of normal plasma Na concentration; and in conscious individuals having free access to water,

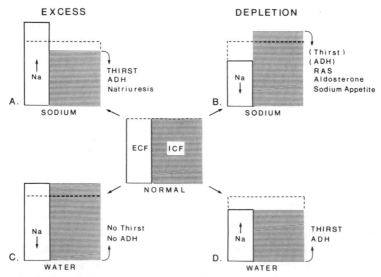

Figure 1 Outline of changes in body fluid distribution and extracellular Na concentration during positive and negative sodium and water balance. Compensatory factors indicated to the right of each diagram. *ADH* = antidiuretic hormone; *ECF* = extracellular fluid compartment; *ICF* = intracellular fluid compartment; *RAS* = the reninangiotensin system. Reprinted with permission from (9).

significant hypernatremia is encountered only if the thirst mechanism is impaired.

By using a sensitive radioimmunological method to determine plasma ADH (arginine vasopressin) and by accurately measuring plasma osmolality, Robertson and associates (58, 60) have disclosed the amazing sensitivity of the enteroceptors responsible for the osmotic control of water balance in man. Performed during various states of hydration, these investigations revealed a close correlation between plasma ADH level and osmolality in healthy adults. Individual variations were seen, but the plasma osmolality during euhydration averaged 287 mOsm/kg with an average plasma vasopressin concentration slightly above 2 pg/ml. ADH secretion of that order involved roughly 50% engagement of the renal capacity to concentrate the urine. A 2% increase in total body water was sufficient to suppress the ADH secretion below the detectable level and, hence, to induce maximal urine dilution. In the opposite direction, the thirst threshold was reached at about 2% deficit of body water (average plasma osmolality 294 mOsm/kg), and this moderate hypovolemic hypernatremia elevated plasma vasopressin to about 5 pg/ml, which was sufficient to induce maximal urine concentration. As pointed out by Robertson et al (60), this implies that the thirst threshold as normally set provides an effective compensation for ADH when the renal action of the hormone can no longer prevent an undue elevation of plasma Na concentration and tonicity. Thus osmoregulatory thirst in man may be regarded as an emergency mechanism that intervenes only when the water in food and anticipatory or habitual drinking, in combination with fully utilized effect of ADH, are insufficient to maintain extracellular Na concentration below a certain level.

Volume Regulation

It is well known that hemorrhagic shock or persistent profuse diarrhea may induce intense thirst in spite of the fact that plasma Na concentration and osmolality remain normal or are even decreased. Furthermore, animals extensively depleted of sodium, having reduced extracellular Na concentration and osmolality, may increase their water intake and continue to secrete ADH (2). What characterizes these conditions is a pronounced diminution of the ECF volume, which makes it obvious that a volume regulation of water intake and ADH release parallels and complements the osmotic regulation. The dimension of the ECF regulated is evidently the effective circulating blood volume, and both cardiovascular reflexes and the renal renin-angiotensin system (RAS) are apparently involved (see the section below on Mediators of Volume Regulation). However, volume regulation is evidently of negligible importance in normal day-to-day control of water balance and remains subordinate to its osmotic counterpart during moderate fluctuations of the ECF volume. Thus during gradually developing sodium depletion the osmotic regulation initially maintains plasma Na concentration and tonicity at or near normal levels. First at the stage when the osmoregulatory preservation of plasma Na concentration has induced critical hypovolemia, the volume regulation takes precedence at the price of hyponatremia (74). The relative insensibility of the volume regulation is also evident from the facts that thirst is no consistent effect of rather substantial blood loss in man (22), and that more than one fifth of the blood volume needs to be drawn in water-replete mammals before the thirst mechanism becomes activated (33, 38, 64). As regards ADH secretion, studies in man (27, 58) and animals (11, 18, 38) have revealed that about a 10% reduction of the blood volume is required before an increase in plasma ADH can be detected with available radioimmunological methods. However, hypovolemia of this order has been found to lower the osmotic threshold for ADH liberation, and to augment the hormone release at super-threshold levels of plasma osmolality, whereas expansion of the blood volume has been shown to have the opposite effect (18, 58). That this subtle interaction between volume and osmotic regulations also embraces thirst is indicated by the observations that hypovolemia lowers (37), and ECF volume expansion elevates (35) the threshold for drinking in response to intravenous infusions of hypertonic NaCl in the dog.

SENSORS OF OSMOTIC REGULATION

Although afferent impulses may modulate the osmotic regulation of water intake and ADH secretion, clinical observations in man and experimental studies in other mammals have gradually made it evident that this regulation is exerted predominantly by cerebral sensors. One hundred years ago Nothnagel (45) postulated that water intake was regulated by a thirst center in the brain. Nothnagel's report concerned the sudden onset of severe thirst without preceding polyuria (primary polydipsia) in a man subjected to head trauma. Other clinical reports on primary polydipsia of apparently cerebral origin followed (79), but the first definite proof of the brain's involvement in the osmotic control of water balance was provided by Verney (75) in the middle of the present century.

The Osmoreceptor Concept

In conscious hyperhydrated dogs Verney conclusively showed that cerebral sensors participate in the regulation of ADH secretion and are stimulated when the carotid blood osmolality is raised with sodium salts and other cell-dehydrating substances (for instance fructose and sucrose). Since no obvious ADH release was obtained in response to carotid blood hyperosmolality induced with substances that more easily equilibrate with the intracellular fluid (d-glucose and urea), Verney postulated that the sensors in question are primarily excited by a diminution of their own volume, and that a certain degree of sensor activity is maintained in euhydrated individuals by the prevailing plasma tonicity. The latter would explain the presence of a basic ADH secretion during euhydration, and the fact that this secretion subsides in response to excessive water intake. The osmoreceptor concept has exerted a far-reaching influence on subsequent research in the field, and when injections of small amounts of hypertonic NaCl into the medial hypothalamus were found to induce polydipsia in water-replete goats (4), it was regarded as evidence that osmoreceptors are also involved in the regulation of water intake. Later replications of Verney's experiments in the same or other mammalian species have confirmed in every respect the results of his pioneering research on the osmotic regulation of ADH secretion (20, 43) and have revealed a positive correlation between the ADH-releasing and thirst-eliciting effects of various substances used to induce plasma hyperosmolality (43, 47, 71, 81). Suggestive evidence for the osmoreceptor concept is also provided by the elucidative radioimmunological investigations on osmotic regulation of ADH secretion in man briefly discussed above (58, 60). However, the evidence for cerebral osmoreceptors becomes obscured when discussed in relation to presently available knowledge about solute transfer between the blood plasma and the interstitial fluid of the brain. As mentioned, carotid blood hyperosmolality induced with urea, and also with glycerol (20, 47) is ineffective as a stimulus for ADH release and thirst. Yet a blood-brain barrier for these substances considerably delays their passage into the cerebral interstitial fluid (15, 34). Consequently, intravascular administration of hypertonic urea and glycerol solutions dehydrates the brain as a whole. This seems to limit conceivable osmoreceptor locations to sites outside the blood-brain barrier, or to cerebral regions devoid of this barrier. Apparently only the latter possibility needs to be considered, since the sensors involved in the control of water balance are highly susceptible to humoral stimuli and inhibitors administered into the cerebrospinal fluid (CSF) of the lateral and third ventricles.

The Sodium Sensor Concept

Two observations made in the goat—(*a*) that hypertonic sucrose (in contrast to hypertonic NaCl) does not elicit ADH release and thirst when infused into the third ventricle (46), and (*b*) that the antidiuretic and dipsogenic responses to similar infusions of angiotensin II are positively correlated to the Na concentration of the CSF (7) —— originally gave rise to the suggestions that juxtacerebroventricular sodium sensors might be an alternative to osmoreceptors, and that the CSF may function as an indirect route by which alterations in blood plasma composition influence the activity of cerebral sensors controlling water balance (5). Continued investigations in the goat (6) have substantiated the evidence for this sodium sensor concept, as have recent studies in the sheep (42, 43) and rhesus monkey (70). Strongly supporting this idea are the results of experiments in which the CSF Na concentration has been lowered by intracerebroventricular infusions of hypertonic solutions of substances (fructose, sucrose, and mannitol) that elevate the effective (cell-dehydrating) osmolality of the CSF. Such infusions have been found to extinguish the dipsogenic (48) and antidiuretic (49) effects of hypernatremia and plasma hypertonicity, and to inhibit the basic ADH secretion in euhydrated animals (44). These observations appear hard to reconcile with the osmoreceptor theory. They also seem to eliminate the possibility that intracranial sensors regulating water intake and ADH secretion are situated outside the blood-brain barrier. However, the sensors in question may well be located in areas lacking that barrier, or have a position making them accessible both to blood-borne and CSF-borne influences. Such a state of affairs could explain why the intravascular administration of hypertonic urea, although elevating CSF Na concentration by cerebral dehydration (43), does not elicit ADH release and thirst. This fact has recently been considered a near fatal blow to the sodium sensor concept (66). However, cation transporting enzymatic activity seems to be essential for the excitation of cerebral sensors controlling water balance (6). Like deuterium (39) and some other inhibitors of active cation transport, urea effectively blocks hyperosmotic thirst and ADH release when administered into the CSF (62). Provided the substance has that action also from the vascular side of the blood-brain barrier, it could explain the lack of dipsogenic and ADH releasing responses to elevated CSF Na concentration induced by the intravascular administration of hypertonic urea. It must be concluded, however, that the nature of the cerebral sensors regulating water intake and ADH secretion in many respects remains to be elucidated.

Tentative Sensor Location

The mere fact that thirst and ADH secretion are easily affected by changes in the composition of the CSF suggests that sensors governing these functions are located somewhere in the surroundings of the cerebroventricular system. More direct evidence for a close juxtaventricular location is provided by the observation that intracerebroventricular infusions of deuterium (with NaCl added to isotonicity) effectively inhibited dehydrative thirst and the basic ADH secretion of euhydrated goats (39). When administered into the CSF, deuterium and other liquids with almost unlimited passage over the blood-brain barrier attain an exceedingly steep CSF/brain-tissue concentration profile (52). Consequently, if the observed effects of deuterium are due to inhibition of sensor activity, these elements must be located in or very near the ventricular wall. The brain area that deserves particular attention is the anterior wall of the third ventricle (Figure 2). Results of both stimulation and ablation experiments suggest that most sensors regulating ADH release and water intake are located in that area (6). Destruction of it by narrow, medially placed radiofrequency lesions was found to have drastic effects on the water balance of goats (8, 63). These lesions caused complete and persistent absence of thirst even during severe dehydration and hypernatremia (permanent adipsia) and lack of apparent ADH release in response to pronounced dehydration and to the intracarotid infusion of hypertonic NaCl and angiotensin II. An uncompensated, temporary water diuresis, which rapidly induced hypernatremia and hypovolemia, was observed as an acute effect of such lesions. The evidence favoring the idea that most sensors subserving water economy are present in or near the anterior wall of the third ventricle has stimulated speculations concerning the particular structures involved, and the morphological characteristics of the tentative sensors. The circumventricular organs present in this area (the subfornical organ and the organum vasculosum of the lamina terminalis) have received particular attention (23), mainly because they are devoid of a blood-brain barrier. This would make sensors confined to these organs accessible both to blood-borne and CSF-borne stimuli and inhibitors. Cell types in the wall of the third ventricle that also have been discussed as sensor candidates are CSF-contacting neurons (76) and tanocytes (77). The tanocytes, especially, seem structurally well adapted to function as sensors governing water intake and ADH release because these cells provide a morphological connection of CSF, nerve cells, and blood vessels. However, ablation experiments demonstrating that structures in front of the third ventricle are essential for the maintenance of water balance do not prove that the cerebral sensors regulating water intake and ADH secretion are exclusively confined to that part of the brain. An additonal function of the lesioned region may be integration or relaying of relevant impulses from sensors in other parts of the brain or from peripheral receptors. Further-more, from a phylogenetic point of view it appears rather unlikely that the entire population of cerebral sensory elements governing functions of so vital importance as thirst and ADH secretion should be confined to one periventricular area. Indications exist that sensors having these functions are also present at more posterior levels of the cerebroventricular system (6).

MEDIATORS OF VOLUME REGULATION

Changes in the effective circulating blood volume modulate the activity of cardiovascular mechano-receptors and the renal renin release. Conse-quently, reduction or increase in the effective amount of circulating blood may induce appropriate volume regulatory changes in water intake and ADH secretion both via cardiovascular reflexes and the RAS.

Cardiovascular Reflexes, ADH Secretion and Thirst

Ambiguities remain concerning the relative importance of differently located cardiovascular mechano-receptors in the volume control of water balance. However, the evidence is convincing that both arterial barorecep-tors and left atrial distention receptors exert a tonic inhibition on the neurohypophyseal ADH release (66) and that at least the latter kind of receptors affect the thirst mechanism in a similar manner (23). On the basis of experiments in the dog showing that balloon-inflation of the left atrium induced a diuresis, Henry et al (32) originally proposed that stimulation of distention receptors in this part of the heart inhibits ADH release. This proposal has been verified in similar studies involving determinations of plasma ADH (14, 73). The primary physiological importance of this inhibi-tory effect of cardiac receptor activity may be to counteract an undue expansion of the blood volume, whereas its importance in the defense against hypovolemia appears to be secondary. Thus underfilling of the heart induced by graded hemorrhage in conscious monkeys (11) and goats (38) did not cause significant ADH release until the hypovolemia had progressed

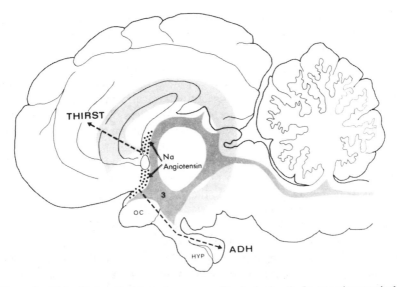

Figure 2 Midsagittal section through a mammalian brain (goat). Juxtacerebroventricular sensors responsible for the osmotic regulation of water intake and antidiuretic hormone (ADH) release are apparently located mainly in the dotted area in front of the third ventricle (3). However, such sensors may also be present at more posterior levels of the cerebroventricular system. *Hyp* = anterior lobe of the pituitary gland; *OC* = optic chiasm. Reprinted with permission from (6).

to a stage when the arterial blood pressure began to fall. This suggests reduced baroreceptor activity as the main cause of the ADH release. Evidence that atrial receptors also exert a tonic inhibition on the cerebral thirst mechanism includes observations that underfilling of the low pressure thoracic circulation elicited angiotensin II independent drinking in the dog (24), and that left thoracic vagosympathectomy lowered the osmotic thirst threshold in that species (69). However, a recent study in the sheep (82) suggests that hypovolemic thirst of cardiac origin may not be solely a release phenomenon. Denervation of the left atrium had no apparent effect on basic and hyperosmotic water intakes but completely abolished hypovolemic drinking. Thus underfilling of the left atrium may act dipsogenically not only by reducing inhibitory input from distention receptors but also by eliciting in some manner afferent nerve activity that stimulates the thirst mechanism.

The RAS, Thirst, and ADH Secretion

To what extent the renal RAS participates in the volume regulation of water intake and ADH secretion is somewhat controversial (31). That the kidney may participate in thirst regulation was originally proposed by Linazasoro et al (40) on the basis of the observation that parenteral administration of renal extract elicited drinking in nephrectomized rats. In the light of the substantial evidence subsequently presented by Fitzsimons and associates (22, 23) it now appears fully established that hypersecretion of renin induced by pronounced hypovolemia can increase the plasma concentration of angiotensin II in rats and dogs to a level at which this octapeptide stimulates the cerebral thirst mechanism. It is less obvious that the same may happen during volume depletion in some other mammalian species and has so far not been demonstrated in man. In the sheep, for instance, even severe Na depletion did not elevate plasma angiotensin II to a level compatible with the carotid blood concentration of exogenous angiotensin II needed to elicit drinking (1). Furthermore, the use of a competitive angiotensin II antagonist (saralasin) showed that the RAS did not to any measurable extent contribute to the drinking of dogs (54), goats (50), and sheep (3) preexposed to water deprivation for two days. However, extreme hyperactivity of the RAS has apparently contributed to intense thirst experienced by some patients suffering from renal failure (61), and abnormally high plasma levels of angiotensin II seem to have acted dipsogenically in patients with renin-secreting Wilm's tumor (67). Studies in animals have shown that ADH release is another centrally mediated effect of angiotensin II (7, 13), but it remains uncertain also whether that effect of the octapeptide has any physiological significance. Intravascular administration of angiotensin II did not cause increased ADH release in man until highly supraphysiological plasma levels were reached, and no correlation was found between plasma ADH and angiotensin II during acute changes of fluid balance in healthy volunteers, or in hyperreninemic patients (51). However, when discussing a conceivable physiological and/or pathophysiological importance of the RAS in the control of water balance, the possibility must be considered that angiotensin II might lower the osmotic stimulus threshold for thirst and ADH release (see below).

A definite answer has so far not been given to the question of whether blood-borne angiotensin stimulates the cerebral thirst and ADH-releasing mechanism(s) directly or indirectly via the CSF. Speaking in favor of the latter possibility are (*a*) the fact that in these respects angiotensin I and II act as efficient stimuli when administered into the lateral and third ventricles (6), and (*b*) the observation made in the sheep that intracerebroventricular administration of saralasin completely extinguished the dipsogenic response to the intracarotid infusion of angiotensin II but did not affect drinking in dehydrated animals (3). The latter finding implies that systemic angiotensin II either elicits thirst via the CSF or acts on cerebral sensors that are affected simultaneously by the CSF and the blood plasma composition. The latter appears more likely since it was recently shown in the rat and the dog that angiotensin I and II did not penetrate from the blood into the CSF unless large amounts of these peptides were administered intravenously (65). However, of interest in this connection is that the choroid plexa (19), and apparently also the ependyma (53), are rich in angiotensin I converting enzyme. It may be that conversion of blood-borne angiotensin I at these sites facilitates the exposure of juxtacerebroventricular sensors to angiotensin II during activation of the RAS. Another intricate question is whether "osmotic" and angiotensin II stimulation of thirst and ADH release is exerted via the same or different cerebral sensors. It has been claimed that the octapeptide and hypernatremia induce drinking via separate cerebral mechanisms (22). Evidence includes the observation that the dipsogenic effects of systemic angiotensin II and hypernatremia simply added to each other in the rat (25). However, speaking in favor of a unitary sensory target is the striking cerebral Na/angiotensin interaction demonstrated in the goat (6). Here intracerebroventricular administration of small amounts of angiotensin II caused a pronounced augumentation of thirst and ADH release in response to elevated CSF Na concentration. This led to the suggestion that the RAS may contribute to the control of water balance by lowering the stimulus threshold of cerebral receptors that are primarily sodium sensitive (5). Later support for that idea includes a study involving radioimmunological determination of urinary ADH excretion in response to intracerebroventricular infusions of angiotensin II and hypertonic NaCl, where a potentiated effect was obtained when both stimuli were applied together (41). Also favoring a unitary sensory target is the observation in the dog that intravenous infusions of ineffective amounts of angiotensin II lowered the thirst threshold to elevated blood plasma Na concentration (36).

In conclusion, to judge from presently available evidence, it appears that angiotensin should be regarded as a reserve expedient in the control of water balance that is used only in conditions associated with large ECF deficits. Perhaps it will be necessary to take a different view when we better understand the importance of the isorenin-angiotensin system that may exist in the brain (21, 26). As yet, however, the very existence of that system remains uncertain (53, 56).

PREABSORPTIVE APPEASEMENT OF THIRST

Thirst is not "permanently" slaked until absorbed water brings the activity of cerebral sensors regulating water intake back to a level below that needed to stimulate drinking. This "permanent" satisfaction of thirst occurs at a somewhat higher degree of body hydration than that present at the thirst threshold, and thereby provides a reserve of water that can be lost without an immediate revival of the urge to drink (23). It is far from obvious that the activity of cerebral sensors regulating water intake also subsides during the reflex temporary appeasement of thirst that takes place in the course of drinking, since the adequate stimulus of the sensors has not yet become reduced by postabsorptive alterations in body fluid composition and volume. It appears more likely that the reflex inhibition from the alimentary canal acts at some synaptic level, and there temporarily prevents sensory information of cerebral origin from reaching other parts of the brain where this information is converted into a conscious urge to drink. Studies in man and experimental animals made relatively long ago revealed that the drinking-induced temporary depression of the thirst drive is mainly exerted from the oropharyngeal region but also from the gastric part of the alimentary canal, implying that a constellation of mechanical, thermal, and chemical factors is involved (22, 79). More recent studies in monkeys indicate that receptors in the duodenum or portal circulation also contribute to the temporary satisfaction of thirst (80). Although no direct evidence exists, it is tempting to speculate that taste receptors, responding specifically to pure water, may contribute to the preabsorptive alleviation of thirst. Such gustatory receptors were originally discovered by Zotterman (83) in the frog and were later demonstrated by recordings of chorda tympani activity in several mammalian species, including the monkey (28). A subsequent study (17) showed that water taste fibers are not present in the human chorda tympani; however, man may have receptors responding to water in other parts of the oropharyngeal region, since afferents conveying impulses from such receptors were recently demonstrated in the superior laryngeal nerve of the rat (68). The temporary appeasement of thirst elicited during drinking obviously fulfills an important physiological mission. Deprived of this inhibitory mechanism man and mammals would yield to excessive drinking each time they became thirsty and would then have to endure the consequence—a profuse water diuresis. A recent study (72) implies that oropharyngeal short-term factors also affect the regulation of ADH secretion. It was shown that the drinking by dehydrated dogs caused an immediate reduction of plasma ADH, which occurred in the absence of diminished plasma osmolality and regardless of whether the imbibed fluid was drained via a gastric fistula or not.

THIRST DISORDERS OF CEREBRAL ORIGIN

Primary Polydipsia

An irresistible craving for water that persists in the absence of known osmotic and nonosmotic thirst stimuli is called primary polydipsia. It has occasionally been reported as a consequence of cerebral (mainly hypothalamic) damage in humans (22, 79), and then seems to have been due to nonspecific, irritative stimulation of neurons or sensors involved in the regulation of water intake. Speaking in favor of that explanation is the observation that electrical stimulation within the hypothalamus may elicit copious, stimulus-bound drinking in animals (10). However, a more common cause of primary polydipsia in humans is psychic disturbance. Psychogenic polydipsia occurs mainly in middle-aged women suffering from acute or chronic psychosis (12) and is sometimes associated with considerably lowered osmotic threshold for ADH release (30, 55, 57). The condition is then potentially life-threatening since the excessive water intake may rapidly induce hyponatremia of such a degree that fatal cerebral and/or pulmonary edemas develop. Although a somatic cause has not been ruled out, it appears likely that this kind of compulsive water drinking is a manifestation of dysfunctioning interaction between superior parts of the limbic system and the hypothalamus.

Adipsia—Hypodipsia, "Essential" Hypernatremia

The term "essential hypernatremia" was introduced twenty years ago by Welt (78) for a marked elevation of plasma Na concentration sometimes observed as the cardinal sign in fully conscious patients with water available *ad lib.* As explanation for the condition Welt suggested an elevation of the stimulus threshold of cerebral osmoreceptors regulating water intake and ADH release. However, subsequent clinical (31) and experimental (8, 63) studies imply that "essential" hypernatremia in man is rather the consequence of cerebral damage that more or less involves the area shown in Figure 2, and to a varying extent affects the mechanism(s) responsible for the osmotic regulation of water intake and ADH release. Hypothalamic damage that severely impairs the osmotic control of water balance may leave the volume regulation of ADH secretion intact (8, 16, 29, 63). It suggests that cardiovascular afferent influence on ADH liberation reaches its final neuronal link (the cells of the supraoptic or paraventricular nuclei) via intracerebral pathways running at some distance from the sensors and neurons that mediate the osmotic regulation of water intake and ADH release.

SUMMARY AND CONCLUSIONS

Here we have reviewed mainly the cerebral regulation of water intake and its relationship with the regulation of the water-retaining antidiuretic hormone (ADH). Much new information of obvious interest has been gained by experiments in conscious animals, by studies in healthy humans, and by clinical investigations. Of particularly great value has been the development of a sensitive radioimmunoassay for determination of plasma ADH (59).

The sketchy picture that emerges in light of this new information is as follows. The osmotic regulation of water intake and ADH secretion is exerted by juxtacerebroventricular sensors apparently mainly located on the anterior border of the third ventricle. These sensors may be accessible both to CSF-borne and blood-borne stimuli and inhibitors, and their activity seems to be correlated to the Na concentration of the ECF rather than to its tonicity. A less sensitive volume regulation of water intake and ADH secretion is effectuated by cardiovascular distention and pressure receptors monitoring the effective circulating blood volume, and in severe volume depletion states also by the renin-angiotensin system (RAS). Afferent impulses from the cardiovascular receptors exert a tonic inhibition of the ADH release by acting upon its final neuronal link (the cells of the supraoptic and paraventricular nuclei). Afferent inflow from these receptors also inhibits thirst to some extent, perhaps by preventing at some synaptic level information from cerebral "thirst" sensors from reaching other parts of the brain where the information is converted into a conscious urge to drink. Therefore, increased cardiovascular receptor activity becomes manifested as elevated osmotic thresholds for ADH liberation and thirst. Severe volume depletion may induce RAS hyperactivity to such an extent that generated angiotensin II stimulates the ADH release and water intake. Demonstrated cerebral Na/angiotensin interaction suggests that this may occur via an angiotensin-induced lowering of the stimulus threshold for the sensors involved in the osmotic control of water balance. Cerebral damage affecting the sensors responsible for the osmotic regulation of water intake and ADH release may result in hypo- or adipsia associated with latent diabetes insipidus, and is apparently the ultimate cause of "essential" hypernatremia.

This fragmentary outline of the cerebral control of water intake is based to a considerable extent upon circumstantial evidence, and is for that reason speculative on many points.

Literature Cited

1. Abraham, S. F., Baker, R. M., Blaine, D., Denton, D. A., McKinley, M. J. 1975. Water drinking induced in sheep by angiotensin—a physiological or pharmacological effect? *J. Comp. Physiol. Psychol.* 88:503–18
2. Abraham, S. F., Coghlan, J. P., Denton, D. A., McDoughall, J. G., Mouw, D. R., Scoggins, B. A. 1976. Increased water drinking induced by sodium depletion in sheep. *Q. J. Exp. Physiol.* 61:185–92
3. Abraham, S. F., Denton, D. A., McKinley, M. J., Weisinger, R. S. 1976. Effect of angiotensin antagonist Sar[1]–Ala[8]-angiotensin II on physiological thirst. *Pharmacol. Biochem. Behav.* 4:243–47
4. Andersson, B. 1953. The effect of injections of hypertonic NaCl-solutions into different parts of the hypothalamus of goats. *Acta Physiol. Scand.* 28:188–201
5. Andersson, B. 1971. Thirst—and brain control of water balance. *Am. Sci.* 59:408–15

6. Andersson, B. 1978. Regulation of water intake. *Physiol. Rev.* 58:582–603
7. Andersson, B., Eriksson, L., Oltner, R. 1970. Further evidence for angiotensin-sodium interaction in the central control of fluid balance. *Life Sci.* 9:1091–96
8. Andersson, B., Leksell, L. G., Lishajko, F. 1975. Perturbations in fluid balance induced by medially placed forebrain lesions. *Brain Res.* 99:261–75
9. Andersson, B. Leksell, L. G., Rundgren, M. 1982. Regulation of body fluids—intake and output. In *Edema*, ed. N. Staub, A. Taylor. NY: Raven Press. In press
10. Andersson, B., McCann, S. M. 1956. Drinking, antidiuresis and milk ejection from electrical stimulation within the hypothalamus of the goat. *Acta Physiol. Scand.* 35:191–201
11. Arnould, E., Czernichow, P., Fumoux, F., Vincent, J.–D. 1977. The effect of hypotension and hypovolaemia on the liberation of vasopressin in the unanesthetized monkey (*Macaca mulatta*). *Pfluegers Arch.* 371:193–200
12. Barlow, E. D., DeWardener, H. E. 1959. Compulsive water drinking. *Q. J. Med.* 28:235–58
13. Bonjour, J. P., Malvin, R. L. 1970. Stimulation of ADH release by the renin-angiotensin system. *Am. J. Physiol.* 218:1155–59
14. Brennan, L. A., Malvin, R. L., Jochim, K. E. 1971. Influence of right and left atrial receptors of plasma concentrations of ADH and renin. *Am. J. Physiol.* 221:273–78
15. Crone, C. 1965. The permeability of brain capillaries to nonelectrolytes. *Acta Physiol. Scand.* 64:407–17
16. DeRubertis, F. R., Michelis, M. F., Beck, N., Field, J. B., Davis, B. B. 1975. "Essential" hypernatremia due to ineffective osmotic and intact volume regulation of vasopressin secretion. *J. Clin. Invest.* 50:97–111
17. Diamant, H., Funakoshi, M., Ström, L., Zotterman, Y. 1963. Electrophysiological studies on human taste nerves. In *Olfaction and Taste*, ed. Y. Zotterman, pp. 193–203. Oxford: Pergamon
18. Dunn, F., Brennan, L., Nelson, A. E., Robertson, G. L. 1973. The role of blood osmolality and volume in regulating vasopressin secretion in the rat. *J. Clin. Invest.* 52:3212–19
19. Erdös, E. G. 1975. Angiotensin I converting enzyme. *Circ. Res.* 36:247–55
20. Eriksson, L., Fernández, O., Olsson, K. 1971. Differences in the antidiuretic response to intracarotid infusions of various hypertonic solutions in the conscious goat. *Acta Physiol. Scand.* 83:554–62
21. Fischer-Ferraro, C., Nahmod, V. E., Goldstein, D. J., Finkielman, S. 1971. Angiotensin and renin in rat and dog brain. *J. Exp. Med.* 133:353–61
22. Fitzsimons, J. 1972. Thirst. *Physiol. Rev.* 52:468–561
23. Fitzsimons, J. T. 1979. The physiology of thirst and sodium appetite. *Monogr. Physiol. Soc. No. 35*
24. Fitzsimons, J. T., Moore-Gillon, M. J. 1980. Drinking and antidiuresis in response to reductions in venous return in the dog: Neural and endocrine mechanisms. *J. Physiol.* 308:403–16
25. Fitzsimons, J. T., Simons, B. J. 1969. The effects on drinking in the rat of intravenous angiotensin, given alone or in combination with other stimuli of thirst. *J. Physiol.* 203:45–57
26. Ganten, D., Minnich, J. L., Granger, P., Hayduk, K., Brecht, H. M., Barbeau, A., Boucher, R., Genest, J. 1971. Angiotensin-forming enzyme in brain tissue. *Science* 173:64–65
27. Goetz, K. L., Bond, G. C., Bloxham, D. D. 1974. Effect of moderate hemorrhage in humans on plasma ADH and renin. *Proc. Soc. Exp. Biol. Med.* 145:277–80
28. Gordon, G., Kitchell, R., Ström, L., Zotterman, Y. 1959. The response pattern of taste fibres in the chorda tympani of the monkey. *Acta Physiol. Scand.* 46:119–32
29. Halter, J. B., Goldberg, A. P., Robertson, G. L., Porte, D. Jr. 1977. Selective osmoreceptor dysfunction in the syndrome of chronic hypernatremia. *J. Clin. Endocrinol. Metab.* 44:609–16
30. Hariprasad, M. K., Eisinger, R. P., Nadler, I. M., Padmanabhan, C. S., Nidus, B. D. 1980. Hyponatremia in psychogenic polydipsia. *Arch. Intern. Med.* 140:1639–42
31. Hays, R. M., Levine, S. D. 1981. Pathophysiology of water metabolism. In *The Kidney*, ed. B. M. Brenner, F. C. Rector, I:777–840. Philadelphia: Saunders
32. Henry, J. P., Gauer, O. H., Reeves, J. L. 1956. Evidence of the atrial location of receptors influencing urine flow. *Circ. Res.* 4:85–94
33. Holmes, J. H., Montgomery, A. V. 1953. Thirst as a symptom. *Am. J. Med. Sci.* 225:281–86
34. Kleeman, C. F., Davson, H., Levin, E. 1962. Urea transport in the central nervous system. *Am. J. Physiol.* 203:739–47

35. Kozlowski, S., Drzewiecki, K., Sobocinska, J. 1968. The influence of expansion of extracellular fluid volume on the thirst threshold. *Bull. Acad. Pol. Sci.* 16:47–51

36. Kozlowski, S., Drzewiecki, K., Zurawski, W. 1972. Relationship between osmotic reactivity of the thirst mechanism and the angiotensin and aldosterone blood levels in the dog. *Acta Physiol. Polon.* 23:417–25

37. Kozlowski, S., Szczepanska-Sadowska, E. 1975. Mechanism of hypovolemic thirst and interactions between hypovolemia, hyperosmolality and the antidiuretic system. In *Control of Drinking*, ed. G. Peters, J. T. Fitzsimons, L. Peters-Haefli, pp. 25–35. Berlin: Springer

38. Larsson, B., Olsson, K., Fyhrquist, F. 1978. Vasopressin release induced by hemorrhage in the goat. *Acta Physiol. Scand.* 104:309–17

39. Leksell, L. G., Lishajko, F., Rundgren, M. 1977. Negative water balance induced by intracerebroventricular infusion of deuterium. *Acta Physiol. Scand.* 100:494–96

40. Linazasoro, J. M., Jiménez Diaz, C., Castro-Mendoza, H. J. 1954. The kidney and thirst regulation. *Bull. Inst. Med. Res. Madrid* 7:53–61

41. Lishajko, F., Appelgren, B., Eriksson, S. 1981. Cerebral sodium/angiotensin interaction studied by RIA-determination of urinary arginine vasopressin in the hydrated goat. *Acta Physiol. Scand.* 111:311–18

42. McKinley, M. J., Denton, D. A., Leksell, L., Tarjan, E., Weisinger, R. S. 1980. Evidence for cerebral sodium sensors involved in water drinking in sheep. *Physiol. Behav.* 25:501–04

43. McKinley, M. J., Denton, D. A., Weisinger, R. S. 1978. Sensors for antidiuresis and thirst—osmoreceptors or CSF sodium detectors? *Brain Res.* 141:89–103

44. McKinley, M. J., Olsson, K., Fyhrquist, F., Liljekvist, E. 1980. Transient vasopressin release and thirst in response to prolonged intracerebroventricular infusions of hypertonic mannitol in saline. *Acta Physiol. Scand.* 109:427–31

45. Nothnagel, H. 1881. Durst und Polydipsie. *Virchows Arch. Pathol. Anat. Physiol.* 86:435–47

46. Olsson, K. 1969. Studies on central regulation of secretion of antidiuretic hormone (ADH) in the goat. *Acta Physiol. Scand.* 77:465–74

47. Olsson, K. 1972. Dipsogenic effects of intracarotid infusions of various hyperosmolal solutions. *Acta Physiol. Scand.* 85:517–22

48. Olsson, K. 1972. On the importance of CSF Na⁺ concentration in central control of fluid balance. *Life Sci.* 11:397–402

49. Olsson, K. 1973. Further evidence for the importance of CSF Na⁺ concentration in central control of fluid balance. *Acta Physiol. Scand.* 88:183–88

50. Olsson, K. 1975. Attenuation of dehydrative thirst by lowering of the CSF [Na⁺]. *Acta Physiol. Scand.* 94:536–38

51. Padfield, P. L., Morton, J. J. 1977. Effects of angiotensin II on arginine-vasopressin in physiological and pathological situations in man. *J. Endocrinol.* 74:251–59

52. Patlak, C. S., Fenstermacher, J. D. 1975. Measurements of dog blood-brain transfer constants by ventriculocisternal perfusion. *Am. J. Physiol.* 229:877–84

53. Ramsay, D. J. 1979. The brain renin angiotensin system: A reevaluation. *Neuroscience* 4:313–21

54. Ramsay, D. J., Reid, I. A. 1975. Some central mechanisms of thirst in the dog. *J. Physiol.* 253:517–25

55. Raskind, M. A., Orenstein, H., Christopher, T. G. 1975. Acute psychosis, increased water ingestion, and inappropriate antidiuretic hormone secretion. *Am. J. Psychiatr.* 132:907–10

56. Reid, I. 1977. Is there a brain renin-angiotensin system? *Circ. Res.* 41:147–53

57. Rendell, M., McGrane, D., Guesta, M. 1978. Fatal compulsive water drinking. *J. Am. Med. Assoc.* 240:2557–59

58. Robertson, G. L., Athar, S. 1976. The interaction of blood osmolality and blood volume in regulating vasopressin secretion in man. *J. Clin. Endocrinol. Metab.* 42:613–20

59. Robertson, G. L., Mahr, E. A., Athar, S., Sinha, T. 1973. Development and clinical application of a new method for the radioimmunoassay of arginine vasopressin in human plasma. *J. Clin. Invest.* 52:2340–52

60. Robertson, G. L., Shelton, R. L., Athar, S. 1976. The osmoregulation of vasopressin. *Kidney Int.* 10:25–37

61. Rogers, P. W., Kurtzman, N. A. 1973. Renal failure, uncontrollable thirst and hyperreninemia. *J. Am. Med. Assoc.* 225:1236–38

62. Rundgren, M., Eriksson, S., Appelgren, B. 1979. Urea-induced inhibition of an-

tidiuretic hormone (ADH) secretion. *Acta Physiol. Scand.* 106:491-92

63. Rundgren, M., Fyhrquist, F. 1978. A study of permanent adipsia induced by medial forebrain lesions. *Acta Physiol. Scand.* 103:463-71

64. Russell, P. J. D., Abdelaal, A. E., Mogenson, G. J. 1975. Graded levels of hemorrhage, thirst and angiotensin II in the rat. *Physiol. Behav.* 15:117-19

65. Schelling, P., Ganten, U., Sponer, G., Unger, T., Ganten, D. 1980. Components of the renin-angiotensin system in the cerebrospinal fluid of rats and dogs with special consideration of the origin and fate of angiotensin II. *Neuroendocrinology* 31:297-308

66. Schrier, R. W., Berl, T., Anderson, R. J. 1979. Osmotic and nonosmotic control of vasopressin release. *Am. J. Physiol.* 236:F321-32

67. Sheth, K. J., Tang, T. T., Blaedel, M. E., Good, T. A. 1978. Polydipsia, polyuria and hypertension associated with renin-secreting Wilm's tumor. *J. Pediatr.* 92:921-24

68. Shingai, T. 1980. Water fibres in the superior laryngeal nerve of the rat. *Jpn. J. Physiol.* 30:305-7

69. Sobocinska, J. 1969. Effects of cervical vagosympathectomy on osmotic reactivity of the thirst mechanism in dogs. *Bull. Acad. Pol. Sci.* 17:265-70

70. Swaminathan, S. 1980. Osmoreceptors or sodium receptors: An investigation into ADH release in the rhesus monkey. *J. Physiol. London* 307:71-83

71. Szczepanska-Sadowska, E., Kozlowski, S. 1975. Equipotency of hypertonic solutions of mannitol and sodium chloride in eliciting thirst in the dog. *Pfluegers Arch.* 358:259-64

72. Thrasher, T. N., Nistal-Herrera, J. F., Keil, L. C., Ramsay, D. J. 1981. Satiety and inhibition of vasopressin secretion after drinking in dehydrated dogs. *Am. J. Physiol.* 240:E394-401

73. Torrente, A. de, Robertson, G. L., McDonald, K. M., Schrier, R. W. 1975. Mechanism of diuretic response to increased left atrial pressure in the anesthetized dog. *Kidney Int.* 8:355-61

74. Valtin, H. 1979. *Renal Dysfunction: Mechanisms Involved in Fluid and Solute Balance.* Boston: Little, Brown

75. Verney, E. B. 1947. The antidiuretic hormone and factors which determine its release. *Proc. R. Soc. London Ser. B.* 135:25-106

76. Vigh, B. 1970. Does the paraventricular organ have a receptor function? *Ann. Endocrinol. Paris* 31:659-63

77. Weindl, A., Joynt, R. J. 1972. Ultrastructure of the ventricular walls. *Arch. Neurol.* 26:420-27

78. Welt, L. G. 1962. Hypo- and hypernatremia. *Ann. Intern. Med.* 56:161-64

79. Wolf, A. V. 1958. *Thirst: Physiology of the Urge to Drink and Problems of Water Lack.* Springfield: Thomas

80. Wood, R. J., Maddison, S., Rolls, E. T., Rolls, B. J., Gibbs, J. 1980. Drinking in rhesus monkeys: Roles of presystemic and systemic factors in control of drinking. *J. Comp. Physiol. Psychol.* 6:1135-48

81. Wood, R. J., Rolls, B. J., Ramsay, D. J. 1977. Drinking following intracarotid infusions of hypertonic solutions in dogs. *Am. J. Physiol.* 232:R88-92

82. Zimmerman, M. B., Blaine, E. H. 1981. Water intake in hypovolemic sheep: Effects of crushing the left atrial appendage. *Science* 211:489-91

83. Zotterman, Y. 1949. The response of the frog's taste fibres to the application of pure water. *Acta Physiol. Scand.* 18:181-89

Ann. Rev. Nutr. 1982. 2:91-111

DEVELOPMENT OF LIPID METABOLISM

Peter Hahn

Centre for Developmental Medicine, Departments of Obstetrics & Gynecology and Pediatrics, University of British Columbia, Vancouver, B.C., Canada

CONTENTS

Eighty years ago Babak (5) reported that very soon after delivery the respiratory quotient (RQ) of the neonate dropped from about 1.0 to below 0.8. This was confirmed 15 years later by Talbot & Benedict (9) and by many others after them. Thus it has been known for some time that the newborn mammal utilizes fat for energy purposes apparently to a greater extent than the fetus and in many cases the adult.

Since space is at a premium only the aspects listed in the table of contents will be covered.

Fatty Acids

In contrast to triglycerides (TG), phospholipids (PL), and cholesterol, there is no doubt that some fatty acids (FA) must be able to cross from mother to fetus in all species since otherwise the newborn would be devoid of essential fatty acids. A persuasive study demonstrated that in a rabbit doe fasted for 2 days between the 26th and 28th day of pregnancy maternal plasma levels of FA and glycerol doubled; the same was found for the fetus, which appeared to deposit the extra fat received from the mother (35, 36, 37, 38, 41). Even more striking is the rapid transfer of FA in the guinea pig (12), in which C^{14} labelled palmitate injected into the maternal circulation

91

0199-9885/82/0715-0091$02.00

appears within 3 min in the fetal blood. The calculated rate of transfer of free fatty acids (FFA) was about 2.2–3.2 μmoles/min to the combined fetuses. FA transfer from mother to fetus could provide all of the triglycerides in the liver (1 g TG for 4 g of liver).

Shapiro et al (140, 141) showed that in post-term rabbits placental transport is impaired; consequently, fetal liver lipid levels decreased and fetal plasma free fatty acid levels increased, suggesting mobilization of fetal fat stores.

Using in vivo techniques, Hudson & Hull (84) showed that fetal rabbit brown fat takes up 8.5 μmoles/g/hr of labelled fatty acids. Rates were much slower in liver and placenta. FA were oxidized to CO_2 in brown fat and incorporated into TG. In liver most of the FA were in TG. In placenta PL also contained the labelled acids.

Hummel et al (86, 87, 88) and Zimmermann & Hummel (162, 163) have quantified the amounts of FFA crossing from mother to fetus in the rat and have estimated the rate of oxidation. They report that fetuses synthesize 0.16 μmoles FA/min/litter and that hence about 50% of the FA are derived from the mother. FA oxidation proceeds at a rate of 0.12 $\pm$ 0.03 μmoles/min/litter. They conclude that about equal amounts of FA are synthesized, oxidized, and transferred from the mother. For a review of FA transport up to 1975 see Hull (85).

The rabbit placenta also possesses a lipoproteinlipase that aids in the transfer of fatty acids derived from maternal TG (38).

The situation is different in sheep. In this animal, transfer of FA is limited (40) as are transfers of ketones (7) and carnitine (72). On the other hand, acetate appears to supply 10% of the energy to fetal lambs (21). However, Noble et al (110, 111) report that transfer of ^{3}H-palmitic acid is fast, whereas that of ^{14}C-linoleic acid is slow. The same 2 acids were used by Elphick et al (40), but their experiment was an acute one using anesthesia, while Noble et al used chronically implanted catheters in unanesthetized ewes. Thus the latter group's results are probably more reliable.

In dogs, starvation of the pregnant animal just before delivery resulted in increased hepatic triglyceride content in the fetal and neonatal liver (103), suggesting increased release and transfer of FA and their esterification in the liver.

Feeding pregnant rats a fat-free diet from the 16th to 22nd day of gestation resulted in a deficiency of linoleic acid in all tissues, again indirectly confirming transfer of FA from mother to fetus (155, 156). Arachidonic acid content in mother, placenta, and fetus was not altered. Arachidonic acid is transferred more rapidly than linoleic acid (118). However, apparently less than 1% of the fatty acids derived from the mother is transported paraplacentally—i.e. from uterine fluid to yolk sac to fetus (163).

Trans- fatty acids (elaidic and linoelaidic) are transported from mother to fetus in the rat at a slow rate; 0.2–1% was taken up by the placenta and about 0.1–0.4% by the fetus. Incorporation into fetal tissues was greater than for cis- acids. Both cis- and trans- acids were found mostly in TG in maternal plasma, in TG and PL in the placenta, and mostly in PL in the fetus. Both linoleic and elaidic acid, but not oleic or linoelaidic acids, are oxidized in the fetus (105).

The amount of transport of FA from mother to fetus in the rat is small, as evidenced by the fact that a 15% corn oil diet, which suppresses maternal hepatic lipogenesis, had no effect on the high rate of FA synthesis in the fetus (104). Nevertheless, the linolenic acid content of *both* fetal and maternal livers trebled. Fasting also raised the polyunsaturated content of fetal and maternal liver. However, maternal fasting does decrease fetal FA synthesis (104). Essential fatty acid deficiency during pregnancy resulted in retarded brain development and a profound reduction in some myelin components (galactolipid, proteolipids) (100). The brain of the fetal rat appears capable of converting linolenic acid to docosahexaenoic acid (22:6 ω3), which may also explain why the fetal brain is not protected from the adverse effect of an imbalance in the linoleic/linolenic acid ratio in the maternal diet (33, 34).

Infusion of glucose into rabbits on the 28th day of pregnancy increased insulin levels in both mother and fetuses and decreased maternal FFA plasma levels without having a strong effect on fetal levels; hence in the infused groups the FFA level in the umbilical vein was twice that in maternal blood, suggesting another source of acids (perhaps the placenta) under these conditions (41).

In humans less is known. Sabata et al (131) reported some dependence of fetal FA plasma levels on maternal levels. As a rule it appears that the rate at which FFA are transferred from mother to fetus is slow (52), although according to Hull (85) all the fat accumulated by the fetus towards the end of gestation may be derived from a transplacental supply of FFA. There is no doubt that some essential fatty acids must be transferred, since they cannot be made by the fetus (50, 51).

That the blood levels of FFA and glycerol rise rapidly after birth, a fact first reported 20 years ago, is still attracting attention. Evidence shows that even in humans the concentration of FFA in the umbilical vein is positively correlated with that in the maternal blood (e.g. 39) and that adipose tissue development in the fetus is dependent on the maternal blood level of FFA (144). In all cases there is a postnatal rise, apparent immediately after delivery (22; but see 3)

Many years ago, Hahn & Koldovsky (74) reported that hepatic levels of glycogen increased in newborn rats fed TG or FFA only. This finding was ascribed to the glycerol in the TG, even though FA had the same effect. Ferre et al (45, 46, 47) have now confirmed this finding and, to a large extent, explained it. They showed that in newborn rats hepatic FA oxidation increases gluconeogenic flux by providing acetyl CoA for pyruvate kinase and NADH to direct the glyceraldehyde-3-phosphate dehydrogenase reaction towards glucose formation. This, of course, brings us back to the importance of carnitine in the peri- and neonatal periods. Apparently the glycogen content of the liver is also important, since if it is high the FA oxidation rate is low (129, 161) and vice versa.

In confirmation of the work of Ferre et al (45, 46), Sabel et al (132) showed that the hypoglycemia of small-for-date newborns could be raised by "fat injection." Feeding milk was only useful if ketones in the serum had attained a certain value. Hence gluconeogenesis could proceed only if fat was being oxidized.

There is thus consensus that fetal levels of FFA are lower than maternal ones but that the actual rate of transfer depends on (a) chain length, (b) desaturation, and (c) the species and age of the fetus (73). Little has been reported between 1975–1980 that alters these conclusions arrived at in the mid-1970s. Similarly, few new reports have appeared concerning the postnatal changes in blood levels of FFA [see (71, 72, 73, 85) for details].

Ketones

It has long been known that pregnant mammals are more prone to ketosis than nonpregnant ones [for review see (136)] and that in human, rat, rabbit, and guinea pig they readily cross the placenta (72). The sheep is the exception. Transplacental passage of β-hydroxybutyrate or acetoacetate in this species is slow or nonexistent (7). The finding that ketogenesis is low in fetal rat liver (26) and that the brain of the newborn rat utilizes ketones in preference to glucose (27) has generated considerable interest. For review of earlier work see (73, 154).

Of particular interest is the fate of ketones produced by the mother and transported to the fetus. Seccombe et al (136) investigated this in some detail and showed that (a) labelled DL-β[3–^{14}C] hydroxybutyrate is rapidly passed from mother rat to her fetuses, (b) it is used for lipid synthesis, and (c) different tissues incorporate it at different rates. Brown adipose tissue contained by far the highest radioactivity, mostly in the triglyceride (75%) fraction (202093 dpm/g against the second highest, lung: 38324 dpm/g). In all other tissues most of the activity was in the phospholipids (44–65%).

Indirect evidence also suggests increased sterol synthesis from acetoacetate in the suckling rat's brain (120, 157, 160). The cytosolic 3-hydroxy-3-methyl-glutaryl CoA synthase in the brain decreases during days 0–21 (119). Ketone utilization by the infant rat brain in vivo has also been demonstrated (19, 24). Benavides et al (8) suggest that the inhibition of 3-hydroxybutyrate dehydrogenase and 3-oxoacid CoA transferase activities by phenylalanine and its metabolites in the suckling rat brain may affect mental development in phenylketonuria. Utilization of ketone bodies for cholesterol and FA synthesis in different parts of the brain is highest in very young rats and greater than that of glucose. The greatest rate of synthesis was found in the brain stem (16).

As shown earlier (26), hepatic ketone production is high in the suckling period of the rat (10, 47) while incorporation of C^{14}-palmitate into lipids is decreased. Blood levels of ketones can be further raised by feeding medium-chain triglycerides (MCT), or long-chain TG (158). In adults rats, MCT feeding is more effective and leads to hypoglycemia.

In sheep, ketones do not cross the placenta (7). However, the fetal liver produces acetoacetate at ever increasing rates as gestational age increases, and there is considerable postnatal rise. This is matched by blood β-hydroxybutyrate levels, which rise from 0.037 pre- to 0.133 μmol/l postnatally and continue rising to high levels (0.4 and higher).

In contrast to adult liver, fetal rat liver (also the brain, placenta and fetal carcass) can oxidize ketones supplied from the mother when the latter is starving (159). Isolated fetal hepatocytes also oxidize ketones. The enzyme 3-oxoacid CoA transferase is present in newborn liver but has little activity in the adult organ (44). Thus the fetal liver is geared to utilize ketones, the suckling liver to make them. The ability of the rat fetus to utilize ketones, *depending on their concentration,* spares glucose and lactate when these are in short supply—e.g. during maternal starvation (138). Similar conditions prevail in baboons (122).

If pregnant rats are fed a 45% corn oil diet for the last 8 days of gestation, ketonemia develops in both mother and fetuses; this has profound effects on the metabolism of the neonatal brain (23). Fetal rat tissues can oxidize ketones in the order placenta, brain, liver, carcass. This is of particular importance during a maternal fast, when a 30–60-fold rise in fetal plasma β-hydroxybutyrate levels can be observed (137, 138, 139). Ketones are also used in preference to glucose for lipid synthesis by the brain of newborn rats (150, 157). In neonatal hypothyroid rats the development of ketone metabolizing enzymes is delayed; the rise and the subsequent decrease occur later (120, 121). In the liver of suckling rats the major site of regulation of ketogenesis involves the disposal of long-chain acylCoA between the esterification and oxidation pathways. The authors suggest that the high levels of cycle AMP in the liver inhibit esterification, thus making possible a maximum rate of ketogenesis (10). The rise in plasma ketone levels after birth starts 4 hr after birth, while plasma FFA and liver carnitine levels rise within 2 hr after birth as soon as the pups consume milk (129).

Twenty-four-hour starvation of the pregnant guinea pig, whose fetuses represent up to 50% of maternal body weight, causes a 5-fold rise in FFA and 8-fold rise in blood ketone levels (56).

Incorporation of ketones into brain lipids (cholesterol, lecithin, gangliosides) develops more slowly in hypothyroid rats than in normal pups and decreases later in life (30). The postnatal rise in blood ketone levels seen in the rat has also been described in man (123). Recently it has been suggested that in man this perinatal rise is due to starvation and can be eliminated by early feeding (3).

Cholesterol

Feeding of cholesterol or cholestyramine to pregnant rats has no effect on fetal cholesterol synthesis (104). It is well established that plasma levels of triglycerides, phospholipids and cholesterol rise rapidly after birth. Considerable attention has been paid recently to the lipoproteins and their cholesterol content (14, 15, 17, 63). At birth, total cholesterol content of the blood is higher in premature than full-term neonates; the same is true for high-density lipoprotein (HDL)- and very low density-low density lipoprotein (VLDL-LDL)-cholesterol content (58, 59, 60). The postnatal rise in total cholesterol content is the same in both groups. Values attained 10 days after birth reach 3.1 mmoles/l or 118 mg/dl regardless of the food consumed, but after that time they increase to higher values in breast fed infants than in babies fed cow's milk or other formulas (86). The cholesterol content of breast milk was not affected by the amount of cholesterol consumed by the mother or the plasma level of this sterol. However, linoleate content of milk was directly proportional to plasma linoleate levels. The plasma cholesterol content of babies decreased as the linoleate content of the milk rose (124).

Feeding a high-cholesterol diet raised maternal plasma cholesterol levels but had no effect on milk or infant serum values. In contrast, phytosterol content of the diet was reflected in both maternal serum and milk and newborn serum (102). At birth, white girls had the highest cholesterol, β-, and α-lipoprotein levels; values were higher for white than for black neonates (18). Thus basic values are already established at birth (49). For discussion see (2, 14, 17).

In small-for-gestational-age newborns, lower values for HDL- and higher ones for LDL-cholesterol were found than in full-term infants (4). Both LDL- and HDL-cholesterol values were higher in prematures. During early postnatal development of normal babies the HDL/VLDL-LDL-cholesterol ratio fell from 1.5 at birth to 0.6 at 3–6 months, with HDL-cholesterol rising by about 60% and VLDL + LDL-cholesterol rising 3.5 times (60). Cord blood has no VLDL (117; but see 17).

Neonatal lipid concentrations have been described in detail for Swedish newborns (77, 78). Others have analyzed lipoprotein and lipid composition in different parts of Norway (64) and have described similar changes in normal newborns (49, 149). A significant correlation was found between the total cholesterol values at birth and values found 3–6 months later; an *inverse* correlation exists between the increase of the first 3–10 days and that in the next 3–6 months for total and VLDL-LDL-cholesterol (60). The conclusion is that in infancy both food and genetic factors control cholesterol levels but that genetic factors predominate later. It was shown many years ago that the postnatal rise in total cholesterol occurs in two steps (114). The first seems to depend on food supply, since it does not occur in infants fed tea with sugar; the second (2–3 days later) occurs even if no food is given.

In postmature rabbit fetuses, blood levels of cholesterol increase from about 90 to 140 mg/dl while in the mother the rise is from about 12 to 40. In normal rabbits blood levels rise to 120 mg/dl in the mother and 180 in the newborn after delivery, whereas TG serum levels are elevated in postmature fetuses only (79, 140).

Serum bile acid levels (lithocholic acid and sulfo-lithocholylglycine) are highest in the newborn (6). They decrease upon the consumption of the first meal in prematures, but rise in full-terms. Adult levels (a 5-fold decrease) are attained only gradually by about one year. In rats there is minimal transfer of bile acids (81).

Newborns of diabetic rats had lower serum cholesterol levels and a smaller cholic acid pool than control pups, whereas the opposite was true for their mothers during pregnancy (80). The strikingly lower serum cholesterol levels in the neonates (13.84 ± 3.3 against 68.38 ± 4.4) deserves special notice.

The postnatal rise in total plasma cholesterol content has been found to occur in all mammalian species examined so far (20, 127) and has been related to the cholesterol content of the milk (125) and of the diet (106, 151). This is probably an oversimplification even though human breast milk contains 20–24 mg/dl while milk formula only 2 mg/dl (59). This is even more strikingly brought home in intravenously fed newborns (and adults) in whom blood total cholesterol content rises up to 500 mg/dl if intralipid is included in the cocktail (63). This occurs within 1–3 days after the start of i.v. feeding. The rise in total cholesterol is directly proportional to the amount of intralipid supplied, whereas HDL-cholesterol levels are decreased and are inversely proportional to the amount of fat infused. The authors calculate that at least 50% of the plasma cholesterol is made by the body. These facts strikingly demonstrate that cholesterol itself, supplied

either orally or intravenously, is not the sole determinant of plasma cholesterol levels. It has been suggested that the ratio of saturated to unsaturated
fatty acid might play a role in the regulation of blood total cholesterol levels
(63). However, other factors are undoubtedly involved. Thus in rats, total
cholesterol levels in 19-day-old animals can be decreased within 24 hr to
less than half the suckling value by feeding a high carbohydrate diet (112);
these values are significantly lower than those found after 24 hr of starvation. Similarly the quantity of milk consumed affects total cholesterol blood
levels. They are elevated in rat pups if only 3 are in the litter compared to
litters of 13–14 (69). It should be mentioned that rats over-fed in infancy
eat more when adult (116).

Interesting relationships exist in the suckling period between blood levels
of total cholesterol and the rate-limiting enzyme of cholesterol synthesis,
3-hydroxy-3-methyl-glutaryl CoA reductase (HMGR). In the rat fetus,
hepatic HMGR shows high activity that is not inhibited by feeding cholesterol to the mother (16). Activity decreases after birth (101, 69). It has been
suggested that the decrease is due to a factor in milk (101). However, no
such factor has been isolated and since it is known that there is an inverse
relationship between blood levels of total cholesterol and hepatic HMGR,
it seems more probable that cholesterol or one of its metabolites, including
VLDL, is responsible. At weaning in the rat, when the high-fat diet of the
suckling period is replaced by the high-carbohydrate rat chow, blood total
cholesterol falls and hepatic HMGR activity rises (101).

Since HMGR is present in most tissues, enabling them to make cholesterol (and other compounds) necessary for growth and differentiation, the
development of its activity in extrahepatic tissues is of interest. Little work
has been done in this area. Attention has been paid to the brain, where
enzyme activity in the rat reaches a maximum on day 3 after birth when
the rate of myelination is at its highest (108, 143) while in the lung activity
is highest prenatally (108).

Even though it has been suggested repeatedly that the gut is a large source
of cholesterol, developmental changes of intestinal HMGR have not been
reported. Results show a steep decline in activity after birth and a rise
after weaning in the rat, and similar changes occur in brown adipose tissue. (75).

Recently it has been suggested, that white adipose tissue plays a special
role in the maintenance of total plasma cholesterol (67), since HMGR
activity in this tissue of obese mice was found to be high, even though the
hepatic enzyme showed low activity. Preliminary results indicated that
HMGR activity in white adipose tissue of suckling rats in a 3-pup litter was
higher than in adipose tissue of suckling rats in a 14-pup litter. Since the
enzyme is inactivated by a protein kinase (probably cyclic AMP sensitive),

it is of interest that the low activity in the intestine of suckling rats can be raised by dephosphorylation (75), suggesting that perhaps the postnatal depression in HMGR activity in liver, brown fat, gut, and lung is related to the well-known increase in blood glucagon levels, which, together with the low blood insulin levels (61), results in elevated activity of adenylcyclase, at least in liver and brown fat (113, 142). This is supported by the changes that occur at weaning to different diets. In rats weaned to a high-carbohydrate diet, blood levels of glucagon and cholesterol decrease together with the hepatic content of cyclic AMP and GMP, while insulin levels rise. Maintenance of the picture seen in suckling rats is found on weaning to a high-fat diet (66).

The regulation of hepatic and perhaps extrahepatic HMGR, however, is not the whole picture. Equally important is the rate at which cholesterol is eliminated into the bile. In the newborn guinea pig (98) the pool size of cholic acid is small and so is its rate of synthesis. The enzyme that commits cholesterol to bile acid synthesis is 7α-cholesterol hydroxylase. Little is known of its postnatal development in any species. In rats, activity in the liver is about the same in the newborn and the 21-day-old animal (107). Unfortunately this tells us nothing about the suckling period. Judging from the activity of HMGR, which according to these authors is twice as high on day 21 as in the newborn, one must assume that the 21-day-old rats were consuming considerable amounts of lab diet. Other data from this paper suggest that 7α-hydroxylase is high in the suckling period, since in older animals it is usually elevated whenever HMGR is depressed.

It has also been suggested that the blood level of HDL-cholesterol is inversely proportional to the incidence of atherosclerosis; the higher level of total cholesterol, the more likely is the occurrence of arterial disease.

In 117 neonates HDL-cholesterol was 25.5 ± 0.9, LDL-cholesterol 30.2 ± 1.0, and total cholesterol 72 ± 1.4 mg/dl. HDL-cholesterol rises by 40–50% in older children, but LDL-cholesterol increases 4-fold to adult levels (62). Obviously in the unfed neonate, chylomicrons are not present (74). Because of the conjectured relationship between HDL-cholesterol levels and atherosclerosis, the effect of age and diet have been examined in experimental animals.

In suckling rabbits, Robert et al (127, 128) found an increase in VLDL and intermediate-density proteins; this contrasts with the hypercholesterolemia found when young weaned rabbits are fed a casein-cholesterol-free diet. Most of the cholesterol in these animals was in the intermediate-density lipoproteins. In sheep (95) a different picture is apparent. At all ages, the main lipoprotein is HDL (76% in the adult),while about 20% is LDL. In the suckling animal both fractions increase, together with the cholesterol and cholesterol ester contents. In the suckling lamb, the transient presence of another lipoprotein in the HDL fraction was reported. In rats (134, 135) HDL-cholesterol levels rise postnatally and rapidly decrease on fat feeding or starvation of prematurely weaned animals. In the suckling rabbit, HDL-cholesterol levels rise from 20 mg/dl two days after birth to 42 mg/dl in the 4th week and fall to 7 mg/dl after weaning. The high VLDL- and LDL-cholesterol levels decreased 10-fold after weaning but rose considerably if casein was added to the diet (127, 128).

In rats, on the other hand, fetal plasma LDL levels were 5-fold higher than in adult animals (135, 136) while VLDL levels were 10-fold lower. HDL levels were 60% those in the adult. About 80% of serum TG are in fetal LDL and 14% in fetal VLDL. Exactly the opposite is true for adult serum.

The intestine of the newborn unsuckled rat contains VLDL in its duodenal villus tip cells. Chylomicrons appear only after suckling in duodenal epithelial cells (11). In the mother rat chylomicron cholesterol does not enter the milk (94).

An important enzyme in cholesterol metabolism and its transport is lecithin-cholesterol acyltransferase (LCAT). The enzyme catalyzes the formation of cholesterol esters from cholesterol and lecithin. It is found to be low in the newborn guinea pig (28) and human (28) and to rise quickly after birth if the newborn are fed milk. Thus in the newborn lamb, 6.7% of labelled cholesterol was esterified; this rose to 9.7% on day 3 but remained unchanged if a nonmilk diet was fed. Similarly, cholesterol esterification in the plasma was 22 μmoles/hr/l in the newborn and 82 three days later if milk was fed, but only 51 on a milk free diet. A large postnatal increase in LCAT in lamb was also reported by Noble et al (111). Frohlich et al (54) found little change in LCAT activity in rats and humans during postnatal development but suggest an inverse relationship between LCAT activity and serum cholesterol.

Adipose Tissue and Obesity

Originally it was proposed that one of the factors causing obesity was the number of cells present in adipose tissue soon after birth (91). This now appears doubtful. Apparently much depends on the origin of the adipose tissue (epididimal, subcutaneous, abdominal, etc). In rats, evidence suggests that adipocytes (probably preadipocytes) can commence multiplying right into adulthood (55, 90). Thus the idea that the young animal or child soon after birth has a fixed number of fat cells in its adipose tissue is probably no longer tenable (65).

However, feeding in the neonatal period can have immediate effects. Formula-fed infants started on solid food before the age of 2 months had more fat at 3 months than those fed formula or breast milk only (48). Two months later this difference had disappeared. In infants of diabetic mothers there was a direct correlation between blood levels of insulin and body fat mass and fat cell weight but not fat cell number (42). These data make it difficult to decide whether the greater fat content of newborns from obese mothers is genetically or environmentally conditioned. A high-carbohydrate diet in pregnant women resulted in 20% obesity in their infants (133); 40% of large-for-gestational-age newborns born to diabetic mothers were obese by 7 years (148) and overweight when adolescents; adequate-for-gestational-age newborns from diabetic mothers did not show this tendency. Kramer (92) showed that breast feeding protects against later obesity.

Some light is shed on the differences between species in a report of G. Alexander (1) on adipose tissue development in the fetal sheep. Fat started to be laid down in the fetus before the 50th day of gestation, and brown fat appeared on day 70. White fat could be found 2 weeks later. Surprisingly, fat regressed considerably after the 115th day of pregnancy. The author suggests that the normal fetal lamb is undernourished for the last 5 weeks of gestation. Supporting this view is the fact that in nutritionally restricted ewes fetal fat content was even lower. Perhaps fetal sheep are able to live off their fat to some extent during the last 5 weeks of gestation.

Human adipose tissue had a fat cell weight of 0.05 μg in the newborn, which increased to 0.25 μg by 9 months (115). For the same cell size, basal lipolysis was greater in infants younger than one year than in older ones. Fat cell size and not fat cell number in newborns is significantly correlated to body fat mass and neonatal plasma insulin levels. These authors conclude that during intrauterine development fat mass expansion occurs almost exclusively by fat cell hypertrophy (43).

A controversy exists over whether early weaning of babies leads to obesity (25, 82, 145). Several factors have been shown responsible for early excessive weight gain, an important one being overconcentrated feeds leading to water deficiency, hyperosmolality, thirst, over-feeding, and overweight. All this can be prevented (at least in Sheffield) by adequate feeding either by breast or with formula. Others have suggested (13) that obesity occurs in children only after they have been overfed for a considerable length of time. Thus one-year-old fat babies remain overweight only if they are further permitted to remain fat and to increase their cell number.

Yet how far early feeding is involved in later obesity is still not clear (25, 30, 48). In contrast to the case with mice (31, 32, 146), genetic factors have not been clearly defined for humans. Undoubtedly the density of the milk plays a role. Thus in the musk shrew, fat content of the milk is 17.5% and the young triple their weight by day 5 after birth (29). It seems that excessive carbohydrate intake in pregnancy can also lead to neonatal obesity (134). Similarly, maternal obesity is reflected in the newborn (152, 153).

Female rats allowed to become obese on a highly palatable high-energy diet did not eat more when lactating (as is usually the case), and 44% of their litters died by the 6th postnatal day. The surviving pups grew more slowly than pups from control mothers (79; see also 130). Overeating in infancy (4 rat or mouse pups against 10 or 16 per litter) also has long-lasting effects. In the overfed group, activities of enzymes of FA synthesis were elevated at 20 weeks—i.e. long after weaning (32). Similarly, blood cholesterol levels were higher in the overfed than the normally fed groups 6 months after birth (P. Hahn, unpublished).

Early Conditioning for Adult Atherosclerosis

In 1951 Gillman & Gillman (57) suggested that the causes of adult atherosclerosis might be found in early childhood. In recent years increased attention has been paid to this idea. It was demonstrated (74) and confirmed later (76) that premature weaning of female rats made them more susceptible to the effects of an atherogenic diet when aged 8 months. Reiser & Sidelman (125) suggested an inverse relationship between the cholesterol content of rat milk and the plasma cholesterol level in adult male rats that had consumed such milk as pups. Unfortunately milk cholesterol content was examined in 2 mother animals only. Weaning rats prematurely (day 18) to a high-fat diet (HF) fed between days 18 and 30 only made them more resistant to the hypercholesterolemic effect of an atherogenic diet when aged 7 months; whereas feeding a high-carbohydrate diet (HC) for these 12 days had the same effects as premature weaning to the laboratory chow in previous experiments (76). Plasma levels of total cholesterol in the animals weaned to the HF diet remained high until day 30, when Purina Chow was offered, but such levels dropped rapidly in 19-day-old rats weaned to the HC diet on day 18.

Thus again there was an inverse relationship between plasma levels of cholesterol in young animals and those in adult rats challenged with an atherogenic diet. Further studies showed that early weaning (day 18) to the HC diet in the rat results in a rapid decrease in plasma glucagon levels and a slower rise in plasma insulin levels (70). This was reflected 8 months later when rats were fed the atherogenic diet by the fact that plasma glucagon levels were increased more in rats weaned to the HF diet than in those weaned to the HC diet. The effects of feeding a HF or HC diet for 12 days between days 18 and 30 can be revealed much sooner with the right technique. These experiments promoted pediatricians to seek a similar phenomenon in humans. Except in one study (147), no effect of early feeding on subsequent plasma cholesterol levels was found (53, 73, 83, 96, 100). These studies all suffer from the same defects: (a) Children were examined between the ages of 1 and 10 years—i.e. they were comparable to very young rats; and (b) they were not challenged with a specific high-fat or high-cholesterol diet. Hence, whether early feeding experience (breast feeding against early weaning) has a late effect in humans has not been effectively examined. [See also (16a) for an evaluation.] Nestel et al (109) also suggest that "the magnitude of the response to dietary cholesterol and fat becomes established early in life."

More recently, Naseem et al (107) showed that even the diet fed to pregnant rats may affect cholesterol metabolism immediately in the fetus and later in the pup. They found that infant rats from mothers fed a high-fat high-cholesterol diet throughout pregnancy and after birth up to day 21 had lower HMGR activity and plasma cholesterol levels than pups from control mothers fed the diet only from day 1 after birth. In other words, prenatal supply of a HF-HC diet had a cholesterol-lowering effect on day 21 postnatally. On the other hand, feeding the control diet from birth to day 21 resulted in *higher* plasma cholesterol levels and hepatic 7α-hydroxylase activity on that day if the experimental diet had been fed during gestation. Note that day 21 is 9 days prior to natural weaning.

The effect of different levels of cholesterol (0–1%) and lard (5–15%) in the diet on maternal plasma and milk cholesterol in rabbit does was examined by Whatley et al (151). In blood, cholesterol levels rose 100-fold (15% lard + 1% cholesterol); in milk they doubled on this diet only. Blood and liver cholesterol levels in suckling pups were elevated but fell to normal after weaning to a low-fat low-cholesterol diet.

The conclusion of a paper by Kris-Elberton et al (93) is definite: "Our work unequivocally refutes the hypothesis that early exposure to exogenous cholesterol protects against subsequent dietary induced hypercholesterolemia in the rats." This is probably a valid conclusion, even though it takes a stand against a premise few investigators have put forward. What has been suggested is that plasma cholesterol levels in infancy are in some way related to these levels in the adult and that early changes in nutrient supply have more permanent effects than was previously thought. This suggestion is borne out in the complex experiments reported by this group. Rat dams were fed 3 diets from the 14th day of gestation: (a) fat free (FF), (b) high-fat high cholesterol with 2% Na cholate (HFHC), and (c) the standard rat diet (S). Milk cholesterol content was more than doubled in the HFHC group but was the same in the other 2 groups (plasma cholesterol in the dams: HFHC, 1120; S, 62; FF, 69 mg/dl). Body weights of the offspring increased more (after weaning) in pups with the HFHC milk than in the other two groups. Feeding a 10% lard diet from days 30–60 resulted in lower plasma cholesterol levels in the group fed the HF diet up to day 30. For reasons that are not clear, a stock diet with 0.5% cholesterol was fed from day 60. On the whole, no differences in plasma cholesterol levels were observed up to day 150, when a diet of 10% lard with 0.5% cholesterol was fed up to day 210. On day 180, but not 210, cholesterol levels were highest in the HF group. Similar results were obtained with a slight variation in the feeding of the infant rats. As a rule, high-cholesterol diets in the suckling periods resulted in lower plasma cholesterol levels in later life (up to day 120); but at day 210, levels were higher in the ones given extra cholesterol when suckling. Finally, some infant rats were artificially reared with or without cholesterol. This resulted in slower growth and (regardless of the cholesterol content of the artificial milk)in higher plasma cholesterol levels than in suckled pups, on days 81 and 111. This experiment supports the unequivocal conclusion of these authors. However, since neonatal undernutrition (artificial feeding in this case) leads to decreased plasma cholesterol levels in infancy (69) it seems possible that perinatal plasma cholesterol levels or some factors other than exogenously supplied cholesterol may be correlated with levels in the adult. This is essentially the conclusion of the authors, who suggest that "the development of a 'normal' metabolic response to exogenous cholesterol in the adult is affected in early life."

It is of interest to note that cholesterol passes from mother rat to fetus only slowly and is without effect on the high rate of its synthesis in fetal liver (16).

It was also shown (107) that hepatic HMGR and 7α-hydroxylase activities may be more sensitive indicators of early nutritional effects than serum cholesterol levels. Thus 52-day-old rats whose dams had been fed a normal diet during gestation and lactation (up to postnatal day 21) were compared with rats from dams fed a HFHC diet during lactation. On day 21 all rats were given this HF diet up to day 52. HMGCoAR was decreased and 7α-hydroxylase activity increased ($p \leq 0.01$) in the group fed the HF diet during lactation, and again the HF diet from day 21 to 52 resulted in higher serum cholesterol and 7α-hydroxylase levels and decreased HMGCoAR activity than when the HF diet was fed during gestation. Thus there remains little doubt that early changes in feeding pattern, even mediated via the mother, can produce long-lasting effects. The question of mechanism remains. Li, Bale & Kottke (97, 99) throw some light on this question using guinea pigs. These are born very mature. They start to eat solid food immediately after birth and hence are not suitable for experiments involving premature weaning. No effect of "early" weaning was noted except a slight ($p \leq 0.05$) decrease in hepatic HMGCoAR in response to a high-cholesterol diet. On the other hand, feeding cholestyramine (1.1% of diet) for 6 weeks after birth made adult animals (aged 105–259 days) more resistant to the hypercholesterolemic effects of a high-cholesterol diet. Such animals, when adult, excreted more bile acids than controls and had higher activities of both hepatic HMGCoAR and 7α-hydroxylase. They also had a larger bile acid pool. Differences between the 2 groups (with or without choles-tyramine for 6 weeks) were more pronounced when a 0.25% cholesterol diet was fed. Feeding cholesterol from the 1st to the 13th postnatal week had little effect on blood cholesterol up to week 25 but did cause a greater excretion of bile acids. Thus it appears that, in guinea pigs at least, choles-terol catabolism is enhanced by treatments in infancy that make the individ-ual more resistant to excessive cholesterol feeding when adult.

Hepatic HMGR activity in adult rats depends on their previous nutri-tional history (126). Animals fed a semipurified diet up to day 60 (but not 35) maintained low HMGR activity even when they ate a commercial diet for 20 days.

Of course, important differences exist among rats, guinea pigs, and hu-mans. Rats are born very premature and are breast fed for at least the first 14 days of postnatal life, whereas guinea pigs eat solid food nearly immedi-ately after birth. Humans lie between these extremes. They are closer to guinea pigs as far as maturity goes, but closer to the rat as far as dependence on the mother is concerned. In addition guinea pigs hardly ever consume cholesterol after weaning; rats and humans do. It is hence difficult to draw any but the most general conclusions from animal experiments.

J. J. Nora (112) suggests that it is possible to identify during childhood the person who will suffer from coronary disease as an adult. Nora stresses the genetic components of the disease but, of course, underlines the possible role of the environment. By identifying those at risk early in life, such an approach would obviate the reduction of butter, milk, and egg intake for the whole population. This "individualization" of treatment (nutritional and otherwise) will undoubtedly replace current all-embracing condemna-tions of certain foods.

Literature Cited

1. Alexander, G. 1978. Quantitative devel-opment of adipose tissue in foetal sheep. *Aust. J. Biol. Sci.* 31:489–503
2. Current infant feeding practices. *Dairy Counc. Dig.* 1980. 51:1–6
3. Anday, E. K., Stanley, C. A., Baker, L., Delivoria-Papadopoulos, M. 1981. Plasma ketones in newborn infants: Ab-sence of suckling ketosis. *J. Pediatr.* 88: 628–30
4. Andersen, G. E., Lifschitz, C., Friis-Hansen, B. 1979. Dietary habits and serum lipids during first 4 years of life-A study of 95 Danish children. *Acta Pe-diatr. Scand.* 68:165–70
5. Babak, E. 1903, 1905. See Ref. 74
6. Barbara, L., Lazzari, R., Roda, A., Al-dini, R., Festi, D., Sama, C., Morselli, A. M., Collina, A., Bazzoli, F., Maz-zella, G., Roda, E. 1980. Serum bile acids in newborns and children. *Pediatr. Res.* 14:1222–25
7. Battaglia, F. C., Meschia, G. 1978. Principal substrates of fetal metabolism. *Physiol. Rev.* 58:499–527
8. Benavides, J., Gimenez, C., Valdivieso, F., Mayor, F. 1976. Effect of phenylala-nine metabolites on the activities of en-zymes of ketone-body utilization in brain of suckling rats. *Biochem. J.* 160: 217–22
9. Benedict, F. G., Talbot, F. B. 1945. See Ref. 74
10. Benito, M., Whitelaw, E., Williamson, D. H. 1979. Regulation of ketogenesis during the suckling-weanling transition in the rat—studies with isolated hepato-cytes. *Biochem. J.* 180:137–44

11. Berendsen, P. B. 1979. Sites of lipoprotein production in the small intestine of the unsuckled and suckled newborn rat. *Anat. Rec.* 195:15–30
12. Bohmer, T., Havel, R. J. 1975. Genesis of fatty liver and hyperlipemia in the fetal guinea pig. *J. Lipid Res.* 16:454–60
13. Bonnet, F. P., Daune, M. R. 1976. Factors affecting the number of subcutaneous adipose cells of the obese child. *Pediatr. Adolesc. Endocrinol.* 1:112–18
14. Boulton, T. J. C., Craig, I. H., Hill, G. 1979. Screening of cord blood low-density-lipoprotein cholesterol in the diagnosis of familial hypercholesterolemia: A study of 2000 infants. *Acta Pediatr. Scand.* 68:363–70
15. Breslow, J. L. 1978. Pediatric aspects of hyperlipidemia. *Pediatrics* 62:510–20
16. Calandra, S., Quartaroli, G. C., Montaguti, M. 1975. Effect of cholesterol feeding on cholesterol biosynthesis in maternal and foetal rat liver. *Eur. J. Clin. Invest.* 5:27–31
16a. Canadian Pediatric Society. 1978. Breast-feeding: what is left besides the poetry. A statement by the nutrition committee. 1978 *Can. J. Publ. Health* 69:13–20
17. Carlson, L. A., Hardell, L. I. 1978. Very low density lipoproteins in cord blood. *Clin. Chim. Acta* 90:295–96
18. Carlson, L. A., Hardell, L. I. 1977. Sex differences in serum lipids and lipoproteins at birth *Eur. J. Clin. Invest.* 7:133–35
19. Carney, S., Morgan, B. 1981. Brain β-hydroxybutyrate utilization in neonatal hypothyroidism. *Fed. Proc.* 40: Abstr. 88
20. Carroll, K. K., Huff, M. W. 1977. Influence of dietary fat and protein on plasma cholesterol levels in the early postnatal period. *Atherosclerosis,* ed. G. W. Manning, M. G. Haust, pp. 638–43. NY: Plenum
21. Char, V. C., Creasy, R. K. 1976. Acetate as a metabolic substrate in the fetal lamb. *Am. J. Physiol.* 230:357–61
22. Christensen, N. C. 1977. Concentrations of triglycerides, free fatty acids and glycerol in cord blood of newborn infants with a birth weight of ≤ 2700 grams. *Acta Pediatr. Scand.* 66:43–48
23. Cornblath, M., Tildon, J. T., Ozand, P. T., Plaut, S. M. 1976. Effect of a high fat diet during pregnancy on neonatal brain metabolism in rats. *Pediatr. Adolesc. Endocrinol.* 1:31–35
24. Dahlquist, G., Persson, B. 1976. The rate of cerebral utilization of glucose, ketone bodies, and oxygen: A comparative in vivo study of infant and adult rats. *Pediatr. Res.* 10:910–17
25. Dine, M. S., Gartside, P. S., Glueck, C. J., Rheines, L., Greene, G., Khoury, P. 1979. Where do the heaviest children come from? A prospective study of white children from birth to 5 years of age. *Pediatrics* 63:1–7
26. Drahota, Z., Hahn, P., Kleinzeller, A., Kostolanska, A. 1964. Acetoacetate formation by liver slices from adult and infant rats. *Biochem. J.* 93:61–65
27. Drahota, Z., Hahn, P., Mourek, J., Trojanova, M. 1965. The effect of acetoacetate on oxygen consumption of brain slices from infant and adult rats. *Physiol. Bohemoslov.* 14:134–38
28. Drevon, C. A., Norum, K. R. 1975. Cholesterol esterification and lipids in plasma and liver from newborn and young guinea pigs raised on milk and non-milk diet. *Nutr. Metabol.* 18:137–51
29. Dryden, G. L., Anderson, R. R. 1978. Milk composition and its relation to growth rate in the musk shrew, *Suncus murinus. Comp. Biochem. Physiol. A* 60:213–16
30. Dubois, S., Hill, D. E., Beaton, G. H. 1979. An examination of factors believed to be associated with infantile obesity. *Am. J. Clin. Nutr.* 32:1997–2004
31. Dubuc, P. U., Willis, P. L. 1979. Postweaning development of diabetes in ob/ob mice. *Metabolism* 28:633–40
32. Duff, D. A., Shell, K. 1976. Induction of hepatic enzyme abnormalities associated with obesity by neonatal overnourishment. *Metabolism* 25:1567–74
33. Dwyer, B., Bernsohn, J. 1979. The incorporation of (1-^{14}C) linolenate into lipids of developing rat brain during essential fatty acid deprivation. *J. Neurochem.* 32:833–38
34. Dwyer, B. E., Bernsohn, J. 1979. The effect of essential fatty acid deprivation on the metabolic transformation of (1-^{14}C) linolenate in developing rat brain. *Biochim. Biophys. Acta* 575:309–17
35. Edson, J. L., Hudson, D. G., Hull, D. 1975. Evidence for increased fatty acid transfer across the placenta during a maternal fast in rabbits. *Biol. Neonate* 27:50–55
36. Elphick, M. C., Hudson, D. G., Hull, D. 1975. The transfer of free fatty acids across the rabbit placenta. *J. Physiol.* 252:29–42
37. Elphick, M. C., Hull, D. 1977. The transfer of free fatty acids across the rabbit placenta. *J. Physiol.* 264:751–66

38. Elphick, M. C., Hull, D. 1977. Rabbit placenta clearing-factor lipase and transfer to the foetus of fatty acids derived from triglycerides injected into the mother. *J. Physiol.* 273:475–87
39. Elphick, M. C., Hull, D., Sanders, R. R. 1976. Concentrations of free fatty acids in maternal and umbilical cord blood during elective caesarean section. *Br. J. Obstet. Gynecol.* 83:539–44
40. Elphick, M. C., Hull, D., Pipkin, F. B. 1979. The transfer of fatty acids across the sheep placenta. *J. Devel. Physiol.* 1:31–45
41. Elphick, M. C., Edson, J. L., Hull, D. 1978. Effect of maternal glucose infusions on fatty acid transport across the placenta in rabbits. *Biol. Neonate* 34:231–37
42. Enzi, G., Inelmen, E. M., Caretta, F., Villani, F., Zanardo, V., DeBiasi, F. 1980. Development of adipose tissue in newborns of gestational-diabetic and insulin-dependent diabetic mothers. *Diabetes* 29:100–4
43. Enzi, G., Inelmen, E. M., Caretta, F., Rubaltelli, F., Grella, P., Baritussio, A., Adipose tissue development "in Utero". *Diabetologia* 18:135–40
44. Fenselau, A., Wallis, K., Morris, H. P. 1975. Acetoacetyl coenzymeA transferase activity in rat hepatomas. *Cancer Res.* 35:2315–20
45. Ferre, P., Pegorier, J. P., Marliss, E. B., Girard, J. R. 1978. Influence of exogenous fat and gluconeogenic substrates on glucose homeostasis in the newborn rat. *Am. J. Physiol.* 234:E129–36
46. Ferre, P., Pegorier, J. P., Williamson, D. H., Girard, J. 1979. Interactions in vivo between oxidation of non-esterified fatty acids and gluconeogenesis in the newborn rat. *Biochem. J.* 182:593–98
47. Ferre, P., Pegorier, J. P., Williamson, D. H., Girard, J. R. 1978. The development of ketogenesis at birth in the rat. *Biochem. J.* 176:759–65
48. Ferris, A. G., Beal, V. A., Laus, M. J., Hosmer, D. W. 1979. The effect of feeding on fat deposition in early infancy. *Pediatr. Res.* 64:397–401
49. Frerichs, R. R., Srinivasan, S. R., Webber, L. S., Rieth, M. C., Berenson, G. S., 1978. Serum lipids and lipoproteins at birth in a biracial population: The Bogalusa heart study. *Pediatr. Res.* 12:858–63
50. Friedman, Z., Danon, A., Stahlman, T., Oates, J. A. 1976. Rapid onset of essential fatty acid deficiency in the newborn. *Pediatrics* 58:640–49
51. Friedman, Z., Shochat, S. J., Maisels, M. J., Marks, K. H., Lamberth, E. L. Jr. 1976. Correction of essential fatty acid deficiency in newborn infants by cutaneous application of sunflower-seed oil. *Pediatrics* 58:650–54
52. Friedman, Z., Danon, A., Lamberth, E. L. Jr., Mann, W. J. 1978. Cord blood fatty acid composition in infants and in their mothers during the third trimester. *J. Pediatr.* 92:461–66
53. Friedman, G., Goldberg, S. J. 1975. Concurrent and subsequent serum cholesterol of breast- and formula-fed infants. *Am. J. Clin. Nutr.* 28:42–45
54. Frohlich, J., Bernstein, V., Bernstein, M. 1975. Lecithin: cholesterol acyltransferase. Initial fractional rates of esterification in human and rat serum during development. *Clin. Chim. Acta* 65:79–82
55. Gaben-Cogneville, A. M., Swierczewski, E. 1979. Studies on cell proliferation in inguinal adipose tissue during early development in the rat. *Lipids* 14:669–75
56. Gilbert, M., Sparks, J., Girard, J., Battaglia, F. 1981. Changes in glucose metabolism during pregnancy induced by fasting in chronically catheterized guinea-pigs. *Fed. Proc.* 40:1360 (Abstr.)
57. Gillman, J., Gillman, T. 1951. *Perspectives in Human Malnutrition.* NY: Greene & Stratton
58. Ginsburg, B. E., Zetterstrom, R. 1977. High density lipoprotein concentrations in newborn infants. *Acta Pediatr. Scand.* 66:39–41
59. Ginsburg, B. E., Zetterstrom, R. 1980. Serum cholesterol concentrations in newborn infants with gestational ages of 28–42 weeks. *Acta Pediatr. Scand.* 69: 587–92
60. Ginsburg, B. E., Zetterstrom, R. 1980. Serum cholesterol concentrations in early infancy. *Acta Pediat. Scand.* 69: 581–85
61. Girard, J. R., Marliss, E. B. 1975. Circulating fuels in late fetal and early neonatal life in the rat. In *Diabetes in Early Life*, ed. R. A. Camerini-Davalos, H. S. Cole, pp. 185–194. NY: Academic. 615 pp.
62. Glueck, C. J., Mellies, M. J., Tsang, R. C., Steiner, P. M. 1977. Low and high density lipoprotein cholesterol interrelationships in neonates with low density lipoprotein cholesterol $\leq$ the 10th percentile and in neonates with high density lipoprotein cholesterol $\geq$ the 90th percentile. *Pediatr. Res.* 11:957–59

63. Griffin, E., Breckenridge, W. C., Kuksis, A., Bryan, M. H., Angel, A. 1979. Appearance and characterization of lipoprotein X during continuous intralipid infusions in the neonate. *J. Clin. Invest.* 64:1703–12

64. Grundt, I., Forsdahl, F., Forsdahl, A. 1976. Cord blood cholesterol, triglyceride, and lipoprotein pattern from two districts in Norway. *Scand. J. Clin. Lab. Invest.* 36:261–64

65. Hager, A., Sjostrom, L., Arvidsson, B., Bjorntorp, P., Smith, U. 1977. Body fat and adipose tissue cellularity in infants: a longitudinal study. *Metabolism* 26:607–14

66. Hahn, P., Skala, J. P., Hassanali, S. 1980. The response of cyclic nucleotide content in liver and brown fat of rats weaned to different diets. *J. Nutr.* 110:330–34

67. Hahn, P. 1980. Cholesterol metabolism in obese mice. *Can. J. Biochem.* 58:1258–60

68. Hahn, P., Kirby, L. 1973. Immediate and late effects of premature weaning and of feeding a high fat or high carbohydrate diet to weaning rats. *J. Nutr.* 103:690–96

69. Hahn, P., Walker, B. I. 1979. Hepatic 3-hydroxy-3-methyl-glutarylCoA reductase response to litter size in suckling rats. *Can. J. Biochem.* 57:1216–19

70. Hahn, P., Girard, J. R., Assan, J., Kervran, A., Koldovsky, O. 1978. Late effects of premature weaning to different diets in the rat. *J. Nutr.* 108:1783–86

71. Hahn, P. 1978. Nutrition of the newborn. In *Perinatal Physiology,* ed. U. Stave, pp. 357–63. NY: Plenum. 851 pp.

72. Hahn, P. 1978. Lipids. See Ref. 71, pp. 397–423.

73. Hahn, P. 1979. Nutrition and metabolic development. In *Human Nutrition,* ed. M. Winick, 1:1–40. NY: Plenum

74. Hahn, P., Koldovsky, O. 1966. *Utilization of Nutrients During Postnatal Development.* Int. Ser. Zool. Div., Vol. 33. NY: Pergamon. 177 pp.

75. Hahn, P., Smale, F.-A. 1982. 3-HMGCoA-reductase in gut and adipose tissue of developing rats. *Can. J. Biochem.* In press

76. Hahn, P., Koldovsky, O. 1976. Late effect of premature weaning on blood cholesterol levels in adult rats. *Nutr. Rep. Int.* 13:87–91

77. Hardell, L. I. 1981. Serum lipids and lipoproteins at birth and in early childhood. *Acta Pediatr. Scand.* Suppl. 285, pp. 1–29

78. Hardell, L. I. 1978. *Serum lipids and lipoproteins at birth and in early childhood.* Doctoral thesis. Uppsala Univ.

79. Harlow, A. C., Roux, J. F., Shapiro, M. I. 1980. Plasma glucose, cholesterol, triglyceride, and glycerol concentrations in the postmature rabbit. *Am. J. Obstet. Gynecol.* 136:500–4

80. Hassan, A. S., Subbiah, M. T. R. 1980. Effect of diabetes during pregnancy on maternal and neonatal bile acid metabolism in the rat. *Proc. Soc. Exp. Biol. Med.* 165:490–95

81. Hassan, A. S., Subbiah, M. T. R. 1980. Bile acids in the fetal rat: effect of maternal bile duct ligation. *Steriods* 36:709–15

82. Himes, J. H. 1979. Infant feeding practices and obesity. *J. Am. Diet. Assoc.* 75:122–25

83. Hodgson, P. A., Ellefson, R. D., Elveback, L. R., Harris, L. E., Nelson, R. A., Weidman, W. H. 1976. Comparison of serum cholesterol in children fed high, moderate, or low cholesterol milk diets during neonatal period. *Metabolism* 25:739–46

84. Hudson, D. G., Hull, D. 1977. Uptake and metabolism of ^{14}C-palmitate by fetal rabbit tissues. *Biol. Neonate* 31:316–23

85. Hull, D. 1975. Storage and supply of fatty acids before and after birth. *Br. Med. Bull.* 31:32–36

86. Hummel, L., Schwartze, A., Schirrmeister, W., Wagner, H. 1976. Maternal plasma triglycerides as a source of fetal fatty acids. *Acta Biol. Med. Germ.* 35:1635–41

87. Hummel, L., Schirrmeister, W., Zimmermann, T. 1975. Transfer of maternal plasma free fatty acids into the rat fetus. *Acta Biol. Med. Germ.* 34:603–5

88. Hummel, L., Zimmermann, T., Wagner, H. 1978. Quantitative evaluation of the fetal fatty acid synthesis in the rat. *Acta Biol. Med. Germ.* 37:229–32

89. Deleted in proof

90. Kazdova, L., Fabry, P. 1975. *Cell Impairment—Aging Development Adv. Exp. Med. Biol.* 53:247–56

91. Knittle, J. L., Hirsch, J. 1968. Effect of early nutrition on the development of rat epididymal fat pads. *J. Clin. Invest.* 47:2091–98

92. Kramer, M. S. 1980. Do breast feeding and delayed solids protect against later obesity? *Pediatr. Res.* 14: Abstr. 463

93. Kris-Etherton, P. M., Layman, D. K., Van Zyl York, P., Frantz, I. D. 1979. The influence of early nutrition on the

serum cholesterol of the adult rat. *J. Nutr.* 109:1244–57

94. Kris-Etherton, P. M., Frantz, I. D., Jr. 1980. The contribution of chylomicron cholesterol to milk cholesterol in the rat. *Proc. Soc. Exp. Biol. Med.* 165:502–7

95. Leat, W. M. F., Kubasek, F. O. T., Buttress, N. 1976. Plasma lipoproteins of lambs and sheep. *Q. J. Exp. Physiol.* 61:193–202

96. Laskarzewski, P., Morrison, J. A., DeGroot, I., Kelly, K. A., Kellies, M. J., Khoury, P., Glueck, C. J. 1979. Lipid and lipoprotein tracking in 108 children over a four-year period. *Pediatrics* 64:584–91

97. Li, J. R., Bale, L. K., Kottke, B. A. 1980. Effect of neonatal modulation of cholesterol homeostasis on subsequent response to cholesterol challenge in adult guinea pig. *J. Clin. Invest.* 65:1060–68

98. Li, J. R., Subbiah, M. T. R., Kottke, B. A. 1979. Hepatic 3-hydroxy-3-methylglutaryl coenzyme A reductase activity and cholesterol 7α-hydroxylase activity in neonatal guinea pig. *Steroids* 34:47–55

99. Li, J. R., Bale, L. K., Subbiah, M. T. R. 1979. Effect of enhancement of cholesterol degradation during neonatal life of guinea pig on its subsequent response to dietary cholesterol. *Atherosclerosis* 32:93–98

100. McKenna, M. C., Campagnoni, H. R. 1979. Effect of pre- and postnatal essential fatty acid deficiency on main development. *J. Nutr.* 7:1195–204

101. McNamara, D. J., Quackenbush, F. W., Rodwell, V. W. 1972. Regulation of hepatic 3-hydroxy-3-methylglutaryl coenzyme A reductase: developmental pattern. *J. Biol. Chem.* 247:5805–10

102. Mellies, M. J., Ishikawa, T. T., Gartside, P., Burton, K., MacGee, J., Allen, K., Steiner, P. M., Brady, D., Glueck, C. J. 1978. Effects of varying maternal dietary cholesterol and phytosterol in lactating women and their infants. *Am. J. Clin. Nutr.* 31:1347–54

103. Miettinen, E.-L. 1981. Effect of maternal canine starvation on fetal and neonatal liver metabolism. *Am. J. Physiol.* 240:E88–94

104. Miguel, S. G., Abraham, S. 1976. Effect of maternal diet on fetal hepatic lipogenesis. *Biochim. Biophys. Acta* 424:213–34

105. Moore, C. E., Dhopeshwarkar, G. A. 1980. Placental transport of trans fatty acids in the rat. *Lipids* 15:1023–28

106. Mott, G. E., McMahan, C. A., McGill, H. C. Jr. 1978. Diet and sire effects on serum cholesterol and cholesterol absorption in infant baboons (*Papio cynocephalus*). *Circ. Res.* 43:364–371

107. Naseem, S. M., Khan, M. A., Jacobson, M. S., Nair, P. P., Heald, F. P. 1980. The influence of dietary cholesterol and fat on the homeostasis of cholesterol metabolism in early life in the rat. *Pediatr. Res.* 14:1061–66

108. Ness, G. C., Miller, J. P., Moffler, M. H., Woods, L. S., Harris, H. B. 1979. Perinatal development of 3-hydroxy-3-methylglutaryl coenzymeA reductase activity in rat lung, liver and brain. *Lipids* 14:447–50

109. Nestel, P. J., Poyser, A., Boulton, T. J. C. 1979. Changes in cholesterol metabolism in infants in response to dietary cholesterol and fat. *Am. J. Clin. Nutr.* 32:2177–82

110. Noble, R. C., Shand, J. H., Bell, A. W. 1979. Fetal to maternal transfer of palmitic and linoleic acids across the sheep placenta. *Biol. Neonate* 36:113–18

111. Noble, R. C., Crouchman, M. L., Moore, J. H. 1975. Plasma cholesterol ester formation in the neonatal lamb *Biol. Neonate* 26:117–21

112. Nora, J. J. 1980. Identifying the child at risk for coronary disease as an adult: A strategy for prevention. *J. Pediatr.* 97:706–14

113. Novak, M., Wieser, P. B., Buch, M., Skala, J. 1979. Cyclic adenosine monophosphate dependent protein kinase in adipose tissue of newborn infants. *Pediatr. Res.* 13:626–31

114. Novak, M., Kohn, R., Vinsova, N. 1959. See Ref. 74,

115. Nyberg, G., Mellgren, G., Smith, U. 1976. Human adipose tissue in culture. IV. Effect of age on cell size and lipolysis. *Acta Pediatr. Scand.* 65:313–18

116. Oscai, L. B., McGarr, J. A. 1978. Evidence that the amount of food consumed in early life fixes appetite in the rat. *Am. J. Physiol.* 235:R141–44

117. Parwaresch, M. R., Radzun, H.-J. 1978. Lack of very low density lipoproteins in cord blood. *Clin. Chim. Acta* 83:295–96

118. Pascaud, M., Rougier, A., Delhaye, N. 1977. Assimilation of ^{14}C-linoleic acid by the rat fetus. *Nutr. Metab.* 21:310–16

119. Patel, T. B., Clark, J. B. 1978. Acetoacetate metabolism in rat brain. Development of acetoacetyl-coenzyme A deacylase and 3-hydroxy-3-methylgluta-

ryl-coenzymeA synthase. *Biochem. J.* 176:951–58

120. Patel, M. S., Owen, O. E. 1977. Development and regulation of lipid synthesis from ketone bodies by rat brain. *J. Neurochem.* 28:109–14

121. Patel, M. S. 1979. Influence of neonatal hypothyroidism on the development of ketone-body-metabolizing enzymes in rat brain. *Biochem. J.* 184:169–72

122. Paton, J. B., Levitsky, L. L., Fisher, D. E., DeLannoy, C. W. 1979. Fetal-maternal gradient for ketone bodies in the baboon: dissociation of fetal ketone body and oxygen uptake. *Pediatr. Res.* 13:Abstr. 927

123. Persson, B., Gentz, J. 1976. The pattern of blood lipids and ketone bodies during the neonatal period, infancy and childhood. *Acta Pediatr. Scand.* 55:353–60

124. Potter, J. M., Nestel, P. J. 1976. The effects of dietary fatty acids and cholesterol on the milk lipids of lactating women and the plasma cholesterol of breast-fed infants. *Am. J. Clin. Nutr.* 29:54–60

125. Reiser, R., Sidelman, Z. 1972. Control of serum cholesterol homeostasis by cholesterol in the milk of the suckling rat. *J. Nutr.* 102:1009–16

126. Reiser, R., Henderson, G. R., O'Brien, B. 1977. Persistence of dietary suppression of β-hydroxy-β-methylglutaryl coenzyme A reductase during development of rats. *J. Nutr.* 107:1131–38

127. Roberts, D. C. K., Huff, M. W., Carroll, K. K. 1979. Influence of diet on plasma cholesterol concentrations in suckling and weanling rabbits. *Nutr. Metab.* 23:476–86

128. Roberts, D. C. K., Huff, M. W., Carroll, K. K. 1979. Plasma lipoprotein changes in suckling and weanling rabbits fed semi-purified diets. *Lipids* 14:566–71

129. Robles-Valdes, C., McGarry, J. D., Foster, D. W. 1976. Maternal-fetal carnitine relationships and neonatal ketosis in the rat. *J. Biol. Chem.* 251:6007–12

130. Rolls, B. J., Rowe, E. A., Fahrback, S. E., Agius, L., Williamson, D. H. 1980. Obesity and high energy diets reduce survival and growth rates of rat pups. *Proc. Nutr. Soc.* 39:51A

131. Sabata, V., Lausmann, S., Wolf, H. 1970. Materno-fetale Stoffwechselbeziehungen. In *Stoffwechsel der Neugeborene,* pp. 9–27 Stuttgart: Hippokrates

132. Sabel, K. G., Olegard, R., Hillingsson, K., Mellander, M., Karlberg, P. 1979. Impaired fatty acid oxidation and in-creased gluconeogenic plasma substrates in SGA newborns with hypoglycemia. Improvement after injection of lipids. *Pediatr. Res.* 13:72

133. Schampheleire, I. De, Parent, M. A., Chatteur, C. 1980. Excessive carbohydrate intake in pregnancy and neonatal obesity: study in Cap Bon, Tunisia. *Arch. Dis. Childh.* 55:521–26

134. Schlag, B., Winkler, L. 1978. Konzentration und Zusammensetzung der Serumlipoproteinklassen der fetalen Ratte. *Acta Biol. Med. Germ.* 37:233–37

135. Schlag, B., Winkler, L. 1978. Untersuchungen zur Entwicklung der Serumlipoproteinverhaltnisse vom Fetalstadium bis zum Erwachsenenalter der Ratte. *Acta Biol. Med. Germ.* 37:239–44

136. Seccombe, D. W., Harding, P. G. R., Possmayer, F. 1977. Fetal utilization of maternally derived ketone bodies for lipogenesis in the rat. *Biochim. Biophys. Acta* 488:402–16

137. Shambaugh, G. E. III., Mrozak, S. C., Freinkel, N. 1977. Fetal fuels. I. Utilization of ketones by isolated tissues at various stages of maturation and maternal nutrition during late gestation. *Metabolism* 26:623–35

138. Shambaugh, G. E. III, Koehler, R. R., Yokoo, H. 1978. Fetal fuels. III: ketone utilization by fetal hepatocyte. *Am. J. Physiol.* 235:E330–37

139. Shambaugh, G. E. III, Koehler, R. R., Freinkel, N. 1977. Fetal fuels. II. Contributions of selected carbon fuels to oxidative metabolism in rat conceptus. *Am. J. Physiol.* 233:E457–61

140. Shapiro, M. I., Roux, J. F., Harlow, A., Masse, D. 1979. Placental uptake and transfer of lipid in the postterm rabbit. *Am. J. Obstet. Gynecol.* 133:713–17

141. Shapiro, M. I., Roux, J. F. 1977. Lipid transport and metabolism in the postterm rabbit. *Am. J. Obstet. Gynecol.* 129:171–77

142. Skala, J., Novak, E., Hahn, P., Drummond, G. 1972. Adenyl cyclase, cyclic AMP, proteinkinase, phosphorylase, phosphorylase kinase and glycogen. *Int. J. Biochem.* 3:229–38

143. Sudjic, M. M., Booth, R. 1976. Activity 3-hydroxy-3-methylglutaryl-coenzyme A reductase in brains of adult and 7-day-old rats. *Biochem. J.* 154:559–60

144. Szabo, A. J. 1976. Fetal adipose tissue development: relationship to maternal free fatty acid level. See Ref. 61, pp. 167–76

145. Taitz, L. S. 1976. Relationship of infant feeding patterns to weight gain in the first weeks of life. *Adipose Child. Pediatr. Adolesc. Endocrinol.* 60–65

146. Thurlby, P. L., Trayhurn, P. 1978. The development of obesity in preweanling ob/ob mice. *Br. J. Nutr.* 39:397–402

147. Valadian, I., Reed, R. B., Taylor-Halvorsen, K. 1979. Breast feeding during infancy and serum cholesterol levels in the young adult. In *Diet and atherosclerosis in pediatrics. Proceedings of an international Symposium,* ed. C. C. Roy, pp. 254–68 . Montreal: Univ. Montreal

148. Vohr, B. R., Lipsitt, L. P., Oh, W. 1979 Obesity in children of diabetic mothers with reference to birth size. *Pediatr. Res.* 13: Abstr. 22

149. Walker, A. R. P., Walker, B. F. 1978. High high-density-lipoprotein cholesterol in African children and adults in a population free of coronary heart disease. *Br. Med. J.* 2:1336–38

150. Webber, R. J., Edmond, J. 1979. The in vivo utilization of acetoacetate, D-(-)-3-hydroxybutyrate, and glucose for lipid synthesis in brain in the 18-day-old rat. *J. Biol. Chem.* 254:3912–20

151. Whatley, B. J., Green, J. B., Green, M. H. 1981 Effect of dietary fat and cholesterol on milk composition, milk intake and cholesterol metabolism in the rabbit. *J. Nutr.* 111:432–41

152. Whitelaw, A. 1977. Infant feeding and subcutaneous fat at birth and at one year. *Lancet* 2:1098–99

153. Whitelaw, A. G. L. 1976. Influence of maternal obesity on subcutaneous fat in the newborn *Br. Med. J.* 1:985–86

154. Williamson, D. H. 1975. Regulation of the utilization of glucose and ketone bodies by brain in the perinatal period. See Ref. 61, pp. 195–202

155. Winkler, L., Schellhorn, P., Zimmermann, T., Goetze, E. 1977. Der Einfluss fettfreier Diat auf den Gehalt und die Synthese von Arachidonsäure in der feto-plazentaren Einheit der Ratte. *Acta Biol. Med. Germ.* 36:221–30

156. Winkler, L., Schlag, B., Franke, S., Kessner, Ch., Maess, J., Pautzke, M., Goetze, E. 1979. Der Einfluss fettfreier Diat während der letzten Schwangerschaftswoche auf den Linol- und Arachidonsäuregehalt der Organlipide des Feten und der Plazentalipide der Ratte. *Acta Biol. Med. Germ.* 38:611–17

157. Yeh, Y.-Y., Streuli, V. L., Zee, P. 1977. Ketone bodies serve as important precursors of brain lipids in the developing rat *Lipids* 12:957–64

158. Yeh, Y.-Y., Klein, L. B., Zee, P. 1978. Long and medium chain triglycerides increase plasma concentrations of ketone bodies in suckling rats. *Lipids* 13:566–71

159. Yeh, Y.-Y., Streuli, V. L., Zee, P. 1977. Relative utilization of fatty acids for synthesis of ketone bodies and complex lipids in the liver of developing rats. *Lipids* 12:367–74

160. Yeh, Y.-Y., 1980. Partition of ketone bodies into cholesterol and fatty acids in vivo in different brain regions of developing rats. *Lipids* 15:904–7

161. Yeh, Y.-Y., Zee, P. 1979. Fatty acid oxidation in isolated rat liver mitochondria. *Arch. Biochem. Biophys.* 199:560–69

162. Zimmermann, T., Hummel, L. 1978. Studies on the fatty acid synthesis in maternal and fetal rats. *Acta Biol. Med. Germ.* 37:223–27

163. Zimmermann, T., Hummel, L., Pielka, E., Zimmermann, A., Wagner, H. 1978. Studies on the paraplacental free fatty acid transport in rats. *Acta Biol. Med. Germ.* 37:245–48

Ann. Rev. Nutr. 1982. 2:113–32

RECENT TRENDS IN CARBOHYDRATE CONSUMPTION

Thomas A. Anderson

Department of Pediatrics, University of Iowa, Iowa City, Iowa 52242

CONTENTS

INTRODUCTION

The amount and type of carbohydrate consumed by a specified population group is related to degree of affluence. As may be seen from Figure 1, much of the world's population subsists on diets providing 75–80% of energy from carbohydrate. As per capita income increases, less carbohydrate is eaten and the ratio of complex carbohydrates to simple sugars also decreases. Composition of the various dietary carbohydrates is influenced by the sophistication of food technology and marketing.

In the national food supply carbohydrate currently contributes 45%, fat 43%, and protein 12% of the energy content (27), whereas in 1909 the comparable percentages were 56%, 32%, and 12%, respectively (14). As is discussed below, the Dietary Goals (59) published by a Senate committee in 1977 suggested a return to a diet containing greater amounts of complex carbohydrate and less refined sugar and fat. The Dietary Goals provided the basis for negotiations resulting in the joint issuance by the Departments of Agriculture and Health, Education and Welfare (now Health and Human Services) of the Dietary Guidelines for Americans (68). Much controversy

113

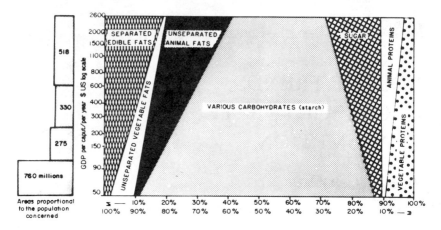

Figure 1 Calories derived from fats, carbohydrates, and proteins as percentage of total calories according to the income of the countries (1962) (correlation based on 85 countries) (38).

has surrounded the publication of both the Dietary Goals and the Dietary Guidelines. The seven recommendations included in the Dietary Guidelines concerned the need to eat a variety of foods; maintenance of ideal body weight; avoidance of excessive intakes of saturated fat, cholesterol, sugar, sodium, and alcohol; and encouragement of increased intakes of complex carbohydrates and fiber. Future trends in carbohydrate consumption would probably have been influenced by the continued promotion of these dietary guidelines; however, free distribution of the recommendations was sharply curtailed in the spring of 1981 because of budget cutbacks and a decision to reduce direct federal involvement in human nutrition. The impact of the dietary guidelines and the subsequent controversy upon intake of various carbohydrates by the American consumer is not known.

Because of the importance of nutrient interaction, one cannot discuss the health aspects of consuming a particular mix of carbohydrates without some consideration of the influence of other dietary components. The quantities of carbohydrate in a "typical American diet" may not be conducive to prevention of the nutrition-related degenerative diseases of greatest public health significance (59, 10, 63, 20), especially in view of the relatively high intake of saturated fat. However, a number of nutritionists doubt that changing the composition of the current US diet would significantly alter the prevalence of coronary heart disease, hypertension, or diabetes (3, 13, 19, 18).

The composition of dietary carbohydrate in the present-day US diet is influenced by a number of factors, some of which are not directly controlled by the consumer. This is true particularly of the technologic and economic considerations that determine the type and amount of sweeteners added to processed foods.

LIMITATIONS IN ESTIMATING INTAKE OF SPECIFIC CARBOHYDRATES

Sources of Data

Obtaining accurate estimates of intake of various foods and determining specific nutrient content of foods selected from a complex and continually changing food supply are not easy tasks. Application of appropriate sampling statistics, interviewer techniques, and computerized data banks of food ingredient and nutrient content is required.

UNITED STATES DEPARTMENT OF AGRICULTURE (USDA) ECO-NOMIC RESEARCH SERVICE (ERS)   The USDA-ERS compiles annual per capita consumption data for approximately 350 foods and for major food categories. These data are derived by dividing estimates of food "disappearance" into civilian wholesale distribution channels by the total civilian population (21). Such disappearance data include food consumed in homes, in eating places, and as snacks purchased from retail stores and vending machines, as well as foods wasted in these places, lost in distribution, used in feeding pets, or put to other uses. Estimates of consumption are likely to be exaggerated for all foods, but particularly for those most subject to these latter considerations.

Year-to-year comparison of these data provides useful information about average per capita consumption at one time and in establishing trends in consumption over a period of time. They do not tell us what people actually eat nor do they provide insight into age, sex, income, or geographic differences in average per capita consumption of various foods.

USDA-AGRICULTURAL RESEARCH SERVICE (ARS)   The USDA-ARS has over the past 40 years conducted large-scale surveys of household food consumption in a representative sample of the US population and, in 1965 (65) and 1977 (66), has surveyed individual food consumption during a 24-hr period. (The current designation for the agency responsible for collection and analysis of these data is Human Nutrition Information Service, Consumer Nutrition Center.) Household food consumption data on quantities of foods used during a specified period are in general agreement with USDA-ERS estimates of per capita food consumption. Nutrient intake has been calculated from the data collected.

Surveys of food consumption by individuals permit inferences about average consumption by the total sample and also by users of a specific food.

From these data it is possible to evaluate various demographic and socioeconomic characteristics of food intake by individuals. Burk & Pao (5) have reviewed the methodology used in large scale surveys of household food procurement and individual diets.

SURVEY OF GENERALLY RECOGNIZED AS SAFE (GRAS) SUBSTANCES
A subcommittee of the National Research Council, National Academy of Sciences, sent questionnaires to food manufacturers inquiring about the usual and maximum usage levels of GRAS substances added to processed foods (33). Possible human intake of these substances was estimated using Market Research Corporation of America records of frequency of consumption of various food items and USDA data on sizes of meal portions of these foods. Many assumptions were made that resulted often in overstating intakes. In 1972, the Food and Drug Administration (FDA) entered into a contract with the Federation of American Societies for Experimental Biology (FASEB) to conduct an evaluation of the health aspects associated with the use of GRAS food ingredients. This evaluation was conducted by the Select Committee on GRAS Substances (SCOGS). A summary of the problems surrounding consideration of the safety of GRAS substances used in foods has been prepared by SCOGS (56).

THE HEALTH AND NUTRITION EXAMINATION SURVEY (HANES)
1971–74   HANES includes findings on dietary intake of calories and selected nutrients based on a recall of food consumption over a 24-hr period (1). A probability sample of the US population 1–74 years of age provided dietary intake data by age, sex, race, and income level.

TEN-STATE NUTRITION SURVEY 1968–70   The dietary component of the Ten-State Nutrition Survey 1968–70 (7) provided data on 24-hr recall of food consumption for selected subsamples of the US population and for households in five states with relatively low per capita income and five states with higher per capita income. A series of standards were developed to evaluate dietary intake by various age groups.

PRESCHOOL NUTRITION SURVEY 1968–70   The Preschool Nutrition Survey 1968–70 (36) provided data on nutritional status of a probability sample of preschool children in the United States. A two-day record of food intake was collected in the home by trained interviewers. Information on food habits and methods of food preparation was also compiled.

FDA TOTAL DIET STUDY   For the past 20 years estimates of pesticide, heavy metal, and radionuclide content of the total diet have been based on the collection of 117 foods divided into twelve composites for analysis. In 1974, the 20 collections, representing adult food intake, were increased to 30 with the addition of 10 collections representative of infant and toddler food intake. Analysis of selected minerals was also initiated at that time. Recent changes in the program have reduced the number of collections to 4, but sampling will include separate analysis of 234 foods (37).

TRADE ASSOCIATIONS   Per capita consumption and sales figures for specific foods and food ingredients are prepared by a wide variety of trade associations. These reports are sometimes published in trade journals and occasionally in the scientific literature, but many are unpublished.

Estimates of Intakes

Reasonably accurate per capita estimates of consumption of a specific unprocessed food (e.g. potatoes) or of a broad group of foods (e.g. grain products) can be obtained through the use of disappearance data. Trends in per capita consumption of these foods can also be evaluated with reasonable accuracy.

The 24-hr recall method of estimating intake of specific foods has proven useful in arriving at intake estimates for groups of people but has limited accuracy in providing information about usual intakes of individuals since the period over which the interview was conducted may have been atypical. Because individuals eat less than their usual intake one half of the time, dietary surveys consistently overestimate inadequate intakes of certain nutrients that may not be consumed each day.

Accurate estimates of intake of specific carbohydrates are further complicated by the high percentage of total food intake consumed away from the home and in the form of processed foods. The recollection that a piece of coffeecake was consumed at breakfast does not reveal much about specific carbohydrate content. The product is likely to contain lactose, starch, and one or more sweeteners but the amounts cannot usually be determined from information supplied by the manufacturer or food service. Some carbohydrate ingredients, such as sugar used in yeast doughs, are changed or lost during processing.

Analytical Data

In the traditional proximate analysis of a food (22) carbohydrate content is estimated by difference after water, ether extract, crude protein, ash, and crude fiber contents have been determined. It is now recognized that the crude fiber determination dissolves significant amounts of cellulose, hemicellulose, and lignin (72), thus underestimating fiber and overestimating carbohydrate content calculated by difference. Further inaccuracies can arise if nitrogen-containing carbohydrates contribute to estimates of protein when nitrogen is determined and the factor N X 6.25 is utilized, or if carbohydrates present in glycolipids are calculated as part of ether extract.

Identification of specific carbohydrates contained in a food requires the application of sophisticated chemical, biochemical, or physical methods (41). Relatively few foods have been analyzed in this fashion, and most data banks do not contain accurate data on the carbohydrate content of foods.

The reducing properties of saccharides are often used to estimate sugar content of a food. Jenness (23) points out that analysis of milk lactose content usually represents the sum of the actual lactose and the lactose equivalent of the reducing power of the oligosaccharides. A human milk sample reported to contain 7 gm of lactose per 100 ml might actually contain 6.5 gm lactose and 1 gm of oligosaccharides with an average size of- tetrasaccharides and reducing power equivalent to about 0.5 gm of lactose. Thus this chemical method is of limited usefulness in analyzing for specific sugars.

TRENDS IN CONSUMPTION OF SPECIFIC CLASSES OF CARBOHYDRATES

Carbohydrates are among the most important structural components of plants and are a major contributor to the energy stored in seeds and tubers. Although carbohydrates are present in lower concentrations in animal tissue, they are ubiquitous constituents of most mammalian milks and in various substituted forms are present in all cell membranes, ground substance, connective tissue, nucleic acids, and in many enzymes and hormones.

The food industry utilizes many purified and chemically modified carbohydrates that have been extracted from natural sources. Many of these are added to foods for their functional characteristics rather than their nutritional value.

In nature, carbohydrates exist in many stereo configurations and structural forms that may be significantly altered during food processing and storage or during isolation and purification processes. Therefore, trends in consumption of naturally occurring carbohydrates will be considered separately from those in consumption of refined, processed carbohydrates added to foods. Carbohydrates may be classified into three major groups—monosaccharides, oligosaccharides (carbohydrates that upon hydrolysis yield 2–15 monosaccharides), and polysaccharides. In the following discussion, naturally occurring substituted carbohydrates are treated as a separate class.

Naturally Occurring Carbohydrates

MONOSACCHARIDES   Although at least 200 different monosaccharides are known to occur in nature, relatively few are of dietary significance. Those of greatest nutritional importance are aldoses (e.g. glucose, galactose, mannose, xylose) or ketoses (e.g. fructose) containing five or six carbon atoms. Glucose and fructose, the two most abundant naturally occurring monosaccharides, contributed an estimated 9.4% of total sugar content of the food supply in 1970 and 20.2% in 1980 (Table 1). The marked increase in consumption of these two sugars during the past ten years is the result of increased use of various forms of corn sweeteners. Fruits are generally thought to provide the greatest concentrations of naturally occurring glucose and fructose, but as indicated in Table 2, certain vegetables such as carrots, squash, and snap beans also provide substantial amounts.

Polyhydroxy alcohols may be formed by reduction of monosaccharides: xylitol from xylose, sorbitol from glucose or fructose, and mannitol from mannose or fructose. These sugar alcohols are widely distributed in fruits, berries, and mushrooms and are of interest because of their sweet taste, relatively low cariogenicity, and such functional characteristics as moisturizing, texturizing, and dispersing.

OLIGOSACCHARIDES   Lactose and sucrose are the major dietary disaccharides, contributing approximately equally to the intake of naturally occurring sugars (26). Dairy products and fruits, respectively, are the principal sources of these carbohydrates in their naturally occurring form. Lactose is the most important dietary carbohydrate during early infancy for breast-fed infants and those fed milk-based formulas. In children 5–12 years of age Morgan & Zabik (32) reported that milk provides approximately 20% of total sugar intake.

Table 1   Sugars in the US food supply, selected years[a]

	Total sugars (gm/day)	Individual sugars (%)					
		Fructose	Glucose	Lactose	Maltose	Sucrose	Unclassified
1909–1913	157	4.0	3.5	13.5	1.1	64.8	13.1
1950	197	2.4	5.5	14.1	1.5	63.6	12.9
1960	192	2.5	5.4	14.4	1.7	62.8	13.2
1970	204	2.4	7.0	12.5	2.8	61.8	13.5
1980[b]	214	7.4	12.8	10.3	3.5	51.2	14.8

[a] Prepared by R. M. Marston, Home Economist, US Dept. Agriculture, Human Nutrition Information Service, Consumer Nutrition Center, Hyattsville, MD 20782. Personal communication. 1981.
[b] Preliminary.

Table 2 Free sugars in foods[a]

Foods	Total solids (%)	Glucose	Fructose	Sucrose	Maltose	Raffinose	Stachyose
Fruits							
Apple	15.96	7.3	37.8	23.7			
Apricot	14.44	12.0	8.9	40.4			
Peach	12.79	7.1	9.2	54.1	0.9		
Pear	13.58	7.0	49.9	11.9	2.3		
Plum	17.97	19.4	8.5	27.5	0.8		
Vegetables							
Beet	11.19	1.6	1.4	54.6			
Carrot	12.00	7.1	7.1	35.3			
Sweet Corn	22.69	1.5	1.4	13.4			
Squash (winter)	13.08	7.3	8.9	12.3			
Sweet potato	22.53	1.5	1.3	15.0			
Legumes							
Lima bean	26.74	0.1	0.3	9.7		2.5	2.2
Snap bean	7.79	13.9	15.4	3.2		1.4	2.4
Pea (Alaska)	25.54		0.3	11.7		0.2	0.2

[a] Adapted from (60).

The marked decline in lactose in the US food supply over the past 20 years (Table 1) reflects reduced milk consumption. Per capita yearly consumption of yogurt has increased ten-fold over the past 20 years, from 0.26 lbs/capita in 1960 to 2.59 lbs/capita in 1979. Yearly per capita consumption of cheese has doubled over this same time interval (8.2 lbs to 17.5 lbs). However, increased intakes of reduced fat milks, yogurt, and cheese (29) have not compensated entirely for the decline in whole fluid milk intake.

The reduction in sucrose in the food supply over the past ten years is mostly due to its replacement by corn sweeteners (Table 1). The percentage of sucrose from natural sources has undoubtedly increased because of this shift in usage. The increased content of maltose in the food supply is also the result of increased use of corn sweeteners.

Approximately 85% of the total sugars in the food supply can be characterized as specific mono- and disaccharides. The remaining 15% remain unclassified because of inadequate information about the specific sugars present in foods known to contain simple carbohydrates.

The trisaccharide, raffinose, and the tetrasaccharide, stachyose, are components of legumes (Table 2); hence, dietary intake is dependent upon intake of legumes. Metabolism of tri- and tetrasaccharides by colonic bacteria contributes to the flatulence often associated with consumption of legumes (11).

The remarkable resurgence of interest in breast feeding in the United States (28) has resulted in a change in oligosaccharide intake by nursing infants. Human milk oligosaccharides have not been precisely quantitated;

however, the concentration of larger oligosaccharides (penta- to tetradecasaccharides) may range from 40–200 mg/100 ml (15, 31) and that of tri- and tetrasaccharides is as high as 1 g/100 ml in mature milk and 2.5 g/100 ml in colostrum (31). The concentration of oligosaccharides in cow milk is only about 100 mg/100 ml (30) and hence the intake of formula-fed infants is much lower than that of breast-fed infants.

POLYSACCHARIDES   Cellulose is the most ubiquitous polysaccharide in nature, but its dietary significance, and that of other components of dietary fiber (hemicellulose, gums, mucilages, pectins) in man is largely limited to its effects on gastrointestinal motility, absorption of nutrients, and gut microflora. Amylose and amylopectin are the two forms of starch that occur widely as the reserve carbohydrate of tubers, seeds, grains, and many fruits. Since the beginning of record keeping by the USDA in 1909, the amount of these polysaccharides in the food supply has decreased approximately 30%, largely due to decreased intake of potatoes and grain products (14).

Most animal cells contain glycogen—i.e. glucose polymers in chains that are more highly branched than those of amylopectin. Although approximately 70% of the protein in the food supply is obtained from animal sources (14), glycogen does not provide a significant contribution to dietary polysaccharide intake, partly because most animals are killed in the fasted state, resulting in relatively low glycogen content of muscle; and liver, the organ with the highest glycogen content, is not a widely consumed food item.

SUBSTITUTED CARBOHYDRATES   A wide variety of carbohydrates are found as components of glycoproteins, glycolipids, mucopolysaccharides, DNA, and RNA. These sugars may be aminated, N-acetylated, carboxylated, methoxylated, or substituted by other groups such as sulfate or phosphate. A nine-carbon straight-chain sugar, neuraminic acid and its N-acetylated derivative, sialic acid, are also important cell constituents. Cell-membrane carbohydrates in the form of glycoproteins and glycolipids are thought to be involved in cellular adhesion and recognition (40). Excellent reviews of the biochemistry of glycoproteins (61) and of glycolipids (12) are available.

The monosaccharide ribose and its deoxy derivative make up approximately one third of the RNA and DNA molecules. Thus carbohydrate is centrally involved in the genetic expression and protein metabolism of every cell.

Little is known about the intestinal absorption and subsequent metabolism of substituted carbohydrates. Pectin, a methoxylated polygalacturonic acid, is not thought to be absorbed by man, although it can influence the

absorption of various nutrients (e.g. cholesterol, iron). Glucosamine is estimated to represent approximately 9% of the nonprotein nitrogen in human
milk, but its metabolic fate is unknown (17). Nitrogen-containing oligosaccharides in human milk are believed to be part of the bifidus factor (16)
responsible for the fact that the gut microflora of breast-fed infants are
predominantly lactobacilli, whereas *E. coli* is the dominant bacterial species
in the gut of formula-fed infants.

Substituted carbohydrates do not make up a significant percentage of
total carbohydrate intake, but their presence in the diet is important because
of their influence on various physiologic processes.

Refined Carbohydrates Added to Foods

When carbohydrates are added to foods they are commonly purified, partially digested, or modified in some manner to influence appearance, taste,
or functional properties. Sucrose, corn starch hydrolysates, and substituted
and nonsubstituted carbohydrates in semipurified form are referred to as
refined carbohydrates.

SUCROSE   Extraction and purification of sucrose from sugar cane or sugar
beet involve complex chemical processes resulting in a crystalline product
of high purity. From data presented in Table 3 it is apparent that sucrose

Table 3   Sweetener composition (67)

Sweetener	Yearly per capita consumption of caloric and noncaloric sweeteners (lbs.)			
	1960	1970	1980	1990[a, b]
Sucrose	98	102	86	74
Corn sweeteners				
dextrose	4	5	4	4
corn syrup	8	13	18	21
high-fructose				
corn syrup		1	19	37
Total	12	19	41	62
Minor caloric[c]	2	1	1	
Total	112	122	128	136
Noncaloric				
sweeteners[d]	2	6	7	

[a] S. Kolodny, Vice President, Economic Research, American Sugar Division, Amstar
Corporation, 1251 Avenue of the Americas, New York, NY 10020. Personal communication to L. J. Filer, Jr., University of Iowa, 1980.
[b] Estimate.
[c] Includes honey and other syrups.
[d] Sugar sweetness equivalent—assumes saccharin is 300 times as sweet as sugar and
cyclamate is 30 times as sweet as sugar. Cyclamate food use was banned by FDA effective in 1970.

currently provides approximately two thirds of the total refined caloric sweetener intake. Its contribution has declined over the past 20 years and is expected to decline further during the next 10 years because of the greater market share of various forms of corn sweeteners.

Substantial controversy exists regarding effects of the intake of so-called "empty calories" in the form of sucrose on the dietary habits and nutritional status of children. Sucrose is no longer added to strained fruits and fruit juices produced by the manufacturers of baby food in the United States, and other food processors have reduced use of sugar in their products largely in response to greater consumer interest in lower calorie foods.

LACTOSE   Purified forms of lactose are used in a wide variety of food products. Commercially prepared milk-based infant formulas provide more than one half of the carbohydrate in the form of added lactose. The addition of fat-free milk solids to low fat milks serves as a source of added lactose for other age groups.

CORN SWEETENERS   Acid and/or enzymatic hydrolysis of corn starch yields a broad range of compounds with varying degrees of sweetness. Sweetness of corn starch hydrolysates increases with the completeness of hydrolysis. Changes in the mono- and oligosaccharide content of a corn syrup that occur as hydrolysis of the starch becomes more complete are shown in Figure 2. Because fructose is sweeter than sucrose, the production of high-fructose corn syrups, through the action of glucose isomerase on corn starch hydrolysates, has increased markedly during the past ten years (Table 3). It is projected that by 1990 corn sweeteners will provide approximately 45% of total refined caloric sweetener intake.

MODIFIED FOOD STARCHES   Starches that have been oxidized, acid hydrolyzed, gelatinized, or chemically cross-linked and/or stabilized are known as modified food starches. Many such starches exhibit properties desirable in food processing. Most of these starches are derived from corn but some are from wheat, milo, or tapioca. Waxy corn and milo are genetic variants composed almost entirely of amylopectin, whereas the starch from normal cereal grains is composed of 15–30% amylose with the remainder amylopectin. In 1971, modified food starches accounted for approximately one half of the total starch used by food processors (58).

A number of questions have been raised about the safety of adding modified starches to foods. Certain of the reagents that were at one time used in the process of modifying starches were demonstrated to be mutagenic in tests with microorganisms or carcinogenic in tests with rodents (70). Modified starches prepared with these reagents, although not demonstrated to be mutagenic or carcinogenic for any organism, are no longer

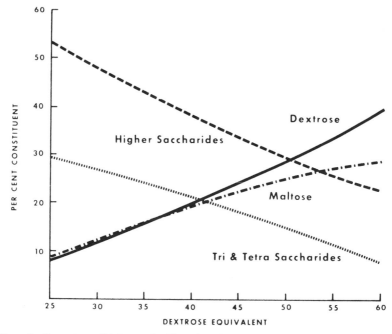

Figure 2   Percentage of higher saccharides, tri- and tetrasaccharides, maltose, and glucose in acid-hydrolyzed corn syrup with dextrose equivalency from 25 to 60 (35).

used in foods. In 1978, the Committee on Nutrition of the American Academy of Pediatrics (8) concluded that use of modified food starch then used in infant foods was justified, that their use was not associated with clinical problems, and that they did not appear to interfere with the bioavailability of trace elements. However, the subsequent opinion of SCOGS was more cautious, concluding that additional data on safety of a number of these modified starches would be desirable (58).

MISCELLANEOUS CARBOHYDRATES   A wide variety of other purified and semipurified carbohydrates are added to foods, usually for organoleptic purposes unrelated to the nutritional value of the product. Estimated intake of several carbohydrates listed as GRAS substances is shown in Table 4. Although total intake of these compounds is not great when expressed as a percentage of total carbohydrate intake, the statistic of interest is the increase in estimated usage of several of these carbohydrates during the past ten years.

Increased usage of sorbitol and mannitol is associated with their relatively low cariogenicity and their desirable functional characteristics in food processing. Various forms of cellulose are added to low-calorie foods, ice

Table 4   Estimated yearly per capita intake of selected GRAS food substances

	SCOGS estimated yearly intake (g)	Increase in food use 1970:1960	Reference
Gums	87	3	42, 43, 46, 47, 48, 49, 54
Agar agar	1	2	51
Carageenan	11	2	50
Alginates	5	—	52
Pectin	18	—	57
Sorbitol	29	7	44
Mannitol	7	10	45
Dextrins	66	—	55
Cellulose	18	7	53
Modified food starches	254	—	58

cream, and to those foods with artificially increased amounts of dietary fiber.

EFFECT OF FOOD PROCESSING ON CARBOHYDRATE

Carbohydrates present in fresh, unprocessed foods may be significantly altered in chemical structure and digestibility by processing and/or storage. Changes due to storage may be demonstrated by the reduction of sweetness of sweet corn as the simple sugars present at the time of picking are enzymatically converted to starch. The ripening process of fruits results in accumulation of simple sugars and of the esters that provide the distinctive aroma and flavor of the mature fruit.

The "shelf life" of processed foods is influenced by many factors. Staling of baked goods results from complex changes in degree of hydration of carbohydrates as well as from their interaction with other ingredients. Rate of staling can be inhibited through the use of a wide variety of food additives (56). Carbohydrates in acidic processed foods may be changed after prolonged storage into dehydration, condensation, or fragmentation compounds that differ markedly from the starting ingredients (60).

Maillard Reaction

The nonenzymatic browning (Maillard) reaction (39) is important in the production of desirable colors and flavors in baked goods. This reaction occurs through the complexing of reducing sugars with free amino groups present in amino acids and proteins. The brown color of bread crust, breakfast cereals, and other baked products is associated with a decrease in the bioavailability of the amino acids (usually lysine) involved in the reaction. One might anticipate that this reaction would occur more readily in processed foods containing corn sweeteners as a replacement for sucrose.

Lactulose

The synthetic disaccharide, lactulose, consisting of one galactose and one fructose moiety, is formed in commercial processing of cow milk by the alkaline enolization of the glucose moiety of lactose to fructose. Human subjects have no disaccharidase that will split lactulose, and its effect on the gastrointestinal tract of a normal individual is therefore similar to that of lactose consumed by a lactase-deficient individual.

Lactulose is known to exert a laxative effect if given in sufficient quantity (6). Presumably the laxative action is mediated through the osmotic properties of the molecule when it reaches the colon and through the products of bacterial degradation of the molecule. Lactulose has been utilized as a therapeutic agent in reducing the extent of hyperammonemia in portal-systemic encephalopathy (9). Adachi & Patton (2) have reported that the lactulose content of evaporated milk may be as high as 940 mg/100 ml.

CARBOHYDRATE INTAKE—DIETARY SIGNIFICANCE

The trend has been toward decreased intakes of total carbohydrate, starch, and naturally occurring sugars (particularly lactose) and increased intakes of refined sugars (particularly in the form of corn sweeteners). The public health significance of these changes in carbohydrate usage has been hotly debated among nutritionists, dietitians, food technologists, and consumer groups. At one extreme are those who maintain that no national food supply has ever provided more variety, greater safety, or better nutrition than ours, and who cite statistical evidence of improved general health and increased longevity. According to this group, health is achieved by selecting a wide variety of foods to assure a nutritionally adequate diet and by avoiding excess energy intake (13).

This optimistic appraisal of the current food supply and the ability of the average American to make wise food choices is not accepted by many nutritionists and consumer groups. Concern is expressed that the food industry is producing foods containing empty calories and additives of questionable safety, formulated with little attention to nutritional value.

A report has been issued by a Task Force evaluating the evidence relating six dietary factors to the nation's health (71). One of the Consensus Statements dealt with the relationships between carbohydrate intake and disease

(4), noting no evidence that (*a*) the body can somehow distinguish a glucose molecule obtained from the digestion of starch from that obtained from digestion of simple sugars, (*b*) the body can distinguish a sucrose molecule obtained from fruit from that obtained from table sugar, (*c*) complex carbohydrates and "naturally occurring" sugars contain components that are missing from refined sugars and that either prevent deficiency disorders or are otherwise beneficial to health, and (*d*) refined sugars may contain harmful substances or lead to harmful effects when consumed in relatively large quantities. The Consensus Statement also found little proof that sugar consumption is associated with any health hazard except dental caries.

Although dental caries is not a nutritional disease per se, it is a major public health problem and should not be viewed with the laissez-faire attitude so common among nutritionists. The Preschool Nutrition Survey (36) found an average of 5.8 defective tooth surfaces in white children and 8.5 such tooth surfaces in black children between five and six years of age. Among persons 45–64 years old the combined effects of dental caries and periodontal disease have produced an adult population 37% of whom are edentulous in one or both dental arches (69).

The high incidence of dental caries among the US population almost suggests that this major public health problem is accepted as an inevitable consequence of eating. Insufficient effort has been devoted toward increasing awareness that occurrence of dental caries is increased by the frequent consumption throughout the day of sweet food retained in the mouth long enough to reduce pH below the point where enamel demineralization occurs.

Trends in consumption of various carbohydrates have been accompanied by many other changes in composition of the food supply and in eating habits. Since the period 1909–1913 the percentage of calories in the US diet provided from fat has increased while the contribution of carbohydrate to total caloric intake has decreased (14). Traditional family meals have been replaced, in part, by between-meal snacks and by meals eaten away from the home.

As shown in Table 5, total sucrose intake obtained through household use in 1980 was only 25% compared to 68% in 1909–1913. The decrease in sugar used in the household would be even greater if the contribution of corn sweeteners were included (i.e. expressed as a percentage of total refined sugars) in Table 5. The net result of decreased household use of sugar is that more than 75% of sugar usage can be controlled only by the decision not to purchase a food item to which sugar has been added.

The increasing consumption of sugar-containing beverages (Table 6) has led to an increased intake of sucrose from this source (Table 5) and increased intakes of various corn sweeteners. These figures represent disappearance intake, and since some individuals consume no soft drinks, others

128   ANDERSON

Table 5 Refined sucrose usage (% of total)[a]

	Household use	Processed foods	Beverages	Other[b]
1909–1913	68	21	5	6
1950	39	41	11	9
1960	34	43	14	9
1970	25	47	24	4
1980[c]	25	43	28	4

[a] Prepared by R. M. Marston, Home Economist, US Dept. Agriculture, Human Nutrition Information Service, Consumer Nutrition Center, Hyattsville, MD 20782. Personal communication. 1981.
[b] Includes use by eating and drinking places, institutions, and the military.
[c] Preliminary.

must consume large quantities. In one day in Spring 1977 (66) 40% of 1–2-year-old children surveyed consumed soft drinks with an average intake of 9 oz/day (272 12-oz containers per year). Average daily soft drink consumption for all children (users and non-users) in this age group was about 3.5 oz. Surveys by the USDA (64) indicate that in the highest consumption category, 10% of the people consume 1.5–3.5 times as much as the remaining 90%. Even if concern is limited to that 1% of the population with greatest intakes of a particular food, more than 2.25 million individuals are involved.

Increasingly sophisticated technology in food processing has resulted in use of semipurified ingredients to produce novel organoleptic qualities. As these foods have gained greater consumer acceptance, dietary fiber content of the food supply has been reduced by approximately one third since 1909–1913. (14).

The factors contributing to development of food habits have been little studied. It is generally assumed that food habits are formed early in life and once formed are difficult to change. If these assumptions are correct, guidance in use of sweetened foods must be provided during early life. Younger age groups have higher than average intakes of cariogenic foods (24).

Table 6 Estimated annual per capita consumption of soft drinks (34)

Year	Per capita (12-oz. containers)
1909	11
1950	105
1960	128
1970	242
1980	410

A comparatively recent influence in shaping food habits has been the advertising of foods on television. Manoff (25) has estimated that more than 50% of the money spent on television food advertising concerns foods that have known or potential adverse effects on health. Over 50% of the total advertising expenditure during one weekend on four Chicago television stations in 1975 was devoted to promotion of nonnutritive beverages (59).

Many social factors influence wise selection of nutritious foods from an abundant food supply composed of a high percentage of continually changing processed foods. New product development often emphasizes convenience and unique organoleptic properties. Product proliferation quickly occurs when a new food gains consumer acceptance. Food advertising often appears to be weighted toward those products providing perceived advantages other than nutritional value. With respect to consumer economics, almost 30% of the adult population are functionally illiterate (59). Clearly, intelligent use of the vast array of foods produced by the food industry requires a degree of knowledge that may not be currently possessed by a significant portion of the population.

Figure 3 illustrates the 70-year trend in consumption of various carbohydrates. The increase in percentage of total carbohydrate provided by sugars has been accompanied by an increase in refined, processed sugar intake and a decrease in sugar obtained from naturally occurring sources. Increased use of sugar has been associated with increased consumption of soft drinks and low-fiber snack foods.

A pattern of dietary carbohydrate consumption similar to that of the period 1909–1913 has been proposed as part of the controversial Dietary Goals (Figure 3). Such a pattern would require foods to be less highly processed and of higher fiber content, and soft drink consumption to de-

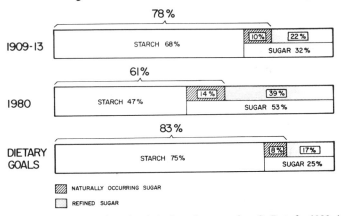

Figure 3   Per capita consumption of carbohydrate (percent of total). Data for 1909–1913 and 1980 adapted from (26). Percentage of naturally occurring sugars in Dietary Goals estimated from 1909–1913 ratio of naturally occurring sugar : total sugar (1:3).

cline. It has been estimated that the energy input into the US food supply approximates 10 kcal for each kcal of food consumed (62). Less energy input would result in lower food cost, and this fact alone may exert pressure toward change in the direction suggested.

A food supply composed of fewer processed foods and foods with higher starch and fiber content would be less cariogenic. Selection of foods more compatible with the carbohydrate composition suggested in the Dietary Goals would require the exercise of parental responsibility with possible ramifications beyond improvement of the dental health of the nation's children.

It would be difficult to take issue with recommendations and conclusions of the Food and Nutrition Board of the National Academy of Sciences in the booklet *Toward Healthful Diets* (13). Unfortunately, many Americans now do not select a nutritionally adequate diet of dairy products, meats or legumes, vegetables and fruits, and cereals and breads in the amounts necessary to maintain appropriate weight for height. To expect wider acceptance of this practice may be unrealistic. On the other hand, it is held by some that the Dietary Goals would encourage not only the proper use of the existing food supply but also broader concerns for traditional meanings of foods and the manner of their consumption, for energy conservation, and for the value of individual responsibility for health.

Literature Cited

1. Abraham, S., Carroll, M. D., Dresser, C. M., Johnson, C. L. 1979. *Dietary Intake Source Data, United States 1971–74.* Washington DC: Dept. HEW Publ. No. (PHS) 79–1221. pp. 2–421
2. Adachi, S., Patton, S. 1961. Presence and significance of lactulose in milk products: a review. *J. Dairy Sci.* 44: 1375
3. American Medical Association Council on Scientific Affairs. 1979. Concepts on nutrition and health. *J. Am. Med. Assoc.* 242:2335–38
4. Bierman, E. L. 1979. Carbohydrates, sucrose, and human disease. *Am. J. Clin. Nutr.* 12(Suppl.):2712–22
5. Burk, M. C., Pao, E. M. 1976. *Methodology for Large-Scale Surveys of Household and Individual Diets. Home Econ. Res. Rpt. No. 40.* Washington DC: USGPO. 88 pp.
6. Bush, R. T. 1970. Lactulose: an ideal laxative for children. *New Zeal. Med. J.* 71:364–65
7. Center for Disease Control. 1972. *Ten-State Nutrition Survey, 1968–70,* part V. Atlanta, GA: Dept. HEW Publ. No. (HSM) 72–8133. 340 pp.
8. Committee on Nutrition. 1978. *Review of Safety and Suitability of Modified Food Starches in Infant Foods.* Evanston, IL: Am. Acad. Pediatr.
9. Conn, H. O., Leevy, C. M., Vlahcevic, Z. R., Rodgers, J. B., Maddrey, W. C., Seeff, L., Levy, L. L. 1977. Comparison of lactulose and neomycin in the treatment of chronic portal-systemic encephalopathy. *Gastroenterology* 72: 573–83
10. Connor, W. E. 1979. Too little or too much: the case for preventive nutrition. *Am. J. Clin. Nutr.* 32:1975–78
11. Cristofaro, E., Mottu, F., Wuhrmann, J. J. 1974. Involvement of the raffinose family of oligosaccharides in flatulence. In *Sugars in Nutrition,* ed. H. L. Sipple, K. W. McNutt, 20:313–36. NY: Academic Press. 768 pp.
12. Fishman, P. H., Brady, R. O. 1976. Biosynthesis and function of gangliosides. *Science* 194:906–15
13. Food and Nutrition Board. 1980. *Toward Healthful Diets.* Washington DC: Nat. Acad. Sci./Nat. Res. Counc. 24 pp.

14. Gortner, W. A. 1975. Nutrition in the United States, 1900 to 1974. *Cancer Res.* 35:3246–53
15. Grimmonprez, L., Montreuil, J. 1975. Isolement et étude des propriétés physico-chimiques d'oligosaccharides du lait de femme. *Biochimie* 57:695–701
16. György, P. 1974. Effect of carbohydrates on intestinal flora. See Ref. 11, 14:215–26
17. Hambraeus, L. 1977. Propietary milk versus human breast milk in infant feeding. *Pediatr. Clin. North Am.* 24:17–36
18. Harper, A. E. 1978. Dietary goals—a skeptical view. *Am. J. Clin. Nutr.* 31: 310–21
19. Harper, A. E. 1980. "Healthy people": critique of the nutrition segments of the Surgeon General's report on health promotion and disease prevention. *Am. J. Clin. Nutr.* 33:1703–12
20. Hegsted, D. M. 1978. Dietary goals—a progressive view. *Am. J. Clin. Nutr.* 31:1504–9
21. Hiemstra, S. 1968. *Food Consumption, Prices, Expenditures. U.S. Dept. Agric., Econ, Res. Serv., Agric. Econ. Rpt. 138.* 193 pp.
22. Horwitz, W., Chichilo, P., Reynolds, H., eds. 1970. Animal feed. In *Official Methods of Analysis of the Association of Official Analytical Chemists,* 7:122–38. Washington DC: Assoc. Official Analyt. Chem. 1015 pp. 11th ed.
23. Jenness, R. 1979. The composition of human milk. *Semin. Perinatol.* 3: 255–39
24. Le Bovit, C. 1978. Who eats the sweets? *Natl. Food Rev.* 4:62–63
25. Manoff, R. K. 1972. *Intl. Cong. Nutr., 9th,* pp. 256–77
26. Marston, R. M., Peterkin, B. B. 1980. Nutrient content of the national food supply. *Natl. Food Rev.* 9:21–25
27. Marston, R. M., Welsh, S. O. 1981. Nutrient content of the national food supply. *Natl. Food Rev.* 13:19–22
28. Martinez, G. A., Nalezienski, J. P. 1979. The recent trend in breast-feeding. *Pediatrics* 64:686–92
29. Milk Industry Fnd. 1980. *1980 Milk Facts.* Washington DC: Milk Industry Fnd. 30 pp.
30. Montreuil, J., Antony, N., Descamps, J. 1963. The glycoproteins of human and cow's milk. *Ann. Biol. Anim. Biochim. Biophys.* 3:(Hors Sér 1) 129–33
31. Montreuil, J., Mullet, S. 1960. Étude des variations des constituants glucidiques du lait de femme au cours de la lactation. *Bull. Soc. Chim. Biol.* 42: 365–77

32. Morgan, K. J., Zabik, M. E. 1981. Amount and food sources of total sugar intake by children ages 5 to 12 years. *Am. J. Clin. Nutr.* 34:404–13
33. National Research Council, Committee on Food Protection. 1972. *A Comprehensive Survey of Industry on the Use of Food Chemicals Generally Recognized as Safe (GRAS).* Washington DC: Natl. Acad. Sci.
34. National Soft Drink Association. 1981. *Sales Survey of the Soft Drink Industry. NSDA 1980.* Washington DC: Natl. Soft Drink Assoc. 16 pp.
35. Newton, J. M. 1970. Corn Syrups. In *Symposium Proceedings.* Washington DC: Corn Refiners Assoc., Inc. 13 pp.
36. Owen, G. M., Kram, K. M., Garry, P. J., Lowe, J. E., Lubin, A. H. 1974. A study of nutritional status of preschool children in the United States, 1968–1970. *Pediatrics* 53:597–646
37. Pennington, J. 1980. Total diet study results and plans for selected minerals. *FDA Bylines* 10:179
38. Périssé, J., Sizaret, F., Francois, P. 1969. The effect of income on the structure of the diet. *FAO Nutr. Newsl.* 7:1–9
39. Reynolds, T. M. 1969. Nonenzymic browning sugar-amine interactions. In *Symposium on Foods: Carbohydrates and Their Roles,* ed. H. W. Schultz, R. F. Cain, R. W. Wrolstad, 12:219–52. Westport, CT: AVI Publ. Co., Inc. 458 pp.
40. Roseman, S. 1975. Sugars of the cell membrane. *Hosp. Pract.* 10:61–70
41. Schultz, H. W., Cain, R. F., Wrolstad, R. W., eds. 1969. Advances in analytical methodology. See Ref. 39, Sect. III:133–204
42. Select Committee on GRAS Substances. 1972. *Evaluation of the Health Aspects of Carob Bean Gum as a Food Ingredient. SCOGS-3.* Bethesda, MD: Life Sci. Res. Off., FASEB. 10 pp.
43. Select Committee on GRAS Substances. 1972. *Evaluation of the Health Aspects of Gum Tragacanth as a Food Ingredient. SCOGS-4.* Bethesda, MD: Life Sci. Res. Off., FASEB. 10 pp.
44. Select Committee on GRAS Substances. 1972. *Evaluation of the Health Aspects of Sorbitol as a Food Ingredient. SCOGS-9.* Bethesda, MD: Life Sci. Res. Off., FASEB. 10 pp.
45. Select Committee on GRAS Substances. 1972. *Evaluation of the Health Aspects of Mannitol as a Food Ingredient. SCOGS-10.* Bethesda, MD: Life Sci. Res. Off., FASEB. 8 pp.

46. Select Committee on GRAS Substances. 1973. *Evaluation of the Health Aspects of Gum Ghatti as a Food Ingredient. SCOGS-12.* Bethesda, MD: Life Sci. Res. Off., FASEB. 7 pp.

47. Select Committee on GRAS Substances. 1973. *Evaluation of the Health Aspects of Guar Gum as a Food Ingredient. SCOGS-13* Bethesda, MD: Life Sci. Res. Off., FASEB. 12 pp.

48. Select Committee on GRAS Substances. 1973. *Evaluation of the Health Aspects of Gum Arabic as a Food Ingredient. SCOGS-1.* Bethesda, MD: Life Sci. Res. Off., FASEB. 16 pp.

49. Select Committee on GRAS Substances. 1973. *Evaluation of the Health Aspects of Sterculia Gum as a Food Ingredient. SCOGS-5.* Bethesda, MD: Life Sci. Res. Off., FASEB. 13 pp.

50. Select Committee on GRAS Substances. 1973. *Evaluation of the Health Aspects of Carrageenan as a Food Ingredient. SCOGS-6.* Bethesda, MD: Life Sci. Res. Off., FASEB. 16 pp.

51. Select Committee on GRAS Substances. 1973. *Evaluation of the Health Aspects of Agar-Agar as a Food Ingredient. SCOGS-23.* Bethesda, MD: Life Sci. Res. Off., FASEB. 14 pp.

52. Select Committee on GRAS Substances. 1973. *Evaluation of the Health Aspects of Alginates as Food Ingredients. SCOGS-24.* Bethesda, MD: Life Sci. Res. Off., FASEB. 14 pp.

53. Select Committee on GRAS Substances. 1973. *Evaluation of the Health Aspects of Cellulose and Certain Cellulose Derivatives as Food Ingredients. SCOGS-25.* Bethesda, MD: Life Sci. Res. Off., FASEB. 26 pp.

54. Select Committee on GRAS Substances. 1975. *Evaluation of the Health Aspects of Gum Guaiac as a Food Ingredient. SCOGS-64.* Bethesda, MD: Life Sci. Res. Off., FASEB. 16 pp.

55. Select Committee on GRAS Substances. 1975. *Evaluation of the Health Aspects of Dextrin and Corn Dextrin as Food Ingredients. SCOGS-75.* Bethesda, MD: Life Sci. Res. Off., FASEB. 17 pp.

56. Select Committee on GRAS Substances. 1977. Evaluation of health aspects of GRAS food ingredients; lessons learned and questions unanswered. *Fed. Proc.* 36:2519–62

57. Select Committee on GRAS Substances. 1977. *Evaluation of the Health Aspects of Pectin and Pectinates as Food Ingredients. SCOGS-81.* Bethesda, MD: Life Sci. Res. Off., FASEB. 19 pp.

58. Select Committee on GRAS Substances. 1979. *Evaluation of the Health Aspects of Starch and Modified Starches as Food Ingredients. SCOGS-115.* Bethesda, MD: Life Sci. Res. Off., FASEB. 100 pp.

59. Senate Select Committee on Nutrition and Human Needs. 1977. *Dietary Goals for the United States.* Washington DC: US GPO. 83 pp. 2nd ed.

60. Shallenberger, R. S. 1974. Occurrence of various sugars in foods. See Ref. 11, 5:67–80

61. Sharon, N., Lis, H. 1981. Glycoproteins: research booming on long-ignored, ubiquitous compounds. *Chem. Eng. News* 59:21–44

62. Steinhart, J. S., Steinhart, C. E. 1974. Energy use in the U.S. food system. *Science* 184:307–16

63. The Surgeon General's Report on Health Promotion and Disease Prevention. 1979. *Healthy People.* Washington DC: Dept. HEW Publ. No. 79–55071

64. US Dept. Agriculture. 1960. *High Consumption of Foods.* Washington DC: USGPO

65. US Dept. Agriculture. 1972. *Food and Nutrient Intake of Individuals in the United States, Spring 1965. Household Food Consumption Survey 1965–66, Rpt. No. II.* Washington DC: USGPO 289 pp.

66. US Dept. Agriculture. 1980. *Food and Nutrient Intakes of Individuals in 1 day in the United States, Spring 1977. Nationwide Food Consumption Survey 1977–78, Preliminary Rpt. No. 2.* Washington DC: USGPO. 121 pp.

67. US Dept. Agriculture. 1981. Sugar and sweetener—outlook and situation. *Sugar and Sweetener Rep.* 6:40

68. US Dept. Agriculture and Dept. Health, Education and Welfare. 1980. *Nutrition and Your Health—Dietary Guidelines for Americans.* Washington DC: USGPO. 20 pp.

69. US Dept. Health, Education, and Welfare. 1979. *Dental Manpower Fact Book.* Hyattsville, MD: Dept. HEW Publ. No. (HRA) 79–14. 106 pp.

70. van Duuren, B. L., Goldschmidt, B. M., Katz, C., Seidman, I., Paul, J. S. 1974. Carcinogenic activity of alkylating agents. *J. Natl. Cancer Inst.* 53:695–700

71. Van Itallie, T. B., ed. 1979. Report of the Task Force on the evidence relating six dietary factors to the nation's health. *Am. J. Clin. Nutr.* 12(Suppl.):2621–748

72. van Soest, P. J. 1978. Dietary fibers: their definition and nutritional properties. *Am. J. Clin. Nutr.* 31:S12–S20

Ann. Rev. Nutr. 1982. 2:133–50

XYLITOL AND DENTAL CARIES

Kauko K. Mäkinen and Arje Scheinin

Institute of Dentistry, University of Turku, SF-20520 Turku 52, Finland

CONTENTS ....

INTRODUCTION

All forms of dental caries are due to microorganisms (1). Numerous studies have thus been conducted in order to identify and define these organisms (2). Such studies have also considered the influence of dietary carbohydrates (sugars in general and sucrose in particular) as substrates on which microbes could form the entire range of noxious metabolites that play a key role in dental hard tissue destruction and the formation of dental caries.

Recently, however, a parallel line of research suggested that the cariogenicity of various carbohydrate sweeteners may vary within extreme limits, implying that several of these substances were low- or noncariogenic.

133

0199-9885/82/0715-0133$02.00

In the case of xylitol, a pentahydric sugar alcohol, anticariogenic properties were suggested (3).

The chemical properties of xylitol have been reviewed (4). Its most important properties in relation to dental caries are: (a) open-chain structure; (b) absence of reducing carbonyl groups, a fact that renders xylitol (and sugar alcohols in general) chemically less reactive than the corresponding aldoses and ketoses; (c) the shorter "length" of the xylitol molecule when compared with that of hexitols; (d) the similarities in the configuration at various C-atoms with common sugars; and (e) The ability of xylitol (and several other sugar alcohols) to form complexes with certain metal cations (Ca^{2+}, for example) or compounds containing these metal atoms. These properties of xylitol affect the metabolisms of both microbial and mammalian species. The fitness of xylitol as a sucrose substitute is also based on its ubiquity in nature (4–6), its established safety in moderate, peroral human use (7–10) and its participation as a normal intermediate in human metabolism—e.g. in the glucuronate-xylulose cycle (4).

In this review we survey xylitol's anticariogenic aspect, with particular regard to xylitol-induced effects in the animal model and as observed in clinical caries trials. Furthermore, we view the background of these mechanisms in terms of microbiological observations, physico-chemical effects in plaque and saliva, influence on enzymatic activities, and biochemical effects.

THE ANIMAL MODEL

With one exception (11), experimental studies in rats demonstrated an extremely low caries rate in relation to a xylitol-containing diet (12–21). Total substitution of xylitol for sucrose in the diets of rats resulted in caries scores comparable to (22) or lower than (20) those of sugar-free controls.

Partial substitution of xylitol for dietary sucrose is considered a more realistic approach than total substitution. The results from such experimental studies are contradictory; sucrose supplemented with xylitol did not result in a caries reduction (12, 23), although the severity scores were significantly lower in some experimental groups (23). On the other hand, alternate feeding of sucrose and xylitol was associated with low increment scores (19, 24). Of particular interest was the experiment of Gey & Kinkel (25), in which rinsing with a xylitol solution after sucrose-containing meals decreased the cariogenicity of the diet. Similarly, dentinal caries in rats, produced by exposure to sucrose, was significantly reversed by a xylitol-supplemented diet (26, 27). Not merely a bland noncariogenic agent, xylitol was found to exert a genuinely therapeutic action against caries (27).

The animal model has permitted experimentation that for various ethical, logistic, and economic reasons is not possible in human subjects (28, 21).

Such studies suggest extreme differences between the cariogenicity of sucrose and xylitol. Despite certain limitations preventing direct translation to human caries, ingenious animal models are expected to contribute to the understanding of cariostatic mechanisms.

CLINICAL CARIES TRIALS: TURKU SUGAR STUDIES

So far, experimental information on xylitol's effect on human caries derives from two clinical trials. Four other studies are in progress; the results from these WHO clinical-trial/field-studies in Thailand, French Polynesia (2 studies), and Hungary are expected in 1982–1984.

Two-Year Clinical Trial

The first study (29) involved almost complete substitution of sucrose (S) by fructose (F) or xylitol (X) during a period of 2 years. In addition to the clinical and radiographic registrations of dental caries, biochemical and microbiological investigations were carried out in order to monitor oral and general health and to identify eventual side effects.

The initial population consisted of 125 subjects, mean age 27.6 years. The subjects were divided partly on individual preference basis into three groups. The S-group comprised 35, the F-group 33, and the X-group 52 subjects, the latter group rendered oversize in case some of its members quit the experiment. During the study 10 subjects discontinued or were otherwise excluded. Only in one case was this due to osmotic diarrhea in relation to xylitol consumption; the other cases were due to difficulties in adhering to the strict dietary regimen, to other personal reasons, and in three cases —two in the S-group and one in the F-group—to excessive caries incidence. The final results were thus based on 115 individuals.

Initially no significant differences were observed with regard to age, sex, number of primary and secondary carious surfaces, filled tooth surfaces, extracted teeth, or the DMFS-index. During the trial, dental conditions were registered on eight occasions, the frequent inspections being due to the potential need for early diagnosis, treatment, and termination of participation in cases of adverse reaction. The clinical and radiographic registrations were utilized for calculating the reversals in diagnosis between the examinations, and the resulting net change. The positive reversals involved a change in diagnosis from an intact to a carious or filled surface, or, when considering an increment in size, from a white spot lesion to a defect. A negative reversal indicated a corresponding change in the opposite direction. Consequently net increment was expressed as new carious surfaces—i.e. positive minus negative reversals, according to the recommendations of the FDI

Commission on Classification and Statistics for Oral Conditions (30).

According to the clinical and radiographic registrations, carried out without knowledge of the experimental group, a highly significant reduction (exceeding 85%) was found in the X-group when compared to the S-group after one year of the dietary regimen. After two years the increment in the number of decayed, missing, and filled tooth surfaces was 7.2 in the S-group, 3.8 in the F-group, and 0.0 in the X-group. The caries incidence was also expressed in combined quantitative and qualitative terms, by considering in addition to the increment in terms of the conventional DMFS-index also the changes in lesion size and the incidence of secondary caries. Irrespective of the way of expressing the caries increment rate in qualitative, quantitative, or combined terms, the reduction in the caries incidence in the X-group exceeded 85%, (30% in the F-group) in comparison to the S-group.

One-Year Intake of Chewing Gum

In the second study (31) the initial population comprised 102 subjects, mean age 22.2 years. The registration of dental conditions was carried out clinically and radiographically (29). Before the study, dietary habits were analyzed (32). The population was divided randomly into the future S- and X-groups.

The subjects were instructed to maintain their regular dietary habits and oral hygiene procedures. Instructions were further given to consume between three and seven sticks of chewing gum per day (sucrose- or xylitol-sweetened for S- and X-groups, respectively, and to keep a complete record of the consumption during the projected study year.

The final results were based on 100 subjects. Initially there were no significant differences between the groups with regard to the experimental variables, except that the number of missing teeth was slightly but significantly higher among the females in the X-group than in the S-group. This feature was considered to have no influence on the results obtained. The consumption of chewing gum, calculated as average number of sticks per day, was 4.0 in the S-group and 4.5 in the X-group, the difference between the groups being insignificant. The frequency of sucrose consumption, calculated before and during the study as the sum of the S-containing products ingested in liquid and solid form, at and between meals, was 4.24 times per subject per day in the S-group and 4.94 in the X-group.

The caries incidence rate was calculated in terms of the conventional DMFS-index, as well as in combined quantitative and qualitative terms corresponding to those used in the two-year clinical trial discussed above (29). Regardless of measurement mode, the reduction of the caries increment rate in the X-group (chewers of xylitol gum) was 82% greater than that of the S-group.

DISCUSSION OF THE TRIALS AND FURTHER FINDINGS

Some of the inherent weaknesses of the first trial (29) were overcome in the second study. In the latter, for example, a total substitution of sucrose through fructose or xylitol was not attempted, and subjects were assigned to their groups on a random basis. Other weaknesses in the experimental design—e.g. a young, homogeneous age group would have been advantageous—remain common to both studies. However, the solidity of the above long-term trials may rest on the general arrangement, the independently assessed clinical and radiographic findings being supplemented by a number of biochemical and microbiological assays of plaque and saliva, and follow-up studies monitoring the health of the subjects.

The assessment of caries in terms of quantitative and qualitative reversals, and particularly the evaluation of changes in size of buccally located carious lesions through stereomicroscopic registration (33) has been criticized, mainly because this use of unconventional methods renders comparison with other studies difficult.

In fact, the values originating from the microscopic registrations were not included in the results so far published (29, 30). These findings will be utilized in conjunction with a planimetric evaluation of incipient caries (34). We emphasize, however, that the caries increment rate in these trials was presented in regular terms, the increment of the DMFS-index being based solely on clinical and radiographic registrations of caries. The changes in number and size of lesion, as evaluated clinically and radiographically for primary and secondary caries, were presented separately. An attempt was thus made to depict the total quantitative and qualitative development, in order to add dimensions that otherwise escape attention. The conventional DMFS-index does not provide a complete description of the total quantitative development, as the incidence of secondary caries remains obscured by such tooth surfaces already being considered as filled. Data pertaining to the microscopic evaluation of the buccal lesions were not included in the results so far presented (29, 31) but will be published separately in conjunction with a planimetric analysis of the findings of the above studies (34).

Other trials on sugar substitutes invariably indicate significant caries reductions in comparison to sucrose. Most such studies concern the replacement of sucrose with polyols and mixtures of these—i.e. sorbitol (35–39) and Lycasin (40). Caries activity also decreased when sucrose was replaced by an equimolecular mixture of fructose and glucose (41). The reduction thus achieved, especially during the second year of the trial, resulted in an overall development markedly similar to that observed with fructose substitution (29).

The results from the above trials were reviewed in terms of duration, age and number of subjects, compound and vehicle used, frequency of intake, and caries reduction in relation to groups exposed to known or *ad libitum* intake of sucrose (42). A detailed comparison seems unjustified, and we emphasize the need for further controlled clinical trials of sufficient duration, preferably through large-scale field studies in young, high-caries-prevalence populations.

The fundamental reasoning for sugar substitution is based on the concept of replacing sucrose, particularly in foodstuffs proven to be highly cariogenic. In addition to the many studies containing circumstantial evidence for the cariogenicity of sucrose, the strong covariation between sucrose consumption and caries scores, this property is further inferred from studies where definite variations in the intake of refined carbohydrates occurred (43, 44). Recently, dietary restriction of sugar was found not only to enhance other methods but to be the most effective single method of caries prevention, an essential part of a regimen to achieve a caries-free state (45). Thus the very low incidence of dental caries in relation to xylitol consumption requires special consideration. It may be argued that the effect in the 2-year feeding study was achieved through virtually complete omission of dietary sucrose. However, partial substitution of sucrose by xylitol achieved the same low caries incidence rate as that recorded in connection with total substitution, indicating that xylitol may possess a therapeutic, caries-inhibitory effect (3). It seems unlikely, however, that such mechanisms could be demonstrated beyond doubt by negative reversals in clinical caries trials. Nevertheless, the results from three recent studies indicate that xylitol may enhance natural defence mechanisms. Xylitol influenced lesion formation and remineralization by means of physicochemical effects (46). Regression of fissure caries was observed in rats fed xylitol-supplemented diets (27). Remineralization/rehardening due to xylitol-supplemented diets was reported in bovine enamel in subjects with rampant caries. Such development occurred particularly in predemineralized enamel (47).

EFFECT OF XYLITOL ON QUANTITY OF PLAQUE

Dental plaque forms as a gelatinous organized structure on the teeth, which consists mostly of microorganisms imbedded in an extracellular matrix of salivary, microbial and dietary origin (48–51). The amount and growth rate of dental plaque in the human depend on factors determined by the oral hygiene, dietary habits, and genetic properties of the individual. Dental plaque is involved in both the initiation and propagation of dental caries. Sucrose and other common, soluble carbohydrates consisting of C_6-units usually enhance plaque growth (48, 49). Partial substitution of dietary sucrose with xylitol for a period of 4 or 5 days on reduced oral hygiene decreased the plaque fresh weight by 50% (52, 53). A similar reduction in plaque fresh weight was obtained after 2- or 3-day consumption of chewing gum containing about 50% xylitol (54–56). The visible plaque index decreased in children given a xylitol-sorbitol mixture (1 : 0.67) in the form of gum arabic pastils and chewing gums for a period of two weeks (57) and after the use of chewable xylitol pastils for a period of two months (58).

In another partial-substitution study 1-month use of xylitol-sweetened chewing gums significantly reduced the amount of dental plaque (59). These results were obtained by determining the plaque fresh weight and clinical plaque indexes by conventional methods. Application of planimetric, computerized methods supported these findings (60). In the 1-year chewing gum trial (31), the consumption of xylitol-sweetened (49%) chewing gum significantly reduced the plaque index scores compared with corresponding consumption of sucrose-sweetened gums (61). Thus daily doses of xylitol amounting to 3–15 g may significantly reduce the growth of dental plaque provided that the consumption of sucrose is not simultaneously increased.

Plaque registrations were also performed in the 2-year Turku sugar studies. The results (62) were identical to those obtained both in the short-term and partial-substitution studies mentioned above. The human clinical trials so far carried out thus suggest that (a) it is possible to reduce plaque growth by up to 50% and (b) even partial substitution for sucrose may be sufficient. We emphasize, however, that mixtures of sucrose and xylitol should be avoided; substitution here means replacement of sucrose candies and chewing gums with those containing xylitol as the only sweetener (with possible small additions of sorbitol, mannitol, or Lycasin).

EFFECT OF XYLITOL ON THE GROWTH OF ORAL MICROORGANISMS

The Turku sugar studies provided information about the effects of dietary xylitol on human plaque flora (61, 63, 64). Replacement of dietary sucrose with xylitol did not affect the proportions of major microbial categories in saliva and dental plaque. The acidogenic and aciduric oral flora were, however, reduced (63). The consumption of a xylitol diet significantly lowered the incidence of *Streptococcus mutans,* a potent cariogenic organism (64). Similar results were obtained in the 1-year chewing gum trial; the use of xylitol-sweetened chewing gums was associated with decreased coloni-forming unit values on Rogosa S. L. agar (61).

Several short-term in vivo and in vitro experiments have supported the microbiological findings of the Turku sugar studies. For example, Gehring and coworkers demonstrated both the poor fermentability of xylitol by rat and hamster oral microorganisms (65) and the absence of *Str. mutans* in the dental plaque of rats fed xylitol (66). Plaque grown during sucrose feeding, however, harbored these organisms. Other authors have confirmed (*a*) the unfermentability or very low fermentability of xylitol by *Str. mutans* and other oral microorganisms and (*b*) the reduced incidence of *Str. mutans* in combination with plaque inhibition during xylitol consumption (67–78).

Some additional studies on the effect of xylitol on isolated cultures deserve consideration. The metabolism of several simple carbohydrates was studied with five different xylitol-metabolizing streptococcal strains from the rat oral cavity (75). The amounts of carbohydrates metabolized were smallest with xylitol and sorbitol, and considerably larger with mannitol and fructose. By far the highest levels of CO_2 were measured in the presence of glucose, while for some reason sucrose was not metabolized by these isolated strains at all. The results confirmed the small metabolic capacity of these microorganisms to use xylitol (75). The oral cavity of rats and hamsters may harbor microorganisms capable of breaking down xylitol at a low rate (65). In rats these are enterococcoid germs and *Proteus* sp., in hamsters short gram-negative rods. The metabolism of polyols by these organisms is, however, slow and forms little acid. Metabolism of xylitol was the poorest (65). Another strain of *Str. mutans,* as well as *Actinomyces viscosus,* neither fermented nor utilized xylitol (74). The little acid formed by a further strain of *Str. mutans* may have stemmed partly from the fermentation of proteinaceous ingredients of the medium used (79).

Although the above-mentioned studies have demonstrated the poor or nil fermentability of xylitol by human oral microorganisms, the existence of a transport mechanism of xylitol into some bacterial cells suggests that xylitol-utilizing microorganisms do occur (4, 80). In some cases xylitol may be transported through a system primarily serving other functions. In *Aerobacter aerogenes* (a non-oral strain) there is an active transport system for D-arabitol, which also acts on xylitol (81). Other related cases have been previously discussed (4, 82).

In view of these findings it is anticipated that occasional low fermentability of xylitol will be displayed in human dental plaque. A few such cases were revealed in the Turku sugar studies (61, 64) and in one in vitro experiment (82). However, the slow fermentation rate demonstrated in vitro does not indicate that similar decomposition will occur to any sizable extent in the oral cavity. In oral biology, it may be desirable to consider the *relative* fermentability of dietary carbohydrates by plaque microorganisms. The available literature indicates that the relative fermentability of xylitol in the human oral cavity is very low indeed. It can be regarded microbiologically as an almost inert compound in the human dental plaque.

METABOLIC PROPERTIES OF DENTAL PLAQUE AS AFFECTED BY XYLITOL

Dental plaque does not contain specific recognition sites for xylitol to any significant extent (71) and the incorporation of radioactively labeled xylitol into plaque microoganisms is nil or very slow (Figure 1) (69, 71, 83, 84).

The metabolic inertness of xylitol in the human dental plaque leads, however, to indirect consequential phenomena, especially if the daily consumption levels of xylitol equal the normal consumption levels of six-carbon sugars. For example, during the consumption of large amounts of xylitol in place of sucrose, the plaque microorganisms become deprived of a preferred substrate and start to synthesize extracellular proteolytic enzymes for

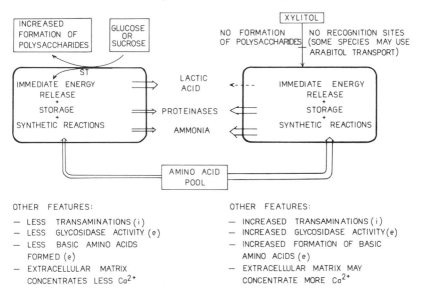

Figure 1 Summarizing, schematic presentation of some biochemical reactions occurring in dental plaque during the consumption of a predominantly hexose-based diet or a xylitol diet. The bacterial cells (shown by the heavy lines) typically represent those of a cariogenic strain of *Str. mutans* in the logarithmic phase of growth. The biochemical phenomena indicated occur during habitual consumption of the diets indicated, with daily consumption levels of xylitol exceeding 10–20 g. The thickness of the arrows indicate the relative activities or concentrations of enzymes and metabolites, respectively; e = extracellular; i = intracellular; ST = sugar transport.

the hydrolysis of the proteins and peptides of the medium. The cells of *Streptococcus mutans* that were maintained in a medium containing xylitol instead of glucose showed no uptake of ^{14}[C(U)]-xylitol, but exhibited strong increase in the extracellular proteinase activity (84). Xylitol behaved as an inert carbohydrate with respect to the increases in the extracellular proteinase activities. This finding was assumed to be associated with a general increase in protein metabolism upon starvation of a fermentable carbohydrate (glucose). Similar increases in the proteinase activities occurred in whole saliva and dental plaque when high quantities of xylitol were habitually consumed (62). Because of the nonspecificity of the proteinases discovered (62, 83), they may attack salivary proteins and peptides in vivo. In fact, increased proteinase activity against denatured hemoglobin was found in whole saliva of human subjects consuming high amounts of xylitol (62). Since saliva is rich in glycoproteins, it is understandable that the activity levels of certain plaque glycosidases also increased during habitual xylitol consumption (62). The above reactions of dental plaque were found to be associated with increased transamination rates (62) and sorbitol dehydrogenase levels (85). The increase of sorbitol dehydrogenase activity in plaque may be due to the simultaneous presence of xylitol and sorbitol in the chewing gums used (85). In no case has any significant xylitol dehydrogenase activity been detected in the whole saliva or plaque of subjects habitually consuming xylitol. The activity of this enzyme was nil in most samples (62, 70, 85).

Striking differences between the sucrose- and xylitol-consuming subjects were found in the activity levels of invertase-like enzymes obtained from whole saliva and dental plaque; the consumption of xylitol reduced this enzyme activity significantly (62, 85, 86). Another important and related metabolic consequence is the decreased production of lactic acid in plaque in the presence of xylitol (62, 85). All these metabolic events may be related to the fact that, during sucrose consumption, gluconeogenetic enzymes are no longer necessary. The nitrogen and protein metabolism is thereby reduced. When sucrose is replaced with xylitol, there is an increased search for metabolizable proteinaceous nutrients of the medium (saliva and plaque extracellular phase), with a concomitant increase in the general nitrogen metabolism. There is no evidence that these metabolic changes of plaque would be detrimental to the oral tissues. Some of these phenomena, like the increase in the size of the amino acid pool (87) and the decrease in the production of lactic acid in plaque, are factors that should be included in the explanation of the effect of xylitol on dental caries. The increase of the amino acid pool renders higher deamination rates possible, thereby increasing the concentration of ammonia (58, 62, 87). The presence of glucose in the medium of *Str. mutans* reduced the free amino acid pool (88). Addition of protein hydrolysates to the medium enlarged the pool. The above biochemical features are summarized in Figure 1.

In contrast with xylitol, the hexitols, sorbitol and mannitol, are readily metabolized by plaque streptococci, almost exclusively by glycolysis (Embden-Meyerhof pathway) (4, 89, 90).

The suitability of a dietary carbohydrate as a sucrose substitute can also be demonstrated by intraoral wire-telemetry. This method revealed that neither xylitol chewing gum nor xylitol mouthwash produced a pH drop of plaque (79, 91–93), whereas with readily fermentable carbohydrates rapid reduction in pH values occurred. pH-Telemetry has thus demonstrated the nonacidogenic nature of xylitol in human use.

EFFECT OF XYLITOL ON SALIVARY PARAMETERS

The consumption of a xylitol diet increased lactoperoxidase (LPO) activity in human (94) and monkey (95) parotid or submandibular saliva. A similar finding was made with the α-amylase of monkey parotid saliva (96). Detailed studies with human parotid saliva in the authors' laboratories suggested that peroral xylitol slightly increased the secretion of sialic acid or sialoproteins (86, 95–97) and sulphate (85, 95) in saliva. The elevated sulphate levels may be due to raised secretion of sulphated polysaccharides.

The possibility that dietary carbohydrates may influence the concentration of salivary enzymes was shown by Walker more than 55 years ago (98). That xylitol consumption may increase the activity levels of salivary LPO is interesting in view of the participation of the LPO-system in defense mechanisms (99–101). The action of this system also requires the presence of SCN^-. A few studies have indicated that the consumption of large amounts of xylitol was associated with increased levels of salivary SCN^- (62, 86). Therefore, in order to elucidate the effects of dietary sugars on the activity of the LPO-system one may have to determine not only the enzyme activity or concentrations but also the levels of the auxiliary compounds (SCN^- and H_2O_2) and reaction products ($OSCN^-$). Use of xylitol in the form of mouthwash or chewing gum caused a quick increase in the pH value of whole saliva (93). Since this pH response occurs within 120 sec following stimulation of saliva, it is possible that basic equivalents rapidly appear in saliva not only from plaque but from the oral mucosa as well (97). These findings thus suggest that dietary xylitol exerts selective effects on the consumption of saliva.

MICROBIAL ADAPTATION

The microbial ecosystem of the oral cavity has been largely affected by carbohydrates that are based on common six-carbon structures and are easily soluble in water. During evolution, such carbohydrates became ecological chemodeterminants just as the common amino acids became determinants in the nitrogen and protein metabolism of oral microorganisms. The easily soluble, common dietary sugars (e.g. glucose, fructose and sucrose), starches and related common six-carbon compounds (including sorbitol and mannitol) and their multiples are effectively metabolized by cariogenic species. These facts must therefore be considered when discussing possible microbial adaptations enabling clinically meaningful acidogenic breakdown of xylitol in plaque. The Turku sugar studies (63, 64) revealed no such adaptation nor was any significant adaptation detected after 4.5 years of continous consumption of xylitol (70).

Earlier studies had indicated that adaptation enabled dental plaque microorganisms to utilize xylitol as a carbon source (67, 84). It was discovered later that the plaque microorganisms started instead to exploit extracellular, chiefly salivary and dietary proteins, peptides, and amino acids as sources of energy, as discussed above. Thus no sizable adaptation to use xylitol has been found. Microbial adaptation to use xylitol may be an uneconomic way to gain energy. This situation may be particularly true for oral microorganisms.

The slow decomposition of xylitol by oral bacteria may also be based on the use of other, preexisting transport systems rather than on the appearance of specific new xylitol transport mechanisms. In yeasts that actively ferment pentose sugars (4), the situation may be different. Therefore, it is advisable in future long-term trials to arrange microbiological follow-up studies to check this matter. The Turku feeding studies indicated that the consumption of a xylitol diet reduced the incidence of oral *Candida* (63). The current literature suggests that the almost complete lack of xylitol fermentation in human dental plaque is genetically fixed, for reasons of evolutionary expediency.

COMPLEXING OF POLYOLS WITH METAL IONS

Complexing of multivalent cations with polyoxygen systems has been exploited in technology and biology, but has received virtually no attention in oral biology. Cyclic polyhydroxy compounds (e.g. the cyclitols and sugars) complex rather strongly with various multivalent cations (102–104). The site of specificity of complexation of the various alditols shows that the strength of complex formation is strongly dependent on the configuration of the ligand. Using Pr [III], the following order of preferential configuration with respect to complex formation in aqueous solution has been given: xylo > threo > arabino (lyxo) > glycerol > erythro, ribo (102–104). Although these results were obtained with Pr^{III}, they are probably applicable to isosteric cations such as Na^{I} and Ca^{II}.

Sugar alcohols like xylitol, sorbitol, and mannitol form complexes with calcium salts, and the precipitation of calcium proteinates in saliva strongly depends on the type of the polyol used (105). Application of these chemical aspects to oral biology has only recently been considered, and it is not possible at this stage to indicate to what extent such phenomena contribute to the non- and anticariogenicity of xylitol in humans. The plaque of subjects consuming polyol-containing chewing gums contained more calcium than plaque collected from the same subjects before the use of chewing gums (85). Whether this calcium was present in plaque owing to its complexation with xylitol or sorbitol remains to be elucidated. Such calcium, however, would be available for remineralization of Ca-deficient lesions at the interphase of dental plaque.

The proposed therapeutic effect of xylitol (29, 31) in the dental caries of humans should be viewed against the following facts: (*a*) Xylitol causes nil or minimal decrease in plaque pH; (*b*) xylitol increases the formation and/or secretion of basic equivalents in the oral cavity; and (*c*) xylitol affects the precipitation of Ca-proteinates in saliva and itself forms complexes with Ca^{2+}. Other factors may also participate in the rehardening of carious lesions. One such factor, still incompletely understood, is the redox state of plaque extracellular fluid and saliva following xylitol administration. Further findings from the authors' laboratory suggest that the presence of xylitol in a 6% sucrose-containing medium strongly decreases the ratio of insoluble polysaccharides to water-soluble polysaccharides in plaque. Consideration of these effects may facilitate understanding of the long-term human clinical trials (29, 31).

CONCLUSIONS AND CONSIDERATIONS

A massive reduction of the increment rate of dental caries was observed with total and partial substitution of dietary sucrose by xylitol. Similar results were obtained in experimental studies, as reviewed in the initial sections of this paper.

These findings must be viewed as natural consequences of the microbiological and biochemical properties of xylitol. These include the stimulation of salivary secretion; elevation of certain electrolyte concentrations of oral fluid; increase of buffering of saliva, and increase or maintenance of high pH levels in oral fluid and plaque; lack of suitability for microbial metabo-

146 MÄKINEN & SCHEININ

lism; influence on enzymatic activities; and also the increase of certain amino acids of oral fluid. Peroral xylitol stimulates a number of existing defense mechanisms against caries. Strict sugar restriction over an extended time undoubtedly leads to a massive caries reduction. In view of biologic and behavioral preferences for sweets, however, restriction of sucrose intake without suggestion of alternatives is a recommendation that lies somewhere between hypocrisy and malpractice. In cases of rampant caries, extremely caries-susceptible tooth structure, sucromania, and reduced salivary secretion rate, the strategy of substitution should thus be considered and applied.

Literature Cited

1. Socransky, S. S. 1979. Criteria for the infectious agents in dental caries and periodontal disease. *J. Clin. Periodontol.* 6:16–21
2. Loesche, W. J. 1976. Chemotherapy of dental plaque infections. *Oral Sci. Rev.* 9:65–107
3. Scheinin, A., Mäkinen, K. K., eds. 1975. *Turku Sugar Studies, Acta Odontol. Scand.* 33: (Suppl. 70) 1–351
4. Mäkinen, K. K. 1978. Principles of the use of xylitol in medicine and nutrition with special consideration of dental aspects. *Experientia* 30: (Suppl.) 1–160
5. Washüttl, J., Riederer, P., Bancher, E. 1973. A qualitative and quantitative study of sugar alcohols in several foods. *J. Food Sci.* 38:1262–63
6. Mäkinen, K. K., Söderling, E. 1980. A quantitative study of mannitol, sorbitol, xylitol and xylose in wild berries and commercial fruits. *J. Food Sci.* 45: 367–71
7. Huttunen, J. K., Mäkinen, K. K., Scheinin, A. 1975. Turku sugar studies. XI. Effects of sucrose, fructose and xylitol diets on glucose, lipid and urate metabolism. *Acta Odontol. Scand.* 33: (Suppl. 70) 239–45
8. Mäkinen, K. K. 1976. Long-term tolerance of healthy human subjects to high amounts of xylitol and fructose: general and biochemical findings. *Int. J. Vitam. Nutr. Res.* 15: (Suppl.) 368–80
9. Mäkinen, K. K., Ylikahri, R., Söderling, E., Mäkinen, P.-L., Scheinin, A. 1982. Turku sugar studies. XXII. A reexamination of the subjects. *Suppl. Int. J. Vitam. Nutr. Res.* 22:9–28
10. Mäkinen, K. K., Ylikahri, R., Mäkinen, P.-L., Söderling, E., Hämäläinen, M. 1982. Turku sugar studies. XXIII. Comparison of metabolic tolerance in human volunteers to high oral doses of xylitol and sucrose after long-term regular consumption of xylitol. *Suppl. Int. J. Vitam. Nutr. Res.* 22:29–51
11. Navia, J. M., Lopez, H., Fischer, J. S. 1974. Caries promoting properties of sucrose substitutes in foods: mannitol, xylitol and sorbitol. *J. Dent. Res.* 53: (Spec. Iss. A, No. 611) 207
12. Mühlemann, H. R., Regolati, B., Marthaler, T. M. 1970. The effect on rat fissure caries of xylitol and sorbitol. *Helv. Odontol. Acta* 14:48–50
13. Karle, E. J., Büttner, W. 1971. Kariesbefall im Tierversuch nach Verabreichung von Sorbit, Xylit, Lycasin und Calcium-Saccharosephosphat. *Dtsch. Zahnärztl. Z.* 26:1097–1108
14. Grunberg, E., Beskid, G., Brin, M. 1973. Xylitol and dental caries. Efficacy of xylitol in reducing dental caries in rats. *Int. J. Vitam. Nutr. Res.* 43: 227–32
15. Brin, M., Miller, O. N. 1974. In *Sugars in Nutrition,* ed. H. L. Sipple, K. W. McNutt, pp. 590–606. NY: Academic. 768 pp.
16. Karle, E. J., Gehring, F. 1975. Wirkung der Zuckeraustauschstoffe Fruktose, Sorbit und Xylit auf Kariesbefall und Plaqueflora der Ratte. *Dtsch. Zahnärztl. Z.* 30:356–63
17. Karle, E., Gehring, F. 1976. A gnotobiotic assay to determine the cariogenicity of xylitol-fermenting microorganisms. *Caries Res.* 10:249
18. Narkates, A. J., Navia, J. M., Bates, D. 1976. Rat caries studies with xylitol-cornstarch containing diets. *J. Dent. Res.* 55: (Spec. Iss., No. 455) 175
19. Moll, R., Büttner, W. 1978. Caries incidence in the rat following partial substitution of sucrose by xylitol. *Caries Res.* 12:119

20. Mühlemann, H. R., Schmid, R., Noguchi, T., Imfeld, T., Hirsch, R. S. 1977. Some dental effects of xylitol under laboratory and *in vivo* conditions. *Caries Res.* 11:263–76

21. Gehring, F., Karle, J. E. 1978. Cariogenicity of L-sorbose compared with xylitol and sucrose in animal studies. *Caries Res.* 12:118–19

22. Karle, E. J. 1977. Die Kariogenität von Xylit in Tierversuch. *Dtsch. Zahnärztl. Z.* 32:S89–95

23. Mundorff, S., Bibby, B. 1977. Xylitol-sucrose effects on enamel dissolution and rat caries. *J. Dent. Res.* 56: (Spec. Iss. B, No. 339) 136

24. Green, R. M., Leach, S. A. 1977. Effect of xylitol dietary supplements on caries in the rat. *J. Dent. Res.* 56: (Spec. Iss. A, No. 207) 94

25. Gey, F., Kinkel, H. T. 1978. Topical application of xylitol and other sucrose substitutes after restricted cariogenic meals. *J. Dent. Res.* 57: (Spec. Iss. A, No. 147) 111

26. Leach, S. A., Green, R. M. 1979. Effect of xylitol-supplemented diets on the incidence of fissure caries in rats. *Caries Res.* 13:95–96

27. Leach, S. A., Green, R. M. 1980. Effect of xylitol-supplemented diets on the progression and regression of fissure caries in the albino rat. *Caries Res.* 14:16–23

28. Huxley, H. G. 1978. In *Proc. Methods of Caries Prediction, Spec. Suppl. Microbiol. Abstr.,* ed. B. G. Bibby, R. J. Shern, pp. 211–16. Washington DC: IRL

29. Scheinin, A., Mäkinen, K. K., Ylitalo, K. 1975. Turku sugar studies. V. Final report on the effect of sucrose, fructose and xylitol diets on the caries incidence in man. *Acta Odontol. Scand.* 33: (Suppl. 70) 67–104

30. Horowitz, H. S., Baume, L. J., Backer-Dirks, O., Davies, G. N., Slack, G. L., eds., COCSTOC (Comm. Classif. Stat. Oral Condit.). 1973. Principal requirements for controlled clinical trials to caries preventive agents and procedures. *Int. Dent. J.* 23:506–16

31. Scheinin, A., Mäkinen, K. K., Tammisalo, E., Rekola, M. 1975. Turku sugar studies. XVIII. Incidence of dental caries in relation to 1-year consumption of xylitol chewing gum. *Acta Odontol. Scand.* 33: (Suppl. 70) 307–16

32. Nizel, A. E. 1972. *Nutrition in Preventive Dentistry: Science and Practice,* pp. 371–73. Philadelphia: Saunders. 506 pp.

33. Von der Fehr, F. R., Löe, H., Theilade, E. 1970. Experimental caries in man. *Caries Res.* 4:131–48

34. Rekola, M. 1980. Planimetry of incipient caries as affected by xylitol consumption. *J. Dent. Res.* 59: (Spec. Iss. B, No. 189) 934

35. Slack, G. L., Millward, E., Martin, W. J. 1964. The effect of tablets stimulating salivary flow on the incidence of dental caries. A two-year clinical trial. *Brit. Dent. J.* 116:105–8

36. Møller, I. J., Poulsen, S. 1973. The effect of sorbitol-containing chewing gum on the incidence of dental caries, plaque and gingivitis in Danish school-children. *Commun. Dent. Oral Epidemiol.* 1:58–67

37. Bánóczy, J., Esztári, I., Hadas, E., Marosi, I., Fözy, L., Szántó, S. 1978. Einjährige Erfahrungen mit Sorbit in klinischen Längsschnitt-Versuch. *Dtsch. Zahnärztl. Z.* 33:701–5

38. Bánóczy, J., Hadas, E., Esztári, I., Marosi, I. 1979. Two-year clinical results with sorbitol. *Caries Res.* 13:90

39. Bánóczy, J., Hadas, E., Esztári, I., Marosi, I., Fözy, L., Szántó, S. 1980. Dreijährige Erfahrungen mit Sorbit im klinischen Längsschnitt-Versuch. *Kariesprophlaxe* 2:39–46

40. Frostell, G., Blomlöf, L., Blomqvist, T., Dahl, G. M., Edward, S., Fjellström, A., Henrikson, C. O., Larje, O., Nord, C. E., Nordenvall, K. J. 1974. Substitution of sucrose by Lycasin® in candy. "The Roslagen Study". *Acta Odontol. Scand.* 32:235–54

41. Frostell, G., Blomqvist, Th., Bruner, P. O., Dahl, G. M., Fjellström, A., Henrikson, C. O., Larje, O., Nord, C.-E., Nordenvall, K.-J., Wik, O. 1982. Reduction of caries in pre-school children by sucrose restriction and by substitution with invert sugar—The Gustavsberg study. *Acta Odontol. Scand.* 39: 333–47

42. Scheinin, A. 1978. Sugar substitutes in relation to the incidence of clinical and experimental caries. *Pharmacol. Ther. Dent.* 3:95–100

43. Gustafsson, B. E., Quensel, C. E., Lanke, L. S., Lundqvist, C., Grahnén, H., Bonow, B. E., Krasse, K. 1953. The Vipeholm dental caries study. The effect of different levels of carbohydrate intake on caries activity in 436 individuals observed for five years. *Acta Odontol. Scand.* 11:232–364

44. Harris, R. 1963. Biology of the children of Hopewood House, Bowral, Australia. IV. Observations of dental caries

experience extending over five years (1957–1961). *J. Dent. Res.* 42:1387–98

45. McDonald, S. P., Cowell, C. R., Sheiham, A. 1981. Methods of preventing dental caries used by dentists for their own children. *Brit. Dent. J.* 151:118–21

46. Arends, J. 1982. Influence of xylitol on solubility complex formation of apatites. *Caries Res.* 16: In press

47. Scheinin, A., Scheinin, U., Glass, R. L., Kallio, M.-L., Söderling, E. 1981. Xylitol-induced changes of enamel microhardness in the human mouth. *J. Dent. Res.* 60: (Spec. Iss. A, No. 817) 514

48. Mäkinen, K. K. 1972. The role of sucrose and other sugars in the development of dental caries. *Int. Dent. J.* 22:363–86

49. Mäkinen, K. K. 1974. Sugars and the formation of dental plaque. In *Sugars in Nutrition*, ed. H. L. Sipple, K. W. McNutt, pp. 645–87. NY: Academic. 768 pp.

50. Dawes, C. 1968. The nature of dental plaque, films, and calcareous deposits. *Ann. NY Acad. Sci.* 153:102–19

51. Schroeder, H. E., de Boever, J. 1970. The structure of microbial dental plaque. In *Dental Plaque,* ed. W. D. McHugh, pp. 49–75. Dundee, Scotland: Thompson. 298 pp.

52. Scheinin, A., Mäkinen, K. K. 1971. The effect of various sugars on the formation and chemical composition of dental plaque. *Int. Dent. J.* 21:302–21

53. Scheinin, A., Mäkinen, K. K. 1972. Effect of sugars and sugar mixtures on dental plaque. *Acta Odontol. Scand.* 30:235–57

54. Mouton, C., Scheinin, A., Mäkinen, K. K. 1975. Effect on plaque of a xylitol-containing chewing-gum. A pilot study. *Acta Odontol. Scand.* 33:27–31

55. Mouton, C., Scheinin, A., Mäkinen, K. K. 1975. Effect on plaque of a xylitol-containing chewing-gum. A clinical and biochemical study. *Acta Odontol. Scand.* 33:33–40

56. Mouton, C., Scheinin, A., Mäkinen, K. K. 1975. Effect of a xylitol chewing gum on plaque quantity and quality. *Acta Odontol. Scand.* 33:251–57

57. Harjola, U., Liesmaa, H. 1979. Effects of polyol and sucrose candies on plaque, gingivitis and lactobacillus scores. *Acta Odontol. Scand.* 36:237–42

58. Pakkala, U., Liesmaa, H., Mäkinen, K. K. 1981. The use of xylitol in the control of oral hygiene in mentally retarded children. *Proc. Finn. Dent. Soc.* 77: 271–77

59. Rekola, M., Läikkö, I., Anttinen, H., Scheinin, A., Mäkinen, K. K. 1980. Die Wirkung von xylit- und sorbithaltigen Kaugummis auf Plaque und Speichel. Teil I: Klinische Aspekte. *Kariesprophylaxe* 2:21–27

60. Rekola, M. 1981. Comparative effects of xylitol- and sucrose-sweetened chew tablets and chewing gums on plaque quantity. *Scand. J. Dent. Res.* 89: 463–69

61. Larmas, M., Scheinin, A., Gehring, F., Mäkinen, K. K. 1975. Turku sugar studies. XX. Microbiological findings and plaque index values in relation to 1-year use of xylitol chewing gum. *Acta Odontol. Scand.* 33: (Suppl. 70) 321–36

62. Mäkinen, K. K., Scheinin, A. 1975. Turku sugar studies. VII. Principal biochemical findings on whole saliva and plaque. *Acta Odontol. Scand.* 33: (Suppl. 70) 129–71

63. Larmas, M., Mäkinen, K. K., Scheinin, A. 1975. Turku sugar studies. VIII. Principal microbiological findings. *Acta Odontol. Scand.* 33: (Suppl. 70) 173–216

64. Gehring, F., Mäkinen, K. K., Larmas, M., Scheinin, A. 1975. Turku sugar studies. X. Occurrence of polysaccharide-forming streptococci and ability of the mixed plaque microbiota to ferment various carbohydrates. *Acta Odontol. Scand.* 33: (Suppl. 70) 223–37

65. Gehring, F. 1974. Mikrobiologische Aspekte zur Kariogenität von Zuckern und Zuckeraustauschstoffen. *Dtsch. Zahnärztl. Z.* 29:769–71

66. Karle, E., Gehring, F. 1975. Wirkunge der Zuckeraustauschstoffe Fruktose, Sorbit und Xylit auf Kariesbefall und Plaqueflora der Ratte. *Dtsch. Zahnärztl. Z.* 30:356–63

67. Mäkinen, K. K. 1972. Enzyme dynamics of a cariogenic streptococcus: The effect of xylitol and sorbitol. *J. Dent. Res.* 51:403–8

68. Mäkinen, K. K., Ojanotko, A., Vidgren, H. 1975. Effect of xylitol on the growth of three oral strains of *Candida albicans. J. Dent. Res.* 54:1239

69. Mäkinen, K. K. 1976. Microbial growth and metabolism in plaque in the presence of sugar alcohols. In *Proc. Microbial Aspects in Dental Caries, Spec. Suppl. Microbiol. Abstr.,* ed. H. M. Stiles, W. J. Loesche, T. C. O'Brien, II:521–38. Washington DC:IRL 580 pp.

70. Mäkinen, K. K., Virtanen, K. K. 1978. Effect of 4.5-year use of xylitol and sorbitol on plaque. *J. Dent. Res.* 57:441–46

71. Mäkinen, K. K., Rekola, M. 1976. Xylitol-binding in dental plaque. *J. Dent. Res.* 55:900-4
72. Gehring, F. 1971. Saccharose und Zuckeraustauschstoffe im mikrobiologischen Test. *Dtsch. Zahnärztl. Z.* 26:1162-71
73. Gülzow, H.-J. 1974. Vergleidende Untersuchungen über den Abbau von Xylit im menschlichen Speichel. *Dtsch. Zahnärztl. Z.* 29:772-75
74. Noguchi, T., Mühlemann, H. R. 1976. The effect of some carbohydrates on *in vitro* growth of *Streptococcus mutans* and *Actinomyces viscosus. Schweiz. Mschr. Zahnheilk.* 86:1361-70
75. Gehring, F., Gülzow, H.-J. 1977. Beitrag zum mikrobiellen Xylitabbau. *Dtsch. Zahnärztl. Z.* 32:580-82
76. Hoerman, K. C. 1979. Enumeration of *Streptococcus mutans* in human dental plaque after chewing gum sweetened with xylitol and sucrose. *Pharmacol. Therap. Dent.* 4:11-19
77. Rölla, G., Oppermann, R. V., Waaler, S. M., Assev, S. 1981. Effect of aqueous solutions of sorbitol-xylitol on plaque metabolism and on growth of *Streptococcus mutans. Scand. J. Dent. Res.* 89:247-50
78. Semlinger, E. 1977. *Vergleichende biochemische Untersuchungen über den anaeroben Abbau von Xylit durch Plaquesmikroorganismen des Menschen.* Academic thesis, Friedrich-Alexander-Univ., Erlangen-Nürnberg. Germany. 43 pp.
79. Toors, F. A., Herczog, J. I. B. 1978. Acid production from a nonsugar licorice and different sugar substitutes in *Streptococcus mutans* monoculture and pooled plaque-saliva mixtures. *Caries Res.* 12:60-68
80. Demetrakopoulos, G. E., Amos, H. 1978. Xylose and xylitol. *Wld. Rev. Nutr. Diet.* 32:96-122
81. Wu, T. T., Lin, E. C. C., Tanaka, S. 1968. Mutants of *Aerobacter aerogenes* capable of utilizing xylitol as a novel carbon. *J. Bacteriol.* 96:447-56
82. Gallagher, I. H. C., Fussell, S. J. 1979. Acidogenic fermentation of pentose alcohols by human dental plaque microorganisms. *Arch. Oral Biol.* 24:673-79
83. Knuuttila, M. L. E., Mäkinen, K. K. 1981. Extracellular hydrolase activity of the cells of the oral bacterium *Streptococcus mutans* isolated from man and grown on glucose or xylitol. *Arch. Oral Biol.* 26:899-904

84. Knuuttila, M. L. E., Mäkinen, K. K. 1975. The effect of xylitol on the growth and metabolism of *Streptococcus mutans. Caries Res.* 9:188-89
85. Mäkinen, K. K., Läikkö, I., Rekola, M., Scheinin, A. 1980. Die Wirkung von Xylit und Sorbit auf die Biochemie der Plaque. *Kariesprophylaxe* 3:103-13
86. Mäkinen, K. K., Kölling, D., Mäkinen, P.-L. 1981. Effect of high dosage of xylitol and sucrose on the biochemical properties of whole saliva in human volunteers after long-term regular consumption of xylitol. *Proc. Finn. Dent. Soc.* 77:262-70
87. Mäkinen, K. K., Lönnberg, P., Scheinin, A. 1975. Turku sugar studies. XIV. Amino acid analysis of saliva. *Acta Odontol. Scand.* 33: (Suppl. 70) 277-86
88. Krzeminski, Z. 1975. Free amino acid pools of cariogenic streptococci. *J. Dent. Res.* 54:183
89. Brown, A. T., Wittenberger, C. C. 1973. Mannitol and sorbitol catabolism in *Streptococcus mutans. Arch. Oral Biol.* 18:117-26
90. Dallmeier, E., Bestmann, H.-J., Kröncke, A. 1970. Über den Abbau von Glukose und Sorbit durch Plaques-Streptokokken. *Dtsch. Zahnärztl. Z.* 25:887-98
91. Hassel, T. M. 1971. pH-Telemetrie der interdentaler Plaque nach Genuss von Zucker und Zuckeraustauschstoffen. *Dtsch. Zahnärztl. Z.* 26:1145-54
92. Imfeld, Th. 1977. Evaluation of the cariogenicity of confectionary by intra-oral wire-telemetry. *Helv. Odontol. Acta* 21:1-28
93. Mühlemann, H. R., Schmid, R., Noguchi, T., Imfeld, T., Hitsch, R. S. 1977. Some dental effects of xylitol under laboratory and *in vivo* conditions. *Caries Res.* 11:263-76
94. Mäkinen, K. K., Tenovuo, J., Scheinin, A. 1976. Xylitol-induced elevation of lactoperoxidase activity in human saliva. *J. Dent. Res.* 55:652-60
95. Mäkinen, K. K., Bowen, W. H., Dalgard, D., Fitzgerald, G. 1978. Effect of peroral administration of xylitol on exocrine secretions of monkeys. *J. Nutr.* 108:779-89
96. Mäkinen, K. K. 1978. The use of xylitol in nutritional and medical research with special reference to dental caries. In *Proc. Sweeteners and Dental Caries, Spec. Suppl. Feeding, Weight & Obesity Abstr.* ed. J. H. Shaw, G. G. Roussos, pp. 193-224. Washington DC:IRL 403 pp.

150   MÄKINEN & SCHEININ

97. Mäkinen, K. K. 1978. Biochemical findings in exocrine secretions in relation to peroral administration of xylitol. In *Xylitol*, ed. J. N. Counsell, Ch. 6. Barking, England: Appl. Sci. Publ. 191 pp.
98. Afonsky, D. 1961. *Saliva and its Relation to Oral Health*, p. 154. Alabama: Univ. Alabama Press. 785 pp.
99. Morrison, M., Steele, W. F. 1968. In *Biology of the Mouth*, ed. P. Person, pp. 89–110. Washington DC: Am. Assoc. Adv. Sci. 301 pp.
100. Björck, L. 1977. *Studies on the antibacterial effect of the lactoperoxidase system on some gramnegative bacteria.* Academic thesis, Landbrukshögskolan, Uppsala, Sweden.
101. Reiter, B. 1978. Review of the progress of dairy science: Antimicrobial systems in milk. *J. Dairy Res.* 45:131–47
102. Angyal, S. J. 1973. Complex formation between sugars and metal ions. *Pure Appl. Chem.* 35:131–46
103. Angyal, S. J., Davies, K. P. 1971. Complexing of sugars with metal ions. *J. Chem. Soc. Chem. Commun.* 500–1
104. Kieboom, A. P. G., Spoormaker, T., Sinnema, A., van der Toorn, J. M., van Bekkum, H. 1975. ^{1}H-NMR study of the complex formation of alditols with multivalent cations in aqueous solutions using praseodymium[III] nitrate as shift reagent. *Rec. J. R. Neth. Chem. Soc.* 94:53–59
105. Söderling, E., Mäkinen, K. K. 1982. Precipitation of human salivary Ca-proteinates in the presence of simple carbohydrates in vivo. *J. Dent. Res.* 61: (Spec. Issue. No. 265) 208

Ann. Rev. Nutr. 1982. 2:151–77

NUTRITION AND IMMUNITY:The Influence of Diet on Autoimmunity and the Role of Zinc in the Immune Response

*Mary Ann Hansen, Gabriel Fernandes, and Robert A. Good**

Memorial Sloan-Kettering Cancer Center, 1275 York Avenue, New York, NY 10021

INTRODUCTION

The effect of nutrition on immunity is manifold. Any single dietary category, be it protein, carbohydrate, fat, individual vitamins, or trace elements, taken in quantities either too large or too small, may cause metabolic abnormalities. These metabolic disturbances can, in turn, affect the well-being of the whole organism and/or a part of the whole, such as the immune system.

Many reviews have been published in the last two decades that amply document the adverse effect of either over- or undernutrition on all aspects of immune function (52, 53, 94, 140, 141, 199). In this chapter, we focus on the effect of diet on autoimmune diseases—including the major disease processes associated with aging—and on the role of a single nutrient, the trace element zinc, in the complex immune systems of man and animal.

It has been shown in experimental animals that diet influences the frequency and severity of several diseases associated with aging. For example, rats fed an unrestricted diet have been more susceptible to malignant, renal, myocardial, and prostatic disease (188) than have those fed a variety of fixed diets. Longevity of experimental animals of several species has also been

*This work was supported by grants from the Molin Foundation, the Zelda R. Weintraub Cancer-Fund, grants AI-19495, NS-18851, AG-03592, and AG-00541, the McConnell Foundation, and the Pew Memorial Trust.

0199-9885/82/0715-0133$02.00

influenced by many variables,including composition of the experimental diet, the quantity consumed, the time of life during which the experimental diet is imposed, duration of the experimental feeding period, and the sex and particular strain of the animal.

Dietary manipulation can, in fact, yield quite spectacular results. Ross, for example, reports that rats exposed to severe dietary restriction from the time of weaning to the time of death have lived to be more than 1800 days old (188), a life span equivalent to approximately 180 years in humans.

I. DIET AND AUTOIMMUNITY

Normal individuals, humans or animal, are immunologically tolerant to self and thus do not form antibodies to fight against native cells. When this aberration does occur, any of several autoimmune diseases may result. These range from the systemic lupus erythematosus to organ-specific diseases such as thyroiditis. It has been noted that autoantibodies occur more frequently in all people, both normal and diseased, as they grow older, an indication that self-tolerance tends to break down during the aging process. It is not surprising, then, that autoimmune disease should be found primarily among the middle-aged and elderly. The etiologies of autoimmune diseases are heterogenous, but the various autoimmune diseases do have many pathological changes in common, including glomerulonephritis, arthritis, and vasculitis. Pericarditis, pleuritis, dermatitis, and/or neuropathy can also be present. Less frequently seen is gonadal failure (211).

Two major factors have been identified in the pathogenesis of autoimmune disease: genetic (e.g. increased susceptibility to infection) and environemntal (e.g. exposure to potential pathogens), both of which can influence immune function (126, 160).

New Zealand Black (NZB) mice have provided investigators with a classic model for study of autoimmune disease (8, 22, 212). At an early age (3–4 months) these animals develop a Coombs positive hemolytic anemia, which in old age is accompanied by renal disease and failure similar to the type found in humans with lupus erythematosus. NZB mice are also prone to develop malignancies of the lymphoid system and other organs.

A related strain of mice, the (NZBxNZW)F_1 hybrid (B/W), is also unusually susceptible to autoimmune disease. Although hemolytic anemia is not a serious problem for them, they do develop a renal disease much like that seen in NZB mice and lupus patients. This lethal disease involves circulating free DNA, DNA-anti-DNA immune complexes and irregular deposits of DNA, complement, and immunoglobulin found in the glomeruli in the capillary basement membranes and on the epithelial side of the basement membranes.

Table 1 Comparison of spleen and thymus weights of NZB mice on normal and low-protein diets

| Age (months) | No. of mice | Spleen[a] Mg ± S.E. | | p[b] value | Thymus (mg) ± S.E. | | p value |
		Normal protein[c]	Low protein[d]		Normal protein[c]	Low protein[d]	
3–4	8	404 ± 35	397 ± 50	ns	174 ± 9	221 ± 27	ns
7–10	10	744 ± 132	425 ± 57	<.02	66 ± 10	136 ± 12	<.001

[a] Relative weights (100 gm. body weight).
[b] Student T-test.
[c] 22%
[d] 6%

A xenotrophic virus, originally described by Levy & Pincus (126) and later extensively studied by Levy (125), has been implicated in the autoimmune disease observed in both the NZB and B/W mice. Tables 1 and 2 show, in addition, early peaking (at three months of age) and decline (3–5 months) of immunologic function in both strains. By 8–12 months of age, at which time the autoimmune disease usually becomes apparent, many immune functions have all but disappeared.

Fernandes et al (62, 64) became interested in the effect of nutrition on autoimmune disease when they observed that two commercial diets, varying in relative fat and protein content (see Table 3), influenced the health and life span of NZB mice in quite different ways. The diet relatively high in fat and low in protein was associated with increased body weight and breeding capacity, more autoantibodies (largely IgG and IgA) on red cell surfaces, and anemia associated with reticulocytosis. The sera of these animals also contained more DNA antibodies. Compared to the mice on the

Table 2 Induction of GVH reaction by spleen cells of 9 month old mice with or without hemolytic anemia[a]

Protein (%)	Mean body wt. (g)	Mean spleen wt. (mg)	Mean thymus wt. (mg)	Mean hematocrit (%)	Coombs test	Mean spleen index	Positive tested
22	50.7	325	7	50.8	—	1.46	5/8
6	25.0	87	32	49.5	—	2.02	7/7
22	47.7	725	5	40.6	+[c]	0.97	1/7
6	25.7	210	25	38.4	+[c]	1.78	6/6

[a] Each (NZBxA)F$_1$ 8 day-old litter was divided into five groups of 7–10 each and injected with spleen cells (10 × 10^6 I.P.) from individual mice with defined disease. Controls (Fifth Group) were not injected.

[b] Student T-Test indicates significance of <.01 level between animals on Diet I and Diet II.

[c] Highly positive.

Table 3 Effect of diets with varying amounts of fat and protein on autoimmune-prone NAB mice

Test	Sex	Age	High fat/low protein (g)[a]	Low fat/high protein (g)[b]	p = <
1. Average body weight	M	9 mos.	53.9	43.8	0.001
2. Total number young (mean)	F		241	171	
3. Hemolytic anemia	M	12 mos.	8/8[c]	13/15	0.02
4. Longevity/days SE	M		295 ± 21	456 ± 15	0.001
	F		305 ± 21	367 ± 18	0.05
5. Reticulocyte count % of 500 rbc	M	12 mos.	67.2 ± 9	22.8 ± 5	0.001
6. % Coombs positivity	M	6 mos.	93.7	62.5	0.01
	M	12 mos.	100	93.3	ns
7. Mean hematocrit % SE	M	12 mos.	31.2 ± 2	37.0 ± 1	0.02
8. Mean white blood cell count/mm³	M/F	12 mos.	13,021 ± 2,869	6,950 ± 622	0.02
9. Hemagglutinating AB titers to SRBC (log 2)					
primary, day 10	M/F	9 mos.	10.5 ± 0.9	11.6 ± 0.2	ns
secondary, day 20			13.2 ± 0.5	12.4 ± 0.2	ns
10. GvH capacity (MSI SD)	M/F	11 mos.	1.10 0	1.67 ± 0	
	M/F	2 mos.		2.03 ± 0	
11. Target cell lysis—% Cr release					
C3H tumor cells	M/F	11 mos.	33	63	
A-strain sarcoma cells	M/F	11 mos.	0	15	
12. Autoantibodies at surface of red blood cells	M/F	11 mos.	greater number, greater variety	no IgA	

[a] 11 % fat, 17% protein
[b] 4.5% fat, 23% protein
[c] Number of animals affected/total number surviving animals

second diet, which was higher in protein and lower in fat, the first group had inferior tumor immunity, a lesser capacity to induce graft-vs-host reactions (GVHR), and a shorter life span.

In a later experiment, Fernandes et al (59) studied the effects of varying the amount of dietary protein, using again the NZB mouse for the experimental model. In this instance a low protein, normal caloric diet helped the animals maintain vigorous immune function longer than controls fed a normal protein, normal caloric diet. Immunoparameters tested included tumor immunity, ability to induce GVHR, the ability to produce antibodies to sheep red blood cells (SRBC), and the mitogenic response of splenic lymphocytes. Longevity was not significantly affected in this experiment.

When dietary protein and/or calorie intake was restricted for the B/W mouse, dissimilar results were obtained (60). It can be seen from Table 4 that protein restriction did not significantly prolong life, whereas calorie restriction did, and to a striking degree for both males and females. In this experiment, B/W hybrids fed a low calorie diet lived twice as long as controls fed a normal diet. Subsequent studies revealed that all of the immune functions that usually fade with age in the B/W mice were much more vigorous in the calorie-restricted animals (54). These included such basic immune functions as cell-mediated cytotoxicity to allogeneic tumor cells, antibody response to sheep red blood cells, and the ability to initiate GVHR. Most recent reports have indicated, however, that for this strain of mouse, dietary fat is also a crucial variable (106). Animals fed a low caloric diet containing a relatively high proportion of fat have developed all the pathological signs—i.e. autoimmune disease, glomerular lesions, and early involution of immune function—regularly seen in mice fed more calories but a lower proportion of fat. Animals fed a low fat diet lived significantly longer than did controls (106). Diets low in the amino acids phenylalanine and tyrosine have also prevented the development of autoimmune kidney disease and doubled the life span of the B/W mouse, particularly the female (45). Similarly, Hurd et al (105a) interfered with development of this disease by restricting essential fatty acids, and Beach et al prevented and/or delayed the onset of these autoimmunities in autoimmune-prone mice by restricting dietary intake of Zn^{2+} (14a).

That diet is capable of influencing the health and longevity of B/W mice after the autoimmune process is underway has been demonstrated by Friend et al (70). They observed that protection from immune nephritis could be achieved either by moderately restricting protein consumption from the time of weaning or by implementing calorie restriction at a later time—i.e. at 4-5 months of age. In these animals, autoimmune activity can be detected in the form of antinuclear antibodies as early as 2 months of age, while evidence of the lupus-like renal disease syndrome becomes manifest by 4 months.

Table 4   The influence of low calorie intake on survival time of (NZB X NZW) F_1 mice

	Diet		Mean survival time/days	
	Protein %	Calories/day	Female	Male
1.	22 (normal)	20 (normal)	317	350
2.	22	10	550	770+
3.	6	20	306	487
4.	6	10	481	700+
5.	22[a]	20	331	488
6.	22[a]	10	547	700+
7.	22[b]	20	318	440
8.	22[b]	10	467	557

[a] Low unsaturated fat
[b] High unsaturated fat

It has been shown (191) that a low calorie diet that prolongs the life of the B/W mouse inhibits the formation of immune complexes and their deposition in vital organs. In this experiment three groups of mice were fed different diets (ordinary lab chow *ad lib,* special diet with 20 cal/day, or special diet with 10 cal/day). Circulating immune complexes (CIC) were measured by the Raji cell radioimmunoassay at 3, 9, 12 and 18 months. No significant differences were found at any age in CIC levels of animals fed regular lab chow and those fed 20 cal/day. At three months, CIC levels were normal for all three groups. At the nine month point an increase was noted in the CIC levels of both sexes in each dietary group. Highest CIC values were found in animals fed regular lab chow at 12 months. Most of these animals died soon thereafter. Mice on the low calorie diet, however, had, at 12 months, CIC values significantly lower than those of either other group. Male mice on the low calorie diet had, at 18 months, lower CIC values than at 12 months, while the control female mice died in the interim between 12–18 months. Those few female control mice still living at 18 months that had been fed the higher calorie diets maintained high levels of CIC.

Inhibition of Other Disease by Dietary Restriction

When dietary restrictions have been applied to other strains of mice not so susceptible to autoimmune disease, or to rats, varying results have been obtained. In 1939, McCay reported that growth-retarded rats subjected to a calorie-restricted diet for periods of 300, 500, 700, and 1000 days all lived longer than did controls fed a normal diet throughout. Other investigators have reported that varying levels of protein restriction had no effect on the longevity of female Sprague-Dawley rats (154). A low calorie diet has not significantly prolonged the life of DBA/2 (see Table 5) or C3H mice. DBA/2 mice, however, have responded favorably to protein restriction begun at the time of weaning. Such a diet has significantly prolonged their life (60).

Table 5   The influence of a low protein diet on longevity of the DBA/2 mouse

Diet		Mean survival time/days		20% survival (days)		Longest survival (days)	
Percentage of protein	Cal/day	Female	Male	Female	Male	Female	Male
22	20	434 ± 53	420 ± 33	650+	524	650+	560
22	10	414 ± 26	357 ± 40	512	444	560	498
6	20	525 ± 46	625 ± 46	650+	650+	650+	650+
6	10	429 ± 46	525 ± 29	550	650	600	650+

C3H female mice, which are prone to develop spontaneous mammary adenocarcinoma, do not do so when fed from weaning a diet restricted in calories (61, 214, 228). Spleen cells from C3H mice restricted to 10 cal/day responded more vigorously to T cell lectins PHA and Con A than did spleen cells from mice fed a conventional diet containing 16 cal/day. The primary PFC response of the calorie-restricted animals, however, was significantly reduced (2091 PFC/spleen vs 10,131 PFC/spleen) four days after immunization with SRBC. In contrast, the secondary PFC response was equivalent in both groups. When spleen cells from both groups were injected into lethally X-irradiated mice, a larger number of PFC/10^6 cells was generated from spleens of calorie-deprived donors. By measuring DNA synthesis in vivo, a suppressor effect was found in spleen cells of calorie-deprived mice. These experiments demonstrated that thymic-dependent cell function, as well as suppressor cell function, remains vigorous in spite of moderate calorie restriction. The interesting possibility that the increased suppressor cell activity observed in the calorie-restricted animals might also be suppressing directly the development of mammary cancer was raised. But, of course, enhancement of immunity by a low caloric diet might also result in an increased specific immunity to tumors (i.e. an antithesis of the "suppressor effect").

More recent studies, however, have shown that the primary effect of calorie restriction in this model comes from the reduction of the fat content of the diet. C3H animals fed low caloric diets with a high proportion of fat have had a high incidence of breast cancer, while those fed a low calorie, low fat diet were largely tumor-free (81).

Good et al (81) have shown that, in C3H mice, restriction of calories and fat inhibit the development and maturation of B type RNA virus particles in mammary cells. The dietary restrictions required to inhibit breast cancer in C3H mice, although perhaps delaying the onset of estrus, permit estrus cycling in an apparently normal fashion. Such diets also appear to permit conception and reproduction. Recently, following a lead from a group studying at the Lilly Laboratories (246) who showed that dihydroepidandrosterone (DHEA) inhibited weight gain at a certain level, Schwartz has employed DHEA to inhibit mammary tumor development in C3H mice (198). DHEA both inhibited weight gain in the mice and completely inhibited mammary adenocarcinoma development in female mice of this strain. Thus it seems likely that both tumor development and weight gain can be inhibited by intake of DHEA. What remains to be determined is whether the DHEA is operating to reduce breast cancer through influence on assimilation or metabolism of food, or through a more direct influence and change in the mammary tumor cells.

Dietary restriction has also exerted dramatic influences on the mice of the very short-lived *kd/kd* mutant strain (128). Mice of the strain bearing this autosomal recessive trait live extremely short lives because they develop progressive nephronophthesis and renal failure. They usually die by 240 days of age. Such animals also develop autoimmune hemolytic anemia relatively early in life, which progresses as they grow older. Calorie restriction from the time of weaning prevents the development of interstitial nephritis, the progressive glomerular and tumular damage, and the autoimmunity that characterizes such mice (63). Whereas the great majority of putatively well-fed mice died of renal failure by 240 days of age, none of the group fed a restricted diet, reduced in total calories by approximately one third that given the controls, had died by 240 days. Changing half of the animals to the higher calorie intake at 240 days of age led to the rapid development of autoimmunity, interstitial nephritis, nephronophthesis, and death within 60 days. By contrast, all the mice that were continuously fed the low calorie intake survived beyond 300 days, and well over half of them lived to two years. For this strain also, total calories seemed a crucial variable. Protein, on the other hand, was not so important, since feeding diets of widely different protein compositions, ranging from 6% to 20% of the diet, did not alter the outcome of their genetically determined disease. Thus, for this strain, as for certain other autoimmune-prone strains studied, calories and fat especially and, to a much lesser extent, protein are crucial variables in determining length of life (63).

Another autoimmune-prone strain of mice, MRL/1pr, was similarly studied in our laboratories. In these mice, development of autoimmunity, apparent immunocomplex-based renal-vascular disease, a dramatic lymphoproliferative disorder, and early death are all strikingly delayed or inhibited entirely by restriction of dietary calorie intake from the time of weaning (55, 56). The vigor of immunity functions is also maintained by restricting the diet, and the animals' life spans are at least doubled.

Thus in several especially short-lived inbred strains of mice, autoimmune phenomena, diseases based on autoimmunity and immune dysfunction, vascular disease, renal disease, immunodeficiency occurring with aging, and even serveral forms of cancer in mice and rats can be very much inhibited by dietary restrictions imposed both early and later in life (70).

These findings indicate that nutritional factors can exert profound influences on immunity functions and immunoregulatory mechanisms, and can inhibit pathologic perturbations that occur with aging in mice and rats. Whether these leads can be exploited and applied to the prevention of diseases of aging that occur relatively early in life in certain humans depends, we believe, on thorough analysis of the cellular, endocrinological, and molecular bases of these most extraordinary influences of diet. We are optimistic that such leads can, indeed, be exploited to greatly prolong health in humans who, like the short-lived autoimmune-prone mice, so regularly sicken and die with the same kinds of diseases of aging that plague these short-lived autoimmune-prone mice. The latter include cellular and humoral immunodeficiencies and consequent increased susceptibility to infection, autoimmunity and autoimmune diseases, hyalinizing renal disease, vascular diseases including arteriosclerosis and atherosclerosis, and amyloidosis. It is to be hoped that mechanisms like those found to underlie dietary prevention of the autoimmune diseases in experimental models may also permit manipulations that will make possible improved treatment or prevention of diseases associated with aging in humans.

T Cell Immunodeficiencies in Malnutrition—A Paradox

In parallel studies, which had been initiated by field observation in Egypt, Uganda, Thailand, and Austrialia, a paradox relating to nutrition and immunity was encountered. In most circumstances, protein or protein-calorie malnutrition (PCM) in the field was accompanied by profound immunodeficiency involving both T cell-mediated immunity and humoral immunity.

Paradoxically, although many antibody responses are deficient in PCM children, Ig levels were not always depressed. Indeed, in many circumstances Ig levels were elevated in children suffering from PCM (81). It is of special concern that in so-called protein calorie malnutrition in field studies, T cell-mediated immunity is usually severely depressed (81). Deficiencies of complement and defects of the effector cellular functions may also be observed in patients with PCM (81). By contrast and paradoxically, in all species studied, especially mice, guinea pigs, rats, and even monkeys, protein or protein-calorie restriction actually increased certain cell-mediated immunodeficiencies. Cell-mediated immunological functions that were actually enhanced by chronic protein or protein-calorie restriction in mice include proliferative responses to T-cell phytomitogens, delayed hypersensitivity, allograft rejection, tumor immunity, and MIF production. By contrast, these studies showed a depression of antibody production reflected by reduction in formation of antibody-producing cells in mice when protein, or protein and calories, were restricted. Whereas most cellular immunity functions were enhanced by dietary restriction in all species studied, antibody production was depressed in almost a linear diet dose-dependent fashion. The paradox to be resolved then was: Why, in contrast to these experimental findings, do protein and protein-calorie malnutrition in humans lead so regularly to profound cell-mediated immunodeficiency?

At least a partial resolution of this apparent paradox has come from the studies of the influence of zinc on immunity function (57, 197). Much of the cell-mediated immunodeficiency seen in the protein malnutrition and

PCM syndromes in humans appears to be attributable to concomitant deficiencies of intake of the element zinc (77, 79), under the circumstances that produce protein and protein-calorie malnutrition in the field. This deficiency does not exist when the circumstances of protein or protein-calorie deficiency are produced in the laboratory (58).

II. THE ROLE OF ZINC IN THE IMMUNE RESPONSE

Two "experiments of nature," one in animals, the other in humans, have provided evidence that adequate supplies of zinc are essential to the development and maintenance of a healthy immune system, particularly the cell-mediated arm of the system. A46 mutant cattle of the Dutch Friesian type inherit an inability to absorb zinc properly. Apparently healthy at birth, within the first few weeks of life they begin to show common signs of the disease, among them lethargy, a scruffy coat with patches of alopecia, tender skin lesions around body orfices and acral areas, bowed hind legs, joint pain, growth arrest, and extreme susceptibility to infection. Supplementary zinc treatment will bring complete and rapid remission, but in the absence of zinc therapy, the calves die at an early age, most of the deaths being due to infection (7, 24, 25, 152, 237).

Postmortem examination of these animals reveals a thymus that is strikingly small and involuted, as well as a generally hypoplastic lymphatic system. Immunological studies (24) have shown that affected calves had normal levels of IgA but significant elevation of IgG_1, IgG_2, and IgM. There was no lymphopenia but increased numbers of large immature lymphocytes. Early antibody response to tetanus toxoid was normal in the sick animals, but late phases of the primary response, measured on days 28 and 42, were diminished. Cell-mediated immune responses against DNCB and tuberculin tests were impaired. Thus, while the cell-mediated immune response is severely impaired in these animals, humoral immunity remains relatively intact. All of the above-mentioned immunological abnormalities in the A46 animals could be corrected, as were other signs of the disease, by adequate amounts of zinc given either orally or parenterally.

Clinical Studies

Acrodermatitis enteropathica (AE) is the human analog of the disease found in A46 cattle. First signs appear during infancy, often at the time of weaning, and include, in part, skin lesions on body extremities and around the orifices, diarrhea and anorexia, alopecia, severe growth retardation, mental disturbances that take the form of extreme irritability, withdrawal and/or lethargy, and easy susceptibility to infection (21, 40, 97–99). Supplementary oral zinc, usually 150 mg given thrice daily in divided doses, can quickly correct all evidence of disease, but without treatment morbidity and mortality are high and death is most often due to infection.

Few precise immunological investigations of children with AE have been undertaken. When done, defective immune structure or function has been found. Autopsy exams have revealed thymuses that were undersized (112, 226), grossly absent (185), or depleted of lymphocytes (162). Lymphocytes obtained from a child dying from AE had decreased responses in vitro to stimulation with PHA (48). Several studies have demonstrated diminished or absent delayed hypersensitivity responses (12, 42, 87, 88, 156, 218). More than 50% of AE patients tested had normal levels of IgG, IgM and IgA, but some deficiencies have been reported (17, 107, 112, 162, 219). Depressed cellular chemotaxis of monocytes in vitro has been reported for three patients with AE (240), an abnormality subsequently corrected with zinc therapy.

Patients with AE suffer from a wide array of complaints, many of them similar to those found in children with severe PCM. And, indeed, there is much shared territory between the two groups (77, 146, 147, 153). Anorexia, a ubiquitous finding in AE patients, who almost always are severely underweight and sometimes described as marasmic, leads to some degree of PCM. PCM patients, in turn, are almost always found with low levels of zinc in their blood (26, 77–80, 120, 123, 194, 233, 247).

Several factors, in addition to low intake of dietary zinc, have been suggested as reasons for the presence of zinc deficiency in children with PCM. These include low levels of plasma proteins, among them albumin and transferrin, which are necessary for the transport of zinc; further intestinal loss of plasma protein or zinc due to diarrhea; metabolic changes caused by infection or stress that result in decreased levels of serum zinc (165, 194, 231); and/or a high dietary intake of zinc-binding fibers or phytate, which reduce the bioavailability of oral zinc (158, 183).

Golden & Golden have been first to study the relationship between zinc and immunoincompetence so regularly found in malnourished children. They found that the thymic atrophy associated with PCM could be reversed when treated with supplementary dietary zinc acetate (80). A subsequent study showed a significant negative correlation between plasma zinc levels in malnourished children and the efficacy of topical zinc sulfate in enhancing the delayed hypersensitivity response (79).

The extreme PCM seen in underdeveloped areas of the world or in chronically ill patients is only one of many examples of an acquired secondary zinc deficiency (see Table 6). Gastrointestinal disorders that cause malabsorption or excess excretion of zinc and/or intake of foods or drugs that chelate zinc and thus hinder its absorption, are other means by which

Table 6 Some means by which zinc deficiency is acquired

Cause or associated condition	References
1. Dietary/nutritional cause	
a. Excess phytate, fiber	150, 175, 183
b. Kwashiorkor[a] + other PCM states	77–80, 105, 123, 233, 247
c. "Marginal" undernutrition	91, 93, 192
d. Infants on formula with no added zinc	111, 230
e. Vegetarian diet	19, 69
2. Gastrointestinal problems	
a. Intestinal mucosal disease[a]	144, 206
b. Malabsorption syndrome	90, 132, 142, 229
c. Intestinal bypass	10, 75, 239
d. Cholecystectomy	216, 238
e. Crohn's disease	130, 204
f. Celiac sprue	205
g. Short bowel syndrome	203
3. Iatrogenic causes	
a. Drugs	
oral contraceptives	90
penicillamine	122
corticosteroids	65, 101
b. Total parenteral nutrition	16, 23, 104, 114–116, 159, 178, 196, 203, 207, 220, 235, 245
c. Major surgery or trauma	20, 75, 89, 127
4. Genetic or congenital defects	
a. Acrodermatitis enteropathica	13, 151
b. Down's syndrome	18, 90, 145
c. Cystic fibrosis	44, 90, 109
5. Infectious disease	50, 90, 127, 165, 202, 227
6. Hematological disease	
a. Hemolytic anemia	174, 200
b. Sickle cell anemia	176, 177
c. Pernicious anemia	187
d. Leukemia	42, 50
e. Hodgkin's disease	1, 11, 76
7. Renal problems	
a. Nephrotic syndrome	221
b. Renal failure	37, 90, 135–139, 186
c. Renal dialysis	9, 90
d. Renal transplants	48
8. Liver disease	
a. Cirrhosis	47, 187, 209, 210, 223–229, 236
b. Other	90

Table 6 *(Continued)*

Cause or associated condition	References
9. Miscellaneous	
a. Pregnancy and lactation	90, 102, 110, 187, 192
b. Alcohol abuse	100, 131, 133, 209, 217, 238, 242
c. Severe burns	28, 36, 39, 103, 124, 157, 173
d. Diabetes mellitus[a]	5, 168, 169, 215
e. Pancreatic defect	242
f. Neoplastic disease[a]	2, 41, 50, 74, 187, 196a, 242
g. Blood loss due to parasitic infection	175, 193
h. Anorexia nervosa	29, 49
i. Psoriasis[a]	82, 83, 171, 172, 244
j. Rheumatoid arthritis	84, 119, 170
k. Myocardial infarction and other heart problems	50, 90, 126
l. Thalassemia	174
m. Lupus erythematosus	129
n. Severe hypogammaglobulinemia	27, 38

[a] denotes inconsistent findings

one can become zinc-deficient. Metabolic conditions resulting from severe burns, surgery, infection, or chronic abuse of alcohol can create a zinc-deficient state. Zinc deficiency is also seen in liver disease, prolonged total parenteral feeding when inadequate amounts of zinc have been added to the solutions, some cancers, and blood loss due, for example, to parasitic infestation.

An acquired zinc deficiency may, in fact, be much more prevalent than commonly realized (3). Recent studies of zinc status in apparently normal Americans have shown that the zinc content of the average American diet may be borderline (91, 92, 230). Currently, the recommended daily allowance for zinc is 15 mg for adults (66), but this allowance is predicated on both normal bioavailability of the zinc ingested and on normal metabolism. Sandstead (192) reported that in the United States those most at risk of consuming too little zinc in their daily diet included some infants (particularly those on a formula unfortified with zinc), pregnant women, teenage and college women on self-selected diets, institutionalized people, and many living on low income diets.

Immunologic studies of patients suffering from iatrogenic zinc deficiency due to inadequate total parenteral nutrition are of special interest because these patients are not simultaneously deficient in either protein or calories. Different reports have found very low levels of IgG (207), impaired skin hypersensitivity (161, 164), decreased numbers of T cells (161), and a depressed response in vitro to mitogenic stimulation (161, 164). All of these abnormalities returned to normal after zinc therapy.

Low levels of serum zinc have also been found in patients with severe hypogammaglobulinemia and one with idiopathic pulmonary fibrosis (38). Oral zinc therapy, in the absence of any other treatment, was associated with an improved lymphoproliferative response to antigens and mitogens in these patients. T and B cell number, including T cells bearing receptors for IgG and IgM, was normal both before and after zinc therapy. Zinc treatment did nothing to improve immunoglobulin levels, but thymopoietin levels, which were low initially, returned to normal in several instances.

In our laboratories, abnormal blood zinc levels have been found in cancer patients, most often when undernutrition was also present (74). Epitheliomas of the head and neck region, which interfere with food intake, were accompanied by low levels of zinc, but not cancer of the breast (73). Immunodeficiencies observed in patients with head or neck cancer were corrected by oral zinc therapy (74). Certain malignancies, however, such as Hodgkin's disease, are associated with low levels of serum zinc that cannot be explained by a dietary deficiency of the trace metal. In these instances abnormal zinc metabolism must be suspected.

The biochemical importance of zinc in the body environment began to be elucidated years ago when it was discovered that zinc was a necessary component of the carbonic anhydrase found in red blood cells (117, 118). Today we know that the proper structure and/or function of more than 90 metalloenzymes depends on the presence of zinc. Included among those metalloenzymes, in addition to carbonic anhydrase, are alkaline phosphatase and many involved in RNA and DNA synthesis, such as thymidine kinase, DNA polymerase and DNA-dependent RNA polymerase (184). With its active participation in protein synthesis and cell division, zinc may be especially important during life stages involving rapid growth and division of cells, such as pregnancy, infancy, and adolescence.

The immune system also depends on rapid proliferation of cells in order to be effective, and it is therefore not surprising to find that, in zinc-deficient men and animals, the function of the immune system is impaired. It has been shown that white blood cells are rich in zinc (222). While red blood cell zinc accounts for 75% of the zinc in whole blood, plasma zinc for 22%, and white blood cell zinc for only 3%, an individual leukocyte contains approximately 25 times the amount of zinc as does a single erythrocyte.

It has likewise been demonstrated that lymphoid cell surface receptors are sensitive to zinc. In vitro addition of small amounts of zinc chloride to lymphocytes derived from both healthy donors and cancer patients has enhanced spontaneous formation of rosettes with SRBC (134). Several studies have attested to the mitogenic effect of zinc when added to lymphocytes in vitro, either by itself or in addition to PHA (6, 15, 31, 72, 95, 96, 121, 166, 167, 182, 189, 190, 243). Zinc is, in fact, the only known naturally occurring lymphocyte mitogen to be found in the body. Recent experiments have demonstrated, however, that its success as a stimulant is dependent on the presence of monocytes (189). It is also apparently an age-dependent phenomenon. Rao et al (182) have reported that lymphocytes derived from young people had more of an enhanced mitogenic response to zinc than did cells derived from older subjects.

Animal Studies

Severe involution of the thymus and other lymphoid tissues have been found in many species of zinc-deficient animals (Table 7). Other aspects of the immune response, particularly those associated with cell-mediated immunity, have also been adversely affected. Circulating thymic hormone levels have been markedly low in A/J mice following three weeks of a zinc-deficient diet. By experimental week number 17, they had disappeared altogether (108). This was promptly corrected, however, when the animals were replenished with zinc. Progressive loss of relative and absolute number of Thy-1.2 cells, with a proportionate increase in the relative number of cells bearing Fc receptors, have been noted in the spleen of mice and rats experimentally deprived of zinc (30, 57).

Investigators have speculated that raised levels of plasma cortisol may contribute to the deterioration of the immune system, as adrenal glands are enlarged in zinc-deprived animals (179, 180), and it is known that the

Table 7   Studies of the thymus in zinc-deficient animals

Animal	Nutritional status	Thymic atrophy present	Reference
A46 cattle	Low weight	+	24, 25
Pigs	Low weight	+	201, 241
Piglets	Low weight	+	143
Rats	Low weight	+	30, 179, 180
S/D rats	Low weight	$-^a$	51
Mice	Low weight	+	57
Mice	Not mentioned; presumed to be low	+	14
BALB/c mice	Low weight	+	71
A/J mice	Low weight	+	213
A/J mice, young adults	Low weight	+	68
Mice, adult	Low weight	+	67

[a] On zinc-supplemented diet, these animals had enlargement of thymus and spleen.

thymus and lymph nodes are adversely affected by hyperadrenocortical activity (45, 195, 234). Recent studies with adrenalectomized mice, however, have established that the depletion of thymic hormone seen in zinc-restricted animals is not due to pituitary adrenal hyperactivity (108a). There are many additional reports of cell-mediated immune irregularities in zinc-deficient animals. Some of these observations include an abnormal migration of circulating lymphocytes (71), an increased number of immature T cells (155), and a diminished mitogenic response in vitro to PHA (85, 163) that could be restored, in one instance, by adding levamisole, an immunostimulatory agent, to the culture (86). Fernandes et al (57) have reported that zinc restriction in mice has a differential effect on T killer cell activity. They noted reduced natural killer cell activity, a normal antibody-dependent cell-mediated cytotoxic response to chicken erythrocytes, and a depressed allogenic cytotoxic T cell response to EL-4 tumor cells after in vivo immunization. Several studies have demonstrated defective T helper cell funtion as well (30, 57, 68, 213).

The humoral immune response of animals experimentally deprived of zinc from weaning has remained more normal than has the cell-mediated response. Activated B cells have proliferated and produced antibody despite exposure to extended periods of zinc restriction (68). In this particular experiment, cells of zinc-restricted mice produced normal numbers of IgM plaques in response to SRBC, but very low levels of IgG, or indirect (T dependent) plaques when compared to control values. Other mice, however, deprived of zinc since the first day of birth (most experiments have initiated zinc restriction at the time of weaning) had dramatically diminished direct splenic plaque-forming cell responses to SRBC. These animals also had highly irregular immunoglobulin levels, with no detectable IgM, $IgG_{2\alpha}$ and IgA, but greatly elevated serum levels of IgG_1 (14).

Individual complement component activity has been influenced, either inhibited or enhanced, by the addition of different levels of zinc chloride in vitro (148, 149). It was thought that zinc had to be present as a reactant during the activation and/or the binding step of each component in order to have an effect (148). Phagocytosis can also be affected by varying levels of cellular zinc in both animals (33–35, 113, 165) and humans (208, 232). It has been suggested that zinc regulates macrophage function through a direct effect on the plasma membrane (32–34) and through its influence on enzymes involved in phagocytic activity (248). Zinc is also able to stimulate macrophage spreading in vitro (181) and to inhibit lysosomal activity (4). Macrophages of rats and guinea pigs have migrated in vitro at a rate inversely proportional to the level of dietary zinc. That is, cells from animals on a low zinc diet migrated most, while those from animals on a high zinc diet migrated the least (248).

Table 8 The immune response in AE and other zinc-deficient states of man and animal

Immunoparameter	Acquired zinc deficiency in humans			A 46 mutant in cattle	Experimental animals deprived of zinc
	Acrodermatitis	PCM	Other		
I. HUMORAL IMMUNITY		Less affected than CMI		Less affected than CMI	Less affected than CMI
B cell number	Generally intact but may be low	Often N	Often N	Normal	Often normal
Immunoglobulins	Generally normal				
IgM	Variable; 55% N	N or ↑	Variable	↑	Highly irregular when Zn^- diet imposed at birth. By 4 wks, no IgM, IgG_2a or IgA; greatly elevated IgG_1 in outbred mice.
IgG	Variable; 62% N	N or ↑	Variable	↑ ($IgG_1 + 2$)	
IgA	Variable; 57% N	↑ or N		↑	
Secretory IgA		Low			
Antibody response					
T independent		Variable; often N		Early response N	Near normal
T dependent		Impaired	Impaired	Late response ↓	Impaired
Autoimmune activity	Some				
II. CELLULAR IMMUNITY	Impaired	Impaired	Impaired	Impaired	Impaired
T cell number	Variable	Reduced	Variable, usu. impaired	Reduced; ↑ no. of large immature lymphocytes	Reduced
T cell function					
Suppressor cell	??	Impaired?	Impaired	?	Impaired
Killer cell					Impaired in vivo; N in vitro with zinc
Helper		Impaired	Impaired	Impaired	Impaired
Delayed hypersensitivity	Impaired	Impaired	Impaired		Impaired
In vitro lymphocyte transformation					
PHA	Variable	Usu. low	Usu. impaired	Reduced; ↑ no. of large immature lymphocytes	Impaired, N or ↑
Con A			Impaired		Impaired
Specific antigens		Low	Impaired		Impaired
Lymphokine production					

SUMMARY

Nutrition exerts profound influence on immunological functions effecting both cell-mediated (humoral) and T cell-mediated (cellular) immune functions. Even the interaction of the immune systems can be profoundly influenced by restrictions or excesses of dietary constituents. In experimental systems where it is possible to control precisely the influence of specific nutriments, development and expression of autoimmune diseases and the associated immunodeficiencies of aging can be delayed by restrictions of dietary protein, protein and calories, fat, zinc, or even essential fatty acids. Tumor immunities likewise can be affected and sometimes even enhanced by restriction of protein, calories, or protein and calories, an influence associated with major delay in development of the experimental cancers— e.g. breast cancer. T cell-mediated immunodeficiencies associated with clinically apparent protein or protein calorie malnutrition are often attributable not to the major nutriment deficiencies per se but to accompanying zinc deficiency, a finding reflecting the vital role of zinc in many immunological functions. Dietary zinc deficiency appears to be responsible, at least in part, for the immunodeficiency that is so regularly associated with certain human cancers, such as epidermoid cancers of the head and neck region.

Literature Cited

1. Addink, N. W. H., Frank, L. J. P. 1955. Zinc in relation to cancer. *Naturwissenschaften* 42:419–20
2. Addink, N. W. H., Frank, L. J. P. 1959. Remarks apropos of analysis of trace elements in human tissues. *Cancer* 12:544–51
3. Aggett, P. J., Harries, J. T. 1979. Current status of zinc in health and disease states. *Arch. Dis. Child.* 54:909–17
4. Aleksandrowicz, J., Astaldi, G., Bodzon, A., Lisiewicz, J., Mysliwiec, D., Sasiadek, U., Strycharska, M., Walewskaczyzewska, M. 1976. Trace elements and immunologic defects: zinc deficiency and activity of lysosomal acid phosphatase in lymphocytes of mice. *Boll. Ist. Sieroter. Milan* 55:195–200
5. Alexander, F. W. 1979. The role of zinc in childhood diabetes mellitus. *Proc. Nutr. Soc.* 38:106A
6. Alford, R. H. 1970. Metal cation requirements for phytohemagglutinin transformation of human peripheral blood lymphocytes. *J. Immunol.* 104:698–703
7. Andresen, E., Basse, A., Brummerstedt, E., Flagstad, T. 1973. Zinc and the immune system in cattle. *Lancet* 1:839–40

8. Andrews, B. S., Eisenberg, R. A., Theofilopoulos, A. N., Izui, S., Wilson, C. B., McConahey, P. J., Murphy, E. D., Roths, J. B., Dixon, F. J. 1978. Spontaneous murine lupus-like syndromes: clinical and immunopathological manifestations in several strains. *J. Exp. Med.* 148:1198–1215
9. Atkin-Thor, E., Goddard, B. W., O'Nion, J., Stephen, R. L., Kolff, W. J. 1978. Hypogeusia and zinc depletion in chronic dialysis patients. *Am. J. Clin. Nutr.* 31:1948–51
10. Atkinson, R. L., Dahms, W. T., Bray, G. A., Jacob, R., Sandstead, H. H. 1978. Plasma zinc and copper in obesity and after intestinal bypass. *Ann. Intern. Med.* 89:491–93
11. Auerbach, S. 1965. Zinc content of plasma, blood and erythrocytes in normal subjects and in patients with Hodgkin's disease and various hematologic disorders. *J. Lab. Clin. Med.* 65:628–37
12. Baird, K. H. 1949. Unusual syndrome associated with Candica albicans infection. *Pediatrics* 4:730–34
13. Barnes, P. M., Moynahan, E. Y. 1973. Zinc deficiency in acrodermatitis enteropathica: multiple dietary intoler-

ance with synthetic diet. *Proc. R. Soc. Med.* 66:327–29

14. Beach, R. S., Gershwin, M. E., Hurley, L. S. 1980. Growth and development in postnatally zinc-deprived mice. *J. Nutr.* 110:201–11

14a. Beach, R. S., Gershwin, M. E., Hurley, L. S. 1981. Nutritional factors and autoimmunity. I. Immunopathology of zinc deprivation in New Zealand mice. *J. Immunol.* 126:1999–2006

15. Berger, N. A., Skinner, A. M. 1974. Characterization of lymphocyte transformation induced by zinc ions. *J. Cell. Biol.* 61:45–55

16. Bernstein, B., Leyden, J. J. 1978. Zinc deficiency and acrodermatitis after intravenous hyperalimentation. *Arch. Dermatol.* 114:1070–72

17. Beyer, P., Wasmer, A., Peter, M., Malfroy, M. L. 1966. Acrodermatitis enteropathica. Observation chez un enfant de 2 ans présentant une carence en beta 2A globulines. *Pediatrie* 21:677–86 (in French)

18. Bjorksten, B., Back, O., Gustavson, K. H., Hallmans, G., Hagglof, B., Tarnvik, A. 1980. Zinc and immune function in Down's syndrome. *Acta Paediatr. Scand.* 69:183–87

19. Bodzy, P. W., Freeland, J. H., Eppright, M. A., Tyree, A. 1977. Zinc status in the vegetarian. *Fed. Proc.* 36:1139 (Abstr.)

20. Bottomley, R. G., Cornelison, R. L., Jacobs, L. A., Lindeman, R. D. 1969. Zinc metabolism following acute tissue injury in man. *J. Lab. Clin. Med.* 74:852 (Abstr.)

21. Brandt, T. 1936. Dermatitis in children with disturbances of the general condition and the absorption of food elements. *Acta Dermatol. Venereol.* 17:513–46

22. Braverman, I. M. 1968. Study of autoimmune disease in New Zealand mice. 1. Genetic features and natural history of NZB, NZY and NZW strains and NZB/NZW hybrids. *J. Invest. Dermatol.* 50:483–99

23. Brazin, S. A., Johnson, W. T., Abramson, L. J. 1979. The acrodermatitis-like syndrome. *Arch. Dermatol.* 115:597–99

24. Brummerstedt, E., Andresen, E., Basse, A., Flagstad, T. 1974. Lethal trait A46 in cattle: immunological investigations. *Nord. Vet. Med.* 26:279–93

25. Brummerstedt, E., Flagstad, T., Basse, A., Andresen, E. 1971. The effect of zinc on calves with hereditary thymus hypoplasia (lethal trait A46). *Acta Pathol. Microbiol. Scand.* A79:686–87

26. Burger, F. J. 1974. Changes in the trace element concentration in the sera and hair of kwashiorkor patients. In *Trace Element Metabolism in Animals,* ed. W. G. Hoekstra, J. W. Suttie, H. E. Ganther, W. Mertz, 2:671–74. Baltimore: University Park Press

27. Caggiano, V., Schnitzler, R., Strauss, W., Baker, R. K., Carter, A. C., Josephson, A. S., Wallach, S. 1969. Zinc deficiency in a patient with retarded growth, hypogonadism, hypogammaglobulinemia and chronic infection. *Am. J. Med. Sci.* 257:305–19

28. Carr, G., Wilkinson, A. W. 1975. Zinc and copper urinary excretion in children with burns and scalds. *Clin. Chim. Acta* 61:199–204

29. Casper, R. C., Kirschner, B., Sandstead, H. H., Jacob, R. A., Davis, J. M. 1980. An evaluation of trace metals, vitamins and taste function in anorexia nervosa. *Am. J. Clin. Nutr.* 33:1801–8

30. Chandra, R. K., Au, B. 1980. Single nutrient deficiency and cell-mediated immune responses. *Am. J. Clin. Nutr.* 33:736–38

31. Chesters, J. K. 1972. The role of zinc ions in the transformation of lymphocytes by phytohemagglutinin. *Biochem. J.* 130:133–39

32. Chvapil, M. 1976. Effect of zinc on cells and biomembranes. *Med. Clin. North Am.* 60:799–812

33. Chvapil, M., Stankova, L., Bernhard, D. S., Weldy, P. L., Carlson, E. C., Campbell, J. B. 1977. Effect of zinc on peritoneal macrophages in vitro. *Infect. Immun.* 16:367–73

34. Chvapil, M., Stankova, L., Zukoski, C. 1977. Inhibition of some functions of polymorphonuclear leukocytes by in vitro zinc. *J. Lab. Clin. Med.* 89:135–46

35. Chvapil, M., Zukoski, C. F., Hattler, B. G., Stankova, L., Montgomery, D., Carlson, E. C., Ludwig, J. C. 1976. Zinc and cells. In *Trace Elements in Health and Disease: Zinc and Copper,* ed. A. S. Prasad, D. Oberleas, 1:269–81. NY: Academic Press

36. Cohen, I. K., Schecter, P. J., Henkin, R. I. 1973. Hypogeusia, anorexia and altered zinc metabolism following thermal burn. *J. Am. Med. Assoc.* 223:914–46

37. Condon, C. J., Freeman, R. M. 1970. Zinc metabolism in renal failure. *Ann. Intern. Med.* 73:531–36

38. Cunningham-Rundles, S., Cunningham-Rundles, C., Dupont, B., Good, R. A. 1980. Zinc-induced activation of hu-

man B lymphocytes. *Clin. Immunol. Immunopathol.* 16:115–122

39. Cuthbertson, D. P., Fell, G. S., Smith, C. M., Tilstone, W. J. 1972. Metabolism after injury. I. Effects of severity, nutrition and environmental temperature on protein, potassium, zinc and creatine. *Br. J. Surg.* 59:925–31

40. Danbolt, N., Closs, K. 1942. Acrodermatitis enteropathica. *Acta Dermatol. Venereol.* 23:127–69

41. Davies, I. J. T. 1972. Plasma-zinc concentration in patients with bronchogenic carcinoma. *Lancet* 1:149

42. Delves, H. T., Alexander, F. W., Lay, H. 1973. Copper and zinc concentration in the plasma of leukaemic children. *Br. J. Haematol.* 24:525–31

44. Dodge, J. A., Yassa, J. G. 1978. Zinc deficiency syndrome in a British youth with cystic fibrosis. *Br. Med. J.* 1:411

45. Dougherty, T. F. 1952. Effect of hormones on lymphatic tissue. *Physiol. Rev.* 32:379–401

46. Dubois, E. L., Strain, L. 1973. Effect of diet on survival and nephropathy of NZB/NZW hybrid mice. *Biochem. Med.* 7:336–42

47. Ecker, R. I., Schroeter, A. L. 1978. Acrodermatitis and acquired zinc deficiency. *Arch. Dermatol.* 114:937–39

48. Ellis, L. 1978. Serum zinc levels and urinary zinc excretion in patients with renal transplants. *Clin. Chim. Acta* 82:105–11

49. Endre, L., Zoltan, K., Kalman, G., Szabo, E. 1977. The role of zinc deficiency and immunopathological changes in the pathogenesis of acrodermatitis enteropathica. *Orv. Hetil.* 118:2033–35 (In Hungarian)

50. Esca, S. A., Brenner, W., Mach, K., Gschnait, F. 1979. Kwashiorkor-like zinc deficiency syndrome in anorexia nervosa. *Acta Dermatol. Venereol. Stockh.* 59:361–64

51. Falchuk, K. H. 1977. Effect of acute disease and ACTH on serum zinc proteins. *N. Engl. J. Med.* 296:1129–34

52. Fang, M., Kilgore, L., Lei, K. Y. 1978. Effects of zinc deficiency on dental caries and immune responses in rats. *Fed. Proc.* 37:584 (Abstr.)

53. Faulk, W. P. 1975. Effects of malnutrition on the immune response in humans: a review. *Trop. Dis. Bull.* 72:89–103

54. Faulk, W. P., Demaeyer, E. M., Davies, A. J. S. 1974. Some effects of malnutrition on the immune response in man. *Am. J. Clin. Nutr.* 27:638–46

55. Fernandes, G., Friend, P., Yunis, E. J., Good, R. A. 1978. Influence of dietary restriction on immunologic function and renal disease in (NZB X NZW)F1 mice. *Proc. Natl. Acad. Sci. USA* 75:1500–4

56. Fernandes, G., Good, R. A. 1979. Alterations of longevity and immune function of B/W and MRL/1 mice by restriction of dietary intake. *Fed. Proc.* 38:1370 (Abstr.)

57. Fernandes, G., Nair, M., Onoe, K., Tanaka, T., Floyd, R., Good, R. A. 1979. Impairment of cell-mediated immunity functions by dietary zinc deficiency in mice. *Proc. Natl. Acad. Sci. USA* 76:457–61

58. Fernandes, G., West, A., Good, R. A. 1979. Nutrition, immunity, and cancer —a review. Part III: Effects of diet on the diseases of aging. *Clin. Bull. MSKCC* 9:91–106

59. Fernandes, G., Yunis, E. J., Good, R. A. 1976. Influence of protein restriction on immune functions in NZB mice. *J. Immunol.* 116:782–90

60. Fernandes, G., Yunis, E. J., Good, R. A. 1976. The influence of diet on survival of mice. *Proc. Natl. Acad. Sci. USA* 73:1279–83

61. Fernandes, G., Yunis, E. J., Good, R. A. 1976. Suppression of adenocarcinoma by the immunological consequences of calorie restriction. *Nature* 263:504–7

62. Fernandes, G., Yunis, E. J., Jose, D. G., Good, R. A. 1973. Dietary influence on antinuclear antibodies and cell-mediated immunity in NZB mice. *Int. Arch. Allergy Appl. Immunol.* 44:770–82

63. Fernandes, G., Yunis, E. J., Miranda, M., Smith, J., Good, R. A. 1978. Nutritional inhibition of genetically determined renal disease and autoimmunity with prolongation of life in *Kd/Kd* mice. *Proc. Natl. Acad. Sci. USA* 75:2888–92

64. Fernandes, G., Yunis, E. J., Smith, J., Good, R. A. 1972. Dietary influence on breeding behaviour, hemolytic anemia, and longevity in NZB mice. *Proc. Soc. Exp. Biol. Med.* 139:1189–96

65. Flynn, A., Pories, W. J., Strain, W. H., Hill, O. A., Fratianne, R. B. 1971. Rapid serum-zinc depletion associated with corticosteroid therapy. *Lancet* 2:1169–72

66. Food and Nutrition Board. 1974. *Recommended Dietary Allowance.* Washington DC: Natl. Acad. Sci. 8th rev. ed.

67. Fraker, P. J., DePasquale-Jardieu, P., Zwickl, C. M., Luecke, R. W. 1978. Regeneration of T-cell helper function in zinc deficient adult mice. *Proc. Natl. Acad. Sci. USA* 75:5660–64

68. Fraker, P. J., Haas, S. M., Luecke, R. W. 1977. Effect of zinc deficiency on the immune response of the young adult A/J mouse. *J. Nutr.* 107:1889–95

69. Freeland-Graves, J. H., Ebangit, M. L., Hendrikson, P. J. 1980. Alterations in zinc absorption and salivary sediment zinc after a lacto-ovo-vegetarian diet. *Am. J. Clin. Nutr.* 33:1757–66

70. Friend, P. S., Fernandes, G., Good, R. A., Michael, A. F., Yunis, E. J. 1978. Dietary restrictions early and late: effects on the nephropathy of the NZB X NZW mouse. *Lab. Invest.* 38:629–32

71. Frost, P., Chen, J. C., Rabbani, I., Smith, J., Prasad, A. S. 1977. The effect of zinc deficiency on the immune response. In *Zinc Metabolism: Current Aspects in Health and Disease,* ed. G. J. Brewer, A. S. Prasad, pp. 143–50. NY: Alan R. Liss, Inc.

72. Gallagher, K., Matarazzo, W., Gray, I. 1978. Trace metal modification of lymphocyte transformation in vitro. *Fed. Proc.* 37:377

73. Garofalo, J. A., Ashikari, H., Lesser, M. L., Menendez-Botet, C., Cunningham-Rundles, S., Schwartz, M. K., Good, R. A. 1980. Serum zinc, and the Cu/Zn ration in patients with benign and malignant breast lesions. *Cancer* 46:2682–85

74. Garofalo, J. A., Erlandson, E., Strong, E., Lesser, M., Gerold, F., Spiro, R., Schwartz, M., Good, R. A. 1980. Serum zinc, serum copper, and the Cu/Zn ratio in patients with epidermoid cancers of the head and neck. *J. Surg. Oncol.* 15:381–86

75. Garofalo, J. A., Strong, E., Good, R. A. 1979. Zinc deficiency and intestinal bypass procedures. *Ann. Intern. Med.* 90:990 (Letter)

76. Gobbi, P. G., Scarpellini, M., Minoia, C., Pozzoli, L., Perugini, S. 1978. Plasma zinc levels in Hodgkin's disease. Evaluation of 37 cases. *Haematologica* 63:143–55

77. Golden, B. E., Golden, M. H. N. 1979. Plasma zinc and the clinical features of malnutrition. *Am. J. Clin. Nutr.* 32:2490–94

78. Golden, B. E., Golden, M. H. N. 1979. Zinc deficiency during recovery from malnutrition. *J. Nutr.* 24:32 (Abstr. #88)

79. Golden, M. H. N., Golden, B. E., Harland, P. S. E. G., Jackson, A. A. 1978. Zinc and immunocompetence in protein-energy malnutrition. *Lancet* 1:1226–28

80. Golden, M. H. N., Golden, B. E., Jackson, A. A. 1977. Effect of zinc on thymus of recently malnourished children. *Lancet* 2:1057–59

81. Good, R. A., Fernandes, G., West, A. 1979. Nutrition, immunity and cancer —a review. Part I.: Influence of protein or protein-calorie malnutrition and zinc deficiency on immunity function. *Clin. Bull. MSKCC* 9:3–12

82. Greaves, M. W. 1972. Zinc and copper in psoriasis. *Br. J. Dermatol.* 86:439–40

83. Greaves, M. W., Boyde, T. R. C. 1967. Plasma zinc concentrations in patients with psoriasis, other dermatosis and venous ulcerations. *Lancet* 2:1019–20

84. Grennan, D. M., Knudson, J. M. L., Dunckley, J., MacKinnon, M. J., Myers, D. B., Palmer, D. G. 1980. Serum copper and zinc in rheumatoid arthritis and osteoarthritis. *N. Z. Med. J.* 91:47–50

85. Gross, R. L., Osdin, N., Fong, L., Newberne, P. M. 1979. Depressed immunological function in zinc-deprived rats as measured by mitogen response of spleen, thymus, and peripheral blood. *Am. J. Clin. Nutr.* 32:1260–65

86. Gross, R. L., Osdin, N., Fong, L., Newberne, P. M. 1979. In vitro restoration by levamisole of mitogen responsiveness in zinc deprived rats. *Am. J. Clin. Nutr.* 32:1267–71

87. Guimaraes, O. P., Viana, R. 1959. Enteropathic acrodermatitis—presentation of a case. *J. Pediat. (Rio)* 24:352–64 (in Spanish)

88. Guiraldes, E., Sorensen, R., Gutierrez, C., Cofre, P., Gonzalez, B. 1975. Zinc sulphate for acrodermatitis enteropathica. *Lancet* 2:710–11

89. Hallbook, T., Hedelin, H. 1978. Changes in serum zinc and copper induced by operative trauma and effects of pre- and post-operative zinc infusion. *Acta Chir. Scand.* 144:423–26

90. Halsted, J. A., Smith, J. C. Jr. 1970. Plasma zinc in health and disease. *Lancet* 1:322–24

91. Hambidge, K. M., Hambidge, C., Jacobs, M., Baum, J. D. 1972. Low levels of zinc in hair, anorexia, poor growth, and hypogeusia in children. *Pediatr. Res.* 6:868–74

92. Hambidge, K. M., Walravens, P. A. 1976. Zinc deficiency in infants and preadolescent children. In *Trace Ele-*

ments in Human Health and Disease, ed. A. S. Prasad, D. Oberleas, pp. 21–31. NY: Academic Press

93. Hambidge, K. M., Walravens, P. A., Brown, R. M., Webster, J., White, S., Anthony, M., Roth, M. L. 1976. Zinc nutrition of preschool children in the Headstart program. *Am. J. Clin. Nutr.* 29:734–38

94. Hansen, M. A., Fernandes, G., Yunis, E. J., Cooper, W. C., Jose, D. G., Kramer, T., Good, R. A. 1981. Infection in the special host: the severely malnourished host. In *Immunology of Human Infection,* ed. A. J. Nahmias, R. O'-Reilly. NY: Plenum. In press

95. Hart, D. A. 1978. Effect of zinc chloride on hamster lymphoid cells: mitogenicity and differential enhancement of lipopolysaccharide stimulation of lymphocytes. *Infec. Immun.* 19:457–61

96. Hart, D. A. 1979. Augmentation of zinc ion stimulation of lymphoid cells by calcium and lithium. *Exp. Cell. Res.* 121:419–25

97. Heite, H.-J., Ody, R. 1965. Die Acrodermatitis Enteropathica im Lichte der Häufigkeitsanalyse. *Hautarzt* 16:529–34 (In German)

98. Heite, H.-J., Ody, R. 1966. Die Acrodermatitis Enteropathica im Lichte der Häufigkeitsanalyse. *Hautarzt* 17:1–7 (In German)

99. Heite, H.-J., Ody, R. 1966. Die Acrodermatitis Enteropathica im Lichte der Häufigkeitsanalyse. *Hautarzt* 17: 49–53 (In German)

100. Helwig, H. L., Hoffer, E. M., Thielen, W. C., Alcocer, A. E., Hotelling, D. R., Rogers, W. H., Lench, J. 1966. Urinary and serum zinc levels in chronic alcoholism. *Am. J. Clin. Pathol.* 45:156–59

101. Henkin, R. I., Metet, S., Jacobs, J. B. 1969. Steroid dependent changes in copper and zinc metabolism. *J. Clin. Invest.* 48:38A

102. Henkin, R. I., Schecter, P. J., Hoye, R., Mattern, C. F. T. 1971. Idiopathic hypogeusia with dysgeusia, hyposmia and dysosmia: a new syndrome. *J. Am. Med. Assoc.* 217:434–40

103. Henzel, J. H., DeWeese, M. S., Lichti, E. I. 1970. Zinc concentrations in healing wounds. *Arch. Surg.* 100:349–57

104. Holbrook, I. B., Milewski, P. J., Clark, C., Shipley, K. 1980. Low serum zinc and long-term intravenous feeding. *Am. J. Clin. Nutr.* 33:1891–92

105. Holt, A. B., Spargo, R. M., Iveson, J. B., Faulkner, G. S., Cheek, D. B. 1980. Serum and plasma zinc, copper and iron concentrations in Aboriginal communi-ties of North Western Australia. *Am. J. Clin. Nutr.* 33:119–36

105a. Hurd, E. R., Johnston, J. M., Okita, J. R., MacDonald, P. C., Ziff, M., Gilliam, J. N. 1981. Prevention of glomerulonephritis and prolonged survival in New Zealand black/New Zealand white F1 hybrid mice fed an essential fatty acid-deficient diet. *J. Clin. Invest.* 67:476–85

106. Ibrahim, A. B., Gardner, M. B., Levy, J. A. 1980. Influence of dietary fat on immune complex disease and immunologic function. *Fed. Proc.* 39:4554 (Abstr.)

107. Idriss, Z. H., der Kaloustian, V. M. 1973. Acrodermatitis enteropathica. *Clin. Pediatr.* 12:393–95

108. Iwata, T., Incefy, G. S., Tanaka, T., Fernandes, G., Menendez-Botet, C. J., Pih, K., Good, R. A. 1979. Circulating thymic hormone levels in zinc deficiency. *Cell. Immunol.* 47:100–5

108a. Iwata, T., Incefy, G. S., Tanaka, T., Fernandes, G., Menendez-Botet, C. J., Pih, K., Good, R. A. 1979. Circulating thymic hormone levels in zinc deficiency. *Cell. Immunol.* 47:100–5

109. Jacob, R. A., Sandstead, H. H., Solomons, N. W., Rieger, C., Rothberg, R. 1978. Zinc status and vitamin A transport in cystic fibrosis. *Am. J. Clin. Nutr.* 31:638–44

110. Jameson, S. 1976. *Effects of Zinc Deficiency in Human Reproduction. Acta Med. Scand.* Suppl. 593:1–64. Linkoping: Linkoping Univ. Dissertations #37

111. Johnson, P. E., Evans, G. W. 1978. Relative zinc availability in human breast milk, infant formulas, and cow's milk. *Am. J. Clin. Nutr.* 31:416–21

112. Julius, R., Schulkind, M., Sprinkle, T., Rennert, O. 1973. Acrodermatitis enteropathica with immune deficiency. *J. Pediatr.* 83:1007–11

113. Karl, L., Chvapil, M., Zukoski, C. F. 1973. Effect of zinc on the viability and phagocytic capacity of peritoneal macrophages. *Proc. Soc. Exper. Biol. Med.* 142:1123–27

114. Katoh, T., Igarashi, M., Ohhashi, E., Ohi, R., Hebiguchi, T., Seiji, M. 1976. Acrodermatitis-like eruption associated with parenteral nutrition. *Dermatologica* 152:119–27

115. Kay, R. G., Tasman-Jones, C. T. 1975. Zinc deficiency and intravenous feeding. *Lancet* 1:605

116. Kay, R. G., Tasman-Jones, C., Pybus, J., Whiting, R., Black, H. 1976. A syndrome of acute zinc deficiency during

total parenteral alimentation in man. *Ann. Surg.* 4:331–40

117. Keilin, D., Mann, T. 1939. Carbonic anhydrase. *Nature* 144:442–43

118. Keilin, D., Mann, T. 1940. Carbonic anhydrase. Purification and nature of the enzyme. *Biochem. J.* 34:1163

119. Kennedy, A. C., Fell, G. S., Rooney, P. J., Stevens, W. H., Dick, W. C., Buchanan, W. W. 1975. Zinc: its relationship to osteoporosis in rheumatoid arthritis. *Scand. J. Rheum.* 4:243–45

120. Khalil, M., Kabiel, A., El-Khateeb, S., Aref, K., El Lozy, M., Jahin, S., Nasr, F. 1974. Plasma and red cell water and elements in protein-calorie malnutrition. *Am. J. Clin. Nutr.* 27:260–67

121. Kirchner, H., Ruhl, H. 1970. Stimulation of human peripheral lymphocytes by Zn^{2+} in vitro. *Exp. Cell Res.* 61:229–30

122. Klingberg, W. G., Prasad, A. S., Oberleas, D. 1976. Zinc deficiency following penicillamine therapy. In *Trace Elements in Human Health and Disease,* ed. A. S. Prasad, D. Oberleas, 1:51–65. NY: Academic

123. Kumar, S., Rao, K. S. J. 1973. Plasma and erythrocyte zinc levels in protein calorie malnutrition. *Nutr. Metabol.* 15:364–71

124. Larson, D. L., Maxwell, R., Abston, S., Dobrkovsky, M. 1970. Zinc deficiency in burned children. *Plast. Reconstr. Surg.* 46:13–21

125. Levy, J. A. 1974. Autoimmunity and neoplasia—possible role of C-type viruses. *Am. J. Clin. Pathol.* 62:258–80

126. Levy, J. A., Pincus, T. 1970. Demonstration of biological activity of a murine leukemia virus of New Zealand black mice. *Science* 170:326–27

127. Lindeman, R. D., Bottomley, R. G., Cornelison, R. L. Jr., Jacobs, L. A. 1972. Influence of acute tissue injury on zinc metabolism in man. *J. Lab. Clin. Med.* 79:452–60

128. Lyon, M. R., Hulse, E. V. 1971. An inherited kidney disease of mice resembling human nephronophthisis. *J. Med. Genet.* 8:41–48

129. McCall, J. T., Goldstein, N. P., Smith, L. H. 1971. Implications of trace metals in human disease. *Fed. Proc.* 30:1011 (Abstr.)

130. McClain, C., Soutor, C., Zieve, L. 1980. Zinc deficiency: a complication of Crohn's disease. *Gastroenterology* 78:272–79

131. McClain, C. J., Van Thiel, D. H., Parker, S., Badzin, L. K., Gilbert, H. 1979. Alterations in zinc, vitamin A and retinol binding protein in chronic alcoholics: a possible mechanism for night blindness and hypogonadism. *Alcoholism (NY)* 3:135–41

132. MacMahon, R. A., Lemoine, P. M., McKinnon, M. C. 1968. Zinc treatment in malabsorption. *Med. J. Aust* 2:210–12

133. McDonald, J. T., Margen, S. 1980. Wine versus ethanol in human nutrition. IV. Zinc balance. *Am. J. Clin. Nutr.* 33:1096–1102

134. McMahon, L. J., Montgomery, D. W., Guschewsky, A., Woods, A. H., Zukoski, C. F. 1976. In vitro effects of ZnCl on spontaneous sheep red blood cell (E rosette) formation by lymphocytes from cancer patients and normal subjects. *Immunol. Commun.* 5:53–57

135. Mahajan, S. K., Gardiner, W. H., Abbasi, A. A., Briggs, W. A., Prasad, A. S., McDonald, F. D. 1978. Abnormal plasma and erythrocyte zinc distribution in uremia. *Trans. Am. Soc. Artif. Intern. Organs* 24:50–54

136. Mahajan, S. K., Prasad, A. S., Lambujon, J., Abbasi, A. A., Briggs, W. A., McDonald, F. D. 1979. Improvement of uremic hypogeusia by zinc. *Trans. Am. Soc. Artif. Intern. Organs* 25:443–48

137. Mahajan, S. K., Prasad, A. S., Rabbani, P., Briggs, W. A., McDonald, F. D. 1979. Zinc metabolism in uremia. *J. Lab. Clin. Med.* 94:693–98

138. Mahajan, S. K., Prasad, A. S., Lambujon, J., Abbasi, A. A., Briggs, W. A., McDonald, F. D. 1980. Improvement of uremic hypogeusia by zinc: a double blind study. *Am. J. Clin. Nutr.* 33:1517–21

139. Mansouri, K., Halsted, J. A., Gombos, E. A. 1970. Zinc, copper, magnesium and calcium in dialyzed and nondialyzed uremic patients. *Arch. Intern. Med.* 125:88–93

140. Mata, L. J. 1971. Nutrition and infection. *Protein Advis. Grp. Bull.* 11:18–21

141. Mata, L. J. 1975. Malnutrition-infection interactions in the tropics. *Am. J. Trop. Med. Hyg.* 24:564–74

142. Meyer, G. 1979. Intestinal bypass and zinc. *Ann. Intern. Med.* 90:278 (Letter)

143. Miller, E. R., Luecke, R. W., Ullrey, D. E., Baltzer, B. V., Bradley, B. L., Hoefer, J. A. 1968. Biochemical, skeletal, and allometric changes due to zinc deficiency in the baby pig. *J. Nutr.* 95:278–86

144. Mills, P. R., Fell, G. S. 1979. Zinc and

inflammatory bowel disease. *Am. J. Clin. Nutr.* 32:2172–73

145. Milunsky, A., Hackley, B. M., Halsted, J. A. 1970. Plasma, erythrocyte and leukocyte zinc levels in Down's syndrome. *J. Ment. Defic. Res.* 14:99–105

146. Montagnani, A. 1964. L'Acrodermatitis enteropatica. Suoi rapporti con il m. celiaco ed il kwashiorkor. *Dermatol. Int. (Napoli)* 15:210–24 (In Italian)

147. Montagnani, A. 1966. Rapporti tra acrodermatite enteropatica, morbo celiaco e kwashiorkor. *Dermatol. Int. (Napoli)* 5:55–58 (In Italian)

148. Montgomery, D. W., Chvapil, M., Zukoski, C. F. 1979. Effects of zinc chloride on guinea pig complement component activity in vitro: concentration dependent inhibition and enhancement. *Infect. Immun.* 23:424–31

149. Montgomery, D., Don, L., Zukoski, C., Chvapil, M. 1974. The effect of zinc and other metals on complement hemolysis of sheep red blood cells in vitro. *Proc. Soc. Exp. Biol. Med.* 145:263–67

150. Morris, E. R., Ellis, R. 1980. Effect of dietary phytate/zinc molar ratio on growth and bone zinc response of rats fed semipurified diets. *J. Nutr.* 110:1037–45

151. Moynahan, E. J. 1974. Acrodermatitis enteropathica: a lethal inherited human zinc deficiency disorder. *Lancet* 2:399–400

152. Moynahan, E. J. 1975. Zinc deficiency and cellular immune deficiency in acrodermatitis enteropathica in man and zinc deficiency with thymic hypoplasia in Freisian calves: a possible genetic link. *Lancet* 2:710 (Letter)

153. Moynahan, E. J. 1976. Zinc deficiency and disturbances of mood and visual behaviour. *Lancet* 1:91

154. Nakagawa, I., Sasaki, A., Kajimoto, M., Fukuyama, T., Suzuki, T., Yamada, E. 1974. Effect of protein nutrition on growth, longevity and incidence of lesions in the rat. *J. Nutr.* 104:1576–83

155. Nash, L., Iwata, T., Fernandes, G., Good, R. A., Incefy, G. S. 1979. Effect of zinc deficiency on autologous rosette-forming cells. *Cell. Immunol.* 48:238–43

156. Neimann, N., Pierson, M., Manciaux, M., Vert, P. 1963. Acrodermatitis enteropathica. *Ann. Pediatr.* 39:13–18

157. Nielsen, S. P., Jemec, B. 1968. Zinc metabolism in patients with severe burns. *Scand. J. Plast. Reconstr. Surg.* 2:47–52

158. O'Dell, B. L., Savage, J. E. 1960. Effect of phytic acid on zinc availability. *Proc. Soc. Exp. Biol. Med.* 103:304–6

159. Okada, A., Takagi, Y., Itakura, T., Satani, M., Manobe, H., Iida, Y., Tanigaki, T., Iwasaki, M., Kasahara, N. 1976. Skin lesions during intravenous hyperalimentation: zinc deficiency. *Surgery* 80:629–35

160. Oldstone, M. B. A., Dixon, F. J. 1969. Pathogenesis of chronic disease associated with persistent lymphocytic choriomeningitis viral infection. I. Relationship of antibody production to disease in neonatally infected mice. *J. Exp. Med.* 129:483–99

161. Oleske, J. M., Westphal, M. L., Shore, S., Gorden, D., Bogden, J. D., Nahmias, A. 1979. Zinc therapy of depressed cellular immunity in acrodermatitis enteropathica. Its correction. *Am. J. Dis. Child.* 133:915–18

162. Pass, R. F., Johnston, R. B. Jr., Cooper, M. D. 1974. Agammaglobulinemia with B lymphocytes in a neonate with acrodermatitis enteropathica. *Am. J. Dis. Child.* 128:251–53

163. Pekarek, R. S., Powanda, M. C., Hoagland, A. M. 1977. Effect of zinc deficiency on the immune response of the rat. *Fed. Proc.* 36:859 (Abstr.)

164. Pekarek, R. S., Sandstead, H. H., Jacob, R. A., Barcome, D. F. 1979. Abnormal cellular immune responses during acquired zinc deficiency. *Am. J. Clin. Nutr.* 32:1466–71

165. Pekarek, R. S., Wannemacher, R. W. Jr., Beisel, W. R. 1972. The effect of leukocytic endogenous mediator (LEM) on the tissue distribution of zinc and iron. *Proc. Soc. Exp. Biol. Med.* 140:685–88

166. Phillips, J. L., 1978. Uptake of transferrin-bound zinc by human lymphocytes. *Cell. Immunol.* 35:318–29

167. Phillips, J. L., Azari, P. 1974. Zinc transferrin, enhancement of nucleic acid synthesis in phytohemagglutinin stimulated human lymphocytes. *Cell. Immunol.* 10:31–37

168. Pidduck, H. G., Wren, P. J. J., Price-Evans, D. A. 1970. Plasma zinc and copper in diabetes mellitus. *Diabetes* 19:234–39

169. Pidduck, H. G., Wren, P. J. J., Price-Evans, D. A. 1970. Hyperzincuria of diabetes mellitus and possible genetical implications of this observation. *Diabetes* 19:240–47

170. Plantin, L. O., Strandberg, P. O. 1965. Whole-blood concentrations of copper and zinc in rheumatoid arthritis studied by activation analysis. *Acta Rheum. Scand.* 11:30–34

171. Portnoy, B., Molokhia, M. M. 1971. Zinc and copper in psoriasis. *Br. J. Dermatol.* 85:597

172. Portnoy, B., Molokhia, M. M. 1972. Zinc and copper in psoriasis. *Br. J. Dermatol.* 86:205

173. Powanda, M. C., Villarreal, Y., Rodriguez, E., Braxton, G. III, Kennedy, C. R. 1980. Redistribution of zinc within burned and burned infected rats. *Proc. Soc. Exp. Biol. Med.* 163:296–301

174. Prasad, A. S., Diwany, M., Gabr, M., Sandstead, H. H., Mokhtar, N., El Hefney, A. 1965. Biochemical studies in thalassemia. *Ann. Intern. Med.* 62:87–96

175. Prasad, A. S., Miale, A. Jr., Farid, Z., Sandstead, H. H., Schulert, A. R., Darby, W. J. 1963. Biochemical studies on dwarfism, hypogonadism and anemia. *Arch. Intern. Med.* 111:407–28

176. Prasad, A. S., Rabbani, P., Worth, J. A. 1979. Effect of zinc on hyperammonemia in sickle cell anemia subjects. *Am. J. Hematol.* 7:323–27

177. Prasad, A. S., Schoomaker, E. B., Ortega, J., Brewer, G. J., Oberleas, D., Oelshlegel, F. J. 1975. Zinc deficiency in sickle cell disease. *Clin. Chem.* 21: 582–87

178. Principi, N., Giunta, A., Gervasoni, A. 1979. The role of zinc in total parenteral nutrition. *Acta Paediatr. Scand.* 68: 129–32

179. Quarterman, J. 1974. The effects of zinc deficiency or excess on the adrenals and the thymus in the rat. In *Trace Element Metabolism in Animals,* ed. W. G. Hoekstra, J. W. Suttie, H. E. Ganther, W. Mertz, 2:742–44. Baltimore: University Park Press

180. Quarterman, J., Humphries, W. R. 1979. Effect of zinc deficiency and zinc supplementation on adrenals, plasma steroids and thymus in rats. *Life Sci.* 24:177–83

181. Rabinovitch, M., DeStafano, M. J. 1973. Macrophage spreading in vitro. I. Inducers of spreading. *Exp. Cell Res.* 77:323–34

182. Rao, K. M., Schwartz, S. A., Good, R. D. 1979. Age dependent effects of zinc on the transformation response of human lymphocytes to mitogens. *Cell. Immunol.* 42:270–78

183. Reinhold, J. G., Parsa, S., Karimian, N., Hammick, J. W., Ismail-Beigi, F. 1974. Availability of zinc in leavened and unleavened wholemeal wheaten breads as measured by solubility and uptake by rat intestine in vivo. *J. Nutr.* 104:976–82

184. Riordan, J. F. 1976. Biochemistry of zinc. *Med. Clin. N. Am.* 60:661–74

185. Rodin, A. E., Goldman, A. S. 1969. Autopsy findings in acrodermatitis enteropathica. *Am. J. Clin. Pathol.* 51: 315–22

186. Rose, G. A., Willden, E. G. 1972. Whole blood, red cell and plasma total and ultrafiltrable zinc levels in normal subjects and patients with chronic renal failure with and without haemodialysis. *Br. J. Urol.* 44:281–86

187. Rosner, F., Gorfien, P. C. 1968. Erythrocyte and plasma zinc and magnesium levels in health and disease. *J. Lab. Clin. Med.* 72:213–19

188. Ross, M. H. 1976. Nutrition and longevity in experimental animals. *Curr. Concepts Nutr.* 4:43–57

189. Ruhl, H., Kirchner, H. 1978. Monocyte-dependent stimulation of human T cells by zinc. *Clin. Exp. Immunol.* 32:484–88

190. Ruhl, H., Kirchner, H., Bochert, G. 1971. Kinetics of the Zn^{2+} stimulation of human peripheral lymphocytes in vitro. *Proc. Soc. Exp. Biol. Med.* 137: 1089–92

191. Safai-Kutti, S., Fernandes, G., Wang, Y., Safai, B., Good, R. A., Day, N. K. 1980. Reduction of circulating immune complexes by calorie restriction in $(NZBxNZW)F_1$ mice. *Clin. Immunol. Immunopathol.* 15:293–300

192. Sandstead, H. H. 1973. Zinc nutrition in the United States. *Am. J. Clin. Nutr.* 26:1251–60

193. Sandstead, H. H., Prasad, A. S., Schulert, A. R., Farid, Z., Miale, A. Jr., Bassilly, S., Darby, W. J. 1967. Human zinc deficiency, endocrine manifestations and response to treatment. *Am. J. Clin. Nutr.* 20:422–42

194. Sandstead, H. H., Shukry, A. S., Prasad, A. S., Gabr, M. K., Hifney, A. E., Mokhtar, N., Darby, W. J. 1965. Kwashiorkor in Egypt. I. Clinical and biochemical studies, with special reference to plasma zinc and serum lactic dehydrogenase. *Am. J. Clin. Nutr.* 17:15–26

195. Santisteban, G. A., Dougherty, T. F. 1954. Comparison of the influences of adrenocortical hormones on the growth and involution of lymphatic organs. *Endocrinology* 54:130–46

196. Schlappner, O. L. A., Shelley, W. B., Ruberg, R. L., Dudrick, S. J. 1972. Acute papulopustular acne associated with prolonged intravenous hyperalimentation. *J. Am. Med. Assoc.* 219: 877–80

196a. Schwartz, M. K. 1975. Role of trace elements in cancer. *Cancer Res.* 35: 3481–87

197. Schloen, L. H., Fernandes, G., Garofalo, J. A., Good, R. A. 1979. Nutrition, immunity and cancer—a review. Part II. Zinc, immune function and cancer. *Clin. Bull. MSKCC* 9: 63–75

198. Schwartz, A. G. 1979. Inhibition of spontaneous breast cancer formation in female C3H(A$^{vy/a}$) mice by long-term treatment with dehydroepiandrosterone. *Cancer Res.* 37:1129

199. Scrimshaw, N. S., Taylor, C. E., Gordon, J. E. 1968. *Interactions of Nutrition and Infection.* Geneva: World Health Organization

200. Serjeant, G. R., Galloway, R. E., Gueri, M. C. 1970. Oral zinc sulfate in sickle cell ulcers. *Lancet* 2:891–93

201. Shanklin, S. H., Miller, E. R., Ullrey, D. E., Hoefer, J. A., Luecke, R. W. 1968. Zinc requirement of baby pigs on casein diet. *J. Nutr.* 96:101–8

202. Sinha, S. N., Gabrieli, E. R. 1970. Serum copper and zinc in various pathological conditions. *Am. J. Clin. Pathol.* 54:570–77

203. Smith, S. Z. 1977. Skin changes in short-bowel syndrome: kwashiorkor-like syndrome. *Arch. Dermatol.* 113: 657–59

204. Solomons, N. W., Elson, C. O., Pekarek, R. S., Jacob, R. A., Sandstead, H. H., Rosenberg, I. H. 1978. Leukocytic endogenous mediator in Crohn's disease. *Infect. Immun.* 22:637–39

205. Solomons, N. W., Rosenberg, I. H., Sandstead, H. H. 1976. Zinc nutrition in celiac sprue. *Am. J. Clin. Nutr.* 29:371–75

206. Solomons, N. W., Vo-Khactu, K., Sandstead, H., Rosenberg, I. H. 1974. Zinc nutrition in inflammatory bowel disease. In *Fifth World Congress of Gastroenterology Abstracts*, p. 263. Mexico City: Mexican Soc. Gastroenterol.

207. Srouji, M. N., Balistreri, W. F., Caleb, M. H., South, M. A., Starr, S. 1978. Zinc deficiency during parenteral nutrition: skin manifestations and immune competence in a premature infant. *J. Pediatr. Surg.* 13:570–75

208. Stankova, L., Drach, G. W., Hicks, T., Zukoski, C. F., Chvapil, M. 1976. Regulation of some functions of granulocytes by zinc of the prostatic fluid and prostate tissue. *J. Lab. Clin. Med.* 88:640–48

209. Sullivan, J. F., Lankford, H. G. 1962. Urinary excretion of zinc in alcoholism

and postalcoholic cirrhosis. *Am. J. Clin. Nutr.* 10:153–57

210. Sullivan, J. F., Williams, R. V., Burch, R. E. 1979. The metabolism of zinc and selenium in cirrhotic patients during six weeks of zinc ingestion. *Alcoholism (NY)* 3:235–39

211. Talal, N., ed. 1977. *Autoimmunity. Genetic, Immunologic, Virologic and Clinical Aspects.* NY: Academic Press

212. Talal, N., Steinberg, A. D. 1974. The pathogenesis of autoimmunity in New Zealand Black mice. *Curr. Top. Microbiol. Immunol.* 64:79–103

213. Tanaka, T., Fernandes, G., Tsao, C., Pih, K., Good, R. A. 1978. Effects of zinc deficiency on lymphoid tissues and on immune functions of A/Jax mice. *Fed. Proc.* 37:931 (Abstr.)

214. Tannenbaum, S. 1940. The initiation and growth of tumors. Introduction. I. Effects of underfeeding. *Am. J. Cancer* 38:335–50

215. Tarui, S. 1963. Studies on zinc metabolism. III. Effects of the diabetic state on zinc metabolism. A clinical aspect. *Endocrinol. Jpn.* 10:9–15

216. Tengrup, I., Zederfeldt, B. 1979. Serum zinc before and after cholecystectomy in zinc-treated patients. *Acta Chir. Scand.* 145:293–95

217. Thomsen, K. 1978. Zinc, liver cirrhosis and anorexia nervosa. *Acta Dermatol. Venereol.* 58:283

218. Torok, E., Foldes, G., Frank, K., Kereszty, M., Kiss, P., Molnar, A., Revesz, T., Rosner, E., Szigeti, R., Torok, I. 1977. Enteropathic acrodermatitis. *Orvosi Hetilap (Budapest)* 118:1461–66

219. Truckenbrodt, H., Hovels, O., Sitzmann, F. C., Weber, G. 1966. Beitrag zur acrodermatitis enteropathica. *Ann. Paediatr. (Basel)* 207:99–114 (in German)

220. Tucker, S. B., Schroeter, A. L., Brown, P. W. Jr., McCall, J. T. 1976. Acquired zinc deficiency. Cutaneous manifestations typical of acrodermatitis enteropathica. *J. Am. Med. Assoc.* 235:2399–2402

221. Underwood, E. J. 1971. *Trace Elements in Human and Animal Nutrition.* NY: Academic Press. 3rd ed.

222. Vallee, B. L., Gibson, J. G. 1948. The zinc content of normal human whole blood, plasma, leucocytes and erythrocytes. *J. Biol. Chem.* 176:445–57

223. Vallee, B. L., Wacker, W. E. C., Bartholomay, A. F., Hoch, F. L. 1959. Zinc metabolism in hepatic dysfunction. *Ann. Intern. Med.* 50:1077–91

224. Vallee, B. L., Wacker, W. E. C., Bartholomay, A. F., Robin, E. D. 1956. Zinc metabolism in hepatic dysfunction. I. Serum zinc concentrations in Laennec's cirrhosis and their validation by sequential analysis. *N. Engl. J. Med.* 255:403–8
225. Vallee, B. L., Wacker, W. E. C., Bartholomay, A. F., Robin, E. D. 1957. Zinc metabolism in hepatic dysfunction. II. Correlations of metabolic patterns with biochemical findings. *N. Engl. J. Med.* 257:1055–65
226. Van Gool, J. D., Went, K., Zegers, B. J. M. 1976. Acrodermatitis enteropathica and cellular immune deficiency. *Lancet* 1:1085
227. Vikbladh, I. 1951. *Studies on Zinc in Blood,* Vol. II. Lund: Carl Bloms Boktryckeri
228. Visscher, M. B., Ball, Z. B., Barnes, R. H., Sivertsen, I. 1942. The influence of calorie restriction upon the incidence of spontaneous mammary carcinoma in mice. *Surgery* 11:48–55
229. Walker, B. E., Dawson, J. B., Kelleher, J., Losowsky, M. S. 1973. Plasma and urinary zinc in patients with malabsorption syndromes or hepatic cirrhosis. *Gut* 14:943–48
230. Walravens, P. A., Hambidge, K. M. 1976. Growth of infants fed a zinc supplemented formula. *Am. J. Clin. Nutr.* 29:1114–21
231. Wannemacher, R. W. Jr., Dupont, H. L., Pekarek, R. S., Powanda, M. C., Schwartz, A., Hornick, R. B., Beisel, W. R. 1972. An endogenous mediator of depression of amino acids and trace metals in serum during typhoid fever. *J. Infect. Dis.* 126:77–86
232. Wannemacher, R., Pekarek, R. S., Klainer, A., Bartelloni, P., Dupont, H., Hornick, R., Beisel, W. 1975. Detection of a leukocytic endogenous mediator-like mediator of serum amino acid and zinc depression during various infectious illnesses. *Infec. Immun.* 11:873–75
233. Warren, P. J., Hansen, J. D. L., Lehman, B. H. 1969. The concentration of copper, zinc, and manganese in the liver of African children with marasmus and kwashiorkor. *Proc. Nutr. Soc.* 28:6A–7A (Abstr.)
234. Weaver, J. A. 1955. Changes induced in the thymus and lymph nodes of the rat by the administration of cortisone and sex hormones and by other procedures. *J. Pathol. Bacteriol.* 69:133–39
235. Weismann, K. 1979. Intravenous zinc

sulfate therapy in zinc depleted patients. *Dermatologica* 159:171–75
236. Weismann, K., Christensen, E., Dreyer, V. 1979. Zinc supplementation in alcoholic cirrhosis. A double blind clinical trial. *Acta Med. Scand.* 205:361–66
237. Weismann, K., Flagstad, T. 1976. Hereditary zinc deficiency (Adema disease) in cattle, an animal parallel to acrodermatitis enteropathica. *Acta Dermatol. Venereol. (Stokh.)* 56:151–54
238. Weismann, K., Hjorth, N., Fischer, A. 1976. Zinc depletion syndrome with acrodermatitis during long term intravenous feeding. *J. Clin. Exp. Dermatol.* 1:237–42
239. Weismann, K., Wadskov, S., Mikkelsen, H. I., Knudsen, L., Christensen, K. C., Storgaard, L. 1978. Acquired zinc deficiency dermatosis in man. *Arch. Dermatol.* 114:1509–11
240. Weston, W. L., Huff, J. C., Humbert, J. R., Hambidge, K. M., Neldner, K. H., Walravens, P. A. 1977. Zinc correction of defective chemotaxis in acrodermatitis enteropathica. *Arch. Dermatol.* 113:422–25
241. Whitenack, D. L., Whitehair, C. K., Miller, E. R. 1978. Influence of enteric infection on zinc utilization and clinical signs and lesions of zinc deficiency in young swine. *Am. J. Vet. Res.* 39:1447–54
242. Williams, R. B., Russell, R. M., Dutta, S. L., Giovetti, A. C. 1979. Alcoholic pancreatitis: patients at high risk of acute zinc deficiency. *Am. J. Med.* 66:889–93
243. Williams, R. O., Loeb, L. A. 1973. Zinc requirement for DNA replication in stimulated human lymphocytes. *J. Cell. Biol.* 58:594–601
244. Withers, A. F. D., Baker, H., Musa, M., Dormandy, T. L. 1968. Plasma zinc in psoriasis. *Lancet* 2:278
245. Wolman, S. L., Anderson, G. H., Marliss, E. B., JeeJeebhoy, K. N. 1979. Zinc in total parenteral nutrition: requirements and metabolic effects. *Gastroenterology* 76:458–67
246. Yen, T. T., Allen, J. V., Pearson, D. V., Acton, J. M., Greenberg, M. M. 1977. Prevention of obesity in $A^{vy/a}$ mice by dehydroepiandrosterone. *Lipids* 12:409
247. Zain, B. K., Haquani, A. H., Iffat-Un-Nisa. 1978. Serum copper and zinc levels in protein-calorie malnutrition. *J. Trop. Pediatr.* 24:198–99
248. Zukoski, C. F., Chvapil, M., Carlson, E., Hattler, B., Ludwig, J. 1974. Functional immobilization of peritoneal macrophages by zinc. *J. Reticuloendothel. Soc.* 16:6A

Ann. Rev. Nutr. 1982. 2:179-99
Copyright © 1982 by Annual Reviews Inc. A ll rights reserved

METABOLIC EFFECTS OF TOTAL PARENTERAL NUTRITION

P. D. Greig, J. P. Baker, K. N. Jeejeebhoy

Departments of Medicine and Surgery, Toronto General Hospital and University of Toronto, Toronto, Ontario, Canada.

INTRODUCTION

Nutritional support of the sick patient has become increasingly important, particularly in cases of prolonged serious illness. The need for attention to the nutritional requirements of the patients has arisen because improved treatment of sepsis, cardiovascular failure, and fluid and electrolyte abnormalities has allowed patients to survive to a point where nutrition becomes a limiting factor in their further progress. Despite advances in surgical and medical treatment of various disorders of the alimentary tract, the survival of the patient with gastrointestinal disease is often limited by continuing malnutrition as a result of the inability of the patient to eat and/or absorb a normal oral diet. Under such circumstances advances in the field of parenteral nutrition have revolutionized the outcome of these patients.

The objective of nutritional support in the critically ill patient is to restore and maintain adequate nutritional status in the face of illness and inadequate oral nutrition. Central to the understanding of the utilization of parenterally infused nutrients and their effects on body composition is knowledge of the effects of starvation and acute injury on nutritional status.

Effects of Starvation and Trauma on Nutritional Status

The prototypical patient who is the target for parenteral nutrition has an inflamed or injured gastrointestinal tract that prevents the absorption of oral nutrients. In such a patient, starvation results in reduced insulin levels which, in turn, allow the mobilization of free fatty acids from adipose tissue stores to meet the major part of the energy requirements of the patient. However, despite the energy flowing in from adipose tissue stores, protein catabolism continues, resulting in a negative nitrogen balance and wasting

179

0199-9885/82/0715-0179$02.00

of both muscle and viscera. As starvation progresses the increasing utilization of fat for energy tends to minimize the breakdown of protein, but the continuing loss of body protein ultimately results in dysfunction of liver, muscle, and the immune system. The loss of 35–40% of lean body mass during such an illness almost invariably results in death. The Irish hunger strikers of 1981 died in this manner after about 60 days of total starvation.

The septic and traumatized patient loses further protein owing to an increased energy requirement and reduced protein synthesis. In addition, levels of catecholamines and corticosteroids in the injured patient rise enormously. These anti-insulin hormones produce the well-known phenomenon of insulin resistance, one consequence of which is reduced utilization of carbohydrate as an energy source.

Gastrointestinal disease with increased loss of intestinal contents through fistula drainage and diarrhea causes additional antianabolic effects. The loss of intestinal contents results in the depletion of electrolytes and trace elements such as zinc, which may then adversely affect nitrogen balance.

Protein Metabolism

The human body is built around a framework of proteins that are not stored to any appreciable extent in an expendable form. The continued loss of body protein during starvation and/or injury is a major cause of morbidity and mortality resulting from malnutrition and/or trauma. Hence, a major goal of nutritional support has been prevention of further protein loss and restoration of total body protein.

The normal adult has a relatively constant cell population; once each cell is replete with protein, further protein retention cannot occur except in two situations. Additional protein retention occurs in the well-nourished adult when cellular hypertrophy is stimulated (e.g. by exercise of muscle) and during the development of obesity due to surfeit feeding.

However, the depleted adult can increase cellular protein in a manner analogous to that of the growing infant. In such a person the ability to retain nitrogen is more evident than in the normal adult. In depleted patients with hypocaloric feeding about 7.5 mg of nitrogen are retained with every kilocalorie of energy intake (18). As caloric intake increases, the ratio of nitrogen retention to caloric intake decreases such that, when caloric intake exceeds energy requirements, only 1.5 mg of nitrogen are retained per kilocalorie. This is associated with an increase in resting energy expenditure. The tissue laid down at the former ratio is largely composed of protein whereas with the latter ratio the excess energy is stored as body fat. Thus in essentially well-nourished human volunteers, positive nitrogen balance is attained only when a large number of calories are given (45–50 kcal per kg body weight) with 15–16 g nitrogen per day.

During starvation, the obligatory nitrogen loss can be reduced by up to 50% by simply giving amino acids without added energy. Blackburn et al (10) hypothesized that under these circumstances, reduced insulin levels promoted fat mobilization and energy from free fatty acids derived from endogenous fat stores aided protein synthesis from the infused amino acids. They suggested that this protein-sparing effect of amino acid infusions might be of benefit to the post-operative patient. However, although the degree of protein-sparing seen with amino acid infusions was greater than that of isocaloric glucose infusions, there was a significant increase in the blood urea nitrogen associated with the inefficient utilization of the amino acids. In clinical studies of patients following elective surgery, the routine use of amino acids did not improve the overall outcome. In view of their cost, amino acids offered no benefit over the traditional glucose support in the average post-operative patient.

Although both amino acid and glucose infusions have protein-sparing effects in starvation, the main determinant of protein-sparing appears to come from amino acids. In a controlled study of patients undergoing surgical procedures, Greenberg et al (28) assigned subjects to a random protocol consisting of four different regimens—either 5% dextrose alone, amino acids alone (1 g per kg ideal body weight), amino acids with hypocaloric glucose, or amino acids with lipid ($<$ 550 kcal per day). The study suggested that protein-sparing (defined as a reduction in the degree of negative nitrogen balance) resulted from amino acids alone and that the addition of 500–600 nonprotein calories did not influence the outcome. Note that the additional calories given in the study were not sufficient to meet metabolic requirements, and the results cannot be interpreted to mean that additional calories that meet metabolic energy needs may not increase nitrogen retention. The next question was whether it was possible to obtain neutral or positive nitrogen balance without additional energy in depleted patients.

Greenberg & Jeejeebhoy (27) showed that by increasing the amino acid infusion from 0.83 to 1.83 g per kg body weight without added energy, the net nitrogen balance rose from –3.66 g per day to +1.54 g per day. This comparison clearly indicated that high-dose amino acid infusions can effect a positive nitrogen balance even when the results are corrected for the increased blood urea nitrogen. Thus it may be possible to induce a positive or neutral nitrogen balance in depleted and malnourished subjects without the provision of additional calories, provided the amount of protein given is much higher than that required to maintain nitrogen balance with a nonprotein energy intake. The ability to induce a positive nitrogen balance without positive energy balance is contrary to classical teaching but has been confirmed (11) in a comparable patient population.

Other clinical studies with amino acid infusions in starved patients have characterized to a degree this protein-sparing phenomenon. Kaminski et al (37) have quantitated 3-methylhistidine excretion and have shown that amino acid infusions have a predominantly muscle-sparing effect. In addition, Skillman et al (69) have measured an increased albumin synthesis in patients receiving amino acids. Thus it appears that the provision of amino acid substrate both reduces protein catabolism and enhances protein synthesis in the starved patient.

Route of Amino Acid Administration

To determine whether oral amino acids are utilized differently from intravenous ones, keeping all other parameters constant, Patel et al (57) infused casein hydrolysate intravenously and through a nasogastric tube into depleted patients. Nonprotein calories were given intravenously in quantities sufficient to meet metabolic requirements; nitrogen balance and whole blood amino acid profiles were then measured. No difference was noted between the nitrogen balances during the two periods. However, when oral casein was substituted for casein hydrolysate, nitrogen retention was significantly better than with oral or intravenous casein hydrolysate. Comparison of the whole blood aminograms demonstrated a deficiency in sulphur containing and aromatic amino acids with the hydrolysate as compared with whole casein. These findings indicate that the route of administration of protein does not affect its utilization. Similarly, McArdel et al (50) demonstrated similar improvements in nitrogen balance and somatic protein (as measured by 3-methylhistidine excretion) in depleted patients given a 7% amino acid solution with 50% dextrose either intravenously or enterally. They advocated use of the enteral route when possible owing to the ease of handling, and the absence of the elevated glucose and insulin levels that were seen with the intravenous system.

Amino Acid Composition

The amino acid composition is of greater importance than the route of administration, and several authors have set out to determine the ideal amino acid mix. By analyzing the plasma amino acid levels in infants and newborns, Anderson et al (1) determined the amount of infused amino acid that caused an abrupt change in the plasma concentration of that amino acid. (When amino acid infusion exceeds requirements, plasma levels tend to rise abruptly.) Using this technique they have examined a number of mixtures and administration rates and have indicated the combinations likely to provide a balanced input of amino acids. Using a slightly different technique, Winters et al (79) performed a computerized analysis of predicted and observed values of plasma amino acids with different mixtures and have predicted a "growth" mixture that would result in the optimal amino acid pattern in neonates and infants.

The role of the branched-chain amino acids (BCAAs) in nitrogen balance is of particular interest. Buse et al (14) observed that BCAAs are transaminated to the corresponding alpha-ketoacids and alanine. Therefore, it was suggested that BCAA catabolism may play a role in providing muscle with energy during periods of exercise or limited glucose availability. BCAAs specifically stimulate muscle protein synthesis in vitro (24). Postabsorptively, BCAAs constitute a major part of amino acid uptake by leg muscle (77). In fasting human adults, the provision of BCAAs in the form of leucine resulted in a significant reduction in negative nitrogen balance. (63). Wolfe (80) has demonstrated an equivalent nitrogen-sparing effect of an infusion of the 3 BCAAs alone when compared with a balanced amino-acid infusion. Sherwin (63) and Wolfe (80) showed a 2- to 10-fold increase in the plasma level of the BCAA studied, but the glucose response to the infusion was not consistent between studies. At this time, the role of the BCAAs in protein and energy metabolism is not entirely understood, but they appear to be important in promoting nitrogen retention.

Specific amino acids have been used therapeutically in patients with chronic renal failure and hepatic failure. In patients with end-stage renal disease, histidine is an essential amino acid, and dietary supplementation with histidine-replete essential amino acids was associated with positive nitrogen balance and increases in albumin and hematocrit (45). BCAAs appear to have a role in optimal nutrition of the cirrhotic. The depressed levels of the BCAAs and the elevated levels of alanine, tyrosine, methionine, and tryptophane seen in cirrhosis can be normalized with a BCAA-enriched diet. Normalizing the plasma amino acid pattern in patients with liver disease may be of importance in the management of hepatic encephalopathy and the patient's overall nutritional status (20).

Energy Metabolism

Studies by Kinney and his colleagues (42) in the early 1970s suggested that increased energy requirements may follow trauma and injury. Energy requirements may increase with trauma and sepsis by as much as 40–60%, and by 100% in burns. It follows that injured-septic patients may require as much as 4000–6000 kcal per day. However, recalculation of the figures based on Kinney's findings suggest a more modest caloric requirement. For example, if the basal metabolic rate of an adult (approximately 25–28 kcal per kg per day) were increased by 60%, as has been observed in severe sepsis, then the caloric requirement would be approximately 40–45 kcal per kg per day which, in a 70 kg adult, would be no more than 2800–3100 kcal per day. Hence in most very sick patients with sepsis and gastrointestinal disease, one would not expect to exceed this figure. The need in patients with burns is somewhat higher.

Recent determinations of metabolic rates by indirect calorimetry in acutely sick and septic patients have suggested that actual requirements may be even lower. Askanazi et al (5) and Roulet et al (60) showed that the measured metabolic rate was only 13–14% above the expected metabolic rate calculated for these patients by the Harris-Benedict equation. This figure is considerably lower than that suggested by earlier observation. The discrepancy may be explained in part by the fact that, in addition to being stressed, these patients were malnourished and thus had lower initial basal energy requirements.

Is it beneficial to give calories in excess of the requirements in such patients? Giving extra calories may actually be harmful, particularly in the hypermetabolic patient. The evidence for this is provided in the studies of Askanazi et al, who noted two adverse effects when glucose was provided in amounts that significantly exceeded the metabolic rate. First, both urinary norepinephrine execretion and resting energy expenditure rose (5). Second, oxygen consumption and carbon dioxide production increased (7). The provision of excess calories in the form of glucose results in an undesirable respiratory load and an increase in the secretion of antianabolic hormones. In addition, the provision of excess glucose calories is associated with the development of a fatty liver, which may become clinically significant (12, 35, 51) However, all these effects of surfeit feeding were noted when glucose was the only source of nonprotein calories.

Would a mixed calorie source of glucose and lipid be more desirable than glucose only in such patients? Initial studies (46) suggested that lipid had no role in promoting nitrogen retention when given as the only caloric source to acutely ill patients. Subsequently, in a controlled trial of malnourished patients, Jeejeebhoy et al (32) showed that when patients were given a constant infusion of amino acids of 1 g per kg body weight per day together with approximately 60–70 g of glucose to cover minimal glucose requirements, then the additional provision of 40 nonprotein kcal per kg per day either as glucose or as lipid resulted in an equal sparing of nitrogen. Thus lipid calories were found to be equivalent to glucose calories in their effect on protein balance. Although all patients were in positive nitrogen balance throughout the study, the degree of this positive balance was temporarily altered when the patient was switched from glucose to lipid or vice versa. However, after an initial period of two or three days following the change in caloric source, this difference was abolished and the nitrogen balance with the two sources became equivalent again. In addition, it was shown that the equivalent nitrogen balances occurred with extremely different circulating substrate-hormone profiles. The patients receiving all their calories as glucose had high levels of pyruvate and lactate with relatively lower levels of free fatty acid and virtually no ketones. There was a corresponding marked increase in the circulating insulin levels in these patients. In contrast, those receiving most of their nonprotein calories as lipid had lower lactate and pyruvate levels but significantly higher levels of free fatty acids and ketones. Their insulin levels were correspondingly low. This was interpreted as indicating that the depleted patient could adapt to utilize either glucose or lipid as an energy substrate. Thus it was possible to promote nitrogen retention by two very different patterns of hormone response. The most physiologic substrate-hormone profile has been associated with a 50%–50% mixture of lipid and glucose calories.

This comparability of lipid and glucose calories in promoting nitrogen balance in depleted patients has been confirmed by many other investigators (8, 19, 25, 48, 81, 82). There are, however, both metabolic and clinical advantages to be gained with the lipid system. Carpentier et al (15) have demonstrated persistent endogenous fat mobilization during total parenteral nutrition using glucose as the only energy substrate. Askanazi et al (6) have found that the respiratory quotient (RQ) in similar patients ranged from 0.96 to 1.04, implying that glucose was utilized for both oxidation and lipogenesis. Thus, during glucose-based total parenteral nutrition (TPN), both mobilization of fat for oxidation and synthesis of fat from glucose occur together. Moreover, in patients receiving a mixture of lipid and glucose for nonprotein calories, the RQ ranged from 0.85 to 0.89, implying a net oxidation of the fat being infused for energy.

The clinical advantages of lipid relate to the effect of TPN on respiration and body composition. Askanazi et al (6) have measured a 20% increase in CO_2 production and a 26% increase in minute ventilation in patients receiving all nonprotein calories as glucose compared with those receiving the lipid-glucose mixture. MacFie et al (48) assessed the change in body composition in depleted patients receiving TPN using either glucose alone, or glucose plus lipid, as the energy source. Although weight gain was similar in both groups, with glucose alone it was limited to fat and water, while with lipid and glucose it was largely nitrogen. Finally, Messing et al (53, 54) and Jeejeebhoy et al (34) have shown that infusion of lipids did not increase liver fat, while infusing glucose did do so.

The question then arises whether the injured and septic patient utilizes fat oxidation as a source of energy production. Carpentier et al showed that patients who were injured and septic continued to mobilize (15) and oxidize (16) fat despite receiving all their nonprotein calories as carbohydrate. Hence, obligatory fat oxidation appears to be prevalent in patients who are injured and septic. Furthermore, Burke et al (13) showed a limit to glucose utilization in patients with burns who were receiving all their calories as glucose. Only 55% of the energy requirement appeared to be derived from glucose oxidation, implying that the remaining calories were derived from fat oxidation. Hence evidence from two sources suggests that in the injured-septic patient fat oxidation provides a significant part of the energy.

Would giving fat as a source of exogenous calories benefit such hyper-metabolic patients? In order to answer this question, Roulet et al (60) randomly divided critically ill patients into two groups. Each group was studied while receiving 5% glucose/water and again while receiving complete parenteral nutrition (amino acids, energy, electrolytes, vitamins, and trace elements). In one group all the nonprotein calories were given as glucose; the other group received half their nonprotein calories as lipid and half as glucose. The order of the infusions of glucose/water or parenteral nutrition was random, and both groups were given comparable amounts of amino acids and total calories (while receiving parenteral nutrition). The results of this study confirmed the observations of Askanazi et al (6) that giving parenteral nutrition with all nonprotein calories as glucose resulted in a significant increase in carbon dioxide production when compared to the mixture of glucose and lipid. The respiratory load created by the need to dispose of carbon dioxide was significantly reduced when a glucose-lipid mixture was given.

In addition, these injured-septic patients continued to have high plasma free fatty acids even when all the calories were given as glucose. Thus fat mobilization continued in these patients even when all exogenous calories were given in the form of glucose. These observations by Roulet et al (60) agreed with those of Carpentier et al (15) and Askanazi et al (6) and were consistent with those of Burke et al (13). Finally, using ^{14}C-leucine, the glucose-lipid mixture was associated with reduced leucine oxidation and increased protein synthesis in relation to catabolism when compared with glucose as the sole source of nonprotein calories. Hence it appears that the significant benefits of lipid in hypermetabolic patients are reduced carbon dioxide production, reduced leucine oxidation, and improved protein economy.

In summary, septic and hypermetabolic patients continue to mobilize and oxidize endogenous fat for energy, even in the presence of the marked increase in glucose and insulin levels associated with amino acid plus glucose infusions. Morever, there is a limit to the utilization of the glucose infused in these patients. This "insulin resistance" likely results from increased circulating anti-insulin factors such as cortisol and norepinephrine since insulin antibodies are unlikely and an intracellular inhibition of insulin effect has not been measured. It may be possible to overcome the "insulin-resistance" with exogenous insulin; however, the other benefits of lipid as a part of the calorie source make it the preferable alternative. The optimal proportion of lipid to glucose is as yet undetermined, but the provision of 30–50% of calories as lipid has been free of significant side effects and has had the beneficial metabolic effects indicated above.

Essential Fatty Acid (EFA) Deficiency

Certain fatty acids, principally linoleic acid, are essential for the human (30). Linoleic acid, which has 18 carbon atoms and two double bonds, is converted to a longer-chain fatty acid, arachidonic acid, with 20 carbon atoms and four double bonds (tetraene). It appears that, when linoleate is deficient, the same system that elongates the chain of linoleate will use oleate as a substrate and will elongate it to a 20-carbon-atom fatty acid, eicosatrienoic acid, with three double bonds (triene). Since oleate can be synthesized from carbohydrates, there is an alteration in the plasma fatty acid pattern during essential fatty acid deficiency. Linoleic acid and arachidonic acid are both reduced and in their place eicosatrienoic acid appears in the circulation. Holman (30) measured the ratio of eicosatrienoic acid to arachidonic acid as the triene-tetraene ratio and found that elevation of the triene-tetraene ratio was indicative of EFA deficiency.

Prior to the advent of parenteral nutrition, a clinical syndrome of skin rash with appropriate alterations in plasma fatty acid pattern was recognized as indicating EFA deficiency in infants. Adults did not seem to suffer the syndrome because they have sufficient stores of essential fatty acids in their adipose tissue to prevent this deficiency. However, with the advent of parenteral nutrition based on a system of continuous infusion of a fat-free solution, EFA deficiency occurred in adults. EFA deficiency in patients receiving TPN is characterized clinically by a skin rash, reduced plasma levels of linoleate, and an elevated triene-tetraene ratio. These changes were corrected by infusing an intravenous lipid emulsion containing linoleate.

Wene et al (78) recently observed the pattern of EFA deficiency as early as 10 days after starting a fat-free parenteral nutrition, prior to the onset of any clinically observable features. EFA deficiency occurs early in adults receiving TPN because when glucose is infused continuously, high insulin levels block the release of free-fatty acids from adipose tissue stores. Hence plasma fatty acids originate from either exogenously infused lipids or, in the case of fat-free parenteral nutrition, from endogenously synthesized lipids derived from carbohydrates. Since the endogenously synthesized lipids do not include linoleate, the pattern of fatty acids alters rapidly to one seen with EFA deficiency. Hence, during continuous glucose infusion the only way to maintain plasma essential fatty acid levels would be to infuse lipids continuously. Since intravenous lipid can reverse and prevent EFA deficiency, various regimens have been suggested with variable amounts of lipid given either once, twice, or three times a week, but none of these regimens has been tested rigorously. However, the recent indication that lipid would be advantageous as a calorie source has made superfluous the concept of giving lipids only as a source of essential fatty acid.

Is linoleate the only essential fatty acid in the human, or does linolenate also serve as an essential fatty acid? This fatty acid appears to be necessary for proper myelination of the central nervous system in newborn animals and therefore may have to be provided when parenteral nutrition is used in the newborn. However, the exact need for, and role of, this fatty acid in the human remains to be determined.

Electrolytes

The internal environment of a cell largely consists of a number of cations and anions; the principle cations are potassium and magnesium and the principle anions are phosphate and protein. The repletion of cell contents in the malnourished patient depends on providing not only nitrogen but also the other constituents of the cell, mainly the electrolytes potassium, magnesium, and phosphate. It has been shown that in protein-calorie malnutrition there is also a depletion of total body potassium and total body magnesium. A number of metabolic abnormalities will occur during TPN unless these electrolytes are provided. Rudman et al (61) showed, in a very elegant study, that nitrogen balance only became positive during parenteral nutrition when there was a concomitant administration of potassium and phosphate, highlighting the need for electrolytes during parenteral nutrition.

Sodium

This cation is principally distributed in the extracelluar fluid. Its role during parenteral nutrition, apart from its role in maintaining extracellular and circulating volume, lies in the relationship between sodium retention and the provision of calories. When nonprotein calories were given as carbohydrate, sodium was retained, a phenomenon not seen when calories were given as fat (75). It is not surprising therefore that during glucose-based parenteral nutrition, there was a significant and marked gain of weight, most of which could be accounted for by retention of extracellular water (83). This water (and inferentially sodium) retention plays a major part in the dramatic weight gains seen during glucose-based parenteral nutrition. A possible clinical counterpart to this phenomenon may be so-called "refeeding edema." This dramatic picture of fluid gain may occur in severely malnourished patients who are abruptly started on parenteral nutrition, and may be severe enough to result in congestive heart failure. In addition, the interstitial accumulation of sodium and water may interfere with gas exchange at the pulmonary alveolar level and contribute to respiratory failure. In comparison, the weight gain with lipid systems is associated with gain in protein and not water (48). These clinical aspects in malnourished patients should be considered. The patient should be renourished cautiously, particularly avoiding an excess of glucose calories and perhaps by the use of significant amounts of lipid.

Potassium

Potassium is the main intracellular ion. During parenteral nutrition, total body potassium may increase. Body potassium is particularly increased when glucose is the only source of nonprotein calories (49, 67), and MacFie et al have measured a further increase when insulin is added (49) during the administration of parenteral nutrition. On the other hand, when lipid is the major source of calories the increase in body potassium is not as great as with glucose (67). This has been interpreted by some investigators as suggesting that the increase in "body cell mass" as estimated by exchangeable potassium is better with glucose than with lipid (67). Since the objective of these investigators was to increase the "body cell mass" derived from total measurements of total body potassium alone, it is not surprising that this finding was interpreted as indicating the superiority of glucose over lipid as a source of calories. However, further investigation has shown that total body potassium does not reflect total body nitrogen. During the administration of parenteral nutrition with glucose as the main source of calories, the increase in body potassium was not associated with an increase in body nitrogen (52). In addition, MacFie et al (49) have measured an increase in total body potassium without change in nitrogen in patients receiving glucose-based TPN and insulin. This indicates that the rise in body potassium is not a true index of total protein synthesis or total cellular contents, but may reflect an independent increase in potassium due to other processes. Exactly why potassium increases without nitrogen has not been determined, but potassium may be retained with glycogen, or this may reflect a transient intracellular shift of potassium associated with elevated levels of glucose and insulin. From what is known of cell composition it appears that such an increase is not representative of an increase in the cellular mass or cellular contents, since such an increase in cell contents or mass would be expected to be associated with a rise in all cellular constituents. Thus the use of total body potassium as an index of an increase in either the lean body mass or in the total body nitrogen can no longer be considered reliable. This particularly applies to acute changes observed during the administration of parenteral nutrition.

Magnesium

The concentration of magnesium falls when parenteral nutrition is instituted. Using balance studies, Freeman et al (22) have shown that nitrogen balance is not optimal unless magnesium is given concomitantly. It has been suggested that approximately 30 meq should be given per day to optimize nitrogen retention. These findings are not surprising since magnesium is an important intracellular cation and is depleted during protein-caloric malnutrition. As such, the restitution of total cellular contents would be expected to be associated not only with restitution of nitrogen but also of magnesium.

Phosphorus

This major intracellular anion is a constituent of 2–3,diphosphoglycerate (2–3,DPG). Therefore, anabolism of the cell would be expected to be associated with retention of phosphorus together with other intracellular elements such as potassium, magnesium, and protein. During the administration of glucose-based parenteral nutrition, the plasma level of phosphorus rapidly falls as this element is transported into cells under the influence of insulin and glucose. In earlier studies with total parenteral nutrition, Silvas & Paragas (68) showed that the serum phosphorus levels may fall to almost undetectable values; associated with this fall is a clinical syndrome consisting of disorientation, tremors, convulsions and coma, which may be fatal. The hypophosphatemia may be avoided and protein synthesis optimized by the administration of appropriate amounts of phosphorus during parenteral nutrition.

Acid-Base Balance

The administration of some amino acid mixtures is followed by the development of a nonketotic metabolic acidosis with hyperchloremia. When the basic amino acids lysine, histidine, and arginine are administered in their chloride form their metabolism causes an accumulation of hydrogen ions, which together with the chloride results in acidosis and hyperchloremia. However, when these amino acids are administered as acetates the production of hydrogen ion is balanced by concomitant production of bicarbonate from the metabolism of acetate. It has therefore become customary for all amino acid mixtures to be buffered with acetate.

Trace Elements

Trace elements have been recognized as being important in animal nutrition for several years; 15 elements have been identified in this category. In the human the recognition of the value of trace elements has been slow, but with the advent of parenteral nutrition the syndromes of zinc, copper, chromium, and selenium deficiency have been recognized and reported.

Zinc

Zinc is an important element in a number of metallo-enzyme systems. In particular, since it is important for the action of deoxythymidine kinase (58), all cell proliferations require the presence of zinc. It is also important in the maintenance of cellular immunity and delayed hypersensitivity. Finally, zinc is an integral part of insulin as secreted by the pancreas, and its appears that the deficiency of zinc is associated with abnormalities of carbohydrate metabolism.

As far as tissues are concerned, zinc is an integral part of muscle, and under conditions of increased catabolism there is an increased loss of zinc in the urine. During parenteral nutrition in which no zinc was added to the infusate, the plasma zinc levels dropped at a steady rate so that subnormal levels were observed between 2–7 weeks (21, 70). In addition, patients receiving parenteral nutrition without zinc developed a syndrome of redness, scaling, and maculovesicular rash around the nasolabial folds, mouth, and genitalia, together with reddening of the palms and the soles with desquamation (4, 39). Hair loss and a loss of the senses of taste and smell also occurred. The lesions were not unlike those of acrodermatitis enteropathica, which is due to zinc deficiency. The plasma levels of zinc in these patients were grossly decreased, and infusion of zinc reversed the lesions. During this manifestation of zinc deficiency, the skin became infected with staphylococci and fungi, which could not be cleared without giving zinc. In another context, Golden et al (26) noted that children with protein-calorie malnutrition who were anergic could be rendered reactive again simply by the local application of zinc to a site where delayed cutaneous hypersensitivity was being tested. Hence it appears that even in the face of protein-calorie malnutrition zinc deficiency seems to be a paramount cause of the immune deficiencies that are observed.

Copper

Copper is another trace metal with important functions in human metabolism. It is involved in intestinal iron absorption, hemoglobin synthesis, mitochondrial function, collagen metabolism, and is a constituent of oxidase enzymes. Despite the finding (70) that patients receiving total parenteral nutrition without added copper for periods from 1.5–2 weeks had consistently declining levels of plasma copper, clinical manifestations of copper deficiency have been uncommon. Karpel et al (38) described an infant with hypochromic normocytic anemia, neutropenia, and skeletal abnormalities (osteoporosis and metaphyseal irregularity) in association with hypocupremia after 7.5 months on TPN without copper. These abnormalities responded well to the addition of copper. Since then, several cases (9, 17, 76) of adult anemia and neutropenia in association with hypocupremia have been described—all responding to copper supplementation. Thus it appears that clinical manifestations of copper deficiency exist but that plasma levels do not accurately reflect body copper stores, which may still contain sufficient copper to fulfill its metabolic role.

Until recently the copper requirements of TPN had not been determined. Shike et al (65) have found daily requirements to be approximately 300 μg in patients without diarrhea and 500 μg in patients with substantial losses of fluids from the gastrointestinal tract. The dose must be decreased in patients with obstructive jaundice, since copper is excreted via the biliary tract.

Chromium

An organically bound form of chromium called "glucose tolerance factor" appears to be required for optimal glucose absorption and utilization. Although chromium supplementation has been reported to improve glucose tolerance in malnourished children (29, 31) and elderly diabetic subjects (44), in these cases the situation has been complicated by many possible micronutrient deficiencies. Direct evidence for the role of chromium deficiency in human disease was presented by Jeejeebhoy et al (33), who described a patient who developed weight loss, peripheral neuropathy, ataxia, and glucose intolerance associated with low chromium levels in blood and hair after 3.5 years on home-TPN. Glucose intolerance and central nervous system abnormalities associated with low serum chromium levels have also been seen in another patient on long-term TPN (23). In both patients, the abnormal glucose metabolism and neurologic symptoms were rapidly corrected with chromium supplementation to the TPN solution.

The time course in these cases suggests that the human body has large stores of chromium. However, when the stores are depleted, the consequent clinical abnormalities of impaired glucose tolerance and central nervous system symptoms occur, paralleled by decreasing blood levels of chromium. Although chromium balance studies have only been performed on a single patient, it appears that 20 μg of chromium daily prevents chromium deficiency.

Selenium

Selenium is important in muscle metabolism and function. It is an essential component of glutathione peroxidase, which helps prevent oxidative damage to cells by peroxides and free radicals. The necessity of dietary selenium has long been known in animals. A dietary selenium deficiency has been shown to produce white-muscle disease in sheep (2) and an exudative diathesis in poultry (72) when these animals are raised on feed grown in selenium-deficient soil. Despite this, evidence for the role of selenium deficiency in human disease has been slow in coming. It is now suggested that

Keshan disease, a congestive cardiomyopathy occurring in certain rural areas of China, is due to selenium deficiency in locally grown foods and may be prevented by selenium supplementation (3, 40, 41). Recently, Johnson et al (36) have described a case of congestive cardiomyopathy with the pathologic features of Keshan disease, associated with reduced erythrocyte and cardiac selenium and glutathione peroxidase levels in a patient on home-TPN unsupplemented by selenium for 4 years. Van Rij et al (74) have also described a patient from New Zealand (a well-known selenium deficient zone) who developed muscular pain and weakness associated with reduced erythrocyte selenium and glutathione peroxidase activity after receiving selenium-deficient TPN for only 30 days. In this instance, addition of selenium to the TPN solution corrected the symptoms as well as plasma selenium levels within 1 week. However, erythrocyte selenium and glutathione peroxidase levels did not change within this time frame.

It would appear, then, that several factors might influence the development of selenium deficiency including geographical location, preceding diet and nutritional state, excessive GI losses, and duration of selenium-deficient TPN. Balance studies (74) in 6 patients with no selenium supplementation in their TPN solution showed a negative balance with a mean of -10 ± 1.7 μg/day. Although further work is necessary, it seems safe to assume that selenium requirements are somewhat greater than $10\,\mu$g per day.

Vitamins

The precise vitamin requirements in TPN are still not known. Until recently, the provision of vitamins to such patients has been based on oral dosage schedules, and most institutions have used a multiple vitamin preparation in the hopes that it will provide an adequate vitamin supply without toxicity. However, recent research in parenterally fed patients has helped clarify this area.

An investigation of the requirements for the water-soluble vitamins, thiamine (B_1), riboflavin (B_2), pyridoxine (B_6), niacin, pantothenic acid, and ascorbic acid (C) has demonstrated that regular use of a well-known multivitamin infusion (MVI) maintained adequate blood levels of several vitamins including riboflavin and ascorbic acid (56). Kishi et al (43) studied levels of thiamine and pyridoxine in patients receiving TPN and concluded that 5 mg/day of thiamine-HCl and 3 mg/day of pyridoxine-HCl are sufficient for these vitamins—amounts found in most multivitamin preparations. Additionally, Jeejeebhoy et al (34) have reported vitamin intakes and levels in 6 long-term TPN patients, again demonstrating that adequate levels of water-soluble vitamins can be provided by routine multivitamin preparations.

Vitamin B_{12} and folic acid are not provided in many multivitamin preparations. However, vitamin B_{12} has long been used parenterally in patients with pernicious anemia where the daily maintenance dose has already been determined—approximately 3–5 μg per day. Folate deficiency is relatively common in hospitalized patients and, although much larger doses have traditionally been given, Lowry et al (47) have demonstrated the adequacy of as little as 0.69 mg per day of folic acid.

The fat-soluble vitamins are also supplied in many multivitamin preparations. Although the problem of vitamin A toxicity and hypercalcemia has been reported, it is rare. Lowry et al (47) studied vitamin A levels in 40 patients given TPN in hospital and concluded that normal serum vitamin A levels can be maintained using 1500–2000 IU/day. In our home parenteral nutrition patients, withdrawal of vitamin A entirely has not caused low serum levels in 11 patients after 6 months, probably because of substantial body stores. Thus it appears that the margin of error for vitamin A administration is wide but that about 2000 IU/day may be sufficient.

Although vitamin E is supplied by the polyunsaturated fatty acids contained in lipid, Jeejeebhoy et al (34) have shown reduced serum vitamin E levels in long-term TPN patients even with daily lipid infusions. More recently, Thurlow et al (73) have described 10 patients who developed low serum vitamin E levels, in vitro platelet hyperactivity, and in vitro red blood cell hemolysis during TPN. These abnormalities were corrected in 7 patients with 50 mg d,1 α-tocopherol given daily. It appears, then, that at least 50 mg of vitamin E must be supplied daily.

Vitamin K is normally derived from diet and produced by gut bacteria. In a patient receiving TPN the latter source may itself suffice. However, if changes occur in the gut flora (e.g. with antibiotics) this supply may no longer be adequate. In this case weekly supplementation with 10 mg of Synkavite (sodium menadiol diphosphate) seems sufficient.

Investigation of calcium and bone metabolism in patients receiving long-term TPN (64) revealed that with average daily intakes of vitamin D_2 amounting to 250 IU (along with 400 mg calcium and 500–700 mg phosphate), the plasma 25–OH cholecalciferol levels were normal. However, a syndrome of continued calcium loss from the skeleton with a histological picture of increased bone osteoid and reduced calcification of the new osteoid was noted (66). These changes occurred despite the normal levels of 25-OH vitamin D. However, these patients were also found to have low levels of 1,25-dihydroxy vitamin D, perhaps as a result of suppressed secretion of parathormone caused by calcium infusion in the TPN solution. It was tempting to speculate that the changes were due to a deficiency of 1,25-dihydroxy vitamin D. This speculation was not substantiated when trial withdrawal of vitamin D from the infusion caused clinical remission of bone pain and fractures, reduction in the increased bone osteoid, and increase in the area of calcifying new osteoid despite continuing low levels of 1,25-dihydroxy vitamin D. Hence this syndrome is clearly aggravated by giving vitamin D. At present, the needs for this vitamin in TPN have not been established, but the use of vitamin D in short-term TPN is not recommended.

Although the genetic syndrome of biotin-responsive carboxylase deficiency has been known for some time (59, 71), acquired biotin deficiency had until recently been shown to occur only in association with raw egg ingestion (62), the whites of which contain a protein capable of binding biotin intraluminally and preventing its absorption. Despite low plasma biotin levels in 6 long-term home-TPN patients, Jeejeebhoy et al (34) found no pathology. However, Mock et al (55) have recently documented a child who, after 3 months on TPN, developed a clinical syndrome consisting of an exfoliative rash and organic aciduria associated with reduced plasma, whole blood, and urinary biotin concentrations. Resolution of the clinical and biochemical features occurred after biotin supplementation of the TPN. Although still possibly due to a genetic deficiency, the evidence appears strong that this was indeed an acquired defect resulting from previous nutritional deficiency and long-term antibiotic therapy. Despite this, the need for routine biotin supplementation in TPN is still not resolved.

In summary, most vitamins are easily and safely provided to the patient on TPN. However, some controversies still exist. It is our present practice to supply a multivitamin preparation containing all vitamins except A, D, E, and biotin on six out of seven days per week. On the seventh day, vitamins A and D are added in the doses of 1000 IU and 100 IU, respectively. Vitamin E is supplied by the lipid used in the TPN regimen (50% of nonprotein calories), but on the basis of recent information will probably have to be increased. The issue of biotin has not been decided upon as yet.

Acknowledgments

The authors wish to thank Mrs. Janet Chrupala and Ms. J. Whitwell for their secretarial assistance.

Literature Cited

1. Anderson, G. H., Bryan, H., Jeejeebhoy, K.N., Corey, P. 1977. Dose-response relationships between amino acid intake and blood levels in newborn infants. *Am. J. Clin. Nutr.* 30:1110–21
2. Andrews, E. D., Hartley, W. J., Grant, A. B. 1968. Selenium-responsive diseases of animals in New Zealand. *N.Z. Vet. J.* 16:3
3. Anonymous. 1979. Selenium in the heart of China. *Lancet* 2:889–90
4. Arakawa, T., Tamura, T., Igarashi, Y., Suzuki, H., Sandstead, H. H. 1976. Zinc deficiency in two infants during total

parenteral alimentation for diarrhea. *Am. J. Clin. Nutr.* 29:197–204
5. Askanazi, J., Carpentier, Y. A., Elwyn, D. H., Nordenstrom, J., Jeevanandam, M., Rosenbaum, S. H., Gump, F. E., Kinney, J. M. 1980. Influence of total parenteral nutrition on fuel utilization in injury and sepsis. *Ann. Surg.* 191: 40–46
6. Askanazi, J., Nordenstrom, J., Rosenbaum, S. H., Elwyn, D. H., Hyman, A. I., Carpentier, Y. A., Kinney, J. M. 1981. Nutrition for the patient with res-

piratory failure. *Anaesthesiology* 54: 373–77

7. Askanazi, J., Rosenbaum, S. H., Hyman, A. I., Silverberg, P. A., Milic-Emili, J., Kinney, J. M. 1980. Respiratory changes induced by the large glucose loads of total parenteral nutrition. *J. Am. Med. Assoc.* 243:1444–47

8. Bark, S., Holm, I., Hakansson, I., Wretlind, A. 1976. Nitrogen-sparing effect of fat emulsion compared with glucose in the post-operative period. *Acta Chir. Scand.* 142:423–27

9. Bernard, L. Z., Shadduck, R. K., Zeigler, Z., et al 1977. Observations on the anemia and neutropenia of human copper deficiency. *Am. J. Hematol.* 3: 177–85

10. Blackburn, G. L., Flatt, J. P., Clowes, G. H. A., O'Donnel, T. F. 1973. Peripheral intravenous feeding with isotonic amino acid solutions. *Am. J. Surg.* 125:447–54

11. Bozetti, F. 1976. Parenteral nutrition in surgical patients. *Surg. Gynecol. Obstet.* 142:16–20

12. Broviac, J. W., Scribner, B. H. 1972. The artificial gut: two years' experience with total parenteral nutrition in the home. *Gastroenterology* 62:727 (Abstr.)

13. Burke, J. F., Wolfe, R. R., Mullany, C. J., Mathews, D. E., Bier, D. M. 1979. Glucose requirements following burn injury. Parameters of optimal glucose infusion and possible hepatic and respiratory abnormalities following excessive glucose intake. *Ann. Surg.* 190:274

14. Buse, M. G., Biggers, J. F., Friderici, K. H., Buse, J. F. 1972. Oxidation of branched-chain amino acids by isolated hearts and diaphragms of the rat. *J. Biol. Chem.* 247:8085–96

15. Carpentier, Y. A., Askanazi, J., Elwyn, D. H., Jeevanandam, M., Gump, F. E., Hyman, A. I., Burr, R., Kinney, J. M. 1979. Effects of hypercaloric glucose infusion on lipid metabolism injury and sepsis. *J. Trauma* 19:649–54

16. Carpentier, Y. A., Nordenstrom, J., Askanazi, J., Elwyn, D. H., Gump, F. E., Kinney, J. M. 1979. Relationship between rates of clearance and oxidation of ^{14}C-Intralipid in surgical patients. *Surg. Forum* 30:72–74

17. Dunlop, W. M., James, G. W. III, Hume, D. M. 1974. Anemia and neutropenia caused by copper deficiency. *Ann. Intern. Med.* 80:470–76

18. Elwyn, D. H., Gump, F. E., Munro, H. N., Iles, M., Kinney, J. M. 1979. Changes in nitrogen balance of depleted patients with increasing infusions of glucose. *Am. J. Clin. Nutr.* 32:1597–1611

19. Elwyn, D. H., Kinney, J. M., Gump, F. E., Askanazi, J., Rosenbaum, S. H, Carpentier, Y. A. 1980. Some metabolic effects of fat infusions in depleted patients. *Metabolism* 29:125–32

20. Fischer, J. E., Rosen, H. M., Ebeid, A. M., James, J. H., Keane, J. M., Soeters, P. B, 1976. The effect of normalization of plasma amino acids on heptatic encephalopathy in man. *Surgery* 80:77–91

21. Fleming, C. R., McGill, D. B., Berkner, S. 1977. Home parenteral nutrition as primary therapy in patients with extensive Crohn's disease of the small bowel and malnutrition. *Gastroenterology* 73: 1077–81

22. Freeman, J. B. 1977. Magnesium requirements are increased during total parenteral nutrition. *Surg. Forum* 28: 61–62

23. Freund, H., Atamian, S., Fischer, J. E. 1979. Chromium deficiency during total parenteral nutrition. *J. Am. Med. Assoc.* 241:496–98

24. Fulks, R. M., Li, J. B., Goldberg, A. L. 1975. Effects of insulin, glucose and amino acids on protein turnover in rat diaphragm. *J. Biol. Chem.* 250:290–98

25. Gazzaniga, A. B., Bartlett, R. H., Shobe, J. B. 1975. Nitrogen balance in patients receiving either fat or carbohydrate for total intravenous nutrition. *Ann. Surg.* 182:163–68

26. Golden, M. H. N., Golden, B., Harland, P. S. E. G., Jackson, A. A. 1978. Zinc and immunocompetence in protein-energy malnutrition. *Lancet* 1:1226–28

27. Greenberg, G. R., Jeejeebhoy, K. N. 1979. Intravenous protein-sparing therapy in patients with gastrointestinal disease. *J. Parenter. Enter. Nutr.* 3: 427–32

28. Greenberg, G. R., Marliss, E. B., Anderson, G. H., Langer, B., Spence, W., Tovee, E. B., Jeejeebhoy, K. N. 1976. Protein-sparing therapy in post-operative patients: Effects of added hypocaloric glucose or lipid. *N. Engl. J. Med.* 294:1411–16

29. Gurson, C. T., Saner, G. 1971. Effect of chromium on glucose utilization in marasmic protein calorie malnutrition. *Am. J. Clin. Nutr.* 24:1313

30. Holman, R. T. 1968. Essential fatty acid deficiency. In *Progress in Chemistry of Fats and Other Lipids,* ed. R. T. Holman, vol. 9, pt. 2, p. 275. Oxford: Pergamon Press

31. Hopkins, L. L. Jr., Ransome-Kuti, O., Majaj, A. S. 1968. Improvement of im-

paired carbohydrate metabolism by chromium (III) in malnourished infants. *Am. J. Clin. Nutr.* 21:203

32. Jeejeebhoy, K. N., Anderson, G. H., Nakhooda, A. F., Greenberg, G. R., Sanderson, I., Marliss, E. B. 1976. Metabolic studies in total parenteral nutrition with lipid in man. Comparison with glucose. *J. Clin. Invest.* 57:125–36

33. Jeejeebhoy, K. N., Chu, R. C., Marliss, E. B., Greenberg, G. R., Bruce-Robertson, A. 1977. Chromium deficiency, glucose intolerance and neuropathy reversed by chromium supplementation in a patient receiving long-term total parenteral nutrition. *Am. J. Clin. Nutr.* 30:531–38

34. Jeejeebhoy, K. N., Langer, B., Tsallas, G., Chu, R. C., Kuksis, A., Anderson, G. H. 1976. Total parenteral nutrition at home: studies in patients surviving 4 months to 5 years. *Gastroenterology* 71:943–53

35. Jeejeebhoy, K. N., Zorab, W. J., Langer, B., Phillips, M. J., Kuksis, A., Anderson, G. H. 1973. Total parenteral nutrition at home for 23 months without complication and with good rehabilitation. A study of technical and metabolic features. *Gastroenterology* 65:811–20

36. Johnson, R. A., Baker, S. S., Fallon, J. T., Maynard, E. P., Ruskin, J. N., Wen, Z., Keyou, G., Cohen, H. J. 1981. An occidental case of cardiomyopathy and selenium deficiency. *N. Engl. J. Med.* 304:1210–12

37. Kaminski, M. V. Jr., Dunn, N. P., Wannemacher, R. W. Jr., Dinterman, R. E., DeShazo, R., Wilson, W. W., Carlson, D. E. 1977. Specific muscle protein-sparing post-operative dextrose-free amino acid infusions. *J. Parenter. Enter. Nutr.* 1:147–51

38. Karpel, J. T., Peden, W. H. 1972. Copper deficiency in long-term parenteral nutrition. *J. Pediatr.* 80:32–36

39. Kay, R. G., Tasman-Jones, C. 1975. Acute zinc deficiency in man during intravenous alimentation. *Aust. N. Z. J. Surg.* 45:325–30

40. Keshan Disease Research Group of the Chinese Academy of Medical Sciences. 1979. Observations on effect of sodium selenite in prevention of Keshan disease. *Chin. Med. J. Engl.* 92:471–77

41. Keshan Disease Research Group of the Chinese Academy of Medical Sciences. 1979. Epidemiologic studies on the etiologic relationships of selenium and Keshan disease. *Chin. Med. J. Engl.* 92:477–82

42. Kinney, J.M., Long, C. L., Duke, J. H. 1970. Carbohydrate and nitrogen metabolism after injury. In *Energy Metabolism in Trauma*, ed. R. Porter, J. Knight, pp. 103–26. London: Churchill

43. Kishi, H., Nishii, S., Ono, T. 1979. Thiamine and pyridoxine requirements during intravenous hyperalimentation. *Am. J. Clin. Nutr.* 32:332–38

44. Levine, R. A., Streeten, H. P., Doisy, R. J. 1968. Effects of oral chromium supplementation on the glucose tolerance of elderly human subjects. *Metab. Clin. Exp.* 17:114

45. Llach, F. 1977. Current studies of amino acid and keto-acid diets in chronic renal failure. *Dialysis Transpl.* 6:24, 26, 72, 82

46. Long, J. M., Wilmore, D. W., Mason, A. D. Jr., Pruitt, B. A. Jr. 1974. Fat carbohydrate interaction: nitrogensparing effect of varying caloric sources for total intravenous feeding. *Surg. Forum* 25:61–63

47. Lowry, S. F., Goodgame, J. T., Maher, M. M., Brennan, M. F. 1978. Parenteral vitamin requirements during intravenous feeding. *Am. J. Clin. Nutr.* 31:2149–58

48. MacFie, J., Smith, R. C., Hill, G. L. 1981. Glucose or fat as nonprotein energy source? A controlled clinical trial in gastroenterological patients requiring intravenous nutrition. *Gastroenterology* 80:103–7

49. MacFie, J., Yule, A. G., Hill, G. L. 1981. Effect of added insulin on body composition of gastroenterologic patients receiving intravenous nutrition—a controlled clinical trial. *Gastroenterology* 81:285–89

50. McArdle, A. H., Mutch, D., Brown, R. A. 1979. Enteral vs. parenteral nutrition: An assessment of nutritional studies. *J. Parenter. Enter. Nutr.* 3:24 (Abstr.)

51. McDonald, A. T. J., Phillips, M. J., Jeejeebhoy, K. N. 1973. Reversal of fatty liver by Intralipid in patients on total parenteral alimentation. *Gastroenterology* 64:885

52. Mernagh, J. R., McNeill, K. G., Harrison, J. E., Jeejeebhoy, K. N. 1982. Effect of total parenteral nutrition in the restitution of body nitrogen, potassium and weight. *Nutr. Res.* 1(2):149–57 In press

53. Messing, B., Bitoun, A., Galian, J., Mary, H. Y., Goll, A., Bernier, J. J. 1977. La stéatose hépatique au cours de la nutrition parenterale depend-elle de

l'apport calorique glucidique? *Gastroenterol. Clin. Biol.* 1:1015–25

54. Messing, B., Latrive, J. P., Bitoun, A., Galian, A., Bernier, J. J. 1979. La stéatose hépatique au cours da la nutrition parentérale depend-elle de l'apport calorique lipidique? *Gastroenterol. Clin. Biol.* 3:719–24

55. Mock, D. M., deLorimer, A. A., Liebman, W. M., Sweeman, L., Baker, H. 1981. Biotin deficiency: an unusual complication of parenteral alimentation. *N. Engl. J. Med.* 304:820–22

56. Nichoalds, G. E., Meng, H. C., Caldwell, M. D. 1977. Vitamin requirements in patients receiving total parenteral nutrition. *Arch. Surg.* 112:1061–64

57 Patel, D., Anderson, G. H., Jeejeebhoy, K. N. 1973. Amino acid adequacy of parenteral casein hydrolysate and oral cottage cheese in patients with gastrointestinal disease as measured by nitrogen balance and blood aminogram. *Gastroenterology* 65:427–37

58. Prasad, A. S., Rabbani, P., Abbasii, A., Bowersox, E., Fox, M.R.S. 1978. Experimental zinc deficiency in humans. *Ann. Int. Med.* 89:483–90

59. Roth, K., Cohn, R., Yandrasitz, J., Preti, G., Dodd, D., Segal, S. 1976. Beta-methyl-crotonic aciduria associated with lactic acidosis. *J. Pediatr.* 88:229–35

60. Roulet, M., Jeejeebhoy, K. N., Shike, M., Marliss, E. B., Todd, T. R. J., Mahon, W. J., Anderson, G. H., Stewart, S. 1980. Energy and protein metabolism in critically ill, malnourished and septic patients. *J. Parenter. Enter. Nutr.* 4:582 (Abstr.)

61. Rudman, D., Millikan, W. J., Richardson, T. J., Bixler, T. J., Stackhouse, W. J., McGarrity, W. C. 1975. Elemental balances during intravenous hyperalimentation. *J. Clin. Invest.* 55:94–104

62. Scott, D. 1958. Clinical biotin deficiency ("egg white injury"): report of a case with some remarks on serum cholesterol. *Acta Med. Scand.* 162:69–70

63. Sherwin, R. S. 1978. Effect of starvation on the turnover and metabolic response to leucine. *J. Clin. Invest.* 61:1471–81

64. Shike, M., Harrison, J. E., Sturtridge, W. C., Tam, C. S., Bobechko, P. E., Jones, G., Murray, T. M., Jeejeebhoy, K. N. 1980. Metabolic bone disease in patients receiving long-term parenteral nutrition. *Ann. Int. Med.* 92:343–50

65. Shike, M., Roulet, M., Kurian, R., Whitwell, J., Stewart, S., Jeejeebhoy, K. N. 1981. Copper metabolism and requirements in total parenteral nutrition. *Gastroenterology* 81:290–97

66. Shike, M., Sturtridge, W. C., Tam, C. S., Harrison, J. E., Jones, G., Murray, T. M., Husdan, H., Whitwell, J., Wilson, D. R., Jeejeebhoy, K. N. 1981. A possible role of Vitamin D in the genesis of parenteral nutrition-induced metabolic bone disease. *Ann. Int. Med.* 95(5):560–68

67. Shizgal, H. M., Forse, R. A. 1980. Protein and calorie requirements with total parenteral nutrition. *Ann. Surg.* 192: 562–69

68. Silvas, S. E., Paragas, P. D. 1972. Paraesthesias, weakness, seizures and hypophosphatemia in patients receiving hyperalimentation. *Gastroenterology* 62:513–20

69. Skillman, J. J., Rosenoer, V. M., Smith, P. C., Fang, M. S. 1976. Improved albumin synthesis in post-operative patients by amino acid infusion. *N. Engl. J. Med.* 295:1037–40

70. Solomons, N. W., Layden, T. J., Rosenberg, I. H., Vo-Khactu, K., Sandstead, H. H. 1976. Plasma trace metals during total parenteral alimentation. *Gastroenterology* 70:1022–25

71. Sweetman, L., Bates, S. P., Hull, D., Nyhan, W. L. 1977. Propionyl-CoA carboxylase deficiency in a patient with biotin-responsive 3-methyl crotonylglycinuria. *Pediatr. Res.* 11:1144–47

72. Thompson, J. N., Scott, M. L. 1969. Role of selenium in the nutrition of the chick. *J. Nutr.* 97:335

73. Thurlow, P. M., Grant, J. P. 1981. Vitamin E, essential fatty acids and platelet function during total parenteral nutrition. Presented at Am. Soc. Parenter. Enter. Nutr., Fifth Clin. Conf. (Abstr)

74. Van Rij, A. M., Thomson, C. D., Fischer, J. E. 1979. Chromium deficiency during total parenteral nutrition. *J. Am. Med. Assoc.* 241:496–98

75. Veverbrants, E. D., Arky, R. A. 1969. Effects of fasting and refeeding. *J. Clin. Endocrinol.* 29:55–62

76. Vilter, R. W., Bozian, R. C., Hess, E. V. 1974. Manifestations of copper deficiency in a patient with systemic sclerosis on intravenous hyperalimentation. *N. Engl. J. Med.* 291:188–91

77. Wahren, D. J., Felig, P., Hagenfeldt, L. 1976. Effect of protein ingestion on splanchnic and leg metabolism in normal man and in patients with diabetes mellitus. *J. Clin. Invest.* 57:987–99

78. Wene, J. D., Connor, W. E., DenBeusten, L. 1975. The development of essential fatty acid deficiency in healthy men

fed fat-free diets intravenously and orally. *J. Clin. Invest.* 56:127–34

79. Winters, R. W., Heird, W. C., Dell, R. B., Nicholson, J. F. 1977. Plasma amino acids in infants receiving parenteral nutrition. In *Clinical Nutrition Update-Amino Acids,* ed. H. L. Greene, M. A. Holliday, H. N. Munro. Chicago: Am. Med. Assoc.

80. Wolfe, B. M. 1980. Substrate-endocrine interactions and protein metabolism. *J. Parenter. Enter. Nutr.* 4:188–94

81. Wolfe, B. M., Culebras, J. M., Sim, A. J. W., Bull, M. R., Moore, F. D. 1977.

Substrate interaction in intravenous feeding. Comparative effects of carbohydrate and fat on amino acid utilization in fasting man. *Ann. Surg.* 186:518–40

82. Woolfson, A. M., Heatley, R. V., Allison, S. P. 1979. Insulin to inhibit protein catabolism after injury. *N. Engl. J. Med.* 300:14–17

83. Yeung, C. K., Smith, R. C., Hill, G. L. 1979. Effect of an elemental diet on body composition. A comparison with intravenous nutrition. *Gastroenterology* 77:652–57

Ann. Rev. Nutr. 1982. 2:201-27
Copyright © 1982 by Annual Reviews Inc. All rights reserved

IATROGENIC NUTRITIONAL DEFICIENCIES

R. C. Young and J. P. Blass

Departments of Psychiatry & Neurology, Cornell University Medical College, The Burke Rehabilitation Center, White Plains, New York

CONTENTS

201

0199-9885/82/0715-0201$02.00

INTRODUCTION

Clinicians and biologists are most familiar with nutritional deficiencies that result from poor diets or a conditioning illness—e.g. protein-calorie malnutrition in Third World nations, and pernicious anemia, respectively. Diagnosis and specific treatment by health professionals correct the deficiency. It is increasingly apparent, however, that many types of therapy by physicians can provoke nutrient deficiencies. This chapter reviews several categories of such iatrogenic nutrient deficiencies (iatrogenic—induced inadvertently by a physician or his treatment).

Although severe deficiencies have been unintentionally induced during parenteral nutrition and by use of certain new therapeutic diets, this chapter does not review these.

SURGERY

Surgical Stress and Tissue Trauma

Immediately following major surgery there is considerable urinary loss of nitrogen, potassium, magnesium, and zinc (69, 205, 206). Hypercalcuria may result from immobilization, soft tissue injury of surgery, and skeletal trauma due to either surgery or accident (205). Such nutrient losses vary with age, with the nature of the underlying injury, and with site and magnitude of trauma. Poor nutritional status preoperatively may interfere with recovery through impaired wound healing, but postoperative megadoses of vitamins do not protect against surgical complications (73).

Gastric Surgery

B_{12} DEFICIENCY   Removal of the stomach eliminates the source of intrinsic factor and therefore leads to deficiency of vitamin B_{12}. The reported

Table 1   Nutrient deficiencies resulting from gastrectomy

Nutrient	References
Vitamin B_{12}	32, 57, 62, 98, 104, 106, 119, 121, 166–171, 174
Vitamin D and calcium	34, 35, 39, 58, 65, 77, 78, 81, 129, 131, 132, 134–137, 159, 175, 176, 190, 199, 210
Folate	104
Iron	9, 11, 57, 106, 121, 210
Protein	141, 204
Thiamine	20, 26

incidence of B_{12} deficiency following gastrectomy for peptic ulcer disease has ranged from 14 to 57% (32, 57, 98, 106, 174). This variation reflects differences in the surgical procedures used—i.e. anastomosis with duodenum or jejunum and presence or absence of associated vagotomy, as well as differences in the duration of follow-up. Johnson & Hoffbrand (104) studied 223 cases and concluded that as a cause of subsequent B_{12} deficiency the extent of gastric resection is more important than ulcer site, type of anastomosis, or inclusion of vagotomy. The deficiency often does not develop until six years following surgery, and new cases still develop after 10–15 years (32). This long depletion period for development of clincially evident deficiency of vitamin B_{12} is consistent with the earlier observations of Darby et al (55) in patients with pernicious anemia who were permitted to relapse under observation. On the other hand, development of low serum B_{12} postoperatively is not related to age or sex. In Buxton's (32) study, about 5% of gastrectomized patients developed evidence of B_{12} deficiency each year between postoperative years 5 and 15.

Multiple mechanisms may be involved. Most of the gastrectomized patients studied by Mahmud et al (121) and Lous & Swartz (119) displayed normal absorption of crystalline B_{12}, and fewer than 30% had abnormal B_{12} absorption tests indicating deficient intrinsic factor activity. In gastrectomized patients Doscherholmen & Swain (62) demonstrated impaired absorption of B_{12} when the vitamin was fed mixed into eggs, but not of crystalline B_{12}. This observation is consistent with a role of impaired acid and/or pepsin secretion in producing deficient utilization of dietary B_{12}. The effect may be additive with that of intrinsic factor deficiency, when present. Other proposed mechanisms for postgastrectomy B_{12} deficiency include bacterial overgrowth of the small intestine and disturbed enterohepatic circulation.

Buxton et al (32) noted that mean cell volume did not increase until serum B_{12} had fallen. They noted "obvious" macrocytosis in only 3 of 35 post-gastrectomy patients at the time when low B_{12} levels in the blood were documented. Iron nutriture was not examined in this series. Mahmud et al (121), on the other hand, reported "moderate" or "large" numbers of macrocytes in peripheral blood smears of 16 of 22 patients with low serum B_{12}; concomitant deficiency of bone marrow iron stores appeared to prevent the development of frank megaloblastosis.

Roos (166–171) found evidence of neuropathy in 34% of 128 gastrectomized patients after 12 years. The patients had primarily a peripheral sensory neuropathy, often associated with some myelopathy, affective changes, and dementia. Myelopathic signs did not respond to B_{12} replacement therapy. Affective improvement with treatment occurred in the majority of cases with intellectual impairment, but cognitive functioning at follow-up was not documented.

FOLATE   More than 30% of the gastrectomized patients reported by Johnson & Hoffbrand (104) had low folate values. Mean serum folate levels were 30% lower in patients who underwent "radical" gastric resection than those who had partial resections, but this difference was not significant because of scatter in the data. Neither ulcer site, presence or absence of vagotomy, nor type of anastomosis significantly differentiated serum folate levels. No data concerning preoperative diet were reported. The stomach is not thought to have a major role in folate absorption, but there are complex interactions between the metabolism of folate and of B_{12}, that do depend on the gastric mucosa. Thus the pathogenesis of folate deficiency after gastrectomy requires further investigation, including its relationship to preoperative nutriture.

VITAMIN D BONE DISEASE   Metabolic bone disease has been recognized as a late complication of gastric surgery since 1941 (175). By the tenth year following surgery the incidence has been judged to be 5–15% (134–137) to as high as 41% (64). Osteomalacia is the most prevalent syndrome described (9, 129), but osteoporosis has also been noted. Osteomalacia may be clinically apparent, with bone pain, low serum calcium and phosphorus, elevated alkaline phosphatase, and radiologic abnormalities (159). Clinically silent bone disease of moderate severity has, however, frequently been detected by bone biopsy. The disorder is most common after subtotal gastrectomy and gastrojejunostomy (Billroth II) and less common after a Billroth I procedure (78) or after vagotomy with gastric drainage (131, 132, 176, 210). The mechanism of the osteomalacia is controversial. Low 25-hydroxy-vitamin D levels have been detected following gastric surgery. Impaired absorption of vitamin D (190) and response to vitamin D therapy have been reported.

Chalmers (35) and Gertner et al (81) proposed that an important etiologic factor is poor dietary intake of vitamin D due to discomfort induced by eating fatty foods. Gertner found normal absorption of 25-hydroxy-cholecalciferol (25-OHD) in 5 of 6 patients with postgastrectomy osteomalacia but a history of dietary insufficiency in 4 of the 6. Destruction of vitamin D by intestinal bacteria has also been suggested but has not received direct support (199).

Osteoporosis can occur alone or in combination with osteomalacia following gastrectomy (34, 39). Reported incidence increases with increased duration of follow-up; changes become manifest more than six years following operation (58). The effect is also age-related, gastrectomy appearing to enhance age-dependent bone loss (77). These changes have been attributed to decreased calcium absorption and increased fecal excretion.

IRON   Iron deficiency and associated anemia are commonly reported following gastric surgery (9, 11, 57, 106, 210), with rates as high as 44% among men and 84% among women (210) depending on the surgical procedures as well as the measures and criteria applied. In Mahmud's series (121) 87% of gastrectomized patients had decreased bone marrow stores of iron. In addition to defective absorption, hemorrhage and dietary deficiency have been considered to be contributing mechanisms.

THIAMINE   Cases of "wet beriberi" following gastrectomy in alcoholics have been reported by Brigden & Robinson (26) and Bjornsson & Jonsson (20). Alchoholics are at risk for thiamine deficiency and for alcholic cardiomyopathy even without gastrectomy. Since the stomach is not known to play a major role in thiamine absorption, knowledge of the preoperative thiamine nutriture and intake of the vitamin during hospitalization is necessary before assessing the significance of gastrectomy per se on absorption and metabolism of thiamine in these patients with symptoms attributed to thiamine deficiency.

PROTEIN-CALORIE MALNUTRITION   Neale (141) reviewed 27 cases of protein-calorie malnutrition following gastrectomy, in all of which surgery was complicated by contaminated bowel syndrome, pancreatic insufficiency, or anorexia. In a case reported by Waldram (204) surgery was complicated by alcoholism, depression, and poor dentition.

Small Bowel Resection or Bypass

B_{12} DEFICIENCY   Impaired absorption of vitamin B_{12} was noted by Booth & Mollin (23) and Valman (200) following ileal resection, and following jejunoileal bypass by others (12, 107). Best (18) and Baker & Bogoch (13) described subacute combined degeneration of the spinal cord after ileal resection for Crohn's disease followed by folate therapy; low serum B_{12} was documented in both cases. Rodgers et al (162) reported abnormal Schilling tests in 3 of 13 children 10–26 months after replacement of the esophagus with a bowel segment that included colon and terminal ileum; serum B_{12} levels were still normal at that time.

VITAMIN D BONE DISEASE   Osteomalacia has been observed following gastrojejunostomy (93, 144), jejunoileal bypass for morbid obesity (46, 139, 148), and resection of jejunum, ileum, or both (43).
    The incidence of histological osteomalacia was nearly 50% in an un-

Table 2 Nutrient deficiencies resulting from intestinal bypass or resection

Nutrient	References
Vitamin A	27, 164, 208
Vitamin B$_6$	100
Vitamin B$_{12}$	12, 13, 18, 23, 107, 162, 200
Vitamin D and	7, 43, 44, 46, 47, 48, 54, 93, 120,
calcium	139, 144, 148, 164, 177, 185
Vitamin E	164, 208
Thiamine	82
Magnesium	46, 72, 117, 143, 146, 195
Trace metals	8, 130, 209
Carnitine	75, 140
Potassium	59, 83, 120, 151
Carbohydrate	151, 177
Protein	140, 179, 182, 211
Fat	102, 120, 178

selected group of patients 3–6 years after jejunoileal bypass (43). Low plasma 25-OHD concentrations suggest vitamin D malabsorption (44, 159). In addition, low serum 1,25-dihydroxy-vitamin D was documented by Mosekilde et al (139). Malabsorption of bile acid following bypass (54) may play a role in the malabsorption of vitamin D and of enterohepatically circulating 25-OHD (7). Bacterial contamination of the bypassed segment and lack of exposure of the patient to sunlight may also contribute to the deficit. Liver disease occurring after bypass may impair 25-hydroxylation of vitamin D (185). Mild, asymptomatic hypocalcemia occurred in 48% of one series (185) and secondary hyperparathyroidism was observed; bone disease was not found preoperatively in 4 morbidly obese subjects studied.

One to 14 years following jejunal, ileal, or combined resections, osteomalacia occurred in 9 of 25 patients (43). Abnormal bone biopsy occurred often in absence of symptoms or other biochemical or radiologic changes. The authors suggested that preoperative inflammatory bowel disease contributed to the bone changes. A history of poor dietary intake of vitamin D and of little exposure to sunlight were not uncommon, and cholestyramine therapy may also have contributed (see also 46) in some cases. The response to parenteral or oral vitamin D supplements varies (47, 48).

PROTEIN DEFICIENCY   Protein malnutrition frequently follows jejunoileal bypass (140, 179, 182, 211). Moxley et al (140) and White et al (211) reported a pattern of blood amino acid changes commonly seen in protein-calorie malnutrition: Low plasma concentrations of essential amino acids (valine, isoleucine, leucine, phenylalanine, threonine and lysine) as well as of nonessential amino acids (alanine, citrulline, cystine, tyramine, ornithine, and arginine) were associated with rapid weight loss during the first four months after surgery. Plasma levels of glycine and serine were elevated. Following stabilization of weight at 12–36 months after surgery, moderate depression of plasma valine, isoleucine, leucine, lysine, tyramine, ornithine, and arginine persisted. Oral amino acid tolerance tests consistent with impaired absorption immediately postoperatively improved by 12 months. Tryptophan was not measured. Normal blood glucose and liver glycogen and absence of ketones were documented throughout the postoperative course.

Liver disease secondary to the small bowel bypass may contribute to the picture of deficiency. Experimentally, hepatic fatty metamorphosis has been attributed to protein deficiencies. During the immediate postoperative period White et al (211) found that SGOT was elevated in 12 of 18 patients, most of whom had marked hepatic steatosis. By 12–36 months hepatic fat diminished and SGOT normalized. Improved amino acid tolerance with time in these patients was attributed to adaptive increases in absorption.

In 44 bypass patients studied by Shizgal et al (182) by multiple isotope dilution techniques, loss of body cell mass in addition to loss of body fat occurred in 4 cases. Increased extracellular mass, characteristic of protein malnutrition, was documented. Six subjects experienced malaise, anorexia, weakness, hypokalemia, abnormal liver function tests, and frequent hospitalizations. Symptoms remitted and abnormal laboratory values were corrected after infusions of amino acids. A high protein diet was necessary to sustain the remission of symptoms and maintenance of normal body composition.

VITAMINS A, E, AND K   Jejunoileal bypass can lead to deficiencies in these fat soluble vitamins (27, 164, 208). Rogers et al (164) found vitamin A levels of less than 30 μg/dl in 17 of 40 patients (42%) studied an average of 17 months after surgery. Abnormal dark adaptation was documented in 4 of 9 patients at least 18 months after surgery; this responded to oral supplementation. The degree of deficiency did not correlate with the time elapsed since surgery or with dietary intake; the weight of the 4 patients was stable. In the case reported by Wechsler (208), dermatologic changes and night blindness developed two years after surgery and were associated with a serum vitamin A level of 16 μg/dl; both abnormalities responded to administration of vitamin A. Reversible night blindness was reported by Brown et al (27) occurring 3.5 years after surgery; a serum carotene level of 6 μg/dl was found, indicating either severe impairment of absorption or a carotene-free diet.

Vitamin E levels less than 5.0 μg/dl in 18 of 40 patients (45%) were observed by Rogers et al (164); a level of 1.6 μg/dl was reported by Wechsler (208) in a patient who also had low serum β-carotene. The serum vitamin A, β-carotene, and vitamin E levels were not changed by 11 weeks of tetracycline therapy, suggesting that bacterial overgrowth was not the major factor in the deficiency. Prothrombin times were normal in the series of Rogers et al (164), which is consistent with normal bacterial production and colonic absorption of vitamin K.

THIAMINE   A case of "atrophic beriberi" that presented four months following jejunoileal bypass was reported by Glad et al (82). This patient had eaten a low-residue, high-carbohydrate diet to reduce diarrhea and developed symptoms and sign of peripheral motor and sensory neuropathy. Serum thiamine was undetectable and folate was low; B_{12}, vitamin A, riboflavin, and ascorbic acid were normal. Sensory changes essentially remitted with dietary therapy and supplementation with thiamine and other vitamins. After discharge from the hospital the patient failed to comply with instructions concerning dietary supplementation and relapsed, eventually requiring reanastomosis. The authors emphasized the importance of her poor dietary intake in the development of the thiamine deficiency.

CARNITINE   Frohlich et al (75) reported significant decreases in total and free plasma carnitine levels observed six weeks after jejunoileal bypass and persisting after six months. Preoperative values had been in the normal range. The authors suggest that the reduction in plasma carnitine resulted either from dietary inadequacy or secondarily from reduced synthesis from lysine, a deficiency of which can occur immediately after surgery (140).

PYRIDOXINE   Howard et al (100) reported pyridoxine deficiency occurring after jejunoileal bypass. The patient became pregnant 18 months following surgery; despite routine vitamin and iron therapy she developed microcytic, hypochromic anemia and symtoms including insomnia, irritabilty, dizziness, and fatigue after the 32nd month. Plasma pyridoxine was 8.0 ng/ml (normal 30–80), with elevated serum iron and iron binding capacity. The symptoms and anemia responded to oral pyridoxine. The authors suggest that malabsorption, impaired storage, impaired hepatic conversion to pyridoxal phosphate, or increased vitamin demand associated with pregnancy may have been etiologic factors.

TRACE METALS   Atkinson et al (8) demonstrated low plasma zinc and copper levels in patients 1–36 months after bypass surgery. Their patients were apparently asymptomatic, except for one case with immunologic impairment and scrofula; neutropenia exhibited by one patient responded to supplementary copper. Weissman et al (209) described a case of clinically manifest zinc deficiency which occurred one year after bypass; the symptoms included anorexia, vomiting, dermatitis, and apathy. These deficiencies may reflect intestinal malabsorption or increased loss due to malabsorption of bile. It is interesting that morbidly obese subjects of Atkinson et al (8) had significantly low zinc levels preoperatively, which were further lowered postoperatively. Observed preoperative copper levels were significantly higher than normal. Anorexia and disturbed taste sensation from low zinc levels may compound postoperative problems (130).

MAGNESIUM   Magnesium is absorbed along the small intestine, and hypomagnesemia has been reported following small bowel resection (71, 138, 141) as well as after bypass procedures (46, 113, 189). Swenson et al (189) considered magnesium deficiency to be an uncommon complication of bypass, reporting an incidence of less than 2.5% at about three years postoperatively; Compston (46), however, found hypomagnesemia in 6 of 21 patients 3–6 years after surgery. In Nielson & Thaysen's case (138), the patient became symptomatic within days after surgery, showing confusion, apathy, and muscle twitching followed by weakness. Tissue depletion preoperatively may account in part for postoperative deficit, as magnesium deficiency can be a concomitant of both inflammatory bowel disease and thiazide diuretic therapy for obesity. Postsurgical decrease in absorption is said to be proportional to length of small bowel resected or bypassed (195). Oral or parenteral replacement is effective (143, 195).

POTASSIUM LOSS   A common complication of small bowel resection or bypass is hypokalemia, specifically because of diarrhea (59, 83, 102, 120, 151). Oral potassium supplementation should be prescribed routinely following such surgery.

FAT MALABSORPTION   Increased fecal fat loss is routine following bypass or resection (120, 178). It results from decreased transit time, altered metabolism of bile salt, or decreased absorptive surface. Huseman (102) demonstrated a decrease in fatty acid absorption immediately after surgery, followed by some later "adaptive" increases. He also documented a persistent reduction in serum cholesterol attributable to increased bile salt loss and greater synthetic demand for cholesterol.

CALCIUM   Hypocalcemia following small intestinal resection or bypass (120, 177) can lead to tetany (177).

CARBOHYDRATE ABSORPTION   Decreased glucose absorption as reflected by flattened glucose tolerance curves follows small bowel resection (179, 151). The fasting glucose has been reported as normal; the clinical significance of the observed decreased absorption is not evident.

Ureteral Diversion

Anastomosis of the ureters to the bowel can result in metabolic alterations that change nutritional requirements. For instance, it may induce hypochloremic acidosis that alters calcium requirements and leads to bone disease (156). Hyperchloremic acidosis has been described following ureteroileostomy (53, 92, 105) and ureterosigmoidostomy (25, 189). It has been ascribed to bowel uptake of chloride and ammonia and to bicarbonate loss into the gut, compounded by renal damage from hydronephrosis or pyelonephritis. Ferris & Odel (71) observed hyperchloremia in 79% and acidosis in 80% of 141 patients at varying intervals (usually within one year) after ureterosigmoidostomy. Hypocalcemia and hypophosphatemia in conjunction with acidosis have been described following ureterosigmoidostomy (84). These were attributed to utilization of calcium to combine with excess acid, with secondary lowering of serum phosphorus induced by parathyroid hormone. Impaired gut absorption of vitamin D in acidosis has also been reported (115).

Rickets and osteomalacia may follow ureterosigmoidostomy in children (84, 115, 188) and in adults (99, 114, 180), bone changes becoming apparent 2–10 years following surgery. Both renal damage and acidosis may contribute. While some case reports indicate that correction of acidosis alone is sufficient (99, 184), other workers have demonstrated an additional requirement for vitamin D, or the occurrence of vitamin D "resistance" (92). Perry et al (153) described a case of vitamin D "resistant" osteomalacia after ureterosigmoidostomy. Deficiency of renal vitamin D-1 hydroxylase was indirectly demonstrated and attributed to hydronephrosis—effective vitamin D deficiency resulting from the kidney's failure to synthesize the active metabolite.

Stamey (189) stressed the dangers of chronic potassium loss in conjunction with acidosis after ureterosigmoidostomy and the therapeutic difficulties it presents. He attributed the loss of combined osmotic diuresis and colonic secretion of potassium.

Prosthetic Cardiac Valves

In a single report, 18 of 90 patients with prosthetic heart valves were reported to have anemia and low serum iron values, which responded to oral iron supplements (96).

HEMODIALYSIS

Bone Disease

Osteomalacia is a recognized complication of the treatment of chronic renal failure with hemodialysis (67, 152), but its etiology has been uncertain. Hypophosphatemia has been considered as a mechanism, via loss of phosphates through the dialyzer membrane (4, 19, 155). However, the osteomalacia was not prevented or cured by use of a phosphate-enriched dialysate in nonhypophosphatemic patients (70). The condition has not responded consistently to vitamin D_2, 1-OHD, or 1-25-OHD (67, 155, 183), and serum 25-OHD levels are reportedly normal (49). The Newcastle group has suggested that aluminum in dialysate may be responsible for osteomalacia by an unknown mechanism (52, 63, 207). Dialysis dementia, which has also been postulated to reflect aluminum toxicity, appears related epidemiologically to the osteomalacia.

Carnitine Deficiency

Reduction in plasma and muscle carnitine concentrations can accompany hemodialysis (17, 22) and may contribute to the cardiomyopathy sometimes seen with this treatment. Reduction in plasma carnitine concentration may be transient or persistent (15). In some patients a deficit in cellular carnitine concentrating capacity seemed to be present. Reduced synthesis of carnitine was apparent and was probably not part of a general synthetic deficit, since plasma protein concentration was normal. Bohmer et al (22) suggested that a lack of cofactors such as ascorbic acid or ferrous iron, or of a specific protein required for carnitine synthesis (113) might be involved.

Choline Deficiency

Reduced nerve conduction in hemodialysis patients has been related to choline loss (161). Therapy with choline or lecithin has not been systematically investigated.

Potassium Depletion

Chronic potassium depletion has been observed in patients receiving hemodialysis (123, 187). The mechanism has not been elucidated.

Hypovitaminosis

Reduced serum levels of folate have been described in patients undergoing repeated hemodialysis (see 163), as have reduced vitamin B_{12} (173) and megaloblastic hematologic changes. Reduced serum ascorbic acid levels have also been reported (94).

IRRADIATION

Therapeutically administered ionizing radiation frequently results in nausea, vomiting, anorexia, and weight loss. A malabsorption syndrome may result from radiation damage to the small bowel. Villous atrophy, lymphangectasia, steatorrhea, dissacharidase deficiency, and protein-losing enteropathy have been described (197, 198). The effects of radiation enteritis may be exacerbated through inhibition of protein synthesis by chemotherapeutic agents. Recovery is promoted by nutrient repletion and by avoiding resultant food intolerances, for example, to gluten and lactose (61).

DRUGS

The growing literature on effects of a variety of drugs on nutrient status has been summarized elsewhere (40). This review updates current thinking resulting from most recently reported studies. The monographs by Hathcock & Cook (95) and Roe (163), and the review by Ovesen (147) provide extensive background and bibliographies.

In general, acute drug use may have little effect on nutriture, but chronic use of some drugs may have more significant impact on nutrient status. In some instances, chronic use may exacerbate preexisting dietary or conditioned nutrient deficiencies.

Drugs may alter intake, synthesis, absorption, transport, storage, metabolism, or excretion of nutrients. Susceptibility to drug-induced nutrient deficiency may be greater during periods of increased requirements—i.e. during growth, pregnancy, and lactation.

The effect of a given dose of a drug varies among individuals; one may expect similar variation in the effect on nutritional status. Drugs such as diphenylhydantoin, tricyclic antidepressants, and procaine amide are classic examples of drugs the effective concentration of which following a given dosage varies among individuals. Concomitant ingestion of other drugs may also increase or decrease the effective concentrations of medication. From experimental animal data arises the suggestion that nutritional status per se may likewise alter drug metabolism. Genetic heterogeneity in drug metabolizing enzymes seems to be an important basis for interindividual differences; intercurrent diseases also alter drug metabolism. In hepatic and renal diseases there are notable examples of effective drug overdosage.

Primary Folate Antagonists

Dihydrofolate reductase is inhibited by a group of drugs including methotrexate, pyrimethamine, trimethoprim, pentamidine, and triamterene. As a result, administration of these drugs can deplete tissues of tetrahydrofolic

Table 3 Drug nutrient interactions

Nutrient	Drug	References[a]
Vitamin A	mineral oil	
	neomycin	
Vitamin B$_6$	hydralazine	
	isoniazid	80
	L-dopa	
	oral contraceptives	1, 28, 111, 196
	penicillamine	
Vitamin B$_{12}$	biguanides	33
	cholestyramine	
	colchicine	
	neomycin	
	nitrous oxide	3, 56, 116, 127
	oral contraceptives	
	potassium chloride	
Vitamin C	oral contraceptives	
	salicylates	
	tetracycline	
Vitamin D	anticonvulsants	6, 16, 87, 88, 118, 125, 138, 191, 212
	cholestyramine	
	irritant cathartics	74
	mineral oil	
Folate	anticonvulsants	36, 186, 203
	cholestyramine	
	methotrexate	5
	oral contraceptives	14
	pyrimethamine	
	sulfasalizine	
	triamterene	
	salicylates	
	trimethoprim	
Vitamin K	anticonvulsants	109
	cholestyramine	
	coumarin	109, 192
	mineral oil	
	salicylates	
Magnesium	gentamycin	110, 149
	diuretics	64, 66
Niacin	isoniazid	41, 42, 86, 91
Riboflavin	oral contraceptives	142, 202
	chlorpromazine	157, 158
Thiamin	oral contraceptives	142, 202

[a] In addition to the text and the reviews by Roe (163), Ovesen (147), Clark (40) and Hatchcock & Coon (95).

acid and lead to megaloblastic anemias (5), particularly in individuals already low in folate. The potency of these drugs in producing folate antagonism parallels their degree of binding to the enzyme. Methotrexate is the most powerful. Treatment of toxicity with folinic acid (citrovoram factor) has been at least partially effective (24, 194).

Anticonvulsants

Chronic treatment with anticonvulsants such as phenobarbitone, phenytoin, and primadone, singly or in combination, often result in folate deficiency (36, 186), megaloblastic anemia occurring in 0.15–0.75% of patients. Vogel (203) has proposed that drug-induced gingival hyperplasia may be mediated by folate deficiency. The mechanisms involved are unknown. There have been conflicting reports as to whether or not supplementing anticonvulsants with large doses of folate increases seizure frequency in epileptics. Folic acid supplementation has been reported to decrease serum and cerebrospinal fluid concentrations of phenytoin and phenobarbitone (126).

The anticonvulsant drugs disturb metabolism of vitamin D (6, 16, 87, 88, 191). Between 10 and 30% of epileptics on long-term therapy show biochemical or radiologic evidence of impaired vitamin D status; asymptomatic hypocalcemia or hypomagnesemia, increased alkaline phosphatase, as well as osteomalacia on bone biopsy or X-ray have been reported. Such evidences of osteomalacia may occur within several months after initiation of anticonvulsant therapy. Generally, the derangements are mild, clinically manifest bone disease being uncommon. The relationship between small biochemical or radiologic abnormalities and clinical disease is not defined.

Anticonvulsant drugs may induce liver enzymes that metabolize vitamin D or its active metabolites (125). Indirect data consistent with that mechanism are the reduction of serum 25-hydroxycholecalciferol (25-OHD) levels in treated epileptics compared to controls (138, 212), and findings of decreased plasma half-life of vitamin D_3 (125) and increased excretion of polar metabolites in treated epileptics. Multiple anticonvulsants seem to be additive in their effects on liver enzymes. Acetazolamide may accelerate bone changes (122) by inducing metabolic acidosis which favors calcium mobilization. Dietary intake and degree of exposure to sunlight are probably important modifying factors (118).

These radiologic and biochemical changes have been reported to respond to vitamin D (38, 154, 145). Stoffer et al (193) suggest that simply changing anticonvulsants may result in resolution of the abnormalities. Monitoring of epileptics for biochemical or radiologic evidence of early changes of bone disease remains a controversial issue (37, 180).

Klein et al (112) reported a case of cardiomegaly and congestive heart

failure responsive to thiamine in a young child receiving long-term anticonvulsants. It is possible that the primary disorder in this child related to
thiamine metabolism.

Hemorrhagic disease attributed to drug-induced vitamin K deficiency has
been reported in the offspring of mothers treated chronically with phenytoin
(109). This has been attributed to increased vitamin K catabolism due to
enzyme induction. Oral and intravenous supplementation prior to labor has
been suggested. A discussion of drug effects on fetal nutrition and development is beyond the scope of this review; the reader is referred to Roe (163).

Antitubercular Drugs

Isoniazid therapy has long been recognized as inducing peripheral neuropathy due to pyridoxine deficiency, the reported prevalences being as high as
40%. The effect occurs within months after the initiation of therapy. Prophylaxis through co-administration of vitamin B_6 has been demonstrated
(but see 31). Pyridoxine-responsive anemia during isoniazid therapy has
also been reported. Cycloserine, another pyridoxine antagonist, has also
been associated with anemias responsive to the vitamin. Neonatal convulsions responsive to pyridoxine have occurred following maternal isoniazid
treatment (128). The mechanism for such pyridoxine deficiency has been
variously attributed to increased urinary excretion of pyridoxine complexed
with drug or competitive inhibition of pyridoxal phosphate. Direct neural
toxicity by the drug-vitamin complex has been reported (80).

Pellagra is a rare complication of isoniazid therapy in well-nourished
populations, but has been recorded in malnourished tuberculous patients
(41, 42, 86, 91). Proposed mechanisms include impaired niacin synthesis
secondary to pyridoxine deficiency and competitive inhibition by isoniazid
of the coenzyme function of the vitamin. Malabsorption, particularly of
vitamin B_{12}, with resultant megaloblastic anemia has been observed in users
of p-aminosalicylic acid (97).

Oral Contraceptives

The effects of estrogen-containing oral contraceptives (ECOC) on folate
metabolism seem of less clinical import than earlier indicated. The megaloblastic anemia recorded in association with their use (14) is usually attributed to preexisting depletion of folate stores or to other contributing
factors.

Reduction in serum vitamin B_{12} levels has been described during ECOC
use, possibly through redistribution among tissues. The clinical significance,
if any, of this effect is unknown.

Pyridoxine lowering has been reported in 20% of women using ECOC
(28, 111, 196). An association between such reduction and depressive symp-

toms has been suggested (see Roe), as has a relationship with glucose intolerance (1); but definitive evidence is not at hand.

It has been indicated that oral contraceptives may increase requirements of thiamine and riboflavin (142, 202), but clinical significance of the changes observed has not been established. Similarly, decreased plasma and tissue concentrations of ascorbic acid have been recorded in conjuntion with ECOC use without establishing clinical significance; no cases of clinical scurvy have been reported.

Anticoagulants

Coumarins act as vitamin K antagonists. The mechanism of action in the prophylaxis of thrombosis is not established but may involve accumulation of abnormal forms of vitamin K-dependent coagulation factors that are unable to bind calcium (192). A variety of other drugs may potentiate the actions of coumarin through decreased microbial synthesis of vitamin K, decreased absorption, decreased coumarin binding to albumin, inhibition of coumarin metabolism, and decreased synthesis or increased catabolism of vitamin K-dependent clotting factors (see 163).

Oral Hypoglycemic Agents

Metformin, a biguanide drug used for treatment of diabetes, may infrequently cause a selective, reversible deficiency of vitamin B_{12} (33). The mechanism may be a competitive inhibition of absorption or drug inactivation of the vitamin.

Laxatives and Antacids

It long has been established that chronic use of laxatives and antacids may impair absorption. For example, mineral oil impairs absorption of fat-soluble carotene and vitamins A, D, and K. Abuse of phenolphthalein and other laxatives has been associated with factitious diarrhea, protein-losing enteropathy, and malabsorption, including that of vitamin D and calcium (74). Loss of integrity of intestinal epithelial cells or increased peristaltic rate have been put forward as mechanisms for such effects of phenolphthalein (76). Prolonged use of magnesium and aluminum hydroxide antacids has resulted in phosphate depletion and osteomalacia through binding of phosphate in the intestinal lumen (50, 103).

Diuretics

Oral diuretics, including furosemide, ethacrynic acid, and triameterene, induce hypercalcuria; in contrast, the thiazides cause calcium retention. Magnesium deficiency has been associated with administration of thiazides, ethacrynic acid, and furosemide (66). Dyckner & Wester (64) demonstrated that magnesium infusion reduced ventricular ectopy in cardiac patients receiving diuretics. Digitalis may augment diuretic-induced excretion of calcium or magnesium. Diuretics may deplete tissue and serum zinc through increased urinary excretion. Evidence concerning induction of tissue depletion of potassium by diuretics has been critically reviewed by Morgan et al (133), who conclude that most studies suffered from improper matching by age of controls and failure to take account of muscle wasting.

Anesthesia

Prolonged ventilation with nitrous oxide can produce megaloblastic changes in blood and has been associated with neurologic changes resembling the myelopathy and peripheral neuropathy of vitamin B_{12} deficiency (3). Recent animal studies (56, 127) and tissue culture experiments (116) indicate that nitrous oxide interferes with vitamin B_{12} metabolism, inhibiting methylcobalamin synthesis and thus reducing methionine synthetase activity.

Antibiotics

There are recent case reports of renal magnesium wasting and associated hypomagnesemia, hypocalcemia, and hypokalemia in patients treated for months with high doses of gentamycin (110, 149). The biochemical changes seem to occur after a latent period of weeks, and may lead to frank clinical symptoms.

Psychotropic Drugs

Pinto et al (157, 158) have documented an interaction between chlorpromazine and the metabolism of riboflavin, the structure of which resembles that of the drug. Chlorpromazine inhibits incorporation of riboflavin into flavin adenine dinucleotide (FAD) in rat liver, brain, and heart, in part through the inhibition of hepatic flavokinase. Chronic administration of clinically relevant doses increased riboflavin excretion, significantly lowered tissue FAD and flavin mononucleotide (FMN) concentrations, and altered the activity coefficient of the FAD-containing enzyme erythrocyte glutathione reductase. Psychoactive drugs structurally unrelated to riboflavin were ineffective. The tricyclic antidepressants, imipramine and amitriptyline, also alter riboflavin metabolism in rats, but only at very high doses.

Drug Effects on Food Intake

The potential effects of drugs on nutriture through alteration of the amount or character of food intake have received little attention except for those drugs designed as appetite depressants. Widely used drugs such as digitalis may reduce appetite, even at therapeutic levels (91, 160). Drugs may also effect food selection; for example, a reported side effect of amitriptyline, a tricyclic antidepressant, is the induction of carbohydrate craving (150). Several drugs, including allopurinol, affect taste and smell (165). Much wider studies of these phenomena associated with commonly used drugs would be useful.

CONCLUSIONS AND RECOMMENDATIONS

The above discussion catalogs nutritional abnormalities accompanying a number of therapeutic regimens and documents that physicians may impair their patients' nutriture while treating their illnesses. The data suggest several generalizations and recommendations.

Many surgical therapies regularly result in important nutritional complications, the recognition and management of which are an essential part of good surgical care. Nutritional problems are particularly frequent consequences of surgery on the gastrointestinal tract.

Nutritional complications of small bowel bypass are potentially so severe that they limit the benefits of this procedure. Regular laboratory evaluation of the nutritional status of these patients is a necessary part of good care following bypass surgery. Weight loss, neuropathy, cardiac arrhythmias, loss of stamina, or changes in mental status are clinical findings that should alert the physician to potential nutritional problems. Minimum laboratory tests should include hematologic evaluation (complete blood count, smear, packed cell volume, etc), B_{12}, folate, and iron levels, albumin, calcium, phosphorus, alkaline phosphatase, transaminases, and sodium, potassium, chloride, and CO_2. Roentgenologic examination of the bone should be obtained. In patients who develop cardiac disease or neuropathy after bypass, it is prudent to obtain a measure of thiamine nutriture—either blood pyruvate or blood transketolase dependence on thiamine pyrophosphate (29). Other more specialized nutritional evaluations are necessary in patients with persistent problems, but will usually need the resources of a specialized nutrition center laboratory. Gastric bypass may be an attractive alternative to small bowel bypass (90, 124), with potentially less severe sequelae (2, 30, 85).

Gastrectomy, whether partial or complete, places patients at risk for a characteristic series of nutritional problems (32, 121). It is important to remember that vitamin B_{12} deficiency can first present as depression, dementia, or other changes in mental status. Postgastrectomy patients should be followed at least yearly, with careful history and examination, including accurate weight, hematologic evaluation, and studies of iron, B_{12}, and folate.

Loss of bone substance is a major complication of many types of therapy, since it can result from simple immobility (60), as well as more specific mechanisms, notably after surgery on the gastrointestinal tract. Osteoporosis is a major problem of older populations, and its proper management is controversial (68). In particular, the proper role of dietary supplements of calcium and vitamin D is unsettled. Bone films at regular intervals appear indicated in patients after gastrectomy or gut bypass, and dietary supplementation with calcium is warranted (78, 176, 210).

Patients vary markedly in the metabolic effects of drugs, and recommendations for nutrition must be interpreted in light of age, sex, reproductive status, and genetic endownment. Altered nutritional needs directly due to genetic effects have only rarely been documented (21, 172). More extensive data demonstrate the genetic variations in drug metabolism, and consequently in the potential effects of medicines on nutrition. These effects are part of the field of pharmacogenetics (201). Finally, the underlying illness being treated can itself alter nutritional requirements and the effect of the treatment on nutrient status—e.g. a morbidly obese person who undergoes intestinal bypass is in a disadvantaged nutritional state initially.

The clinical significance of many of the demonstrable changes in nutritional levels listed above are obscure, particularly some of those that relate to drug (e.g. contraceptive) use and other medical therapies. Reported abnormalities are often limited to low blood levels of nutrients, the relationships of which to clinical syndromes may not have been established. Drugs prescribed for chronic medication are often for use by people who are chronically ill and therefore already at risk of nutritional deficiency. For instance, psychotropic drugs are appropriately given to people whose behavior, including their feeding behavior, is chronically or recurrently disordered. Schizophrenics may eat bizarre diets, and depressed people characteristically suffer anorexia. Even in a schizophrenic who appears relatively intact on phenothiazines, it is hard confidently to attribute a nutritional disorder to the effects of the phenothiazines. In general, physicians should determine and monitor the nutritional status (by dietary history and applicable biochemical and clinical observations) of chronically ill patients receiving multiple or chronic medications. Bone changes and calcium metabolism should be watched particularly closely. It is reasonable to give pyridoxine to patients on isoniazid, and to give folate to patients who develop laboratory or clinical evidence of complications of anticonvulsant therapy. Routine nutrient supplementation on the basis of drug therapy alone, however, is not generally justified.

Further research to assess the biochemically detectable changes in nutriture induced by drugs is to be encouraged, including especially the appraisal of the clinical significance of laboratory changes. In those instances where the clinical significances and predictibility are established, biochemical assessment of the nutriture at intervals during therapy is beneficial both in the management of the patient and in diagnosis of those signs and symptoms that occur during therapy. Appropriately selected biochemical and physiologic measures of nutriture are useful initially in guiding therapy in patients known to be nutritionally at risk, such as alcoholics, schizophrenics, and individuals with malabsorption or other syndromes that are recognized as diseases that may condition nutritional deficiencies. Although not specifically discussed in this review, these measures likewise are of particular usefulness in identifying instances of hypervitaminoses, such as hypervitaminosis A, carotenemia, hypervitaminosis D, and the like.

In many of the situations discussed in this chapter, nutritional complications are a price for effective therapy. If the therapy is necessary, then the price seems justified. Therapeutic interventions that effect treatment of severe illnesses have inherent potential to cause side effects. The ability to alter physiology for the patient's benefit implies the ability to alter it to the patient's harm. Powerful new therapies enable physicians successfully to treat patients for whom previously nothing effective could be done. The side effects that accompany new regimens, however, complicate their use. Nutritional side effects that can be identified by proper assessment procedures and managed by oral or parenteral supplementation are among the more satisfying of these to manage.

ACKNOWLEDGMENTS

Supported by the Will Rogers Institute, a grant from the General Foods Corporation, and N.I.H. grants NS15125, NS16994 and AA03883.

Literature Cited

1. Adams, P. W., Folkard, J., Wynn, V., Seed, M. 1976. Influence of oral contraception, pyridoxine (vitamin B_6) and tryptophan on carbohydrate metabolism. *Lancet* 1:759–64
2. Adler, J. F. 1977. Gastric and jejunoileal bypass. A comparison in the treatment of morbid obesity. *Arch. Surg.* 112:799–806
3. Adornato, B. T. 1978. Nitrous oxide and vitamin B_{12}. Letter. *Lancet* 2:1318
4. Ahmed, K., Wills, M., Skinner, R., Vorhese, Z., Meinhard, E., Baillod, R. A. 1976. Persistent hypophosphataemia and osteomalacia in dialysis patients not on oral phosphate-binders: response to dihydrotachysterol therapy. *Lancet* 2: 439–42
5. Anderson, J. M., Smith, M. D., Hutchinson, J. 1966. Megaloblastic anemia and methotrexate therapy. *Brit. Med. J.* 2:641–42
6. Anticonvulsant osteomalacia. Editorial. 1976. *Br. Med. J.* 2:13401

7. Arnaud, S. B., Goldsmith, R. S., Lambert, P. W., Go, V. W. I. 1975. 25-Hydroxy vitamin D_3; evidence of an enterohepatic circulation in man. *Proc. R. Soc. Exp. Biol. Med.* 149:570–72
8. Atkinson, R. L., Dahms, W. T., Bray, G. A. 1978. Plasma zinc & copper in obesity and after intestinal bypass. *Ann. Int. Med.* 89:491–93
9. Baird, I. M., Blackburn, E. K., Wilson, G. M. 1959. The pathogensis of anemia after partial gastrectomy. *Q. J. Med.* 28:21–33
10. Baird, I. M., Oleesky, S. 1957. Osteomalacia following gastric surgery. *Gastroenterology* 33:284–91
11. Baird, I. M., Wilson, G. M. 1959. The pathogenesis of anemia after partial gastrectomy. II. Iron Absorption. *Q. J. Med.* 28:35–41
12. Badderley, R. M. 1976. Results of jejuno-ileostomy for gross refractory obesity. *Br. J. Surg.* 63:801–6

13. Baker, S. M., Bogoch, A. 1973. Subacute combined degeneration of the spinal cord after ileal resection and folic acid administration in Crohn's disease. *Neurology* (MINNEAP) 23:40–41
14. Barone, C., Bartoloni, C., Ghirlanda, G., Gentiloni, N. 1979. Megalo-blastic anemia due to folic acid deficiency after oral contraceptives. *Haematologica (Pavia)* 64:190–95
15. Battistella, P. A., Angelini, C., Vergani, L. 1978. Carnitine deficiency induced during haemodialysis. *Lancet* 1:939
16. Bell, R. D., Pak, C. Y., Zerwekh, J., Barilla, D. E., Vasko, M. 1979. Effect of phenytoin on bone & vitamin D. metabolism. *Ann. Neurol.* 5:376–78
17. Bertoli, M., Battistella, O. P., Vergani, L. et al. 1979. Carnitine deficiency induced during hemodialysis. *Second International Congress on Nutrition in Renal Disease.*
18. Best, C. N. 1959. Combined degeneration of spinal cord after extensive resection of ileum in Chron's disease. *Br. Med. J.* 2:862–64
19. Bishop, M. C., Woods, C. G., Oliver, D. O. 1972. Effects of hemodialysis on bone in chronic renal failure. *Br. Med. J.* 3:644–47
20. Bjornsson, O. G., Jonsson, A. 1979. Wet beriberi in an alcoholic after gastrectomy. *Br. J. Clin. Pract.* 33:119–21
21. Blass, J. P., Gibson, G. E., 1979. Genetic factors in Wernicke-Korsakoff syndrome. *Alcoholism* 3:126–34
22. Bohmer, T., Bergrem, H., Eiklid, K. 1978. Carnitine deficiency induced during intermittent haemodialysis for renal failure. *Lancet* 1:126–28
23. Booth, C. A., Mollin, D. L. 1959. The site of absorption of vitamin B$_{12}$ in man. *Lancet* 1:18–21
24. Borrie, P., Clark, P. A. 1966. Meglo-blastic anemia during methotrexate treatment of psoriasis. *Brit. Med. J.* 1: 1339
25. Boyd, J. D. 1931. Chronic acidosis secondary to ureteral transplanation. *Am. J. Dis. Child.* 42:366–72
26. Brigden, W., Robinson, J. 1964. Alcoholic heart disease. *Br. Med. J.* 2: 1283–89
27. Brown, G. C., Felton, S. M., Benson, W. E. 1980. Reversible night blindness associated with intestinal bypass surgery. *Am. J. Ophthalmol.* 89:776–79
28. Brown, R. R., Rose, D. P., Leklem, J. E., Linkswiler, H. M. 1975. Effects of oral contraceptives on tryptophan metabolism & vitamin B requirements in women. *Acta Vitaminol. Enzymol. (Milano)* 29:151–57
29. Brubacher, G., Harnel, A., Ritzel, G. 1972. Transketolase activity, thiamine excretion, and blood thiamine content in man as criteria of vitamin B$_1$ supply. *Int. J. Vitam. Nutr. Res.* 42:190–95
30. Buckwalter, J. A. 1977. A prospective comparison of the jejunoileal and gastric bypass operations for morbid obesity. *World J. Surg.* 1:757–68
31. Burke, G. J., Hlangebeza, T. 1977. Isoniazid-induced pellegra in a patient on vitamin B supplement. *S. Afr. Med. J.* 51:719–20
32. Buxton, R. A., Collins, C. D. 1977. Vitamin B$_{12}$ deficiency following gastrectomy. A long-term follow-up. *Br. J. Clin. Pract.* 31:69–72
33. Callaghan, T. S., Hadden, D. R., Tomkin, G. H. 1980. Megalo-blastic anemia due to vitamin B$_{12}$ malabsorption associated with long-term metformin treatment. *Br. Med. J.* 280:1214–15
34. Caniggia, A., Gennari, C., Cesari, L. 1964. Intestinal absorption of ^{45}Ca and dynamics of ^{45}Ca in gastrectomy osteoporosis. *Acta Med. Scand.* 176:599–606
35. Chalmers, J., Conacher, W. D. H., Gardner, D. L., Scott, P. J. 1967. Osteomalacia—a common disease in elderly women. *J. Bone Joint Surg.* 49:403–23
36. Chanarin, I. 1979. Effects of anticonvulsant drugs. In *Folic Acid In Neurology, Psychiatry & Internal Medicine*, ed. M. I. Botez, E. H. Reynolds, pp. 75–80. NY: Raven Press. 534 pp.
37. Christiansen, C., Radbro, P. 1977. Anticonvulsant osteomalacia. Letter. *Br. Med. J.* 1:439–40
38. Christiansen, C., Radbro, P., Munck, O. 1975. Actions of vitamins D2 & D3 & 25-OHD3 in anticonvulsant osteomalacia. *Br. Med. J.* 2:363–65
39. Clark, C. G., Crooks, I., Dowson, A. A., Mitchell, P. F. G. 1964. Disordered calcium metabolism after Polya partial gastrectomy. *Lancet* 1:734–38
40. Clark, F. 1976. Drugs & vitamin deficiency. *J. Hum. Nutr.* 30:333–37
41. Comaish, J. S., Cooper, M. 1977. Isoniazid-induced pellagra. Letter. *Arch Dermatol.* 113:986–87
42. Comaish, J. S., Felix, R. H., McGrath, H. 1976. Topically applied niacinamide in isoniazid-induced pellagra. *Arch. Dermatol.* 112:70–72
43. Compston, J. E., Ayers, A. B., Horton, L. W., Tighe, J. R., Creamer, B. 1978.

Osteomalacia after small-intestinal resection. *Lancet* 1:9–12

44. Compston, J. E., Creamer, B. 1977. Plasma levels and intestinal absorption of 25-hydroxyvitamin D in patients with small bowel resection. *Gut.* 18: 171–75

45. Compston, J. E., Horton, L. W. 1978. Oral 25-hydroxyvitamin D3 in treatment of osteomalacia associated with ileal resection & cholestyramine therapy. *Gastroenterology* 74:900–2

46. Compston, J. E., Horton, L. W., Laker, M. F., Ayers, A. B., Woodhead, J. S., Bull, H. J., Gazet, J. C., Pilkington, T. R. 1978. Bone disease after jejuno-ileal bypass for obesity. *Lancet* 2:1–4

47. Compston, J. E., Horton, L. W., Laker, M. F., Merrett, A. L., Woodhead, J. S., Gazet, J. C., Pilkington, T. R. 1980. Treatment of bone disease after jejunoileal bypass for obesity with oral 1-alpha-hydroxy-vitamin D3. *Gut.* 21: 669–74

48. Compston, J. E., Horton, L. W., Tighe, J. R. 1979. Treatment of osteomalacia with oral 1-hydroxy vitamin D3 in a patient with malabsorption. *Br. Med. J.* 2:612–14

49. Cook, D. B., Pierides, A. M., Shannon, G. 1977. Seasonal variation of serum 25-hydroxy vitamin D in patients with chronic renal failure treated by regular hemodialysis. *Clin. Chem. Acta* 76: 251–58

50. Cooke, N., Teitelbaum, S., Avioli, L. V. 1978. Antacid-induced osteomalacia & nephrolithiasis. *Arch. Intern. Med.* 138: 1007–9

51. Corrick, R., Ireland, A. W., Rose, S. 1971. Bone abnormalities after gastric surgery. *Ann. Int. Med.* 75:221–25

52. Cournot-Witmer, G., Zingraff, J., Bourdon, R., Drueke, T., Balsan, S. 1979. Aluminum & dialysis bone disease. Letter. *Lancet* 2:795–96

53. Creevy, C. D. 1960. Renal complications after ileal diversion of the urine for non-neoplastic disorders. *J. Urol.* 83: 394–98

54. Danö, P., Lenz, K., Justesen, T. 1974. Bile acid metabolism and intestinal bacterial flora after three types of intestinal shunt operation for obesity. *Scand. J. Gastroenterol.* 9:767–74

55. Darby, W. J., Jones, E., Clark, S. L. Jr., McGanity, W. J., Dutra de Oliveira, J., Perez, C., Kevany, J., le Brocquy, J. 1958. The development of vitamin B_{12} deficiency by untreated patients with pernicious anemia. *Am. J. Clin. Nutr.* 6:513

56. Deacon, R., Lumb, M., Perry, J., Chanarin, I., Minty, B., Halsey, M. J., Nunn, J. F. 1978. Selective inactivation of vitamin B_{12} in rats by nitrous oxide. *Lancet* 2:1023–24

57. Deller, D. J., Richards, W. C. D., Witts, L. J. 1962. Changes in the blood after partial gastrectomy with special reference to vitamin B_{12}. *Q. J. Med.* 31: 71–86

58. Deller, D. J., Begley, M. D. 1963. Calcium metabolism and the bones after partial gastrectomy. I. Clinical features and radiology of the bones. *Aust. Ann. Med.* 12:282–88

59. De Wind, L. T., Payne, J. H. 1976. Intestinal bypass surgery for morbid obesity. *J. Am. Med. Assoc.* 236:2298–301

60. Dietrick, J. E., Whedon, G. D., Shorr, E. 1948. Effects of immobilization upon various metabolic and physiologic functions of normal men. *Am. J. Med.* 4:3–36

61. Donaldson, S. S. et al. 1975. Radiation enteritis in children—a retrospective review. *Cancer* 35:1167–78

62. Doscherholmen, A., Swaim, W. R. 1973. Impaired assimilation of EGG CO 57 vitamin B_{12} in patients with hypochlorydria & achlorhydria & after gastric resection. *Gastroenterology* 64: 913–19

63. Drueke, T. 1980. Dialysis osteomalacia and aluminum intoxication. *Nephron* 26:207–10

64. Dyckner, T., Wester, P. O. 1979. Ventricular extrasystoles & intracellular electrolytes before & after potassium & magnesium infusions in patients on diuretic treatment. *Am. Heart J.* 97:12–18

65. Eddy, R. L. 1971. Metabolic bone disease after gastrectomy. *Am. J. Med.* 50:442–47

66. Editorial: 25 Jan. 1975. Calcium, magnesium & diuretics. *Br. Med. J.* 1: 17C–1

67. Ellis, H. A., Pierides, A. M. et al 1977. DNS: Histopathology of renal osteodystrophy with particular reference to the effects of 1 hydroxy vitamin D_3 in patients treated by long-term hemodialysis. *Clin. Endocrinol.* 7:31–38

68. Exton-Smith, A. N. 1976. The management of osteoporosis. *Proc. R. Soc. Med.* 69:931–34

69. Fell, G. S. et al. 1973. Urinary zinc levels as an indication of muscle catabolism. *Lancet* 1:2080–82

70. Feest, T. G., Ward, M. K., Ellis, H. A., Aljama, P., Kerr, D. 1978. Osteomalacia dialysis osteodystrophy: a

trial of phosphate-enriched dialysis fluid. *Brit. Med. J.* 1:18–20

71. Ferris, O. D., Odel, H. M. 1950. Electrolyte patterns of blood after uterosigmoidostomy. *J. Am. Med. Assoc.* 142:634–35

72. Fletcher, R. F., Henley, A. A., Sammons, H. G., Squire, J. R. 1960. Magnesium deficiency following massive intestinal resection. *Lancet* 1:522–25

73. Flynn, A. et al 1973. Zinc deficiency with altered adrenocortical function and its relation to delayed healing. *Lancet* 1:789–91

74. Frier, B. M., Scott, R. D. 1977. Osteomalacia & arthropathy associated with prolonged abuse of purgatives. *Br. J. Clin. Pract.* 31:17–19

75. Frohlich, J., Hahn, P., Cleator, I. 1980. Changes in plasma carnitine levels after jejunoileal bypass. *Lancet* 1:1085

76. Frame, B., Guiang, H. L., Frost, H. M., Reynolds, W. A., 1971. Osteomalacia induced by laxative (phenolphthalein) ingestion. *Arch. Intern. Med.* 128:794–96

77. Fujita, T., Okuyama, Y., Handa, N., Orimo, H., Ohata, M., Yoshikawa, M., Akiyama, H., Kogure, T. 1971. Agedependent bone loss after gastrectomy. *J. Am. Geriatr. Soc.* 19:840–46

78. Fukuda, M., Shibata, H., Hatakeyama, K., Yamagishi, Y., Soga, J., Koyama, S., Muto, T. 1979. Difference in calcium-metabolism following Billroth-I & Billroth-II procedures for gastric & duodenal ulcers. *Jpn. J. Surg.* 9:295–303

79. Garcia, C. A., Tweedy, J. R., Blass, J. P., McDowell, F. H. 1982. Lecithin and Parkinsonian dementia. In *Approaches to Treatment of Memory Disorders,* ed. S. Corkin, K. L. Davis, J. H. Growdon, R. J. Wurtman. NY: Raven Press. In press

80. Gershoff, S. N. 1976. Vitamin B$_6$. In *Present Knowledge in Nutrition,* pp. 141–61. NY: The Nutrition Foundation, Inc. 605 pp.

81. Gertner, J. M., Lilburn, M., Domenech, M. 1977. 25-hydroxycholecalciferol absorption in steatorrhoea & postgastrectomy osteomalacia. *Br. Med. J.* 1:1310–12

82. Glad, B. W., Hodges, R. E., Michas, C. A., Moussavian, S. N., Righi, S. P. 1978. Atrophic beriberi. A complication of jejunoileal bypass surgery for morbid obesity. *Am. J. Med.* 65:69–74

83. Goldberger, J. H., Cha, C., Hazard, W. L., Randall, H. T. 1976. Jejuno-ileal bypass for morbid obesity: early results

and body composition changes in forty-five patients. *Surgery* 80:493–97

84. Green, R. C., Boyd, J. A. 1959. Rickets secondary to chronic hyperchloremic acidosis in ureterosigmoidostomy. *Am. Med. Assoc. Arch. Int. Med.* 103:807–13

85. Griffin, W. O., Young, V. A., Stevenson, C. C. 1978. A prospective comparison of gastric and jejunoileal bypass procedures of morbid obesity. *Am. Surg.* 186:500–7

86. Griffiths, W. A. 1976. Isoniazid-induced pellagra. *Proc. R. Soc. Med.* 69:313–14

87. Hahn, T. J. 1976. Bone complications of anticonvulsants. *Drugs* 12:201–11

88. Hahn, T. J. 1980. Drug induced disorders of vitamin D and mineral metabolism. *Clin. Endocrinol. Metab.* 9:107–27

89. Hahn, T. J., Halstead, L. R. 1979. Anticonvulsant drug-induced osteomalacia: Alterations in mineral metabolism & response to vitamin D3 administration. *Calcif. Tiss. Int.* 27:13–18

90. Halmi, K. 1980. Gastric bypass for massive obesity. In *Obesity,* ed. A. J. Stunkard, pp. 388–94. Philadelphia: W. B. Saunders

91. Harrington, C. I. 1977. A case of pellagra induced by isoniazid therapy. *Practitioner* 218:716–17

92. Harrison, A. R. 1958. Clinical and metabolic observations on osteomalacia following ureterosigmoidostomy. *Br. J. Urol.* 30:445–62

93. Harwald, B., Krogsgaard, A. R., Louis, P. 1962. Calcium deficiency following partial gastrectomy. *Acta Med. School.* 172:497–503

94. Hasik, J. 1961. Ascorbic acid during the course of extracorporeal dialysis. *Poznan. Towarz. Navk. Wydzial Lekar* 21:161–66

95. Hathcock, J. N., Coon, J. 1978. *Nutrition and Drug Interrelations.* NY: Academic. 927 pp.

96. Heilmann, E., Bender, F., Giulker, H., Bonek, J. 1979. Investigation of iron & folate levels in serum after implantation of heart valve prostheses. (author's trans.) *Herz* 4:298–302

97. Heinivaara, O., Plava, I. P. 1964. Malabsorption of vitamin B$_{12}$ during treatment with para-amino salicylic acid. A preliminary report. *Acta. Med. Scand.* 175:469–71

98. Hines, J. D., Hoffbrand, A. V., Maclin, D. L. 1967. The hematologic complications following partial gastrectomy. *Am. J. Med.* 43:555–60

99. Hossain, M. 1970. The osteomalacia syndrome after colocystoplasty: a cure

with sodium bicarbonate alone. *Br. J. Urol.* 43:243–45

100. Howard, L., Oldendorf, M., Chu, R. 1976. Letter: Pyridoxine deficiency: Another potential sequel of the jejunal-ileal bypass procedure. *N. Eng. J. Med.* 295:733

101. Hull, S. M., Mackintosh, A. 1977. Discontinuation of maintenance digoxin therapy in general practice. *Lancet* 2:1054–55

102. Huseman, B. 1977. Metabolism after jejuno-ileostomy in the treatment of extreme obesity. *Prog. Surg.* 15:77–108

103. Insogna, K. L., Bordley, D. R., Card, J. F., Lockwood, D. A. 1980. Osteomalacia and weakness from excessive antacid ingestion. *J. Am. Med. Assoc.* 244:2544–46

104. Johnson, H. D., Hoffbrand, A. V. 1970. The influence of extent of resection, type of anastomosis, & ulcer site on the haematological side-effects of gastrectomy. *Br. J. Surg.* 57:33–37

105. Johnston, J. H., Rickham, P. P. 1958. Complications following uretero-ileostomy in childhood and the use of cutaneous ureterostomy in advanced lesions. *Br. J. Urol.* 30:437–46

106. Jones, C. T., Williams, J. A., Cox, E. V. et al. 1962. Peptic ulceration. Some heamotological and metabolic consequences of gastric surgery. *Lancet* 2:425–28

107. Juhl, E., Bruusgaard, A., Hippe, E. 1974. Vitamin B_{12} depletion in obese patients treated with jejunoileal shunt. *Scand. J. Gastroenterol.* 9:543–47

108. Keith, D. A., Gallop, P. M. 1979. Phenytoin, hemorrhage, skeletal defects & vitamin K in the newborn. *Med. Hypoth.* 5:1347–51

109. Keith, D. A., Gundberg, C. M., Gallop, P. M. 1980. Phenytoin therapy and hemorrhagic disease. *J. Pediatr.* 97:501–9

110. Kelnar, C. J., Taor, W. S., Reynolds, D. J., Smith, D. R., Slavin, B. M., Brook, C. G. 1978. Hypomagnesaemic hypocalcaemia with hypokalemia caused by treatment with high dose gentamicin. *Arch. Dis. Child.* 53:817–20

111. Kishi, H., Kishi, T., Williams, R. H., Watanabe, T., Folkers, K., Stahl, M. L. 1977. Deficiency of vitamin B6 in women taking contraceptive formulations. *Res. Commun. Chem. Pathol. Pharmacol.* 17:283–93

112. Klein, G. L., Florey, J. B., Goller, V. L., Larese, R. J., Van Meter, Q. L. 1977. Multiple vitamin deficiencies in association with chronic anticonvulsant therapy. Letter. *Pediatrics* 60:767

113. La Badie, J., Dunn, W. A., Aronson, N. N. 1976. Hepatic synthesis of carnitine from protein bound trimethyl-lysine. *Biochemistry* 160:86–95

114. Leite, C. A., Frome, E., Frost, H. M. et al. 1969. Osteomalacia following ureterosigmoidostomy with observations on bone morphology and remodelling rate. *Clin. Orthop.* 49:103–8

115. Levin, E. J., Frank, D. F. 1973. Bone changes following ureteroileostomy. *Am. J. Roentgenol. Radium Ther. Nucl. Med.* 118:347–55

116. Linnell, J. C., Quadros, E. V., Matthews, D. M., Jackson, B., Hoffbrand, A. V. 1978. Nitrous oxide & megaloblastosis: Biochemical mechanism. Letter. *Lancet* 2:1372

117. Lipner, A. 1977. Symptomatic magnesium deficiency after small intestinal bypass for obesity. *Br. Med. J.* 1:148–50

118. Livingston, S., Pauli, L. L. 1976. Letter: Anticonvulsants & rickets—a different view. *Pediatrics* 57:979–80

119. Lous, P., Schwartz, M. 1959. The absorption of vitamin B_{12} following partial gastrectomy. *Acta Med. Scand.* 164:407–17

120. MacLean, L. D. 1976. Intestinal bypass operations for obesity: a review. *Can. J. Surg.* 19:387–98

121. Mahmud, K., Ripley, D., Doscherholmen, A. 1971. Vitamin B_{12} absorption tests. Their unreliability in postgastrectomy states. *J. Am. Med. Assoc.* 216:1167–71

122. Mallette, L. E. 1977. Acetazolamide-accelerated anticonvulsant osteomalacia. *Arch. Intern. Med.* 137:1013–17

123. Mansouri, K., Halsted, J. A., Combos, E. A. 1970. Zinc, copper, magnesium & calcium in dialyzed & nondialzyed uremic patients. *Arch. Intern. Med.* 125:88–93

124. Mason, E. E., Printen, K. J., Blommers, T. J. et al. 1978. Gastric bypass for obesity after ten years experience. *Int. J. Obesity* 2:197–206

125. Matheson, R. T., Herbst, J. J., Jubiz, W., Freston, J. W., Tolman, K. G. 1976. Absorption & biotransformation of cholecalciferol in drug-induced osteomalacia. *J. Clin. Pharmacol.* 16:426–32

126. Mattson, R. H., Gallagher, B. B., Reynolds, E. N., Glass, D. 1973. Folate therapy in epilepsy. A controlled study. *Arch. Neurol.* 29:78–81

127. McKenna, B., Weir, D. G., Scott, J. M. 1980. The induction of functional vitamin B_{12} deficiency in rats by exposure to

nitrous oxide. *Biochem. Biophys. Acta* 628:314–21

128. McKenzie, S. A., MacNab, A. J., Katz, G. 1976. Neonatal pyridoxine responsive convulsions due to isoniazid therapy. *Arch. Dis. Child.* 51:567–68

129. Melick, R. A., Benson, J. A. 1959. Osteomalacia following partial gastrectomy. *N. Engl. J. Med.* 260:976–80

130. Meyer, G. 1979. Intestinal bypass and zinc. *Ann. Int. Med.* 90:278–80

131. Mitchell, A. B., Glass, D., Gill, A. M. 1972. Bone disease after gastrectomy. *Br. Med. J.* 2:164–72

132. Mitchell, A. B., Glass, D., Gill, A. M. 1971. Osteomalacia following vagotomy & pyloroplasty. *Postgrad. Med. J.* 47:233–37

133. Morgan, D. B., Murkinshaw, L., Davidson, C. 1978. Potassium depletion in heart failure & its relation to long-term treatment with diuretics: A review of the literature. *Postgrad. Med. J.* 54: 72–79

134. Morgan, D. B., Hunt, G., Paterson, C. R. 1970. The osteomalacia syndrome after stomach operations. *Q. J. Med.* 39:395–410

135. Morgan, D. B., Paterson, C. R., Pulvertoft, C. N., Woods, C. G., Faumon, P. 1965. Osteomalacia after gastrectomy: A response to very small doses of vitamin D. *Lancet* 2:1089–91

136. Morgan, D. B., Paterson, C. R., Pulvertoft, C. N., Woods, C. G., Faumon, P. 1965. Search of osteomalacia in 1228 patients after gastrectomy and other operations on the stomach. *Lancet* 2: 1085–88

137. Morgan, D. B., Pulvertoft, C. N., Foruma, P. 1966. Effects of age on the loss of bone after gastric surgery. *Lancet* 2:772–73

138. Mosekilde, L., Christensen, M. S., Lund, B., Sorensen, O. H., Melsen, F. 1977. The interrelationships between serum 25-hydroxycholecalciferol, serum parathyroid hormone and bone changes in anticonvulsant osteomalacia. *Acta Endocrinol.* 84:559–65

139. Mosekilde, L., Melsen, F., Hessov, I., Christensen, M. S., Lund, B. J., Lund, B. I., Sorensen, O. H. 1980. Low serum levels of 1,25-dihydroxy vitamin D and histomorphometric evidence of osteomalacia after jejunoileal bypass for obesity. *Gut* 21:624–31

140. Moxley, R. T., Pozefsky, T., Lockwood, D. H. 1974. Protein nutrition & liver disease after jejunoileal bypass for mobid obesity. *N. Engl. J. Med.* 290: 921–26

141. Neale, G. 1968. Protein malnutrition in gastrointestinal disease. *Postgrad. Med. J.* 44:642–45

142. Newman, L. J., Lopez, R., Cole, H. S., Boria, M. C., Cooperman, L. J. 1978. Riboflavin deficiency in women taking oral contraceptive agents. *Am. J. Clin. Nutr.* 31:247–49

143. Nielsen, J. A., Thaysen, E. H. 1971. Acute & chronic magnesium deficiency following extensive small gut resection. *Scand. J. Gastroenterol.* 6:663–66

144. Nordin, B. E. C., Fraser, R. 1956. A calcium infusion test. I. Urinary excretion data for recognition of osteomalacia. *Lancet* 1:823–26

145. Offermann, G., Pinto, V., Kruse, R. 1979. Antiepileptic drugs & vitamin D supplementation. *Epilepsia* 20:3–15

146. Opie, L. H., Hunt, B. G., Finley, J. M. 1964. Massive small bowel resection with malabsorption and negative magnesium balance. *Gastroenterology* 47: 415–17

147. Ovesen, L. 1979. Drugs & vitamin deficiency. *Drugs* 18:278–98

148. Parfitt, A. M., Miller, M. J., Frame, B. et al. 1978. Metabolic bone disease after intestinal bypass for treatment of obesity. *Ann. Int. Med.* 89:193–99

149. Patel, R., Savage, A. 1979. Symptomatic hypomagnesemia associated with gentamycin therapy. *Nephron* 23:50–52

150. Paykel, E. S., Mueller, P. S., De La Verge, P. M. 1973. Amitriptyline, weight gain and carbohydrate craving: a side effect. *Brit. J. Psychiat.* 123:501–7

151. Payne, J. H., DeWind, L., Schwab, C. E., Kern, W. H. 1973. Surgical treatment of morbid obesity. *Arch. Surg.* 106:432–36

152. Pendras, J. P., Erikson, R. V. 1966. Hemodialysis—a successful therapy for chronic renal failure. *Am. Intern Med.* 64:293–311

153. Perry, W., Allen, L. N., Stamp, T. C., Walker, P. G. 1977. Vitamin D resistance in osteomalacia after ureterosigmoidostomy. *N. Engl. J. Med.* 297: 1110–12

154. Peterson, P., Gray, P., Tolman, K. G. 1976. Calcium balance in drug-induced osteomalacia: Response to vitamin D. *Clin. Pharmacol. Ther.* 1:63–67

155. Pierides, A. M., Simpson, W., Ward, M., Ellis, H., Dehvar, J., Kerr, D. 1974. Variable response to long-term 1-hydroxycholecalciferol in haemodialysis osteodystrophy. *Lancet* 1:1092–95

156. Pines, K. L., Mudge, G. H. 1951. Renal

tubular accidosis and osteomalacia. *Am. J. Med.* 11:302–11

157. Pinto, J., Huang, Y. P., Rivlin, R. S. 1982. Inhibition of riboflavin metabolism in rat tissues by chlorpromazine, imipramine and amitriptyline. *J. Clin. Invest.* In press

158. Pinto, J., Wolinsky, M., Rivlin, R. S. 1979. Chlorpromazine antagonism of thyroxine-induced flavin formation. *Biochem. Pharmacol.* 28:597–600

159. Pyrah, L. N., Smith, I. B. 1956. Osteomalacia following gastrectomy. *Lancet* 1:935–37

160. Reidenberg, M. 1980. Drugs in the elderly. *Bull. NY Acad. Med.* 56:703–14

161. Rennick, B., Acara, M., Hysert, P., Mookerjee, B. 1976. Choline loss during hemodialysis. *Kidney Int.* 10:324–26

162. Rodgers, B. M., Talbert, J. L., Moazam, F., Felman, A. H. 1978. Functional & metabolic evaluation of colon replacement of the esophagus in children. *J. Pediatr. Surg.* 13:35–39

163. Roe, D. A. 1976. *Drug Induced Nutritional Deficiencies.* Westport, CT: AVI Publishing Company. 270 pp.

164. Rogers, E. L., Douglass, W., Russell, R. M., Bushman, L., Hubbard, T. B., Iber, F. L. 1980. Deficiency of fat soluble vitamins after jejunoileal bypass surgery for morbid obesity. *Am. J. Clin. Nutr.* 33:1208–14

165. Rollin, H. 1978. Drug-related gustatory disorders. *Ann. Otol.* 87:37–42

166. Roos, D. 1974. Neurological complications in an unselected group of patients partially gastrectomized for gastric ulcer. *Acta Neurol. Scand.* 50:753–73

167. Roos, D. 1977. Electrophysiological findings in gastrectomized patients with low serum B_{12}. *Acta Neurol. Scand.* 56:247–55

168. Roos, D. 1978. Neurological complication in patients with impaired vitamin B_{12} absorption following partial gastrectomy. *Acta Neurol. Scand. Suppl.* 59:1–77

169. Roos, D. 1977. The vibration perception threshold in gastrectomized patients with low serum B_{12}. A clinical & biothesiometric follow-up after intensive B_{12} therapy. *Acta Neurol. Scand.* 56:551–62

170. Roos, D., Willanger, R. 1977. Various degrees of dementia in a selected group of gastrectomized patients with low serum B_{12}. *Acta Neurol. Scand.* 55:363–76

171. Roos, D. 1974. Neurological symptoms & signs in a selected group of partially gastrectomized patients with particular reference to B_{12} deficiency. *Acta Neurol. Scand.* 50:719–52

172. Rosenberg, L. E. 1970. Vitamin-dependent genetic diseases. *Hosp. Pract.* 5:59–66

173. Rostand, S. G. 1976. Vitamin B_{12} levels and nerve conduction velocities in patients undergoing maintenance hemodialysis. *Am. J. Clin. Nutr.* 29:691–97

174. Rygvold, O. 1974. Hypovitaminosis B_{12} following partial gastrectomy by the Billroth II method. *Scand. J. Gastroenterol. Suppl.* 9:57–64

175. Sarasin, C. 1941. Osteomalacia and hypochrome anaemie noch mogen resektion. *Gastroenterologia* 66:182–97

176. Schofield, P. F., Watson-Williams, E. J., Sorrell, V. F. 1967. Vagotomy and pyloric drainage for chronic duodenal ulcer. *Arch. Surg.* 95:615–21

177. Schwartz, H., Jensen, H. 1973. Jejunoileostomy in the treatment of obesity. *Act. Chir. Can.* 139:551–56

178. Schwartz, M. K., Medwid, A., Roberts, K., Sleisenger, M., Randall, H. et al. 1955. Fat and nitrogen metabolism in patients with massive small bowel resections. *Surg. Forum* 6:385–90

179. Scott, H. W. Jr., Law, D. H., Sandstead, H. H., Lanier, V. C. Jr., Younger, R. K. 1970. Jejunoileal shunt in surgical treatment of morbid obesity. *Ann. Surg.* 171:770–82

180. Sherk, H. H., Cruz, M., Stambaugh, J. 1977. Vitamin D prophylaxis & the lowered incidence of fractures in anticonvulsant rickets & osteomalacia. *Clin. Orthop.* 129:251–57

181. Sherman, M. 1953. Bone changes following bilateral ureterosigmoidostomy. *Surg. Gynecol. Obstet.* 97:159–61

182. Shizgal, H. M., Forse, R. A., Spanier, A. H., MacLean, L. D. 1979. Protein malnutrition following intestinal bypass for morbid obesity. *Surgery* 86:60–69

183. Siddiqu, S., Kerr, D. N. S. 1971. Complications of renal failure and their response to dialysis. *Br. Med. Bull.* 27:153–55

184. Silkos, P., Davie, M., Jung, R. T., Chalmers, T. M. 1980. Osteomalacia in uretero-sigmoidostomy: healing by correction of the acidosis. *Br. J. Urol.* 52:61–62

185. Sitrin, M., Meredith, S., Rosenberg, I. H. 1978. Vitamin D deficiency & bone disease in gastrointestinal disorders. *Arch. Intern. Med.* 138:886–88

186. Smith, D. B., Obbens, E. A. 1979. Antifolate-antiepileptic relationships. In *Folic Acid In Neurology, Psychiatry, & Internal Medicine,* ed. M. I. Botez, E.

H. Reynolds, pp. 267–83. NY: Raven Press. 534 pp.

187. Sokal, A., Gral, T., Rubini, M. E. 1967. Some medical problems of chronic hemodialysis. *Calif. Med.* 107:236–46

188. Specht, E. E. 1967. Rickets following ureterosigmoidostomy and chronic hyperchloremia. *J. Bone Joint Surg.* 49:1422–30

189. Stamey, T. A. 1956. Electrolyte imbalance in ureterosigmoidostomy. *Surg. Gynecol. Obstet.* 103:736–58

190. Stamp, T. C. B. 1974. Intestinal absorption of 25-hydroxycholecalciferol *Lancet* 2:121–23

191. Stamp, T. C., Flanagan, R. J., Richens, A., Round, J. M., Thomas, M., Jackson, M., Dupre, P., Twigg, C. A. 1978. Anticonvulsant osteomalacia. In *Endocrinology of Calcium Metabolism*, ed. D. H. Copp, R. V. Talmage, pp. 16–22. Amsterdam: Excerpta Medica

192. Stenflo, J. 1977. Vitamin K, prothrombin, and gammacarboxyglutamic acid. *N. Engl. J. Med.* 296:624–26

193. Stoffer, S. S., Zaka-Ur-Rahman, Meier, D. A., Howker, C. D. 1980. Prompt resolution of osteomalacia by switching from phenytoin to phenobarbital. *Arch. Intern. Med.* 140:852

194. Sullivan, R. D., Miller, E., Sikes, M. P., 1959. Antimetabolite combination cancer chemotherapy. Effects of intraarterial methotrexate-intramuscular citrovacuum factor therapy in human cancer. *Cancer* 12:1248–62

195. Swenson, S. A. Jr., Lewis, J. W., Sebby, K. R. 1974. Magnesium metabolism in man with special reference to jejunoileal bypass for obesity. *Am. J. Surg.* 127: 250–55

196. Tant, D. 1976. Megaloblastic anaemia due to pyridoxine deficiency associated with prolonged ingestion of an oestrogen-containing contraceptive. *Br. Med. J.* 2:979–80

197. Tarpila, S. 1971. Morphological and functional response of human small intestine to ionizing radiation. *Scand. J. Gastroenterol.* 6:48–56

198. Tarpila, S., Jassila, J. 1969. The effect of radiation on the disaccharidase activities of the human small intestinal mucosa. *Scand. J. Clin. Lab. Invest. Suppl.* 23:44–50

199. Thompson, G. R., Lewis, B., Booth, C. C. 1966. Vitamin D absorption after partial gastrectomy. *Lancet* 1:457–58

200. Valman, H. B. 1972. Late vitamin B_{12} deficiency following resection of the ileum in the neonatal period. *Acta Paediatr. Scand.* 61:561–64

201. Vessel, E. S. 1971. Drug metabolism in man. III. Genetic aspects of drug metabolism in man. *Ann. NY Acad. Sci.* 179:514–773

202. Vis, S. C., Love, A. H. 1979. Riboflavin nutriture of oral contraceptive users. *Int. J. Vitam. Nutr. Res.* 49:286–90

203. Vogel, R. I. 1977. Gingival hyperplasia & folic acid deficiency from anticonvulsive drug therapy: a theoretical relationship. *J. Theor. Biol.* 67:269–78

204. Waldram, R. 1973. Syndrome resembling kwashiorkor after partial gastrectomy. *Br. Med. J.* 2:92–93 K

205. Walker, W. F. 1974. Nutrition after injury. *World Rev. Nutr. Dietet.* 19:173–204

206. Walker, W. F., Fleming, L. W., Stewart, W. K. 1968. Urinary magnesium excretion in surgical patients. *Brit. J. Surg.* 55:466–69

207. Ward, M. K., Feest, T. G., Ellis, H. A., Parkinson, I. S., Kerr, D. N. 1978. Osteomalacic dialysis osteodystrophy: evidence for a waterborne aetiological agent, probably aluminium. *Lancet* 1: 841–45

208. Wechsler, H. L. 1979. Vitamin A deficiency following small bowel bypass surgery for obesity. *Arch. Dermatol.* 115:73–75

209. Weismann, K., Wadskov, S., Mikkelsen, H. I. 1978. Acquired zinc deficiency dermatosis in man. *Arch. Dermatol.* 114:1509–11

210. Wheldon, E. J., Venobles, C. W., Johnston, I. D. A. 1970. Late metabolic sequelae of vagotomy and gastroenterostomy. *Lancet* 1:437–41

211. White, J. J., Moxley, R. T., Pozefsky, T., Lockwood, D. H. 1974. Transient kwashiorkor: a cause of fatty liver following small bowel bypass. *Surgery* 75:829–40

212. Winnacker, J. L., Yeager, H., Saunders, J. A., Russell, B., Anast, C. S. 1977. Rickets in children receiving anticonvulsant drugs: biochemical & hormonal markers. *Am. J. Dis. Child* 131:286–90

Ann. Rev. Nutr. 1982. 2:229–48
Copyright © 1982 by Annual Reviews Inc. All rights reserved

CELLULAR FOLATE BINDING PROTEINS; FUNCTION AND SIGNIFICANCE

C. Wagner

Department of Biochemistry, Vanderbilt University and VA Medical Center, Nashville, Tennessee 37203

INTRODUCTION

In recent years a number of proteins from a variety of tissues have been characterized as folate binding proteins. Studies have been made possible by the availability of radioactive folic acid and by the development of simple and rapid methods of separating the free labeled folic acid from that which is protein bound. In practice, the material is incubated in vitro with a trace amount of radioactive folic acid for a short period; the unbound tracer is removed by adsorption with coated charcoal, or by some other method of separating the small folate molecules from the large proteins (gel filtration, dialysis, etc). The protein-bound radioactivity is then counted. Folic acid, however, is not a natural, physiological form of the vitamin. Natural folates are reduced and may carry one-carbon substituents. Moreover, within cells, these folates are predominantly found as the polyglutamate derivatives (Figure 1). Therefore, studies on the binding of the natural forms of folate have been carried out by measuring the ability of the natural, reduced forms to compete with radioactive folic acid for binding to the protein.

This method of in vitro binding has been used successfully to identify a variety of proteins that bind folate rapidly and specifically with high affinity. Alternatively in a few cases, radioactive folic acid has been administered either orally or parenterally to experimental animals for various periods before removal of the tissue. The folate binding proteins are thus labeled in vivo and can be identified by procedures that separate molecules on the basis of size.

The binding proteins identified thus far may be classified as being either extracellular—i.e. in fluids such as milk, serum, cerebrospinal fluid, etc—

229

0199-9885/82/0715-0229$02.00

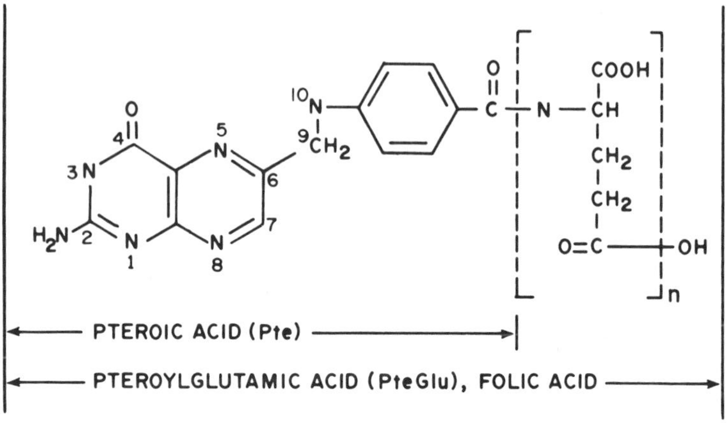

PTEGLU$_5$	PTEROYLPENTAGLUTAMIC ACID (N=5)
H$_4$PTEGLU	5,6,7,8-TETRAHYDROPTEROYLGLUTAMIC ACID TETRAHYDROFOLIC ACID
H$_4$PTEGLU$_5$	5,6,7,8-TETRAHYDROPTEROYLPENTAGLUTAMIC ACID
5-CH$_3$-H$_4$PTEGLU	5-METHYLTETRAHYDROFOLIC ACID
5-HCO-H$_4$PTEGLU	5-FORMYLTETRAHYDROFOLIC ACID
5,10-CH$_2$-H$_4$PTEGLU	5,10-METHYLENETETRAHYDROFOLIC ACID
5,10-CH=H$_4$PTEGLU	5,10-METHENYLTETRAHYDROFOLIC ACID

Figure 1 Structures and nomenclature of the folate derivatives.

or associated with cellular material. It is convenient to subdivide the cellular folate binding proteins further into those that are membrane bound and those that are intracellular and soluble. The membrane-bound folate binding proteins are found associated with membranes of kidney, intestinal epithelium, choroid plexus, and liver as well as the plasma membrane of bacteria. These membrane-associated folate binding proteins can be solubilized by detergents and are believed to participate in the transport of folate derivatives. Two sources of intracellular folate binding proteins have been studied most extensively—those derived from chronic granulocytic leukemia cells and those derived from mammalian liver. The former represent a specialized type of circulating lymphocyte, and the folate binding proteins derived from these cells resemble the folate binding proteins present in serum more closely than those present in liver.

The granulocyte folate binding proteins are, therefore, usually discussed along with the extracellular folate binding proteins. They have been reviewed thoroughly in recent articles (6, 38, 39). Not much more can be added at this time; therefore, I do not consider these binding proteins here except where such discussion is pertinent to those of primary interest. Instead, I confine this review to the membrane-derived and the intracellular folate binding proteins.

MEMBRANE-DERIVED FOLATE BINDING PROTEINS

Mammalian Sources

In 1972, Leslie & Rowe (20) demonstrated that although rat intestinal epithelial cells could not accumulate radioactive folic acid, they could bind it rapidly in a process that was saturable and showed structural specificity for the components of the folate molecule. Reduced folate compounds competed slightly less well for binding of labeled folic acid than oxidized derivatives. The binding of [^{3}H] folic acid to the cell membrane was very tight, and the brush-border fraction of cells labeled by incubation with [^{3}H] folic acid could be isolated with the label still associated. Solubilization of the brush-border membrane fraction with sodium dodecyl sulfate resulted in radioactivity associated with a molecular species greater than 100,000 M_r as well as with smaller molecules having M_r of 24,000 to 16,000.

Selhub & Rosenberg (29) demonstrated the presence of folate binding macromolecules in a membrane preparation from rat kidney that was highly enriched for the brush border. Binding was not measured in a solubilized membrane fraction; however, solubilization of the membrane preparation subsequent to binding of radioactive folic acid demonstrated that the label was associated with the particulate material, rather than the material trapped within vesicles formed by these membrane preparations. The binding of folic acid was saturable with a binding constant, K_b, of 4.2 $\times$ 10^{-11}M and showed specificity for oxidized rather than reduced derivatives. The binding was optimal at pH 6.4–7.7 but was reversible in that endogenous folate could be removed by acid treatment. At pH 9.0, 5-CH$_3$-H$_4$PteGlu was as effective as PteGlu in competing for the binding of labeled folic acid. Selhub & Rosenberg speculated that these folate binding proteins might be involved in the tubular reabsorption of folic acid by the proximal tubule cells of the kidney. There is no doubt that folate conservation by the

kidney is extremely important. It has been shown that soon after administration of radioactive folic acid to mice (26) most of the radioactivity is
found in the kidney. Only later does the majority of the radioactivity appear
in the liver.

The properties of the material studied by Selhub & Rosenberg are similar
to the folate binding protein identified some years earlier by Kamen &
Caston (19). The latter authors isolated a soluble binder from a commercial
preparation of hog-kidney acetone powder. The acetone powder was extracted at acid pH (3.5) at 4°C overnight in the presence of charcoal. This
material bound radioactive folic acid tightly between pH 6.0 and 9.0 but was
dissociated at acid pH. Binding activity was destroyed by trypsin. The
material showed high specificity for H_4PteGlu and 5-CH_3-H_4PteGlu as well
as PteGlu at neutral pH. It had a molecular weight of 35,000 to 40,000 as
determined by gel filtration. The solubility of the material prepared by
Kamen & Caston, as opposed to the particulate nature of the preparations
obtained by Selhub & Rosenberg, may be attributed to the use of acetone
powder as the starting material by the former group. Delipidation brought
about by acetone extraction and the extensive treatment at pH 3.5 may have
resulted in the liberation (and possible modification) of the protein from the
membranes of the kidney tubules.

Indirect evidence that membrane-associated folate binding proteins are
probably concerned with transport was first obtained by Zamierowski &
Wagner (44) in studies performed using the in vivo binding technique. The
distribution of radioactivity in various subcellular fractions of the liver was
measured at time intervals following an intra-peritoneal injection of [^{3}H]
folic acid. At the earliest time (0.5 hr following injection) most of the
radioactivity was present bound to components of the crude nuclear and
microsomal cell fractions. Subsequent purification of these fractions on
sucrose density gradients showed that the radioactivity was bound to the
plasma membrane components of these cell fractions. The radioactive material bound to the plasma membrane fraction after 0.5 hr was dissociated and
shown to be unchanged folic acid. After longer periods the majority of the
folate was bound to proteins in the cytosol and mitochondria (see below).
The folates bound to these latter proteins are primarily reduced and polyglutamate forms. These kinetic studies suggest that the injected folic acid
is first bound to a transport protein in the plasma membrane, and that upon
entering the cell the folic acid is reduced and converted to polyglutamates.

Evidence that a folate-binding protein is located in the choroid plexus was
first obtained from studies designed to investigate transport. The choroid
plexus is a vascular structure in the brain believed to transport substances
selectively between the cerebrospinal fluid and the blood. Chen & Wagner
(5) and Spector & Lorenzo (33) using the choroid plexus from hog and

rabbit, respectively, showed that labeled 5-methyltetrahydrofolate taken up during in vitro incubations was bound to macromolecules. In both these studies, following uptake, the choroid plexus was dispersed by sonication (5) or homogenization (33) and centrifuged at low speed. The radioactivity in the supernatant was bound to a macromolecule. Because of the low speed of centrifugation it was possible that the radioactivity in the supernatant was associated with a membrane component rather than a soluble macromolecule. Spector has extended these studies on the folate-binding protein of the choroid plexus in a series of papers (30–32). Rabbit choroid plexus, previously incubated with radioactive PteGlu or 5-CH_3-H_4PteGlu and homogenized, contained tightly bound radioactivity (31). Treatment of the homogenates with Triton X-100 produced a soluble preparation in which most of the radioactivity was bound to a macromolecule. The binder was insoluble at concentrations of Triton X-100 below 0.02%. The solubilized binder has a M_r of 340,000–400,000 as estimated by chromatography on Sephadex G-200 and Sepharose 4B. The bound folate derivatives were dissociated at acid pH in much the same manner as the folate-binder complex of hog kidney (19). Using an in vitro binding assay in which albumin-coated charcoal was used to separate the free labeled folate from that which was bound, it was shown that the binder had a higher affinity for PteGlu than for 5-CH_3-H_4PteGlu. The protein nature of the macromolecule was indicated by the loss of binding activity after treatment with papain. This folate-binding protein has been presumed to be located in the plasma membrane (30, 32) of the choroid plexus, though data supporting this contention rest largely on the fact that the preparation is particulate and that uptake of folate derivatives by the intact choroid plexus is a carrier-mediated process. Treatment of intact choroid plexus with Pronase, a crude extract of *Streptomyces griseus* having proteolytic activity, decreased the uptake of radioactive folate (30), prompting speculation that the binding protein is on the exterior surface of the structure. The possibility exists, however, that uptake was impaired by nonspecific alteration in membrane structure, though the preparation appeared unaltered under light microscopy and lactic dehydrogenase, a cytosolic enzyme, was not lost by Pronase treatment.

Binding studies carried out with the Triton X-100 solubilized protein from rabbit choroid plexus indicated a tight association between the protein and radioactive folic acid (30). These studies were carried out using equilibrium dialysis and were probably complicated by the micellar nature of the Triton solubulized preparation, which resulted in an extremely long time for equilibrium to be reached ($\sim$ 7 days). The apparent dissociation constant (K_a) of radioactive PteGlu was dependent on the concentration of PteGlu used, being 0.4×10^{-12}M when folate was present at a concentration of .36 × 10^{-9}M, and 46 × 10^{-12}M when folate was present at a concentration of 3.3 × 10^{-9}M.

Sulieman & Spector have recently reported the purification of a folate-binding protein from hog choroid plexus (35). Triton X-100 was used to solubilize the homogenate of choroid plexus. After removal of endogenous folate by acidification, the preparation was placed over an affinity column consisting of folic acid bound to bovine serum albumin that was in turn bound to Sepharose 4B. The binding protein was eluted with an acidic buffer, and subsequent purification steps included chromatography on Sephadex G-200, DEAE-Sephadex, and finally, slab gel electrophoresis. Binding activity was followed by an in vitro charcoal binding assay. The final preparation was purified 6000-fold. The undenatured, but solubilized, binding protein had a M_r of about 200,000 by gel chromatography on Sephadex G-200 and a M_r of about 51,000 upon sodium dodecyl sulfate gel electrophoresis after denaturing in the presence of 2-mercaptoethanol. Binding activity was optimal at pH 7–8 and between 23° and 37°C. Significant binding did take place at 1° and 50°C. Relative binding affinities were measured by the inhibition of the binding of radioactive PteGlu. Both 5-CH_3-H_4PteGlu and H_4PteGlu competed equally for binding of PteGlu while pteroic acid and H_2PteGlu competed less well. Binding activity was also identified in the choroid plexus from a number of mammalian species, including humans. Assuming a one-to-one binding ratio and a molecular weight of 51,000, the highest concentration of the binding protein was found in the choroid plexus of the rat.

A binding protein involved in transport has been identified in the plasma membrane of L-1210 cells (10). These are mouse leukemia cells that can be propagated in an ascites form in mice or in tissue culture. They have been used extensively to study folate transport [see (17) for review]. Such studies have led to the conclusion that L-1210 cells contain two separate systems for the transport of folate compounds: one specific for folic acid and a second specific for 5-CH_3-H_4PteGlu, other reduced folate compounds, and the folate analog, methotrexate. Transport studies that show substrate specificity imply the existence of a protein as part of the "carrier" system.

The binding protein on the surface of L-1210 cells was detected by measuring the binding of radioactive 5-CH_3-H_4PteGlu and methotrexate to intact L-1210 cells at low temperatures (4°C). Under these conditions, little internalization of the bound ligand occurs, while at 37°C transport and metabolism of the substrates may take place. Thus experiments at the two different temperatures enable a comparison of the parameters that affect both binding and transport. Using this method, Henderson et al showed that the inhibition constants (K_i) for binding or transport of labeled 5-CH_3-H_4PteGlu by unlabeled 5-CH_3-H_4PteGlu, aminopterin,

5-HCO-H$_4$PteGlu, methotrexate, and PteGlu were in the same relative order of effectiveness. The absolute values of the K$_i$'s for transport were about 3 times higher than the K$_i$'s for binding, which may be due to the fact that they were performed at different temperatures. Additionally, it was noted that the dissociation constants, K$_d$, measured for binding of labeled 5-CH$_3$-H$_4$PteGlu and methotrexate were 0.11 and 0.35 μM, respectively, which agreed well with the values for the inhibition constants shown by unlabeled 5-CH$_3$-H$_4$PteGlu (0.11 μM) and methotrexate (0.44 μM) for the binding of radioactive 5-(CH$_3$H$_4$PteGlu. The binding was almost completely reversible at 4°C, and inhibition of binding by various anions was in the same relative order of effectiveness as for inhibitors of transport. About 1 pmol of ligand was bound per mg of cell protein, which corresponded to about 8 X 10^4 receptors per cell if there is one ligand per receptor. Although the binding protein of L-1210 cells has not yet been isolated, nor even extracted and measured in an in vitro system, the correlation of properties between binding and transport strongly suggests that this is a component of the transport system. Indeed, the authors are careful to refer to this material as a binding component rather than a binding protein. Further studies by this laboratory on the nature of this component are eagerly awaited.

A folate binder has been extensively characterized in cells of human origin grown in tissue culture. McHugh & Cheng used human KB cells grown in either folate-deficient (D) or folate-replete (R) medium (22). A crude membrane (particulate) fraction bound radioactive PteGlu in vitro at pH 7.5. Prior treatment of the fraction at acid pH followed by incubation at pH 7.5 resulted in greater amounts of bound radioactivity, which led to the conclusion that the latter treatment measured total binding capacity while only free (uncovered) binder was measured unless the covered binding sites were first stripped by acid treatment. Another possible conclusion is that the binding is not reversible at pH 7.5. When grown in deficient medium the amount of folate bound by the crude membrane fraction increased from a total of 1,731 to 8,307 pmole/10^8 cells. In replete medium about 5% of the binding sites were saturated while about half were saturated in deficient medium. This increase in the number of binding sites required growth in deficient medium for at least 2 months.

When intact KB cells from deficient medium were incubated with radioactive PteGlu for various periods of time and the cells then disrupted and separated into a crude membrane fraction and soluble fraction, the amount of PteGlu bound to the membranes was much greater than that present in the soluble fraction and did not increase much with time, whereas the amount of soluble folate did increase. These authors also showed that a considerable fraction (55%) of the soluble radioactivity was associated with a folate polyglutamate fraction (as measured by elution position on a Sephadex G-25 column) after 15 hr incubation of the intact cells with labeled PteGlu. Almost none of the radioactivity bound to membranes appeared to be polyglutamate derivatives at this time. It was not determined how much of the radioactive folate in the soluble fraction was protein bound.

When KB cells grown in deficient medium were incubated with radioactive PteGlu for 16 hr and the crude membrane fractions further separated into plasma membrane, post-mitochondrial (presumably endoplasmic reticulum) membrane, nuclear membrane, and mitochondrial membrane fractions, it was found that most of the radioactivity was associated with the mitochondrial membrane when expressed per mg of protein. On a cellular basis, most of the radioactivity was associated with the plasma membrane. It was not established what form of folate was bound to each of these membrane fractions although it is presumed that it was no longer PteGlu.

McHugh & Cheng (22) also attempted to investigate the specificity of binding by incubating intact KB cells with radioactive PteGlu for 1.5 hr either alone or in the presence of unlabeled analogs. The crude membrane fraction was isolated and the radioactivity was counted. Only those compounds with an intact pteroylglutamate structure inhibited to any significant extent. The experiment was also carried out using a preparation of crude membranes from KB cells solubilized with the non-ionic detergent NP-40. Binding was measured by incubation with labeled PteGlu at 37°C for 15 min. Unbound PteGlu was removed with charcoal and albumin. It was found that $10\text{-}CH_3\text{-}PteGlu$, $H_2PteGlu$, and $H_4PteGlu$ were the most potent inhibitors. Since these experiments were carried out in the absence of reducing agents to protect reduced folate compounds that were added, the results obtained with these compounds should be viewed with caution. The fact that the entire crude membrane fraction was used as a source of the binder makes interpretation even more difficult since the different types of membranes may well have binding proteins with different specificities.

The purifications of a folate binding protein from human placenta was recently reported by Antony et al (1). This material is referred to as a folate receptor by the authors because it was isolated from a particulate, presumably membrane, preparation of placenta and is therefore believed to be involved in the transport of folate. The particulate preparation was solubilized by the use of Triton X-100, and binding activity was measured in vitro using [3H] PteGlu. Unbound radioactivity was separated by adsorption onto dextran-coated charcoal. Purification was accomplished largely through adsorption onto a folic acid affinity column. A purified glycoprotein was obtained after a 61,000-fold purification. This had a molecular weight of about 38,500 as determined by SDS-polyacrylamide gel electrophoresis. Carbohydrate analysis showed that the purified material contained about 12% carbohydrate which was covalently bound. One mole of PteGlu was bound per mole of protein. The binding of PteGlu to the protein was tight, as evidenced by the fact that radioactive PteGlu bound in vitro to the protein did not dissociate during polyacrylamide gel electrophoresis in 0.1% Triton X-100. This tight binding was pH-dependent since endogenous folate was stripped of the crude binder by incubation at pH 3.0.

The purified binding protein had an association constant (K_a) of 3.5 mM^{-1} for PteGlu. The K_a values for 5-HCO-H_4PteGlu and methotrexate were 0.1% and 0.3%, respectively, of the value obtained for PteGlu. Antony et al noted that other reduced folate analoges, H_2PteGlu, H_4PteGlu, and 5-CH_3-H_4PteGlu were less than 90% pure and were unstable during measurement of the K_a. The latter three compounds had K_a values in the range of 5–20% less than that of PteGlu. Such studies indicate a greater affinity of the binding protein for PteGlu than for the natural, reduced folate monoglutamates.

Antiserum raised to the purified binding protein permitted an investigation of the distribution of immunologically similar proteins in various tissues. Immunological cross-reacting material was demonstrated on the membrane of human erythrocytes by an immunofluorescence technique. This antiserum also cross-reacted with both the high- and low-M_r folate binding proteins of human milk (38).

Bacterial Sources

Some of the best evidence that a membrane-associated folate binding protein is involved in transport comes from studies carried out with *Lactobacillus casei*. This microorganism is the one generally used for assay of folates. Much of this has been reviewed recently in detail (17). Briefly, Henderson, Zevely & Huennekens (11, 16) showed that intact cells of *L. casei* rapidly bound radioactive PteGlu at 4°C in a saturable manner. Transport of PteGlu took place at 37°C and required an energy source (16). Compounds such as iodoacetate that block transport had no effect on binding at 4°C. A crude preparation of the folate binding protein was made by Triton extraction of *L. casei* protoplasts. [^{3}H] PteGlu was added to the suspension of protoplasts before Triton extraction, and the radioactivity remained bound to the protein following chromatography on Sephadex G-25. These authors showed that when *L. casei* was grown in media containing various levels of folates, the transport ability was inversely proportional to the folate levels; maximal transport was seen at 2 nM folate, and transport was completely repressed at 1 μM. The binding activity of whole cells and the levels of Triton X-100 solubilized binding protein exactly paralleled the transport activity of the cells grown at different levels of folate. Purification of the folate binding protein from *L. casei* was achieved simply by adsorption to and elution from microgranular silica (Quso G-32) and chromatography on Sephadex G-25 (12). At this point the protein–folic acid complex was pure but was contained in a Triton micelle with an apparent M_r of 220,000. This micelle could be disrupted by chaotropic agents (SCN$^-$ and $C1O_4^-$) and by ethanol, resulting in loss of the bound radioactive folic acid. The protein was pure as judged by polyacrylamide electrophoresis in sodium dodecyl sulfate and had an M_r of 25,000. The amino acid composition was notable for the absence of cysteine and the high levels of methionine, tryptophan, and other nonpolar amino acids. There was no detectable carbohydrate. The ratio of PteGlu to protein in the purified preparation was 1 : 1.

Further studies were carried out using mutants of *L. casei* that were resistant to amethopterin (methotrexate) (13). These cells have a defective transport system for uptake of folic acid and also have a comparable defect in the ability to bind folate. Such results are powerful evidence that the folate binding protein of *L. casei* is involved with the transport of folate into the cell.

INTRACELLULAR FOLATE BINDING PROTEINS

Presence in Erythrocytes

The earliest evidence for the existence of an intracellular folate binding protein is probably the discovery by Iwai, Luttner & Toennies in 1964 (18) that folic acid in human erythrocytes was bound to a macromolecular substance having a M_r of at least 50,000. This was called folate precursor substance and it bound primarily polyglutamates of 5-CH$_3$-H$_4$PteGlu, based upon differential microbiological assay with *L. casei, Streptococcus faecium,* and *Pediococcus cerevisiae.* The macromolecule was purified about 700-fold on DEAE cellulose and was clearly separated from hemoglobin. It could be precipitated with ammonium sulfate and was presumably a protein. The partially purified material contained about 30% of the folate originally present in the red-cell hemolysate. Unfortunately, this work was never followed up, and the nature of the protein in human erythrocytes to which the folate is bound remains unknown.

Evidence for Several Folate Binding Proteins in Liver

In 1974, two papers reported the presence of folate binding proteins in rat liver. The first, by Corrocher et al (8), studied the binding of radioactive folate both in vivo and in vitro. The in vitro experiments were carried out by incubating [^{3}H] folic acid with a crude liver homogenate at room temperature. The mixture was then chromatographed on a column of Sephadex

G-75. About 15% of the radioactivity was bound to two macromolecular species eluting at positions roughly corresponding to that shown by the "Y" and "Z" proteins of liver. These "Y" and "Z" proteins were believed to be involved in the binding of organic anions and were shown to have molecular weights of 44,000 and 10,000, respectively (2). In vivo labeling was carried out by injecting [^{3}H] PteGlu intraperitoneally. After 24 hr the animal was killed, its liver was homogenized and centrifuged, and the supernatant was chromatographed on Sephadex G-75. In this case two peaks of bound radioactivity were seen, one at the void volume of the column and the other corresponding to peak "X." They were not further characterized.

The second paper, by Zamierowski & Wagner (43), also utilized in vivo administration of [^{3}H] PteGlu to label the macromolecular species to which folate was bound. Twenty-four hours after injection of the labeled PteGlu into normal rats a large amount of radioactive folate was shown to be associated with a high molecular weight fraction of liver, kidney, and intestine. Most of the radioactivity was found in the liver. A crude fractionation of the liver into nuclei, mitochondria, microsomes, and cytosol by differential centrifugation showed that most of the bound radioactivity was in the nuclear and cytosol fractions. [The activity bound in the nuclear fraction was subsequently shown (45) to be associated with mitochondria that contaminated this fraction in the procedure originally used for subcellular separation.] Chromatography of the cytosol fraction on Sephadex G-150 columns showed three peaks of bound radioactivity: one that eluted close to the void volume of the column with a M_r of about 300,000, a second with a M_r of about 150,000, and a third with a M_r of about 25,000. When the material in the mitochondrial fraction was chromatographed in a similar way it had a M_r of about 90,000. These folate binding proteins are referred to as FBP-CI, FBP-CII, FBP-CIII, and MFBP. The fact that radioactivity could be dissociated from the macromolecular complex by boiling indicated it was not covalently bound, and microbiological assay with and without conjugase treatment showed that the bound material contained primarily polyglutamate forms. Unbound folate primarily consisted of monoglutamates (they supported the growth of L. casei without prior hydrolysis). Microbiological assay with L. casei and S. faecium also provided some information about the type of folate bound to each of the peaks. FBP-CII (M_r of 150,000) was associated with 5-CH$_3$-H$_4$PteGlu polyglutamates, while little if any 5-CH$_3$-H$_4$PteGlu polyglutamate was found in any of the other peaks. Further characterization of these binding proteins was provided in a subsequent paper (44). The two high molecular weight peaks in the cytosol that contained most of the bound radioactivity (FBP-CI and FBP-CII) and the peak from the mitochondria (MFBP) were shown to be sensitive to trypsin treatment. This together with the fact that binding was destroyed by boiling indicated that they were probably protein. These proteins were able to bind folates in vitro as well as in vivo as long as the proper (i.e. polyglutamate) form of folate was used. A mixture of labeled, biosynthesized, folate polyglutamates was prepared from liver cytosol or mitochondria of animals previously injected with [^{3}H] PteGlu. The cytosol or mitochondria was boiled to denature the protein, centrifuged, and the respective supernatant incubated at 4°C with unlabeled cytosol or mitochondrial extract. Chromatography on Sephadex G-150 resulted in the same pattern of labeled folate binding proteins as was obtained by in vivo labeling.

The possibility that these intracellular folate binding proteins are enzymes involved in folate metabolism was also considered (36, 43–45). Fractions of the Sephadex G-150 column were assayed to determine whether the folate binding proteins co-eluted with any enzymes known to metabolize folate derivatives. These were dihydrofolate reductase (EC 1.5.1.3), methionine synthase (EC 2.1.1.13), glutamate formiminotransferase (EC 2.1.2.5), 5,10-methylenetetrahydrofolate reductase (EC 1.1.1.68), serine hydroxymethyltransferase (EC 2.1.2.1), methylenetetrahydrofolate dehydrogenase (EC 1.5.1.5) and formyltetrahydrofolate synthase (EC 6.3.4.3). In only one case was there any evidence for co-elution of any of these enzymes with any of the binding proteins. The elution position of the low molecular weight binding protein of liver cytosol (FBP-CIII) partially overlapped that of dihydrofolate reductase. This is a minor binding protein and suggests that at least a portion of the folate binding activity may be due to dihydrofolate reductase.

Evidence for a folate binding protein in bovine liver was also provided by Watabe (37). In the course of purifying the enzyme, dihydropteridine reductase (EC 1.6.99.7), it was found that a high molecular weight material contained a folate compound that was apparently $H_4PteGlu_2$. The $H_4PteGlu_2$ was not covalently bound. This material was called tetrahydrofolate ·protein complex and abbreviated as TFPC. It was detected because it catalyzed the transfer of electrons from NADH to reduce cytochrome c in the presence of purified dihydropteridine reductase. The series of reactions are presumed to take place as follows:

$$Protein\text{-}H_4PteGlu_2 + Fe^{3+}\ Cyt\ c \rightarrow Protein\text{-}H_2PteGlu_2 + Fe^{2+}\ Cyt\ c$$

$$Protein\text{-}H_2PteGlu + NADH \xrightarrow{\text{(dihydropteridine reductase)}} Protein\text{-}H_4PteGlu_2 + NAD^+$$

The reduction of Fe^{3+} Cyt c can take place in the presence of dihydropteridine reductase if free (unbound) $H_4PteGlu_2$ is used, and this formed one of the bases for its identification. Other evidence for the form of folate bound as $H_4PteGlu_2$ included growth-promoting behavior in several types of microbiological assays, stability of the compound, chromatographic behavior, and conversion to $H_4PteGlu$ after conjugase action. The TFPC was partially purified and shown to have an estimated M_r of about 70,000 by gel filtration. Although this protein was discovered by virtue of its ability to participate in the reduction of cytochrome c and be reduced in turn by dihydropteridine reducatase, Watabe speculated that it may not necessarily function this way in vivo. The subcellular location of TFPC was not determined, but its size was similar to that of the mitochondrial folate binding protein of rat liver (90,000) found by Zamierowski & Wagner (44). It should be noted (see below) that both $H_4PteGlu_5$ and $H_4PteGlu$ were subsequently found as the folate ligands bound to the mitochondrial protein of rat liver (41).

Characterization of a Folate Binding Protein of Liver Cytosol

The folate binding protein of rat liver cytosol that showed a specificity for $5\text{-}CH_3\text{-}H_4PteGlu$ polyglutamates (FBP-CII) was purified to homogeneity by Suzuki & Wagner (36). It was shown to have a M_r of about 150,000 by gel chromatography and sucrose density gradient centrifugation. Electrophoresis under denaturing conditions showed a single protein band of 32,000 daltons, while amino acid analysis indicated a minimum molecular weight of about 35,000. This suggests the protein is composed of four subunits. When isolated, the purified protein contained endogenous $5\text{-}CH_3\text{-}H_4PteGlu_5$ bound to it. In addition, it was shown that radioactive $5\text{-}CH_3\text{-}H_4PteGlu_5$ was the form of radioactive folate specifically bound in vitro by FBP-CII.

We may speculate on the possible role of FBP-CII in the liver. An enzymatic role for this protein appears to be excluded. FBP-CII in vivo contains bound $5\text{-}CH_3\text{-}PteGlu$ polyglutamates almost exclusively (36). The only two enzymes known to participate in the metabolism of $5\text{-}CH_3\text{-}H_4\text{-}PteGlu_n$ are methionine synthase and 5,10-methylenetetrahydrofolate reductase. Both have been shown to use polyglutamate as well as monoglutamate forms of folate, but both of these enzymes clearly separated from FBP-CII by gel chromatography. The folate substrates are also less tightly bound to these enzymes than $5\text{-}CH_3\text{-}H_4PteGlu_5$ is to FBP-CII.

It is possible to make a circumstantial case for FBP-CII serving a storage role in the liver. The major single form of folate in rat liver is $5\text{-}CH_3\text{-}H_4$ $PteGlu_n$—a form metabolically active only for the synthesis of methionine. In vitamin B_{12} deficiency, folate is trapped in this form because of decreased methionine synthase activity. This is the basis of the methyl trap hypothesis to explain the functional folate deficiency that occurs in pernicious anemia (vitamin B_{12} deficiency) (15, 24). In addition, Scott & Weir have recently speculated on the physiologic function of the "methyl trap" (28) and have suggested that it operates also in folic acid deficiency as well as vitamin B_{12} deficiency. Previous studies carried out by Zamierowski & Wagner measured bound and free folate levels in folate-deficient and pair-fed animals using differential microbiological assay (45). These results showed that during deficiency the free folate pool was most severely depleted (Table 1). The percent of folate in cytosol bound to FBP-CI and FBP-CIII did not change, but the amount bound to FBP-CII increased from 31 to 50%. Likewise, in mitochondria the majority of folate lost during deficiency comes at the expense of the unbound fraction. These data support the hypothesis that $5\text{-}CH_3\text{-}H_4PteGlu_n$ accumulates and the "methyl trap" is in operation during folate deficiency. Thus $5\text{-}CH_3\text{-}H_4PteGlu_n$ is trapped—bound to FBP-CII. Moreover, when radioactive PteGlu was injected into these folate deficient animals, almost all the radioactivity of the cytosol was associated with FBP-CII, in contrast to the situation in normal animals where most of the bound radioactivity of the cytosol is bound to FBP-CI or is not bound at all (45). $5\text{-}CH_3\text{-}H_4PteGlu_5$ is the most abundant single species of all the folate derivatives in rat liver, making up about 31% of the total (27, 34). Liver contains most of the body stores of folates, amounting to about 50% of the total in man (14). Therefore, if $5\text{-}CH_3\text{-}H_4PteGlu_n$ can be considered to be a storage form of folate, then the protein that binds it, FBP-CII, may be a storage protein!

Consistent with this hypothesis is the distribution of FBP-CII in various tissues. A radioimmunoassay was established by Cook & Wagner to measure FBP-CII (7). This permits measurement of the apoprotein regardless of the state of saturation with the ligand. These data showed that the liver

Table 1   Folate levels bound to proteins in rat liver in control and folate deficient animals[a]

Cellular constituent	Column fraction[b]	Control		Deficient	
		Folate[c]	Percent[d]	Folate	Percent
Cytosol	FBP-CI	13.0	18	5.2	18
	FBP-CII	21.8	31	14.1	50
	FBP-CIII	7.8	11	3.2	11
	Unbound	27.8	40	5.9	21
Mitochondria	MFBP	7.5	18	4.1	39
	Unbound	33.3	82	6.5	61

[a] Data taken from (45)
[b] The folate binding proteins were separated by Sephadex G-150 chromatography of the cytosol and the mitochondria.
[c] Values are expressed as ng/ml of the peak fraction isolated as above. Measured by microbiological assay with *L. casei* after conjugase treatment.
[d] Values of percent of total folate in either the cytosol or mitochondrial fractions.

contains much greater levels than the kidney, the next most abundant source. The levels of total folate are also much greater in the liver, though they tend to vary with diet (4). Using the value of FBP-CII as determined by radioimmunoassay, and assuming that four moles of 5-CH$_3$-H$_4$PteGlu$_5$ can be bound per mole of protein (there are four identical subunits per mole), one can calculate that the total binding capacity of FBP-CII in rat liver is about 12 X10^{-3} μmole/g. This is about twice the amount of 5-CH$_3$-H$_4$PteGlu$_5$ normally present and provides significant excess to bind additional folate stores. In addition, although FBP-CII contains less bound folate during an period of folate deficiency, measurement of the FBP-CII by radioimmunoassay showed that the protein itself was not decreased. This indicates that it becomes progressively unsaturated during folate deficiency.

Of further interest is the observation that the level of FBP-CII in both liver and kidney is low in rat embryos (7). The levels increase about ten-fold immediately before birth and may reflect the absence of any need for storage in the fetal tissue since nutrients can be obtained from maternal circulation.

The Folate Binding Protein of Liver Mitochondria

The protein-bound folate of mitochondria, first identified by Zamierowski & Wagner (43) and shown to have a M_r of about 90,000 by chromatography on Sephadex G-150, has recently been found to consist of two closely related enzymes not previously recognized to be involved in folate metabolism. Wittwer & Wagner (41) showed that the chemical structure of the folate ligand bound to the partially purified mitochondrial folate binding protein was H$_4$PteGlu$_5$. H$_4$PteGlu was also bound to the protein, but this is probably a result of conjugase activity since rapid processing decreased the amount of H$_4$PteGlu found. The fact that H$_4$PteGlu was bound permitted the development of a rapid in vitro binding assay to follow purification. When the material eluted from the Sephadex G-150 column was chromatographed on DEAE cellulose, two binding proteins with similar molecular weights were separated. The first was shown to have dimethylglycine dehydrogenase activity (40, 41). It is also capable of oxidizing sarcosine and several other N-methyl amino acids. The second protein was shown to have only sarcosine dehydrogenase activity.

$$\text{Dimethylglycine} \xrightarrow{\text{(Dimethylglycine dehydrogenase)}} \text{Sarcosine} + \text{Formaldehyde}$$

$$\text{Sarcosine} \xrightarrow{\text{(Sarcosine dehydrogenase)}} \text{Glycine} + \text{Formaldehyde}$$

Final purification of dimethylglycine dehydrogenase (EC 1.5.99.2) and sarcosine dehydrogenase (EC 1.5.99.1) to homogeneity was achieved using an affinity column of aminohexyl Sepharose to which 5-HCO-H$_4$PteGlu had been bound. The molecular weights were estimated by polyacrylamide gel electrophoresis in sodium dodecyl sulfate. Dimethylglycine dehydrogenase has a M$_r$ of about 89,000, and sarcosine dehydrogenase has a M$_r$ of about 105,000. Both enzymes are flavoproteins in which the flavin is covalently bound (42). This was shown by the characteristic flavin absorbance spectra of the purified enzymes. Injection of [^{14}C]-labeled riboflavin into rats resulted in the incorporation of the label into both purified enzymes. The radioactive flavin, folate binding activity, as well as enzyme activity copurified with each of the two enzymes. The [14C]flavin bound to each of these enzymes was not dissociated by 6 M urea, sodium dodecyl sulfate, boiling or precipitation with 5% trichloroacetic acid.

The properties of dimethylglycine dehydrogenase have been studied in somewhat more detail than those of sarcosine dehydrogenase, though the reactions carried out by both these enzymes are very similar. The specificity of ligand binding to dimethylglycine dehydrogenase has been determined by competition of unlabeled folate analogs for the binding of [^{3}H]-labeled H$_4$PteGlu. The enzyme displayed the greatest affinity for H$_4$PteGlu$_5$ followed by H$_4$PteGlu, 5-HCO-H$_4$PteGlu, and 5-CH$_3$-H$_4$PteGlu. As a group the reduced folates were bound 100-fold tighter than folic acid or methotrexate. Since 5-CH$_3$-H$_4$PteGlu is more stable than H$_4$PteGlu, radioactive 5-CH$_3$-H$_4$PteGlu was used to determine the equilibrium constant for binding to dimethylglycine dehydrogenase. Two independent methods gave values of 2 μM for the dissociation constant of 5-CH$_3$-H$_4$PteGlu. Values of 0.2 μM and 0.4 μM were calculated for the dissociation constants of H$_4$PteGlu$_5$ and H$_4$PteGlu, respectively; 0.90 moles of 5-CH$_3$-H$_4$PteGlu were bound per mole of enzyme, indicating a one-to-one stoichiometry. Participation of the flavin moiety in the reaction mechanism was demonstrated by the fact that the flavin spectrum was reduced by the substrate of the enzyme.

The involvement of protein-bound H$_4$PteGlu$_5$ (or H$_4$PteGlu) in the mechanism of dimethylglycine dehydrogenase and sarcosine dehydrogenase is suggested in the scheme pictured in Figure 2. Because dimethylglycine dehydrogenase can use both dimethylglycine and sarcosine as substrates, while sarcosine dehydrogenase uses only sarcosine, the same scheme may be used for both enzyme reactions. Electron transfer is shown as occurring first with the production of a Schiff base–type adduct and reduction of the protein bound flavin. If no H$_4$PteGlu is available, the Schiff base may be hydrolyzed to give free formaldehyde. In the presence of bound H$_4$PteGlu, the formaldehyde produced by hydrolysis of the Schiff base may react directly with H$_4$PteGlu to produce 5,10-CH$_2$-H$_4$PteGlu. This reaction is well known to occur non-enzymatically (3). The fact that this does take

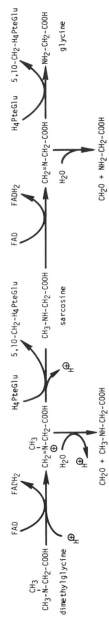

Figure 2   Scheme for the involvement of H₄PteGlu in the mechanism of action of dimethylglycine and sarcosine dehydrogenase.

place was shown by an experiment in which purified dimethylglycine dehydrogenase was equilibrated with $H_4PteGlu$ of high specific radioactivity (42). The radioactive ligand–protein complex was treated with dimethylglycine as substrate for the enzyme. This was followed immediately by the addition of sodium borohydride, which will reduce any $5,10\text{-}CH_2\text{-}H_4PteGlu$ to $5\text{-}CH_3\text{-}H_4PteGlu$. The latter compound is more stable than the former, which dissociates to formaldehyde and $H_4PteGlu$ during chromatography. Radioactive $5\text{-}CH_3\text{-}H_4PteGlu$ was detected in this manner, indicating that formaldehyde produced during the reaction is converted to $5,10\text{-}CH_2\text{-}H_4$ PteGlu on the enzyme as shown in Figure 2. The reaction of enzyme-bound $H_4PteGlu$ with formaldehyde may prevent accumulation of the latter, which may be toxic. The $5,10\text{-}CH_2\text{-}H_4PteGlu$ thus formed may also be available for subsequent reactions in the mitochrondria (e.g. formation of serine).

The role of folate coenzymes in the oxidation of dimethylglycine and sarcosine has been a matter of speculation for over 25 years. Mackenzie (21) found that mitochondria (made permeable with phosphate) incorporated the N-methyl groups of dimethylglycine and sarcosine into carbon 3 of serine in high yield. Free formaldehyde, however, was not incorporated into carbon 3 of serine under these conditions. It was suggested that "active formaldehyde" was the product of dimethylglycine and sarcosine oxidation which could be directly incorporated into serine (21) and that a folate derivative might be involved in some way (21, 25). Dac & Wriston (9) found that folate deficiency did not impair sarcosine oxidation in isolated mitochondria. (Table 1 shows that the protein-bound folate is not readily lost during folate deficiency.) With partially purified sarcosine dehydrogenase, Mell & Huennekens (23) found that $H_4PteGlu$ was not required for the reaction, and the hypothesis that folate was involved in the oxidative demethylation of dimethylglycine and sarcosine was no longer considered tenable. The fact that both of these enzymes were purified by virtue of their ability to bind $H_4PteGlu$ in spite of the fact that the involvement of folate in these reactions was unknown is indeed a tribute to serendipity.

SUMMARY

It appears that specific functions may be assigned to some of the cellular folate binding proteins with some degree of certainty. Those that are membrane bound or derived from membranes probably have a role in transport of folate molecules into the cell. This is in spite of the fact that the localization of this protein to the plasma membrane has been carried out in only a limited number of cases. The role of the folate binding protein of *L. casei* in transport is much clearer. Bacteria provide the opportunity to obtain mutants defective in both transport and binding, and such mutants are more difficult to obtain with mammalian cell lines.

The intracellular folate binding proteins have been discovered so far only in liver. The fact that the folate binding proteins in rat liver mitochondria are two enzymes, dimethylglycine dehydrogenase and sarcosine dehydrogenase, suggests that enzyme activities may eventually be discovered for the other intracellular folate binding proteins. This may not be possible, however, and a reasonably strong case has been made that the folate binding protein of cytosol, FBP-CII, serves in a storage role. Such a storage role is difficult to prove since it depends, in part, on the demonstration that the protein becomes progressively less saturated during deficiency—a situation true also for enzymes.

Literature Cited

1. Antony, A. C., Utley, C., Van Horne, K. C., Kolhouse, J. F. 1981. Isolation and characterization of a folate receptor from human placenta. *J. Biol. Chem.* 256:9684–92
2. Arias, I. M. 1972. Transfer of bilirubin from blood to bile. In *Sem. Hematol.* 9:55–70
3. Blakley, R. L. 1960. Spectrophotometric studies on the combination of formaldehyde with tetrahydropteroylglutamic acid and other hydroxypteridines. *Biochem. J.* 74:71–82
4. Blakley, R. L. 1969. *The Biochemistry of Folic Acid and Related Pteridines.* NY: Wiley
5. Chen, C.-P., Wagner, C. 1975. Folate transport in the choroid plexus. *Life Sci.* 16:1571–81
6. Colman, N., Herbert, V. 1980. Folate binding proteins. *Ann. Rev. Med.* 31:433–39
7. Cook, R. J., Wagner, C. 1981. Measurement of a folate binding protein from rat liver cytosol by radioimmunoassay. *Arch. Biochem. Biophys.* 208:358–64
8. Corrocher, R., DeSandre, G., Pacor, M. L., Hoffrand, A. V. 1974. Hepatic protein binding of folate. *Clin. Sci. Mol. Med.* 46:551–54
9. Dac, L. K., Wriston, J. C. 1958. The cofactor requirements of sarcosine oxidase. *J. Biol. Chem.* 233:222–24
10. Henderson, G. B., Grezelokowska-Sztabert, B., Zevely, E. M., Huennekens, F. M. 1980. Binding properties of the 5-methyltetrahydrofolate/methotrexate transport system in L1210 cells. *Arch. Biochem. Biophys.* 202:144–49
11. Henderson, G. B., Zevely, E. M., Huennekens, F. M. 1976. Folate transport in

Lactobacillus casei: Solubilization and general properties of the binding protein. *Biochem. Biophys. Res. Commun.* 68:712–17
12. Henderson, G. B., Zevely, E. M., Huennekens, F. M. 1977. Purification and properties of a membrane-associated, folate-binding protein from *Lactobacillus casei. J. Biol. Chem.* 252:3760–65
13. Henderson, G. B., Zevely, E. M., Kadner, R. J., Huennekens, F. M. 1977. The folate and thiamine transport proteins of *Lactobacillus casei. J. Supramol. Struct.* 6:239–47
14. Herbert, V., Colman, N., Jacob, E. 1980. Folic acid and vitamin B$_{12}$. In *Modern Nutrition in Health and Disease,* ed. R. S. Goodhart, M. E. Shils, pp. 229–59. Philadelphia: Lea & Febiger
15. Herbert, V., Zalusky, R. 1962. Interrelationship of vitamin B$_{12}$ and folic acid metabolism: Folic acid clearance studies. *J. Clin. Invest.* 41:1263–76
16. Huennekens, F. M., Henderson, G. B. 1975. Transport of folate compounds into mammalian and bacterial cells. In *Chemistry and Biology of Pteridines,* ed. W. Pfleiderer, pp. 179–96. Berlin/NY: de Gruyter. 949 pp.
17. Huennekens, F. M., Vitols, J. S., Henderson, G. B. 1978. Transport of folate compounds in bacterial and mammalian cells. *Adv. Enzymol. Relat. Areas Mol. Biol.* 47:313–46
18. Iwai, K., Luttner, P. M., Toenneis, G. 1964. Blood folic acid studies. Purification and properties of the folic acid precursors of human erythrocytes. *J. Biol. Chem.* 239:2365–69

248   WAGNER

19. Kamen, B. A., Caston, J. D. 1975. Identification of a folate binder in hog kidney. *J. Biol. Chem.* 250:2203–5
20. Leslie, G. I., Rowe, P. B. 1972. Folate binding by the brush border membrane proteins of small intestinal epithelial cells. *Biochemistry* 11:1696–703
21. Mackenzie, C. G. 1955. Conversion of N-methyl glycines to active formaldehyde and serine. In *Amino Acid Metabolism*, ed. W. D. McElroy, H. B. Glass, pp. 684–726. Baltimore: Johns Hopkins Press
22. McHugh, M., Cheng, Y.-C. 1979. Demonstration of a high affinity folate binder in human cell membranes and its characterization in cultured human KB cells. *J. Biol. Chem.* 254: 11312–18
23. Mell, G. P., Huennekens, F. M. 1960. Sarcosine dehydrogenase. *Fed. Proc.* 19:411
24. Noronha, J. M., Silverman, M. 1962. On folic acid, vitamin B_{12}, methionine, and forminimoglutamic acid metabolism. In *Vitamin B_{12} and Intrinsic Factor*, ed. C. Heinrich, pp. 728–36. Stuttgart: F. Enke
25. Sakami, W. 1955. Discussion. In: *Amino Acid Metabolism*, ed. W. D. McElroy, H. B. Glass. Baltimore: Johns Hopkins Press. 790 pp.
26. Sankar, D. V. S., Rosza, P. W. 1972. Metabolism of folate-2-^{14}C in the mammal. *Res. Comm. Chem. Pathol. Pharmacol.* 4:93–113
27. Scott, J. M., Weir, D. G. 1976. Folate composition, synthesis and function in natural materials. *Clin. Haematol.* 5: 547–68
28. Scott, J. M., Weir, D. G. 1981. Hypothesis. The methyl folate trap. *Lancet* II:337–40
29. Selhub, J., Rosenberg, I. H. 1978. Demonstration of high-affinity folate binding activity associated with the brush border membranes of rat kidney. *Proc. Natl. Acad. Sci. USA* 75:3090–93
30. Spector, R. 1977. The effect of Pronase on choroid plexus transport. *Brain Res.* 134:573–76
31. Spector, R. 1977. Identification of folate binding macromolecule in rabbit choroid plexus. *J. Biol. Chem.* 252:3364–70
32. Spector, R. 1979. Affinity of folic acid for the folate-binding protein of choroid plexus. *Arch. Biochem. Biophys.* 194: 632–34
33. Spector, R., Lorenzo, A. V. 1975. Fo-
late transport by the choroid plexus in vitro. *Science* 187:540–42
34. Stokstad, E. L. R. 1979. Overview of folic acid derivatives in animal tissues. In *Folic Acid in Neurology, Psychiatry, and Internal Medicine*, ed. M. E. Botez, E. H. Reynolds, pp. 35–45. NY: Raven Press
35. Sulieman, S. A., Spector, R. 1981. Purification and characterization of a folate binding protein from porcine choroid plexus. *Arch. Biochem. Biophys.* 208: 87–94
36. Suzuki, N., Wagner, C. 1980. Purification and characterization of a folate binding protein from rat liver cytosol. *Arch. Biochem. Biophys.* 199:236–48
37. Watabe, S. 1978. Purification and characterization of tetrahydrofolate-protein complex in bovine liver. *J. Biol. Chem.* 253:6673–79
38. Waxman, S. 1975. Annotation. Folate binding protein. *Br. J. Haematol.* 29:23–29
39. Waxman, S., Schreiber, C., Rubinoff, M. 1978. The significance of folate binding proteins in folate metabolism. In *Advances in Nutritional Research*, ed. H. Draper, 1:55–76. NY: Plenum
40. Wittwer, A. J., Wagner, C. 1980. Identification of folate binding protein of mitochondria as dimethylglycine dehydrogenase. *Proc. Natl. Acad. Sci. USA* 77:4484–88
41. Wittwer, A. J., Wagner, C. 1981. Identification of the folate binding proteins of rat liver mitochondria as dimethylglycine dehydrogenase and sarcosine dehydrogenase. Purification and folate-binding characteristics. *J. Biol. Chem.* 256:4102–8
42. Wittwer, A. J., Wagner, C. 1981. Identification of the folate-binding proteins of rat liver mitochondria as dimethylglycine dehydrogenase and sarcosine dehydrogenase. Flavoprotein nature and enzymatic properties of the purified proteins. *J. Biol. Chem.* 256:4109–15
43. Zamierowski, M. M., Wagner, C. 1974. High molecular weight complexes of folic acid in mammalian tissues. *Biochem. Biophys. Res. Commun.* 60: 81–87
44. Zamierowski, M. M., Wagner, C. 1977. Identification of folate binding proteins of rat liver. *J. Biol. Chem.* 252:933–38
45. Zamierowski, M. M., Wagner, C. 1977. Effect of folacin deficiency on folacin-binding proteins in the rat. *J. Nutr.* 107:1937–45

Ann. Rev. Nutr. 1982. 2:249–76
Copyright © 1982 by Annual Reviews Inc. All rights reserved

CHEMICAL SENSES IN THE RELEASE OF GASTRIC AND PANCREATIC SECRETIONS

Joseph G. Brand

Monell Chemical Senses Center, and Department of Biochemistry, School of Dental Medicine, University of Pennsylvania, Philadelphia, Pennsylvania 19104

Robert H. Cagan

Veterans Administration Medical Center, and Monell Chemical Senses Center, and University of Pennsylvania School of Medicine, Philadelphia, Pennsylvania 19104

Michael Naim

The Hebrew University of Jerusalem, Faculty of Agriculture, Rehovot, 76100, Israel

CONTENTS

249

0199-9885/82/0715-0249$02.00

INTRODUCTION

Within the context of nutrition, the chemical senses—taste (gustation) and smell (olfaction)—function in search, identification, and ingestion of food (70, 108). The complexity of behaviors involved in these functions is appreciable, and the influence of experience leads ultimately to the catalog of information on foods carried within the memory of the organism (6). A less-appreciated function of the chemical senses is their action in triggering digestive processes that anticipate arrival of food in the gut (83, 85, 138). In this context, the chemical senses act as components of a larger group of effects collectively termed cephalic. Cephalic effects result from stimulation of sensory-receptive relay systems in the region of the head and neck. Pavlov (97) used "psychic effects" to denote the cephalic phase. Didactic arguments about the terminology are reviewed by Powley (101). An historical perspective on the study of gastric function and its relationship to eating, emotions, and general health is given in an enjoyable account by Wolf (143).

Stimulation of digestive secretions is classified into cephalic, gastric, and intestinal phases (43, 62, 126). The digestive sequences triggered by the cephalic phase are in the same direction as those triggered by the gastric and intestinal phases. Usually the cephalic-stimulated responses are of smaller magnitude and shorter duration than responses to the gastric and intestinal phases. Nevertheless, it is inappropriate to ignore the cephalic function of the chemical senses, since it could have important consequences for overall digestive efficiency and nutritional well-being.

The digestive effects that result from cephalic reflexes are initiated most reliably by the taste and smell of food. The sight of food and other circumstances associated with eating may also act as stimuli, although these seem to be less potent. Initiation of digestive events by cephalic-phase stimulation depends upon intact vagi (e.g. 3, 12, 64, 74, 97, 103). It is generally assumed that direct neural innervation to the site of secretory activity is responsible for the cephalic-phase effects (12), although for some secretory responses an indirect hormonal relay cannot be ruled out (46, 139; but see 11). With the conscious animal, the cephalic phase can be isolated for experimental study by the technique of sham feeding (30, 97) in which ingested food is diverted to the exterior. This is usually achieved by using an esophageal fistula. With human subjects, sham feeding may be performed simply by having the subject chew and then expectorate the food (63). The latter method, designated "modified sham feeding" (MSF), is experimentally simpler than sham feeding using a fistula, but it omits the action of swallowing. Several experiments (see below) suggest that swallowing may be an important component of the cephalic phase, and caution should be exercised when activation of neural receptors of the pharynx and esophagus is ignored (1).

In each experimental situation, stimuli of the cephalic phase may be varied and controlled to isolate one component from the others, or to combine one or more of these components.

In addition to the stimulus provided by sham feeding, the efferent vagus can be stimulated either directly, by electrical stimulation, or indirectly, by glucose deprivation of the higher vagal centers. The latter can be achieved, for example, by insulin-induced hypoglycemia (50, 56, 65) or by intravenous infusions of 2-deoxy-D-glucose (5, 28, 48). Under normal conditions the efferent vagus is stimulated reflexively either from higher centers of the brain, after the cephalic phase components are activated, or by visceral afferents. Impulses are transmitted from the cortex and subcortical areas to the anterior hypothalamus and then to the medullary vagal centers (14). In the case of gastric secretion, the impulses then proceed via vagal nerves either to oxyntic glands of the fundus, where they stimulate acid and pepsin secretion, or to the neuroendocrine cells of the antrum, where they stimulate the release of gastrin (12).

In this review we focus on the effects of taste and smell on digestive and metabolic reflexes. We emphasize cephalic-stimulated responses leading to gastric, pancreatic exocrine, and endocrine secretions. We indicate the mechanisms operating in these responses and where appropriate suggest future experiments, particularly ones we feel may help clarify the specific role of the chemical senses in nutrition. Other major aspects of the chemical senses have been covered adequately in recent reviews. These include the morphology and ultrastructure of taste (82) and olfactory (40) peripheral structures, the central neuroanatomy of taste (91) and olfactory pathways (121), the biochemical basis of taste and olfaction (15), the neurophysiology of taste cells (110), and the functioning of the chemical senses during aging (113, 114).

CEPHALIC-PHASE EFFECTS ON GASTRIC SECRETION

Control of Secretion

Gastric secretion is regulated by both neural and hormonal mechanisms (12, 62). For the cephalic phase, impulses from the vagal nucleus stimulate secretory cells in the oxyntic glands of the fundus. Gastric distention also causes secretion through local reflex arcs and via vagal afferent and efferent fibers (12, 21, 22, 42, 125). At least in the dog, gastric distention stimulates release of the hormone gastrin from the antrum (21, 22); and in both dog and human, distention potentiates acid secretion (21, 22, 42, 44, 125). Vagal impulses to the antrum stimulate gastrin release, and impulses to the oxyntic gland potentiate the secretory action of gastrin (12). This sequence is not as clear in humans. Grotzinger et al (44) reported that for humans, fundic distention is an adequate stimulus for acid release but a poor stimulus for gastrin release. Even when stomach contents were neutralized during distention, serum gastrin did not rise significantly (44). In a similar study (125), serum gastrin rose only slightly at the highest distention pressures, but no correlation was found between rate of acid secretion and increases in serum gastrin.

Numerous reports employ cephalic-phase stimuli to study gastric secretion. Here we review studies either reporting recent advances in understanding the mechanism for cephalic-phase stimulation or employing variables relevant to the chemical senses. The general observation that the cephalic phase affects gastric secretion dates to the 18th century (143), but credit is usually given to Pavlov for placing this phenomenon on a sound experimental basis. The common pathway used by the cephalic phase to trigger gastric secretion is the vagus nerve; vagotomy abolishes the reflex (12, 14, 30, 43, 62, 64, 97). The neurotransmitter for vagal release of gastric acid is atropine-sensitive (12, 64, 88), and H_2-receptor antagonists cause a marked decrease (80%) in acid secretion (115). Under normal conditions the gastric secretory response to sham feeding appears after a latent period of 5–7 minutes and continues for as long as 3 hours after the food is eaten (78, 97, 106). Maximal secretion in response to sham feeding is reached by around 30 to 45 minutes (64, 78, 106), and stomach distention potentiates the secretory effect caused by sham feeding and prolongs the maximal rate of secretion (106).

A recent report by Konturek et al (64) details the time course of gastric secretion after cephalic-phase stimulation and the effect of atropine. Normal human subjects showed elevated gastric acid and pepsin output after modified sham feeding (MSF). Gastric acid attained a maximal release in normal subjects at the end of the 30 min sham feeding period, reaching 62% of the peak pentagastrin response. Infusion of atropine (20 μg/kg/hr) resulted in almost complete inhibition of basal acid and pepsinogen secretions, while the serum gastrin concentration remained at the pre-atropine level. MSF in atropinized subjects failed to stimulate release of gastric acid or pepsinogen above the pre-MSF level. However, when MSF was superimposed on pentagastrin-induced gastric secretion, acid output was increased compared with simple pentagastrin stimulation, but pepsinogen output was not augmented. In all cases with healthy human subjects, serum gastrin levels did not change with MSF.

Increases in serum gastrin levels with cephalic phase stimulation in humans are not consistently observed (reviewed in 12; see, for example, 64, 80, 131; but also 32, 34). When pH of the gastric contents was not permitted to fall, a distinct increase in serum gastrin was reported with MSF (34).

When atropine was administered in the study by Feldman et al (34), gastric acid and pancreatic polypeptide levels fell in response to sham feeding, but gastrin levels rose. In contrast, with dogs the cephalic phase usually induces serum gastrin increases. Electrical stimulation of the distal ends of the cut vagus reliably increased serum gastrin levels that were usually, but not always, related to gastric acid output (66). These increases in serum gastrin could be blocked by antrectomy or by perfusion of the antrum with acid (66). An apparent independence (or, at least, not strict dependence) of acid and gastrin was recently found in dogs using β_2-agonists with vagal stimulation induced by insulin or 2-deoxyglucose (39).

Hirschowitz & Gibson (48) reported that central vagal excitation induced by 2-deoxyglucose produces a higher level of serum gastrin (and of gastric acid secretion) after fundic vagotomy compared with the intact fundic innervation. The effects after atropine injection in both groups of animals led the experimenters to conclude that the mechanism for gastrin release is not cholinergic. It was found in dogs that low doses of atropine (1.25 μg/kg and 25 μg/kg) enhanced serum gastrin levels in response to food given orally (52). [Gastrin responses in this study (52) could have been due to gastric as well as cephalic stimulation.] Dockray & Tracy (27) report that using sham feeding in dogs, serum gastrin rose soon (4–7 min) after sham feeding began. If intragastric pH was not permitted to fall, serum gastrin was always higher than under unregulated conditions. When the same meal was delivered through a gastric fistula, serum gastrin did not change until after 10 min. Atropine given at 25 μg/kg did not change the meal-stimulated gastrin response but it did abolish the decline in serum gastrin normally observed after 10–20 min. Vagotomy in these animals abolished the early rise in serum gastrin after feeding, but also caused an increase in basal serum gastrin. These investigators (52) concluded that since "high doses of atropine reduced the gastrin response to [normal] feeding, but had little effect on the gastrin response to sham feeding . . . presence of food in the stomach might initiate a cholinergic stimulatory pathway of gastrin release."

In a previous study (23) atropine blocked gastrin release that was initiated by normal eating in the vagotomized dog. In the report of Hirschowitz & Gibson (48), the fundic vagotomized dogs displayed an increase in serum gastrin compared with intact animals when under stimulation by 2-deoxyglucose. Atropine (100 μg/kg), however, completely abolished this elevation. The conclusions from these studies are that fundic vagotomy removes an inhibitory pathway of gastrin release and that the inhibitory neurons are cholinergic. This conclusion is supported by observations that vagal denervation of the oxyntic mucosa led to a food-stimulated increase in gastrin release in both humans (31) and dogs (147). To further confirm this hypothesis, it was recently reported (127) that excision of the fundic mucosa led to an increased release of both gastrin and acid after meal stimulation, suggesting that an inhibitory mechanism directly related to the fundic mucosa was removed. It appears at present that gastrin secretion is under complex control involving both cholinergic and peptide (neurotransmitter) mediation (29, 79).

Effects of Chemical Senses on Secretion

Although the effects of sham feeding on gastric responses are well known, the effect of taste or smell stimuli themselves on gastric secretion is not clearly understood. For example, does a "very palatable" meal increase gastric secretion to levels higher than a "less palatable" meal? Obviously, "palatability" must be determined on an individual basis, since food preferences are not the same for all individuals of a species (6). One widely cited reference directly addressing the effect of the cephalic phase on gastric secretion, but also cautioning a respect for individuality, is that from Pavlov (97). He noted that "the majority of dogs prefer flesh to bread, and correspondingly less [gastric] juice will be produced by sham-feeding with bread than with flesh. Sometimes, however, we find dogs which will devour bread with greater appetite than flesh. In these cases one obtains more and stronger [gastric] juice in sham-feeding with bread than with flesh."

While sham-feeding is known to be a potent stimulant to gastric secretion in humans [and has been suggested as a test for the completeness of vagotomy (33)], few experimental studies have considered the hedonic quality of the food. Those that did employ palatability as a variable have documented results parallel to Pavlov's. An earlier study of Janowitz et al (54) reports volume, total acid, and pepsin secretion from a stomach tube of a human subject who was maintained in caloric equilibrium by introduction of predigested diet into the stomach. In experiments to test the potency of cephalic stimulation, the subject was given one of three meals, randomly presented over several days between 9:00 A.M. and noon, following 10 hours of fasting. One meal consisted of a cereal gruel, a second the standard hospital diet for the day, and the third a meal composed of the subject's unrestricted choice. Because the subject selected this latter meal on the day previous to its administration, she was aware of the contents of the meal before it was presented. In all cases the self-selected meal led to higher levels of acid secretion than the cereal gruel (Figure 1). Parker et al (95) reported that sham feeding of the healthy human subject led to immediate increases in gastric volume secretion and large increases in potassium output. In general the pattern of changes in acid, volume, potassium, sodium, and chloride were similar for both sham feeding and histamine injection. They noted greater changes from basal levels for evening meals than for breakfast

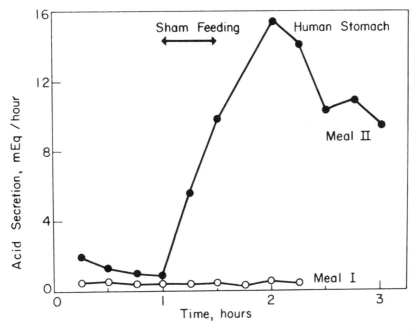

Figure 1   Rate of gastric acid secretion from one human subject vs time for two types of meals. Meal I is a cereal gruel, meal II is composed of the subject's unrestricted choice. Points of meal I are means of 4 experiments, and those of meal II are means of 12 experiments. The figure is reproduced with permission from Davenport (19), page 168 [adapted from Janowitz et al (54)].

meals (both following 12-hr deprivation) and suggested that since the evening meals were composed of the subject's choice, greater gustatory and "anticipatory" cephalic stimuli were responsible.

A recent study (76) using healthy volunteers demonstrated that a solid-liquid meal given orally elicited stronger gastric (acid, pepsin, and volume) responses than a homogenized meal of identical composition delivered intragastrically. The volunteers were unaware of which type meal they would encounter until immediately before the meal was served. Most of the early responses observed in this study to the solid-liquid meal compared with the homogenized meal are probably due to a greater stimulation of the cephalic phase evoked by the former meal's being tasted, smelled, masticated, and swallowed.

A study reporting the relative potency for stimulating gastric secretion between cephalic stimulation and stomach distention has been published by Richardson et al (106). The technique of modified sham feeding (MSF) was employed using an "appetizing" meal consisting of steak, french-fried potatoes, and water. Following a 10 hr fast, all subjects received the same meal;

the MSF lasted 30 min. For control stimulation (no meal) the subject chewed on a plastic tube for 30 min. Under MSF conditions, this meal led to an increase in gastric acid secretion compared to the no-meal condition. Gastric acid output rose significantly within the first sampling period (15 min) using MSF and reached maximal output by 30 min, the end of the MSF period. After this, acid secretion declined (Figure 2A). The amount of acid secreted was approximately 45% of the subject's maximal acid response to histamine.

Distention of the stomach also stimulated gastric acid secretion (106). One of three distention-causing equiosmolar solutions was delivered intragastrically: a NaCl solution, a glucose solution, or a slurry of blended food (steak, bread, butter, water). All three test meals led to acid stimulation, although the food slurry was the most potent stimulator. The onset of acid secretion was delayed after delivery of the food-slurry test meal, not being significantly different from basal levels until 30 min into the test period. If the stomach was first distended by food slurry and then MSF begun, the amount of acid secreted during the first 30 min owing to the MSF was not increased above the nondistended condition. However, acid was secreted for a longer period, lasting beyond the 2-hr collection period. These results point to the importance of cephalically derived increased vagal activity as an initiator of gastric secretion while a meal is being eaten.

In addition to measuring gastric acid secretion, this study (106) also found that serum gastrin was not significantly increased by MSF (Figure 2B). However, distention of the stomach with the food slurry, along with buffering of the stomach contents to pH 5 (to prevent acid-induced inhibition of gastrin release), did give rise to a significant increase in serum gastrin. This increase was not significantly augmented by superimposing MSF onto the intragastric infusion of the food slurry.

One component of the cephalic phase that has received little experimental study is the suspected stimulation of digestive sequences due to smell, to sight of food, or to association with events surrounding food ingestion. Moore & Motoki (80) reported that when subjects were permitted to observe (and presumably smell) the preparation of meals of their choice, gastric acid secretion increased significantly, to 55% of their normal pentagastrin-stimulated response. Blood glucose and gastrin levels were not affected by this procedure. Presumably, however, the subjects in this study could both see and smell the food, so simple anticipation was not the only stimulant. In a previous study (81) with a single subject it was reported that "anticipation" alone was a sufficient stimulus for acid release. A recent study (32) reported that the sight and smell of food and even simply talking about food were sufficient stimuli to initiate gastric secretion. The authors report their results as a combination of all types of stimulation so that effects

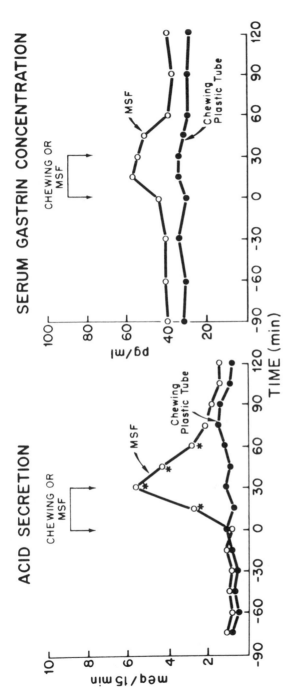

Figure 2 Acid secretion and serum gastrin concentration vs time in human subjects before, during, and after modified sham feeding (MSF) or chewing of a plastic tube. Significantly different (p < 0.05) mean values between the two types of stimulation are indicated as *. Time of chewing and MSF is shown by bracketed arrows. Points are mean values from nine human subjects. Figure is from Richardson et al (106), reproduced with permission of the publisher.

of individual stimuli, such as sight alone or smell alone cannot be determined. They report significant increases in both acid output and serum gastrin concentration after the 30 min sham sessions. The acid output was 28% of the peak acid output to pentagastrin. What is particularly notable about this study, for the purposes of the present review, is that the experimenters requested each subject to list his or her favorite (most appetizing) foods. It was these preselected meals that were either smelled, seen or talked about.

In order to achieve maximal responses to food stimuli, most investigators employ what they believe to be appetizing meals. Only a few studies have examined the effects of foods of varying palatability. This raises a question of what the effect of marginally palatable or even unpalatable foods may be, not only on secretion itself, but also on its duration and character. For example, if stomach distention precedes sham feeding as in the Richardson et al study (106), could unpalatable food in the subsequent sham feeding stage of the experiment truncate the secretion that would normally occur due to distention? Would the rate be altered and would sham feeding with unpalatable food fail to increase the amount of time that secretion was evident? Also, what would be the effect of marginally palatable food or the effect of sham feeding with a food that the subject anticipated as being palatable, but that was adulterated to be unpalatable?

CEPHALIC-PHASE EFFECTS ON EXOCRINE PANCREATIC SECRETION

Control of Secretion

Pavlov was the first investigator to report a convincing cephalic-phase stimulation of exocrine pancreatic flow (97). Since then the effect has been demonstrated several times (7, 84, 92, 93, 104, 109), but its precise nature is still difficult to explain. It is possible that pancreatic exocrine output after cephalic stimulation is due to secondary effects of gastric acid entering the duodenum and thus releasing secretin, to primary effects of cephalically released gastrin, or to direct vagal stimulation of pancreatic exocrine secretory cells (3, 61, 84, 103, 104, 126). An account of the probable mechanisms during the cephalic phase is provided by Solomon & Grossman (126). It is interesting to note that Pavlov (97) was convinced that the increased pancreatic output he observed to sham feeding in dogs was not secondary to a gastric acid effect. His reasoning was based on the time course of the effect. "The latent period of the gastric secretion in dogs has a sharply marked lower limit, and is never less than four and a half minutes. The pancreatic juice, on the contrary, begins to flow 2–3 min after the application of the exciting agency, for example, an acid. In the experiment of teasing the animal by offering it food, the pancreatic flow also generally begins after two to three minutes. This appears to me to point to a direct psychic influence through the secretory nerves of the pancreas . . ." (97).

Some portion of the pancreatic response to cephalic stimulation appears to be due to secondary effects, particularly to hormone release. Especially in dogs, where cephalic stimulation reliably releases gastrin, this argument must be considered, although the physiological relevance of experiments using exogenous gastrin is not yet clear. In the human, large increases in gastrin following cephalic stimulation are not as obvious (see also preceding section), yet a cephalic phase of pancreatic output has been documented. Its magnitude relative to the gastric and intestinal phases has not been directly assessed (126). Other reflexive pathways are well known, often confusing interpretation of cephalic-phase experiments on pancreatic exocrine function; these include gastric vago-vagal reflexes (45, 140) and modifications of hormone release (20, 63, 141).

In dogs, an ingested meal causes a larger volume and protein response than does sham feeding, the latter being responsible for only 10–15% of volume and up to 25% of the normal amount of protein (17). Preshaw et al (104) observed that protein output, volume flow, and bicarbonate output from the pancreas all increased in sham-fed dogs, but acidificiation of the antral pouch with 0.1 N HCl abolished the stimulation of protein release by the pancreas. They concluded that gastrin was a permissive requirement for protein release under these conditions since antral acidification will effectively block gastrin release. However, their surgical procedure for forming an innervated pouch of the pyloric gland may have resulted in partial damage to vagal fibers innervating the pancreas (104, 126). Because the pancreas has vagal innervation, direct vagal stimulation (i.e. not mediated by gastrin) can affect pancreatic output (20, 47, 57, 123). Anticholinergic drugs inhibit the cephalic phase of pancreatic secretion in humans (109), but the site of action of the drugs cannot be determined under the experimental conditions used. Atropine was reported (141) to reduce pancreatic amylase output in response to vagal (electrical) stimulation in the monkey, but complete abolishment of the enzyme release was not observed.

It is assumed that the intestinal phase is quantitatively very important for the pancreatic exocrine response to a meal (20, 103, 126) and that a vago-vagal enteropancreatic reflex (sensitive to atropine and vagotomy) is important for rapid release of pancreatic enzymes (4). Malegalada et al (76) observed that trypsin output of the pancreas in response to two types of meals, a solid-liquid meal (chewed and swallowed) and a homogenized meal (delivered intragastrically) did not differ initially. After one hour, however, the pancreatic output with the homogenized meal had declined faster than that for the solid-liquid meal. However, because the homogenized meal also emptied faster from the stomach, the difference in pancreatic response could have been due to transit time and not to differences in cephalic-phase stimulation.

In order to eliminate the possibility that the pancreatic response to sham feeding was due to gastric acid stimulation of secretin or cholecystokinin, Novis et al (92) used achlorhydric human subjects. They were sham fed (using MSF) a breakfast of their choice, the preparation of which they were permitted to observe (and smell). Sham feeding maintained volume flow and bicarbonate concentration at or slightly above basal levels, while the activities of lipase, trypsin, and chymotrypsin were generally increased. Amylase activity increased in only 2 of the 5 subjects during the sham period. These investigators suggest that the increase in pancreatic protein output was due primarily to vagal stimulation. It was previously reported (67) that pentagastrin could maintain basal pancreatic flow and increase enzyme concentration only slightly. Novis et al (92) concluded that the suggestion of Preshaw et al (104) that gastrin mediates the cephalic phase of pancreatic release in dogs could not explain their results with human subjects. Although a cephalic phase of pancreatic enzyme release exists, the results of Novis et al (92) suggest that it is quantitatively of minor importance.

Effects of the Chemical Senses

Sarles et al (109) report a cephalic phase of pancreatic secretion in humans. Their experimental paradigm varied the type of meal presented to their subjects. When allowing their subjects to see and smell a typical breakfast, they observed an increase in lipase activity, volume output and bicarbonate concentration compared with the condition of having the subjects see and smell a less typical breakfast (steak). When subjects were permitted to chew (but not swallow) the less typical breakfast, lipase volume and bicarbonate increased beyond levels present when subjects simply saw and smelled it. Sarles et al (109) also report that time of day had an effect on their results, early morning being a period of decreased secretory activity. Also, in one anorectic patient no obvious stimulation due to any of the test conditions was observed. These researchers concluded that even though pancreatic release by the cephalic phase is quantitatively small, its effects last long after (1 hr) sham feeding ceases, so that it could play a significant role in augmenting further release during normal eating.

Previous studies (92, 104, 109) employed food as a stimulus for sham feeding-excitation of the cephalic phase. The experiment of Sarles et al (109) suggested that palatability of the food may influence the amount of exocrine pancreatic secretion to cephalic stimulation. Experiments with conscious dogs have shown that both pancreatic flow and protein output can be affected by the palatability of the diet during a sham feeding regimen (7).

In this experiment (7) a basal diet was adulterated with either acceptable or aversive taste stimuli, and the animals generally showed a greater pancreatic response to the acceptable than the aversive diet.

A subsequent study (83, 84) explored the relationship between specific taste stimuli and pancreatic exocrine secretion. Dogs were prepared with gastric and duodenal fistulas for continuous drainage of gastric and intestinal contents. The duodenal fistula permitted direct cannulation of the main pancreatic duct. Taste stimulation was achieved by application with cotton swabs soaked in aqueous taste solutions to the dogs tongue for 6 minutes. Sucrose at a concentration to produce positive acceptance, and quinine sulfate or citric acid at concentrations that produced aversive responses were selected as stimuli. Dog saliva was employed as a control stimulus. During the experiment, the gastric and duodenal fistulas were kept open.

At first, oral stimulation with these substances produced a large increase in both the pancreatic volume and protein output during the 45-min collection (Figure 3). However, after one or two trials with each stimulus with each dog, an increased output no longer occurred. It is probable that the

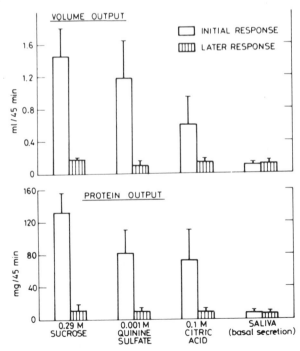

Figure 3   Total pancreatic volume and protein output during 45 min following oral stimulation of 4 dogs with three different taste stimuli using a swab technique. Values are mean ± S.E.M. of 4 experiments for each stimulus during either the initial or later sessions. Figure is adapted from Naim & Kare (83).

dogs associated the initial taste stimulations with anticipated feedings; however, after repeated trials, when food was not forthcoming, they no longer responded. The phenomenon of reduced response (extinction) following repeated trials has not been reported with sham feeding, but the orogastric reflexes, in addition to being excited by taste stimuli, are subject to inhibition by the hypothalamic area (67).

Since swallowing is usually involved with sham feeding in dogs, the same dogs were next given orally 100 ml of taste-stimulus solution mixed with 25 g of cellulose (Figure 4) (84). A pancreatic secretory response, which occurred within 40 min following the 6-min period of sham feeding with the cellulose mix, was restored primarily for a sucrose-cellulose mixture. Oral administration of the less palatable citric acid–cellulose or quinine-cellulose mixtures resulted in low pancreatic output, similar to that for the

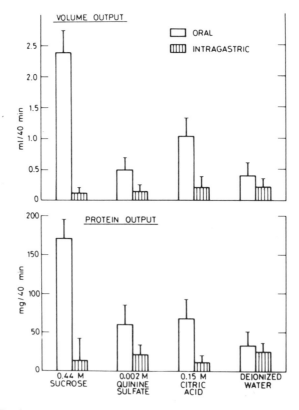

Figure 4   Total pancreatic volume and protein output during 40 min following oral or intragastric administration of taste-cellulose mixtures to 4 dogs. Values are means ± S.E.M. of 6–8 experiments on each dog. Figure is adapted from Naim et al (84).

(control) water-cellulose mixture. Although the gastric and intestinal fistulas remained open, intragastric administrations of the same taste-stimulus cellulose mixtures were performed in order to separate any pregastric factors that affect pancreatic secretion from those due to postingestive stimulation, e.g. the vago-vagal reflex (45, 140). These intragastric experiments resulted in low pancreatic output during the 40 min after administration. It was concluded that chewing and swallowing actions were necessary to trigger the feedback mechanisms that could restore the pancreatic response.

Schwartz et al (119) also found that in humans the cephalic phase of pancreatic polypeptide secretion from the endocrine pancreas was larger and less variable when the food was not only tasted and chewed, but also swallowed. Naim et al (84) concluded that taste stimulation alone is not sufficient to affect pancreatic exocrine secretion, but when coupled with swallowing, palatable taste stimuli exert a greater effect than do unpalatable stimuli on the cephalic phase of pancreatic exocrine secretion. Using a design similar to that of Naim et al (84), Ohara et al (93) reported that the effect of taste stimulation on pancreatic exocrine secretion of Beagle dogs depended upon the carrier used. Statistically significant increases in pancreatic response to orally delivered sucrose-cellulose mixtures compared with water-cellulose stimulation were not found in these dogs. However, the mean for sucrose stimulation was about 18-fold higher than that for water. It is apparent that the individual responses varied markedly among these dogs, not allowing a statistically significant difference in the group data.

Taken collectively, the experimental results of cephalic-phase effects on pancreatic exocrine secretions suggest that the response is quite fragile. When food was presented to human subjects to determine if sight and smell alone are sufficient stimuli for exocrine pancreatic release, little (109) if any (122) secretion was observed. Apparently, the full complement of the cephalic-phase cascade is required for the secretory response, and even then the response is small, although prolonged (76, 84, 109). Since pancreatic polypeptide is also released by the cephalic phase (see below) and has been implicated as an inhibitor of exocrine pancreatic secretion (137), the low secretory response of the exocrine pancreas to cephalic stimulation could be partly due to this inhibition.

CEPHALIC-PHASE EFFECTS ON ENDOCRINE PANCREATIC SECRETION

Insulin and Glucagon

During the past 15 years, many studies have demonstrated that stimulation by specific tastes, by food intake, or by the smell (and sight) of food can lead to a rapid increase in plasma insulin. This is assumed to be a preabsorptive elevation (8–11, 13, 36, 38, 51, 58, 74, 75, 94, 98, 100, 107, 124, 129, 132,

133, 142). Although the studies cited are not exhaustive, they serve as a guide to hypotheses formulated both to document the cephalic-phase response of insulin and to explore the physiologic mechanisms for the preabsorptive insulin release and its nutritional significance. Although the mechanisms are not clearly understood, the phenomenon is clearly demonstrable. Fischer et al (36) and Hommel et al (51) demonstrated that in the conscious dog immunoreactive plasma insulin increases after oral glucose stimulation. Stimulation of the oral cavity with fluids or food seems to be the critical factor, since saccharin solutions (8, 11, 74, 132) and even water (51) are sufficient to initiate this response, suggesting that the rise is a true cephalic effect and not dependent upon the presence of ingested glucose. In addition, drenching the oral cavity of the conscious dog with a topical anesthetic resulted in failure to observe the early rise in plasma insulin with oral glucose as the stimulant (35). As with other cephalic phase–mediated reflexes, the early rise in insulin resulting from oral stimulation can be blocked by atropine (99) or by vagotomy (74, 102, 144).

The effects of vagotomy indicate that direct vagal stimulation should lead to insulin release. It is known, for example, from morphological studies that pancreatic beta-cells receive cholinergic innervation (89), and the implications of neural innervation to the endocrine pancreas have been discussed (105, 145). Experiments performed by Frohman et al (37) and Daniel & Henderson (18) demonstrate that immunoreactive insulin is released following direct vagal stimulation. When the cut right vagal trunk was stimulated electrically (18) a 50% increase in plasma insulin was observed in blood taken from the inferior vena cava. Vagal stimulation did not alter blood glucose levels at any time during the experimental period. After a stimulation period of 10 min, plasma insulin levels remained elevated for about 100 min. These experiments support the hypothesis that the rise in peripheral plasma insulin observed to cephalic phase stimulation is vagally mediated.

Nicolaidis (85) reported hyperglycemia after either oral sucrose or oral saccharin stimulation in anesthetizied, food-deprived rats. He has hypothesized (86) that during food deprivation, anticipatory processes that result in release of endogenous glucose prevail, resulting in early hyperglycemia. Conversely, during *ad libitum* feeding, glucose storage processes predominate, and the early hyperglycemia is not consistently observed. This hypothesis is congruent with the observation that the release of insulin during the first minute of feeding is much smaller in food-deprived rats than in rats fed *ad libitum* (132).

The hyperglycemic hormone glucagon is also released by the cephalic phase, although this phenomenon is not as completely documented as is the cephalic phase–stimulated release of insulin (24, 25, 90). The report of

Nilsson & Uvnäs-Wallensten (90) provides evidence that the sight, smell, and taste of a meal are all effective stimuli for glucagon release in the dog and that the glucagon rise can be abolished by atropine (0.2 mg/kg) injections. The sight and smell of the food (minced boiled beef liver in water) were not as effective stimuli for glucagon release as was sham feeding. That the two apparently opposing hormones, insulin and glucagon, should both be released by the cephalic phase is interesting, yet not too surprising when viewed from the point of regulation and maintenance of the internal milieu. The possible reciprocal modulation by the CNS of release of glucagon and insulin has received some attention and is discussed in a recent review (87).

One question of current interest is whether the release of insulin to sweet taste is innate. Deutsch (26) found that the hypoglycemic effect induced by saccharin injection into rats was reversible by exposing the animals to long-term oral access to saccharin. Based on the results of various studies (9, 36, 85, 129) the preabsorptive insulin release to sweet taste should be innate. Yet the response can be conditioned, being associated with the time of eating [and sensitive to atropine (146)]; it is not observed in response to saccharin in the newborn rat pup, but is observed by the time of weaning (8). More recently, Berridge et al (9) demonstrated that the preabsorptive release of insulin evoked by glucose could be abolished by pairing the taste with LiCl in a conditioned aversion paradigm. This result suggests that experience can alter not only consummatory behavior but neuroendocrine function as well.

The observations of a preabsorptive rise in insulin after cephalic-phase stimulation raises the question of whether the magnitude of the rise is modulated by the "palatability" or "hedonic quality" of the stimulus. Berridge et al (9) showed that even though the stimulus solutions NaCl, saccharin, and glucose were presented to naive rats at preferred levels, only glucose resulted in a preabsorptive insulin response. Solutions shown to be aversive resulted in no preabsorptive release of insulin. [Preference was determined by a catalog of mimetic responses to the stimuli flowed into the oral cavity of the rat (41).]

Other experiments have measured preabsorptive insulin responses to complex foods. Strubbe & Steffens (132) observed an increase in plasma insulin within 1 min after the unanesthetized rat begins consuming a carbohydrate-free, high-fat meal (43% fat: type not specified). Food deprivation was not necessary to observe this effect. When the animals were changed from the carbohydrate-rich food to a "dummy food" (56% paraffin oil, 8% vaseline, 36% cellulose), insulin levels nevertheless rose, although blood glucose did not rise. For the groups of rats fed *ad libitum,* comparison of their data (132) for the carbohydrate-rich and fat-rich diets with the diets composed of dummy foods indicates that the former diets provoked a larger rise in insulin levels. The preabsorptive insulin rise to food can be observed when the blood glucose level does not change. Indeed, only with the food-deprived rat, or when a carbohydrate meal is offered to the rat at any time, is blood glucose significantly elevated (128, 132). Louis-Sylvestre & Le-Magnen (75) reported that quinine-adulterated food led to a decrease in the preabsorptive insulin response compared with nonadulterated food, while food adulterated with 0.2% sodium saccharin resulted in higher levels of preabsorptive insulin release. Based on the amount of food consumed, these researchers report that the saccharin-adulterated diet was preferred to the normal diet, which in turn was preferred to the quinine-adulterated diet.

Could these early neuroendocrine reflexes have physiologic or nutritional significance? As noted in the above sections on digestive secretions, the postabsorptive effects are usually larger in magnitude and duration than their counterpart preabsorptive effects. According to Nicolaidis (86) the sensory-endocrine reflexes take on an optimizing role in the metabolism of nutrients. Oral ingestion of saccharin, for example, improved the anabolic utilization of nutrients administered intravenously (86). A more direct role for the preabsorptive rise in insulin could be in its promotive effect to initiate eating. Prolonged insulin administration can lead to increased food intake (49) and to changes in preference for taste solutions (53, 107). Louis-Sylvestre & LeMagnen (75) discuss the preabsorptive insulin release as an "on transient response." They suggest that the initial insulin release can decrease glucose availability and thereby actually enhance hunger arousal. Palatability modulates this effect by modulating the quantity of preabsorptive insulin released. They further suggest (75) that even though an animal may be satiated on a given food, sampling a different food could initiate a new sequence of insulin release, which in turn would initiate further ingestion. This hypothesis could be a physiologic basis for the observations of LeMagnen (69) on the effect of food variety on intake. The general hypotheses for explaining these observations have been recently discussed (107, 108).

Rodin (107) found that individual human subjects whose eating was most responsive to cues associated with food (such as taste or caloric density) showed the largest insulin release in response to sight and smell of grilling steaks. In previous studies (124, 133) insulin levels were higher after food presentation (sight and smell) in obese subjects than in the non-obese. These investigators suggested that the insulin response might act as an index of appetite. They also pointed out that the response was quite variable and tended to extinguish on the second trial. Fragility of response to certain types of cephalic stimulation for both pancreatic exocrine and endocrine responses has been noted before (84, 119). In a recent experiment (10) rats that displayed the highest degree of cephalic-phase response for preabsorptive insulin release also ate more than those animals showing a lower response. This result is congruent with the observation that ventromedial hypothalamic hyperphagic rats have an exaggerated cephalic phase–stimulated insulin response (102, 128) and that the hyperphagia can be mitigated by vagotomy (102). Recent work has, however, demonstrated that the mitigating effects of vagotomy are modulated by parameters such as completeness of vagotomy, sequence in which vagotomy and the hypothalamic lesions are made, and the type of diets offered to the animals following the lesions (111, 112). These experiments collectively suggest that response to cephalic-phase stimulation could be an indicator of potential dietary obesity.

Pancreatic Polypeptide

In addition to the well-documented release of insulin from the endocrine pancreas by the cephalic phase, the peptide hormone pancreatic polypeptide is also released by cephalic stimuli (2, 116, 118, 119, 134, 135). Pancreatic polypeptide is a 36 amino acid polypeptide bearing little similarity to other polypeptide hormones (16, 59). It is localized to specific endocrine cells of the pancreas (68). Specific functions for pancreatic polypeptide have not been defined, although it has been implicated in a number of gastrointestinal processes (71). For example, it may act as a local regulator of pancreatic exocrine secretion (72). A recent report by Taylor et al (137) demonstrated that pancreatic polypeptide, exogenously administered at levels normally observed after feeding, inhibited exocrine pancreatic output of bicarbonate and protein stimulated by secretin and caerulein. Pancreatic polypeptide may also play a role in satiety (77). The peptide appears to have little regulatory effect on gastric acid secretion, at least as this phenomenon was experimentally investigated using pharmacological initiators of acid secretion (96).

The mechanism of pancreatic polypeptide release by cephalic-phase stimulation involves vagal mediation and is to a large degree cholinergic (2, 116, 118, 134, 135). Using insulin-induced hypoglycemia in normal and duodenal ulcer patients, Schwartz et al (116) demonstrated a reliable increase in serum pancreatic polypeptide following the insulin injection. Atropine injections of 0.03 mg/kg given before insulin reduced the pancreatic polypeptide response. After truncal vagotomy in the ulcer patients, no increase in pancreatic polypeptide was observed to insulin-induced hypoglycemia. Also, basal levels of pancreatic polypeptide in these patients after vagotomy were at levels not significantly different from those in control healthy subjects.

Schwartz et al (116) also report that electrical stimulation of the vagal nerves of anesthetized pigs produces an increase in circulating levels of pancreatic polypeptide. This effect is inhibited 74% after atropine (0.5 mg/kg) injections. Adrenergic alpha and beta blockers (combined phenoxybenzamine and propranolol) had no effect on the increase in circulating levels of pancreatic polypeptide after electrical stimulation. In an isolated perfused pig pancreas (55, 116) acetylcholine infusions increased pancreatic polypeptide concentrations in the perfusate in a graded manner. This effect could be reduced by atropine. These studies provide evidence for vagal control of pancreatic polypeptide release from the pancreas due to cephalic stimulation. They further suggest that since the release of polypeptide by insulin-induced hypoglycemia lasts beyond 180 min, the vagal mechanism may also contribute to the secondary phase of pancreatic polypeptide release.

Release of pancreatic polypeptide while eating a normal meal occurs in two phases: a rapid primary phase (5–30 min) which can be abolished by truncal vagotomy (118) and a longer and larger secondary phase (30 min–6 hr). This larger secondary release is the result of both gastric and intestinal phases (136). The gastric phase is mediated by vago-vagal stimulation via distention (60, 117, 134). The intestinal phase of release of pancreatic polypeptide may be mediated, at least partially, by cholecystokinin since injections of this hormone lead to increases in circulating levels of pancreatic polypeptide in humans (73). Lonovics et al (73) discuss previous studies that failed to demonstrate a CCK effect on pancreatic polypeptide release (e.g. 134) and conclude that those experiments may have employed a hormone solution that was partially or wholly inactivated during the purification process. Taylor et al (135) observed an increase in serum levels of pancreatic polypeptide in dogs given a standard ground beef liver meal. The increase was significantly different from basal (premeal) levels by the first time point of sampling at 30 min. At this point 80% of the maximal amount was already released. Both atropine (25 μg/kg and 100 μg/kg) and truncal vagotomy reduced this response, with the reduction by truncal vagotomy lasting the entire 4 hr period.

A report by Schwartz et al (119) describes cephalic phase–initiated pancreatic polypeptide release in humans with sham feeding. In two groups, healthy subjects and duodenal ulcer patients, a significant increase in pancreatic polypeptide was observed to MSF. Four of the 26 ulcer patients and 2 of the 8 healthy subjects did not show this response to MSF. Pretreating the subjects with atropine (2.5 mg) or benzilonium (1 mg or 2 mg) led to a decrease in resting levels of pancreatic polypeptide (120) and no response to sham feeding. In the duodenal ulcer patient group, 17 individuals had a selective parietal cell area denervation and thus secreted no gastric acid. Pancreatic polypeptide release to MSF was found in 13 of these 17 patients, suggesting that pancreatic polypeptide release is not dependent on gastric acid response.

If instead of modified sham feeding, the subjects were permitted to chew and swallow the food, release of pancreatic polypeptide was enhanced (Figure 5) (119). In this experiment food did not reach the stomach, but was carried through a tube temporarily inserted into the distal part of the esophagus. The pancreatic polypeptide response was not only larger with swallowing but was also less variable. That the swallowing reflex leads to more robust release of pancreatic polypeptide is interesting in light of the observations of Naim et al (84) on cephalic-phase stimulation of the exocrine pancreas. They found that including chewing and swallowing in the stimulatory sequence restored the pancreatic response. While swallowing would appear to influence the cephalic phase of pancreatic exocrine and pancreatic polypeptide release, it apparently adds little to the cephalic phase of gastric acid release (130). No study has yet appeared, as far as we are

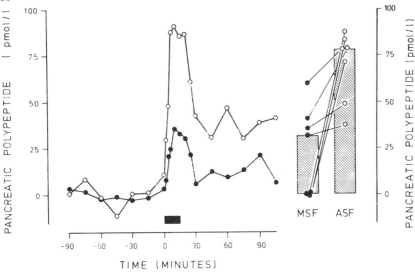

Figure 5   Plasma concentrations of pancreatic polypeptide vs time in 7 human subjects for either normal sham feeding (chewing and swallowing) or modified sham feeding. Normal sham feeding is indicated as (o——o) and "ASF," and modified sham feeding is indicated as (●——●) and "MSF." Sham feeding time is indicated by the length of the horizontal bar beginning at zero minutes. The height of the columns on the right represent the mean of the integrated response over the first 30 min. Individual subject points are indicated for each type of sham feeding. Figure is from Schwartz et al (119), reproduced here with permission of the publishers, Universitetsforlaget.

aware, attempting to determine if the magnitude of the pancreatic polypeptide release is dependent upon the hedonic quality of the food stimulus, or if pancreatic polypeptide can be released by other cephalic-phase stimulants such as odor.

CONCLUSIONS

As components of the cephalic phase, the chemical senses affect digestive and metabolic processes at several levels. Those we reviewed here include gastric acid secretion, exocrine pancreatic secretion and endocrine secretion of gastrin, glucagon, insulin, and pancreatic polypeptide hormone. The primary mediator of cephalic-phase stimuli is the vagus nerve. The responses initiated by the chemical senses have nutritional relevance since they initiate secretions that prepare the organism for digestion and metabolism. The magnitude and duration of these secretions are directly affected by the hedonic status of the stimuli.

ACKNOWLEDGMENTS

We thank Dr. Gary M. Levine and Dr. William J. Snape for critical review of this manuscript.

Literature Cited

1. Abrahamsson, H., Jansson, G. 1969. Elicitation of reflex vagal relaxation of the stomach from pharynx and esophagus in the cat. *Acta Physiol. Scand.* 77:172–78
2. Adrian, T. E., Besterman, H. S., Cooke, T. J. C., Bloom, S. R., Barnes, A. J., Russell, R. C. G., Farber, R. G. 1977. Mechanisms of pancreatic polypeptide release in man. *Lancet* 1:161–63
3. Alphin, R. S., Lin, M. 1959. Effect of feeding and sham feeding on pancreatic secretion of the rat. *Am. J. Physiol.* 197:260–62
4. Bank, S., Cobb, J. S., Marks, I. N. 1970. The effect of pentagastrin and Boots and pure natural (Jorpes) secretin and pancreozymin on pancreatic and gastric function in man. *Abstr. 4th World Cong. Gastroenterol.*, p. 239, Copenhagen.
5. Baume, P. E., Nicholls, A., Barnett, R. A., Room, R. A. 1966. Rat gastric acid secretion in response to graded subcutaneous doses of 2-deoxy-D-glucose. *Am. J. Physiol.* 211:626–28
6. Beauchamp, G. K., Maller, O. 1977. The development of flavor preferences in humans: A review. In *The Chemical Senses and Nutrition*, ed. M. R. Kare,

O. Maller, pp. 292–310. NY: Academic
7. Behrman, H. R., Kare, M. R. 1968. Canine pancreatic secretion in response to acceptable and aversive taste stimuli. *Proc. Soc. Exp. Biol. Med.* 129:343–46
8. Bernstein, I. L., Woods, S. C. 1980. Ontogeny of cephalic insulin release by the rat. *Physiol. Behav.* 24:529–32
9. Berridge, K., Grill, H. J., Norgren, R. 1981. Relation of consummatory responses and preabsorptive insulin release to palatability and learned taste aversions. *J. Comp. Physiol. Psychol.* 95:363–82
10. Berthoud, H. R., Bereiter, D. A., Trimble, E. R., Siegel, E. G., Jeanrenaud, B. 1981. Cephalic phase, reflex insulin secretion. Neuroanatomical and physiological characterization. *Diabetologia* 20:393–401
11. Berthoud, H. R., Trimble, E. R., Siegel, E. G., Bereiter, D. A., Jeanrenaud, B. 1980. Cephalic-phase insulin secretion in normal and pancreatic islet-transplanted rats. *Am. J. Physiol.* 238:E336–40
12. Bonfils, S., Mignon, M., Roze, C. 1979. Vagal control of gastric secretion. In *International Review of Physiology. Vol.*

19. Gastrointestinal Physiology III, ed. R. K. Crane, pp. 59–106. Baltimore: University Park Press

13. Bassett, J. M. 1974. Early changes in plasma insulin and growth hormone levels after feeding in lambs and adult sheep. *Aust. J. Biol. Sci.* 27:157–66

14. Brooks, F. P. 1967. Central neural control of acid secretion. In *Handbook of Physiology,* ed. C. F. Code, 2(Sect.6):805–26. Washington DC: Am. Physiol. Soc.

15. Cagan, R. H., Kare, M. R., eds. 1981. *The Biochemistry of Taste and Olfaction.* NY: Academic

16. Chance, R. E., Lin, F. M., Johnson, M. G., Moon, N. E., Evans, D. E., Jones, W. E., Koffenberger, J. E. 1975. Studies on a newly recognized pancreatic hormone with gastrointestinal activities. *57th Ann. Meet. Endocrine Soc.* 1:265/183A

17. Crittenden, P. J., Ivy, A. C. 1937. The nervous control of pancreatic secretion in the dog. *Am. J. Physiol.* 119:724–33

18. Daniel, P. M., Henderson, J. R. 1967. The effect of vagal stimulation on plasma insulin and glucose levels in the baboon. *J. Physiol.* 192:317–27

19. Davenport, H. W. 1977. *Physiology of the Digestive Tract,* Chicago: Year Book Medical Publishers. 4th ed.

20. Debas, H. T., Konturek, S. J., Grossman, M. I. 1975. Effect of extragastric and truncal vagotomy on pancreatic secretion in the dog. *Am. J. Physiol.* 228:1172–77

21. Debas, H. T., Konturek, S. J., Walsh, J. H., Grossman, M. I. 1974. Proof of a pyloro-oxyntic reflex for stimulation of acid secretion. *Gastroenterology* 66: 526–32

22. Debas, H. T., Walsh, J. H., Grossman, M. I. 1975. Evidence for oxyntopyloric reflex for release of antral gastrin. *Gastroenterology* 68:687–90

23. Debas, H. T., Walsh, J. H., Grossman, M. I. 1976. After vagotomy atropine supresses gastrin release by food. *Gastroenterology* 70:1082–84

24. DeJung, A., Strubbe, J. H., Steffens, A. B. 1977. Hypothalamic influence on insulin and glucagon release in the rat. *Am. J. Physiol.* 233:E380–88

25. Dencker, H., Hedner, P., Holst, J., Tranberg, K. G. 1975. Pancreatic glucagon response to an ordinary meal. *Scand. J. Gastroenterol.* 10:471–74

26. Deutsch, R. 1974. Conditioned hypoglycemia: A mechanism for saccharin-induced sensitivity to insulin in the rat. *J. Comp. Physiol. Psychol.* 86:350–58

27. Dockray, G. J., Tracy, H. J. 1980. Atropine does not abolish cephalic vagal stimulation of gastrin release in dogs. *J. Physiol.* 306:473–80

28. Duke, W. W., Hirschowitz, B. I., Sachs, G. 1965. Vagal stimulation of gastric secretion in man by 2-deoxy-D-glucose. *Lancet* 2:871–76

29. DuVal, J. W., Saffouri, B., Weir, G. C., Walsh, J. H., Arimura, A., Makholouf, G. M. 1981. Stimulation of gastrin and somatostatin secretion from the isolated rat stomach by bombesin. *Am. J. Physiol.* 241:G242–47

30. Farrell, J. I. 1928. Contributions to the physiology of gastric secretion. The vagi as the sole efferent pathway for the cephalic phase of gastric secretion. *Am. J. Physiol.* 85:685–87

31. Feldman, M., Dickerman, R. M., McClelland, R. N., Cooper, K. A., Walsh, J. H., Richardson, C. T. 1979. Effect of selective proximal vagotomy on food-stimulated gastric acid secretion and gastrin release in patients with duodenal ulcer. *Gastroenterology* 76: 926–31

32. Feldman, M., Richardson, C. T. 1981. "Partial" sham feeding releases gastrin in normal human subjects. *Scand. J. Gastroenterol.* 16:13–16

33. Feldman, M., Richardson, C. T., Fordtran, J. S. 1980. Experience with sham feeding as a test for vagotomy. *Gastroenterology* 79:792–95

34. Feldman, M., Richardson, C. T., Taylor, I. L., Walsh, J. H. 1979. Effect of atropine on vagal release of gastrin and pancreatic polypeptide. *J. Clin. Invest.* 63:294–98

35. Fischer, U., Hommel, H., Ziegler, M., Jutzi, E. 1972. The mechanism of insulin secretion after oral glucose administration. III. Investigations on the mechanism of a reflectoric insulin mobilization after oral stimulation. *Diabetologia* 8:385–90

36. Fischer, U., Hommel, H., Ziegler, M., Michael, R. 1972. The mechanism of insulin secretion after oral glucose administration. I. Multiphasic course of insulin mobilization after oral administration of glucose in conscious dogs. Differences in the behaviour after intravenous administration. *Diabetologia* 8:104–10

37. Frohman, L. A., Ezdinli, E. Z., Javid, R. 1967. Effect of vagotomy and vagal stimulation on insulin release. *Diabetes* 16:443–48

38. Goldfine, I. D., Abraird, C., Gruenewald, D., Goldstein, M. S. 1970. Plasma

insulin levels during imaginary food ingestion under hypnosis. *Proc. Soc. Exp. Biol. Med.* 133:274–76

39. Gottrup, F., Lovgreen, N. A., Andersen, D. 1981. Effect of β_2-sympathomimetic on gastrin release, acid secretion, and blood glucose during basal conditions and in response to insulin, 2-deoxy-D-glucose, and feeding in the dog. *Scand. J. Gastroenterol.* 16:673–80

40. Graziadei, P. P. C., Graziadei, G. A. M. 1978. The olfactory system: A model for the study of neurogenesis and axon regeneration in mammals. In *Neuronal Plasticity*, ed. C. W. Cotman, pp. 131–53, NY: Raven Press

41. Grill, H. J., Norgren, R. 1978. The taste reactivity test: I. Mimetic response to gustatory stimuli in neurologically normal rats. *Brain Res.* 143:263–79

42. Grossman, M. I. 1962. Secretion of acid and pepsin in response to distention of vagally innervated fundic gland area in dogs. *Gastroenterology* 42:718–21

43. Grossman, M. I. 1967. Neural and hormonal stimulation of gastric secretion of acid. In *Handbook of Physiology*, ed. C. F. Code, 2(Sect.6):835–63. Washington DC: Am. Physiol. Soc.

44. Grotzinger, U., Rehfeld, J. F., Olbe, L. 1977. Is there any oxyntopyloric reflex for release of gastrin in man? *Gastroenterology* 73:753–57

45. Harper, A. A., Kidd, C., Scratcherd, T. 1959. Vago-vagal reflex effects on gastric and pancreatic secretion and gastrointestinal motility. *J. Physiol.* 148:417–36

46. Henderson, J. R., Jeffreys, D. B., Jones, R. H., Stanley, D. 1976. The effect of atropine on the insulin release caused by oral and intravenous glucose in human subjects. *Acta Endocrinol.* 83:772–80

47. Hickson, J. C. D. 1970. The secretion of pancreatic juice in response to stimulation of the vagus nerves in the pig. *J. Physiol.* 206:275–97

48. Hirschowitz, B. I., Gibson, R. G. 1979. Augmented vagal release of antral gastrin by 2-deoxyglucose after fundic vagotomy in dogs. *Am. J. Physiol.* 236:E173–79

49. Hoebel, G. B., Teitelbaum, P. 1966. Weight regulation in normal and hypothalamic hyperphagic rats. *J. Comp. Physiol. Psychol.* 61:189–93

50. Hollander, F. 1946. The insulin test for the presence of intact nerve fibers after vagal operations for peptic ulcer. *Gastroenterology* 7:607–14

51. Hommel, H., Fischer, U., Retzlaff, K., Knöfler, H. 1972. The mechanism of

insulin secretion after oral glucose administration. II. Reflex insulin secretion in conscious dogs bearing fistulas of the digestive tract by sham-feeding of glucose or tap water. *Diabetologia* 8:111–16

52. Impicciatore, M., Walsh, J. H., Grossman, M. I. 1977. Low doses of atropine enhance serum gastrin response to food in dogs. *Gastroenterology* 72:995–96

53. Jacobs, H. L. 1958. Studies on sugar preference. I. The preference for glucose solutions and its modification by injections of insulin. *J. Comp. Physiol. Psychol.* 51:304–10

54. Janowitz, H. D., Hollander, F., Orringer, D., Levy, M. H., Winkelstein, A., Kaufman, M. R., Margolin, S. G. 1950. A quantitative study of the gastric secretory response to sham feeding in a human subject. *Gastroenterology* 16:104–16

55. Jensen, S. L., Kühl, C., Nielsen, O. V., Holst, J. J. 1976. Isolation and perfusion of the porcine pancreas. *Scand. J. Gastroenterol. Suppl.* 37:57–61

56. Jogi, P., Strom, G., Uvnäs, B. 1949. The origin in the CNS of gastric secretory impulses induced by hypoglycaemia. *Scand. J. Gastroenterol.* 17:212–21

57. Kaminski, D. L., Ruwart, M. J., Willman, V. L. 1975. The effect of electrical vagal stimulation on canine pancreatic exocrine function. *Surgery* 77:545–52

58. Karamanos, B., Butterfield, W. J. H., Asmal, A. C., Cox, B. D., Whichelow, M. J. 1971. The pattern of early insulin response to oral glucose. *Postgrad. Med. J.* 4:(Suppl.)440–43

59. Kimmel, J. R., Hayden, L. J., Pollock, H. G. 1975. Isolation and characterization of a new pancreatic polypeptide hormone. *J. Biol. Chem.* 250:9369–76

60. Knutson, U., Olbe, L. 1973. Gastric acid response to sham feeding in the duodenal ulcer patient. *Scand. J. Gastroenterol.* 8:513–22

61. Kogen, B. E. 1931. Über den Einfluss des bedingten Nahrungsreizes auf die Exkretorische Pankreasfunktion. *Z. Klin. Med.* 117:203–9

62. Konturek, S. J. 1974. Gastric secretion. In *Gastrointestinal Physiology, Vol. 4, Physiology Series One, MTP International Review of Science*, ed. E. D. Jacobson, L. L. Shanbour, pp. 227–64. London: Butterworths

63. Konturek, S. J., Jaworek, J., Tasler, J., Cieszkowski, M., Pawlik, W. 1981. Effect of substance P and its C-terminal hexapeptide on gastric and pancreatic

secretion in the dog. *Am. J. Physiol.* 241:G74–81

64. Konturek, S. J., Kwiecien, N., Obtulowicz, W., Mikos, E., Sito, E., Oleksy, J., Popiela, T. 1978. Cephalic phase of gastric secretion in healthy subjects and duodenal ulcer patients: Role of vagal innervation. *Gut* 20:875–81

65. Korman, M. G., Soveny, C., Hansky, S. J. 1971. Radioimmunoassay of gastrin. The response of serum gastrin to insulin hypoglycaemia. *Scand. J. Gastroenterol.* 6:71–75

66. Lanciault, G., Bonoma, C., Brooks, F. P. 1973. Vagal stimulation, gastrin release, and acid secretion in anesthetized dogs. *Am. J. Physiol.* 225:546–52

67. Langlois, K. J., Lim, R. K. S., Rosiere, G., Steward, D. I., Stumpff, O. L. 1952. Unconditioned orogastric secretory reflex. *Fed. Proc.* 11:88–89

68. Larsson, L.-I., Sundler, F., Hakanson, R. 1975. Immunohistochemical localization of human pancreatic polypeptide (HPP) to a population of islet cells. *Cell Tiss. Res.* 156:167–71

69. LeMagnen, J. 1956. Rôle de l'odeur ajoutée au régime dans la régulation quantitative à court terme de la prise alimentaire chez le rat blanc. *C. R. Soc. Biol.* 150:136–39

70. Lepkovsky, S. 1977. The role of the chemical senses in nutrition. In *The Chemical Senses and Nutrition,* ed. M. R. Kare, O. Maller, pp. 413–27. NY: Academic

71. Lin, T. M., Chance, R. E. 1974. Gastrointestinal actions of a new bovine pancreatic polypeptide (BPP). In *Endocrinology of the Gut,* ed. W. Y. Chey, F. P. Brooks, pp. 143–45. Thorofare, NJ: Charles B. Slack

72. Lin, T. M., Evans, D. C., Chance, R. E., Spray, G. F. 1977. Bovine pancreatic peptide: Action on gastric and pancreatic secretion in dogs. *Am. J. Physiol.* 232:E311–15

73. Lonovics, J., Guzman, S., Devitt, P., Hejtmancik, K. E., Suddith, R. L., Rayford, P. L., Thompson, J. C. 1980. Release of pancreatic polypeptide in humans by infusion of cholecystokinin. *Gastroenterology* 79:817–22

74. Louis-Sylvestre, J. 1976. Preabsorptive insulin release and hypoglycemia in rat. *Am. J. Physiol.* 230:56–60

75. Louis-Sylvestre, J., LeMagnen, J. 1980. Palatability and preabsorptive insulin release. *Neurosci. Biobehav. Rev.* 4 (Suppl. 1):43–46

76. Malagelada, J.-R., Go, V. L. W., Summerskill, W. H. J. 1979. Different gas-

tric, pancreatic, and biliary responses to solid-liquid or homogenized meals. *Dig. Dis. Sci.* 24:101–10

77. Malaisse-Lagae, F., Carpentier, J.-L., Patel, Y. C., Malaisse, W. J., Orci, L. 1977. Pancreatic polypeptide: A possible role in the regulation of food intake in the mouse. *Experientia* 33:915–17

78. Mayer, G., Arnold, R., Feurle, G., Fuchs, K., Ketterer, H., Track, N. S., Creutzfeldt, W. 1974. Influence of feeding and sham feeding upon serum gastrin and gastric acid secretion in control subjects and duodenal ulcer patients. *Scand. J. Gastroenterol.* 9:703–10

79. McDonald, T. J., Nilsson, G., Vagne, M., Ghatei, M., Bloom, S. R., Mutt, V. 1978. A gastrin releasing peptide from the porcine non-antral gastric tissue. *Gut.* 19:767–74

80. Moore, J. G., Motoki, D. 1979. Gastric secretory and humoral responses to anticipated feeding in five men. *Gastroenterology* 76:71–75

81. Moore, J. G., Schenkenberg, T. 1974. Psychic control of gastric acid: Response to anticipated feeding and biofeedback training in a man. *Gastroenterology* 66:954–59

82. Murray, R. G. 1973. The ultrastructure of taste buds. In *The Ultrastructure of Sensory Organs,* ed. I. Friedmann, pp. 1–81. NY: American Elsevier

83. Naim, M., Kare, M. R. 1977. Taste stimuli and pancreatic functions. In *The Chemical Senses and Nutrition,* ed. M. R. Kare, O. Maller, pp. 145–62. NY.: Academic

84. Naim, M., Kare, M. R., Merritt, A. M. 1978. Effects of oral stimulation on the cephalic phase of pancreatic exocrine secretion in dogs. *Physiol. Behav.* 20:563–70

85. Nicolaidis, S. 1969. Early systemic responses to orogastric stimulation in the regulation of food and water balance: Functional and electrophysiological data. *Ann. N.Y. Acad. Sci.* 157:1176–1200

86. Nicolaidis, S. 1977. Sensory-neuroendocrine reflexes and their anticipatory optimizing role on metabolism. In *The Chemical Senses and Nutrition,* ed. M. R. Kare, O. Maller, pp. 123–40, NY: Academic

87. Nicolaidis, S. 1980. Hypothalamic covergence of external and internal stimulation leading to early ingestive and metabolic responses. *Brain Res. Bull.* 5 (Suppl. 4):97–101

88. Nilsson, G., Simon, J., Yalow, R. S., Berson, S. A. 1972. Plasma gastrin and

gastric acid responses to sham feeding and feeding in dogs. *Gastroenterology* 63:51–59

89. Nilsson, G., Uvnäs-Wallensten, K. 1975. Effect of teasing, sham feeding and feeding on plasma insulin concentrations in dog. Hormone and metabolic research. In *Radioimmunoassay: Methodology and Applications in Physiology and in Clinical Studies*, ed. B. Luft, R. Yalow, pp. 91–97. Littleton MA: PSG Publications

90. Nilsson, G., Uvnäs-Wallensten, K. 1977. Effect of teasing and sham feeding on plasma glucagon concentration in dogs. *Acta Physiol. Scand.* 100:248–302

91. Norgren, R. 1976. Taste pathways to hypothalamus and amygdala. *J. Comp. Neurol.* 166:17–30

92. Novis, B. H., Bank, S., Marks, I. N. 1971. The cephalic phase of pancreatic secretion in man. *Scand. J. Gastroenterol.* 6:417–22

93. Ohara, I., Otsuka, S., Yugari, Y. 1979. The influence of carrier of gustatory stimulation on the cephalic phase of canine pancreatic secretion. *J. Nutr.* 109:2098–2105

94. Para-Covarrubias, A., Rivera-Rodriquez, J., Almarez-Ugalde, A. 1971. Cephalic phase of insulin release in obese adolescents. *Diabetes* 20:800–2

95. Parker, J. G., Werther, J. L., Hollander, F. 1963. Gastric cation secretion in a patient with complete esophageal obstruction and permanent gastrotomy. *Am. J. Dig. Dis.* 8:319–29

96. Parks, D. L., Gingerich, R. L., Jaffe, B. M., Akande, B. 1979. Role of pancreatic polypeptide in canine gastric acid secretion. *Am. J. Physiol.* 236:E488–94

97. Pavlov, I. P. 1902. *The Work of the Digestive Glands* (transl. W. H. Thompson). London: Charles Griffin

98. Perley, M. J., Kipnis, D. M. 1967. Plasma insulin responses to oral and intravenous glucose: Studies in normal and diabetic subjects. *J. Clin. Invest.* 46:1954–62

99. Porte, D. Jr., Girardier, L., Seydoux, J., Kanazawa, Y., Posternak, J. 1973. Neural regulation of insulin secretion in the dog. *J. Clin. Invest.* 52:210–14

100. Porter, R. J., Bassett, J. M. 1979. Early insulin release following suckling in neonatal lambs and rabbits. *Diabetologia* 16:201–6

101. Powley, T. 1977. The ventromedial hypothalamic syndrome, satiety and a cephalic phase hypothesis. *Psychol. Rev.* 84:89–126

102. Powley, T. L., Opsahl, C. A. 1974. Ventromedial hypothalamic obesity abolished by subdiaphragmatic vagotomy. *Am. J. Physiol.* 226:25–33

103. Preshaw, R. M. 1974. Pancreatic exocrine secretion. In *Gastrointestinal Physiology, Vol. 4, Physiology Series One, MTP International Review of Science*, ed. E. D. Jacobson, L. L. Shanbour, pp. 265–91. London: Butterworths

104. Preshaw, R. M., Cooke, A. R., Grossman, M. I. 1966. Sham-feeding and pancreatic secretion in the dog. *Gastroenterology* 50:171–78

105. Renold, A. E. 1971. The beta cell and its responses: Summarizing remarks and some contributions from Geneva. *Diabetes* 21:619–31

106. Richardson, C. T., Walsh, J. H., Cooper, K. A., Feldman, M., Fordtran, J. S. 1977. Studies on the role of cephalic-vagal stimulation in the acid secretory response to eating in normal human subjects. *J. Clin. Invest.* 60:435–41

107. Rodin, J. 1978. Has the distinction between internal versus external control of feeding outlived its usefulness? In *Recent Advances in Obesity Research*, ed. G. Bray, 2:75–85. London: Newman

108. Rolls, B. J., Rowe, E. A., Rolls, E. T., Kingston, B., Megson, A., Gunary, R. 1981. Variety in a meal enhances food intake in man. *Physiol. Behav.* 26:215–21

109. Sarles, H., Dani, R., Prezelin, G., Souville, C., Figarella, C. 1968. Cephalic phase of pancreatic secretion in man. *Gut* 9:214–22

110. Sato, T. 1980. Recent advances in the physiology of taste cells. *Prog. Neurobiol.* 14:25–67

111. Sawchenko, P. E., Gold, R. M. 1981. Effects of gastric vs. complete subdiaphragmatic vagotomy on hypothalamic hyperphagia and obesity. *Physiol. Behav.* 26:281–92

112. Sawchenko, P. E., Gold, R. M., Alexander, J. 1981. Effects of selective vagotomies on knife cut–induced hypothalamic obesity: Differential results on lab chow vs high-fat diets. *Physiol. Behav.* 26:293–300

113. Schiffman, S. 1979. Changes in taste and smell with age: Psychophysical aspects. In *Sensory Systems and Communication in the Elderly*, ed. J. M. Ordy, K. Brizzee, pp. 227–46. NY: Raven Press

114. Schiffman, S., Orlandi, M., Erickson, R. P. 1979. Changes in taste and smell with

CHEMICAL SENSES & DIGESTIVE SECRETIONS   275

age: Biological aspects. See Ref. 113, pp. 247–68
115. Schöön, I.-M., Olbe, L. 1977. Effect of cimetidine on cholinergic reflex stimulation of gastric acid secretion in duodenal ulcer patients. In *Cimetidine, Proceedings of the Second International Symposium on Histamine H_2-receptor Antagonists,* ed. W. L. Burland, M. A. Simkins, pp. 207–13. Amsterdam: Excerpta Medica
116. Schwartz, T. W., Holst, J. J., Fahrenkrug, J., Jensen, S. L., Nielsen, O. V., Rehfeld, J. F., Schaffalitzky de Muckadell, O. B., Stadil, F. 1978. Vagal, cholinergic regulation of pancreatic polypeptide secretion. *J. Clin. Invest.* 61: 781–89
117. Schwartz, T. W., Grötzinger, U., Schöön, I.-M., Olbe, L. 1979. Vagovagal stimulation of pancreatic polypeptide secretion by graded distention of the gastric fundus and antrum in man *Digestion* 19:307–14
118. Schwartz, T. W., Rehfeld, J. F., Stadil, F., Larsson, L.-I., Chance, R. E. 1976. Pancreatic-polypeptide response to food in duodenal-ulcer patients before and after vagotomy. *Lancet* 1: 1102–5
119. Schwartz, T. W., Stenquist, B., Olbe, L. 1979. Cephalic phase of pancreatic-polypeptide secretion studied by sham feeding in man. *Scand. J. Gastroenterol.* 14:313–20
120. Schwartz, T. W., Stenquist, B., Olbe, L. Stadil, F. 1979. Synchronous oscillations in the basal secretion of pancreatic-polypeptide and gastric acid. *Gastroenterology* 76:14–19
121. Shepherd, G. M. 1979. *The Synaptic Organization of the Brain.* London: Oxford Univ. Press. 2nd ed.
122. Sinclair, I. S. R. 1956. Observations on a case of external pancreatic fistula in man. *Brit. J. Surg.* 44:250–62
123. Singer, M., Solomon, T. E., Wood, J., Grossman, M. I. 1980. Latency of pancreatic enzyme response to intraduodenal stimulants. *Am. J. Physiol.* 238: G23–29
124. Sjöstrom, L., Garrellick, G., Krotkievski, M., Luyckx, A. 1980. Peripheral insulin in response to the sight and smell of food. *Metabolism* 29:901–9
125. Soares, E. C., Zaterka, S., Walsh, J. H. 1977. Acid secretion and serum gastrin at graded intragastric pressures in man. *Gastroenterology* 72:676–79
126. Solomon, T., Grossman, M. I. 1977. Vagal control of pancreatic exocrine secretion. In *Nerves and the Gut,* ed. F.

P. Brooks, P. W. Evers, pp. 119–29. Thorofare, NJ: Charles B. Slack
127. Soon-Shiong, P., Debas, H. T. 1980. Fundic inhibition of acid secretion and gastrin release in the dog. *Gastroenterology* 79:867–72
128. Steffens, A. B. 1970. Plasma insulin content in relation to blood glucose level and meal pattern in the normal and hypothalamic hyperphagic rat. *Physiol. Behav.* 5:147–51
129. Steffens, A. B. 1976. Influence of the oral cavity on insulin release in the rat. *Am. J. Physiol.* 230:1411–15
130. Stenquist, B., Knutson, U., Olbe, L. 1978. Gastric acid responses to adequate and modified sham feeding and to insulin hypoglycemia in duodenal ulcer patients. *Scand. J. Gastroenterol.* 13: 357–62
131. Stenquist, B., Nilsson, G., Rehfeld, J. F., Olbe, L. 1979. Plasma gastrin concentrations following sham feeding in duodenal ulcer patients. *Scand. J. Gastroenterol.* 14:305–11
132. Strubbe, J. H., Steffens, A. B. 1975. Rapid insulin release after ingestion of a meal in the unanesthetized rat. *Am. J. Physiol.* 229:1019–22
133. Szybinski, Z., Sieradzki, J., Huszno, B. 1975. The cephalic phase of insulin secretion in simple obesity. *Pol. Arch. Med. Wewn.* 53:605–10
134. Taylor, I. L., Feldman, M., Richardson, C. T., Walsh, J. H. 1978. Gastric and cephalic stimulation of human pancreatic polypeptide release. *Gastroenterology* 75:432–37
135. Taylor, I. L., Impicciatore, M., Carter, D. C., Walsh, J. H. 1978. Effect of atropine and vagotomy on pancreatic polypeptide response to a meal in dogs. *Am. J. Physiol.* 235:E443–47
136. Taylor, I. L., Kauffman, G. L., Walsh, J. H., Trout, H., Chew, P., Harmon, J. W. 1981. Role of the small intestine and gastric antrum in pancreatic polypeptide release. *Am. J. Physiol.* 240: G387–91
137. Taylor, I. L., Solomon, T. E., Walsh, J. H., Grossman, M. I. 1979. Pancreatic polypeptide. Metabolism and effect on pancreatic secretion in dogs. *Gastroenterology* 76:524–28
138. Tepperman, J. 1974. Control of carbohydrate and fat metabolism. In *The Control of Metabolism,* ed. J. D. Sink, pp. 35–48. Philadelphia: Pennsylvania State Univ. Press
139. Unger, R. H., Ketterer, H., Dupre, J., Eisentraut, A. M. 1967. The effect of secretin, pancreozymin and gastrin on

insulin and glucagon secretion in anesthetized dogs. *J. Clin. Invest.* 46:630–45

140. Vagne, M., Grossman, M. I. 1969. Gastric and pancreatic secretion in response to gastric distention in dogs. *Gastroenterology* 57:300–10

141. Vega, D. F., Martinez-Victoria, E., Esteller, A., Murillo, A. 1977. Secretion of pancreatic juice in response to nervous and hormonal stimulation in the anaesthetized monkey. *Comp. Biochem. Physiol.* 58A:259–64

142. Wolf, S. 1973. The challenge of methodology in psychosomatic research with notes on the psychic secretion of insulin. *Tex. Rep. Biol. Med.* 31:3–10

143. Wolf, S. 1981. The psyche and the stomach. A historical vignette. *Gastroen-*
terology 80:605–14

144. Woods, S. C., Bernstein, I. L. 1980. Cephalic insulin response as a test for completeness of vagotomy to the pancreas. *Physiol. Behav.* 24:485–88

145. Woods, S. C., Porte, D. Jr. 1974. Neural control of the endocrine pancreas. *Physiol. Rev.* 54:596–619

146. Woods, S. C., Vasselli, J. R., Kaestner, E., Szakmary, G. A., Milburn, P., Vitiello, M. V. 1977. Conditioned insulin secretion and meal feeding in rats. *J. Comp. Physiol. Psychol.* 91:128–33

147. Yamagishi, T., Debas, H. T., Walsh, J. H. 1977. Fundic inhibition of gastrin release. *Gastroenterology* 72:1152 (Abstr.)

Ann. Rev. Nutr. 1982. 2:277–301
Copyright © 1982 by Annual Reviews Inc. All rights reserved

METABOLIC APPROACHES TO CANCER CACHEXIA

David H. Lawson[1,3], *Ann Richmond*[1], *Daniel W. Nixon*[2,3], *Daniel Rudman*[1]

Clinical Research Facility[1], the Winship Clinic for Neoplastic Diseases[2], and the Division of Hematology-Oncology[3], Department of Medicine, Emory University School of Medicine, Atlanta, Georgia 30322

CONTENTS

I. OVERVIEW OF CANCER CACHEXIA

A. Introduction

Progressive wasting, weakness, anorexia, and anemia are frequent complications of neoplastic disease. As the tumor enlarges, the host's muscle mass and adipose mass are depleted; in contrast, the liver, kidney, adrenal glands, and spleen tend to be spared and may actually enlarge. In the early stages, total body protein may be unchanged, although nitrogen is redistributed from muscle to tumor. Later, when anorexia is pronounced, total body protein declines, and other essential nutrients may also be depleted. This syndrome has been extensively studied in both man and rodent (9, 26, 37, 47, 113) but remains poorly understood.

277

0199-9885/82/0715-0277$02.00

B. Prevalence of Clinical Cancer Cachexia

Cachectic cancer patients frequently have not only protein-calorie undernutrition (PCU) but also depletion of vitamins and minerals. Nevertheless, most surveys have concentrated on weight loss, contraction of lean body mass, depletion of fat mass, and hypoproteinemia as indicators of cancer cachexia. This necessity to rely on convenient indicators probably causes a significant underestimation of the problem, in that the metabolic abnormalities presumably responsible for the undernutrition precede appreciable changes in body weight (16). At the time of presentation, 54% of untreated patients with disseminated cancer had lost some weight and 32% had lost greater than 5% of their usual weight in the preceding six months. The frequency of weight loss ranged from 31% for patients with non-Hodgkin's lymphomas of favorable histological pattern to 87% in patients with gastric carcinomas. Whereas only 14% of patients with carcinoma of the breast had lost more than 5% of their usual weight during the preceding six months, 67% of patients with gastric cancer had suffered this degree of weight loss (33). Nixon and co-workers (95) reported that 42% of their patients with widespread cancer had subnormal adipose stores as determined by triceps skin-fold measurements less than 80% of standard (as compared to only 3% of controls), and 19% were less than 60% of standard. None of the healthy control subjects fell below 60% of standard. Fully 88% of these patients had creatinine:height indexes of less than 80% of standard (compared to 28% of controls), and 53% were less than 60% of standard. No controls fell below this level. Serum albumin concentration was subnormal in 31% of these patients. Furthermore, 45% of patients who had lost at least 6% of their premorbid weight also had subnormal serum concentrations of vitamins A and C, and 20% had decreased levels of serum folate.

These studies demonstrate a high frequency of nutritional abnormalities in cancer patients, confirming the widely held clinical impression. However, it must be emphasized that protein-calorie undernutrition (PCU) is not unique to cancer. On the contrary, 30–50% of hospitalized patients presently have some degree of PCU (51), and most chronic, fatal, nonneoplastic diseases terminate in a cachectic state (e.g. chronic disseminated infections, or prolonged insufficiency of heart, lungs, liver, kidneys, or the small intestines).

C. Relationship of Protein-Calorie Undernutrition to Survival in Cancer Patients

Recent studies have documented the association between undernutrition and decreased survival. DeWys and co-workers (33) found that median survival was significantly shorter in patients who had lost weight with most tumor types examined. Further examination revealed that weight loss was also associated with a worse performance status (activity level) in all tumor types except pancreatic and gastric carcinoma. Since performance status has a known relationship to length of survival, the correlation of weight loss with longevity was evaluated within performance-status categories. The adverse effect of weight loss persisted as an independent variable in most patients with a favorable performance-status rating. In the unfavorable performance status group, however, weight loss had a significantly adverse relationship to survival only in patients with nonsmall-cell lung cancer.

Visceral protein and lean body mass depletion (as assessed by serum albumin concentration and creatinine:height index) have a worse prognostic import than adipose depletion (as measured by triceps skin-fold thickness) (95). Twelve of 27 patients (44%) with triceps skin-fold measurements less than 60% of standard died within 70 days of nutritional evaluation compared to 7 of 31 (23%) patients with higher measurements; this difference was not significant. Fifty-three percent (16/30) of patients with serum albumin concentration less than 3.5 gm/dl died within this time period, compared to only 18% (7/39) of patients with higher serum albumin concentrations. Similarly, 56% (18/32) of patients with a creatinine:height index less than 60% of standard died within 70 days of study, compared to only 4% (1/26) of patients with higher values ($p<0.05$).

In 1932, Warren (126) attempted to determine the cause of death in 500 autopsied cancer patients. In 114 cases, the charts documented progressive weakness, wasting and anemia, and at autopsy no other clear cause of death could be discerned. Warren concluded that these 22% of his patients had died of cancer cachexia. He commented that cachexia was also present in many, but certainly not all, of the other patients, and thus could have contributed to death from other causes, such as infection. Other investigators (58) fail to mention undernutrition as a cause of death, while still others list cachexia as the cause of death in about two thirds of cancer patients (45). Thus although there is a general *association* between PCU and survival in cancer patients, a cause and effect relation is not clearly established. Primary PCU is known to affect adversely resistance to some infections, wound healing, and cardiorespiratory, hepatic, and renal functions; these factors probably contribute to cancer mortality. The precise mechanisms by which the cancer cachexia syndrome may cause death in some patients and perhaps contribute to it in others, however, are not completely understood. Consequently, the features of the syndrome that must be reversed to prolong survival are unknown.

D. Postulated Mechanisms for the Development of Cancer Cachexia

In general, people lose weight because of reduced food intake, because of gastrointestinal malabsorption, or because of endogenous metabolic abnormalitites leading to various combinations of impaired protein synthesis, accelerated protein breakdown, or hypermetabolism. An additional mechanism, unique to cancer, for the erosion of lean body mass and adipose tissue even in the absence of weight loss, is the redistribution of protoplasmic elements from host to tumor.

Hypophagia is prominent in rodents and patients with advanced cancer. Although mechanical factors (dysphagia, GI obstruction, ascites) and anorexigenic chemotherapeutic drugs are major contributors, many cancer patients and laboratory animals show pronounced food aversion in the absence of such factors. In the rat, the degree of hypophagia is not regularly correlated with tumor size (40). If the food's nutrient density is reduced by unabsorbable bulk, the hypophagia often becomes demonstrable at an earlier stage. In some cases, feeding activity commences at normal intervals, but is terminated abnormally rapidly. This suggests that responsiveness to preabsorptive signals is intact but satiety signals are hyperactive (90). Abnormalities of taste are also often demonstrable in both rats and patients with cancer (32). The metabolic mechanisms by which tumors depress appetite are unknown (32, 40), but leading possibilities include: (a) abnormal amino acid metabolism, (b) effect on hepatic glucoreceptors believed to influence food intake, and (c) anorexigenic effect of lactic acid or circulating free fatty acids, or bioactive factors released from tumors, including products of necrosis, inflammation and infection.

Gastrointestinal malabsorption occurs frequently in clinical cancer and contributes significantly to the wasting (74). The malabsorption is usually caused either by treatment (resection of a portion of the GI tract, or enteropathic effects of chemotherapeutic drugs or irradiation) or by the metabolic infiltration of mesenteric lymphatics, or by the nonspecific intestinal atrophy caused by semistarvation.

In both rat and man, erosion of muscle and adipose tissue frequently precedes a detectable fall in food intake (26). In undernourished cancer patients, moreover, measured food intake fails to correlate with degree of PCU (14, 28). Finally, when control rats are pair fed with tumorous rats, the atrophy of muscle and adipose mass in the latter exceeds that in the former (40). These observations show that anorexia is only a partial cause of the wasting process. Evidently there are metabolic disturbances within the tumor or within the host tissues, or both, that also contribute. The nature of these metabolic disorders is the focus of the remainder of this review. First, metabolic characteristics of cancer cells themselves are discussed. Then tumor-associated changes in host tissues are mentioned, followed by an overview of metabolic abnormalities at the whole-organism level. Finally, some of the possible mediators of these effects are listed.

II. METABOLIC ABNORMALITIES IN CANCER SUBJECTS

A. Metabolic Characteristics of Cancer Cells

1. "REGULATORY" NUTRIENTS VERSUS "BUILDING BLOCK" NUTRIENTS   The progressive wasting of host tissue contrasts with the often vigorous growth of tumor tissue. Evidently tumor cells can divide (and thus cause tumors to grow) under conditions where host cells atrophy. This growth advantage is responsible for both the atrophy of muscle and adipose tissue during the early phase of some rat cancers, when food intake is not yet depressed, and for the "N trapping" action of tumors. Therefore a discussion of the characteristics of cancer cells that account for or contribute to this growth advantage is in order.

When serum or any one of a large number of nutrients is provided to cultured cells in less than a certain minimum amount, the cells "growth arrest" and enter a stable G1 phase (72). When serum or the limiting nutrient is supplied, growth resumes in a few hours. One of the earliest changes induced by the addition of serum factors to growth-arrested cells is an increase in nutrient uptake. Apparently, a serum factor–nutrient interaction is involved in the control of proliferation of mammalian cells. Holley (53) has proposed that the critical factor is the intracellular concentration of certain key nutrients, and that extracellular nutrients and serum factors exert their effects by altering this intracellular concentration. Since intact organisms maintain the extracellular concentrations of nutrients at a fairly constant level, changes in the levels of the serum factors appear to be the most likely mechanism for growth regulation.

Based on these observations, Holley (53) has further proposed that transformation to the malignant state may result from an alteration in membrane transport such that nutrient uptake is increased. This would result in a decrease in the requirement for serum factors and consequent escape from control by normal growth restraints. Viewed differently, serum factors may act by allowing a cell to divide while exposed to an extracellular concentration of nutrients that is ordinarily unable to support division; transformation may represent alterations in the cell such that this extracellular nutrient concentration is virtually always adequate, and proliferation continues unchecked.

To investigate this hypothesis further, McKeehan and co-workers have developed a system for studying proliferation control in which they hold serum factor concentration constant and vary the extracellular concentration of various nutrients, or hold nutrient concentration stable and vary the extracellular concentration of serum factors, and measure the rate of proliferation (86). Using this system and a normal human lung fibroblast cell line, these investigators have tried to answer this question: "If serum factors act by transiently decreasing the extracellular concentration of nutrients required for proliferation, which specific nutrients are affected?" The extracellular concentrations of sugars, amino acids, purines, and pyrimidines required to support growth were not affected by serum factors. On the other hand, serum factors did affect the required concentration of five nutrients: Ca^{2+}, Mg^{2+}, K^+, P_i, and oxocarboxylic acids (e.g. pyruvate). These "regulatory" nutrients could thus be distinguished from "building block" nutrients (amino acids, choline, glucose, inositol, polyamines, purines, pyrimidines), which, in this system at least, did not appear to be of regulatory significance. Transformation with the SV40 virus resulted in nutrient requirements for proliferation that resembled those of growth factor–stimulated normal cells; thus the transformed cell in this sense resembled the chronically growth factor–stimulated cell. This work suggests that the behavior of the "building block" nutrients is controlled by the interaction between serum factors and "regulatory" nutrients. Nitrogen accumulation by a tumor, then, would reflect the results of this interaction; that is, the cancer cell, with a decreased requirement for "regulatory nutrients," would have a growth advantage over the host tissues and thus would win in the competition for "building block" nutrients.

Another view of the relationship of "building block" nutrients to cell growth comes from the work of Baserga and co-workers (39). By microinjection of fragments of SV40 virus DNA into NIH 3T3 cells, these investigators showed that when some fragments were injected DNA synthesis occurred without the synthesis or accumulation of ribosomal RNA, whereas injection of other fragments induced RNA synthesis but not DNA synthesis. This work suggests that it may be possible to regulate DNA replication and growth in cell size separately, or that a cell could be stimulated to increase in size (hypertrophy), with increased utilization of "building block" nutrients, without dividing. This is in some ways analogous to the finding that the metabolic effects of some insulin-like peptides are separable from their effects on cell division (44). This separation between classical metabolic and "building block" nutrient effects and features of transformation, including proliferation, is also evident in the studies of cancer cells discussed below. The possibility of dissociating these two effects offers some hope that, if these mechanisms are more completely understood, restoration of normal nondividing host cells (e.g. muscle) can be accomplished without stimulating growth in cancer cells.

In the next section, certain aspects of carbohydrate, lipid, and amino acid metabolism of cancer cells are reviewed, with an emphasis on those features that may contribute to the growth advantage of malignant cells or to the overall picture of cancer cachexia.

2. CARBOHYDRATE METABOLISM IN CANCER CELLS   An increase in hexose uptake is frequently associated with the transition from quiescence to the proliferating state (59); therefore, it is not surprising that most transformed cell lines examined have also shown elevated hexose uptake. Although in some systems there is a transformation-specific augmentation of hexose uptake (131), in others there is a clear dissociation between increased hexose uptake and proliferation (6) and transformation (100). Thus enhanced hexose uptake is not a universal feature of malignancy and is neither necessary nor sufficient by itself for the initiation of proliferation.

There are several possible fates of a hexose taken up by a malignant cell, the most prominent of which is utilization for energy production. Weber (129) has demonstrated that many chemically and virally induced neoplasms are characterized by marked increases in the specific activities of the key enzymes of glycolysis (hexokinase, 6-phospho-fructokinase, and pyruvate kinase). Furthermore, in a series of Morris hepatomas, the rate of glycolysis was proportional to the rate of tumor growth. The increased glycolytic activity reflects in part the fact that many tumors express fetal glycolytic (and other) enzymes normally repressed during adult life (61, 132). These fetal isozymes often demonstrate increased glucose avidity and freedom from host control (61, 132). This high rate of glycolysis is not completely abolished by oxygen, as it is in normal cells (Pasteur effect); however, the hypothesis of Warburg (124) that this represents a universal and fundamental defect in respiration in all cancer cells is no longer accepted (132). Increased glycolysis is neither an universal nor a necessary finding in malignancy (59, 100, 132).

Some idea of the complexity of the area of carbohydrate metabolism in cancer cells may be gained from a brief consideration of the enzyme pyruvate kinase. This enzyme catalyzes the formation of pyruvate from phosphoenol pyruvate, with the concurrent generation of ATP from ADP. There are three distinct isozymes of pyruvate kinase (K, L, and M) (60). The normal adult liver primarily expresses the L-type, whereas the K-type is the predominant isozyme of fetal life. The activity of the L-type isozyme was found to be decreased and the activity of the K-type isozyme increased in hepatomas of progressively less differentiation. The K-type isozyme is apparently better able to compete with the mitochondrial respiratory system for available ADP than is the adult L-form, and is not subject to known host control mechanisms. Weinhouse has suggested (132) that this may account for the fact that glycolysis does not stop when the cells are exposed to oxygen, and thus may help explain some of Warburg's observations. Furthermore, pyruvate may play a role in the regulation of cell proliferation beyond its participation in glycolysis (86). The McKeehans' work, mentioned above, suggests that the extracellular concentration of pyruvate and its interaction with serum factors may be important in the regulation of cell division in normal human lung fibroblasts. It is not clear why a cell should have a requirement for a nutrient that is synthesized intracellularly; however, it has been hypothesized that the increased ratio of oxidized to reduced pyridine nucleotide (NAD+/NADH) that results when 2-oxocarboxylic acids are reduced is the link between the extracellular requirement for pyruvate and cellular proliferation (87). It is conceivable that increased glycolysis resulting in increased intracellular pyruvate might lower the extracellular requirement of this nutrient for multiplication and thus, in some systems, facilitate the escape from normal growth controls that is characteristic of malignant cells. On the other hand, Rous sarcoma virus transformation of chick embryo fibroblasts is associated with decreased affinity of pyruvate kinase for the substrate phosphoenol pyruvate and a more rapid inactivation of the enzyme by Mg ATP (41). Thus abnormalities in this enzyme may contribute to two of the observed characteristics of malignant cells, but its behavior in intact cells may vary from cell line to cell line.

The hexoses taken up by a malignant cell may, in addition to participation in the glycolytic pathway, be shunted to the pentose phosphate pathway for the synthesis of both DNA and RNA. Weber has demonstrated increased activity of the primary enzymes of this pathway in Morris hepatomas (129). Still another use of hexoses in malignant cells is glycosylation of membrane proteins and lipids. This area has not been completely evaluated, but there are studies suggesting that hexose uptake does affect membrane glycoproteins (71) and alter cell behavior.

Thus the cancer cell is frequently a high consumer of glucose and a producer of lactate; both functions clearly affect the host. Furthermore, the hexoses utilized by many malignant cells may support proliferation in ways other than the production of energy, ultimately contributing to the growth advantage of these cells. Much work remains to be done in this area.

3. LIPID METABOLISM IN CANCER CELLS   The ability of tumors to synthesize fatty acids varies widely, but in many cases the synthetic rate is felt to be inadequate for replication (115). From such studies has come the belief that tumor cells derive most of their constituent fatty acids from host

tissues. However, tumor cells implanted intraperitoneally in mice maintained on a lipid-free diet for 26 weeks, and clearly showing signs of essential fatty acid deficiency, grow just as well as similar tumor cells injected into adequately nourished animals (2). Furthermore, over 20 cell lines of various types have been successfully adapted to growth in de-lipidized medium, though other cell lines are reported to exhibit a lipid requirement. Thus the fatty acid requirements of tumors and the contribution of host lipids to these requirements are not completely understood, but malignant cells have some ability to adapt to decreased fatty acid availability (102, 115).

Three of the many aspects of lipid metabolism that may impinge on the ability of cancer cells to grow effectively are energy production, cell membrane composition, and abnormalities of cholesterol synthesis. Although many tumors can oxidize fatty acids rapidly, other less well differentiated ones have essentially lost the ability to use them as fuel (19, 31, 132) and have increased requirements for carbohydrate or amino acids as energy sources.

Some of the differences in lipid composition between normal and transformed cells may be related to the stage of differentiation of the cells or to the proliferative state rather than to transformation per se. For example, the lipid composition of blast cells from patients with acute myeloblastic leukemia differs from that of normal neutrophils, but is similar to that of normal immature myeloid cells isolated from the bone marrow (69). Membrane phospholipids of quiescent cells differ from those of proliferating normal or transformed cells in degree of saturation. An increased proportion of unsaturated fatty acids increases the fluidity of the membrane (15, 106), alters the transport of drugs (15) and some nutrients (62) and the exposure of some cell membrane proteins (114), increases the activation of certain membrane enzymes (25), and alters the mobility of cell surface receptors (57), all of which may affect growth. Interestingly, unsaturated fatty acids (linoleic acid) may act directly on both normal and neoplastic mammary epithelium in vitro to promote growth (68), whereas saturated fatty acids are inhibitory. Linoleic acid cannot initiate proliferation in the absence of hormones in this system; rather it augments growth in cells stimulated by the appropriate hormonal factors. The growth-promoting effect of the unsaturated fatty acids may result from their incorporation into cell membranes, perhaps with resultant increased availability of hormone receptors. The extent to which dietary unsaturated fatty acids contribute to this is unclear.

There is increasing interest in the cholesterol metabolism of malignant cells (20). Loss of feedback control of cholesterol is a frequent occurrence in the malignant cell lines examined to date (73, 101). Such abnormalities may account for many of the other anomalies of malignant cell proliferation

(73). Although much interest in the past has centered on the role of cholesterol in the cell membrane, recent evidence (101) suggests that increased hydroxymethylglutaryl (HMG) CoA reductase activity in transformed cells may promote cell division by providing mevalonate, a cholesterol precursor, rather than through an effect of cholesterol per se. HMG CoA reductase activity consistently rises just before increased DNA synthesis in BHK-21 transformed fibroblasts in the S phase. Blockage of the increased HMG CoA reductase activity prevents the entry of the cells into S phase, an effect that is reversible by the provision of exogenous mevalonate.

4. AMINO ACID METABOLISM IN CANCER CELLS   There are interesting differences in the uptake of amino acids by transformed cells, proliferating normal cells, and quiescent normal cells (99). Growth and transformation are associated with increased uptake of some amino acids due to an increase in V_{max}, with no change in apparent K_m. These characteristics usually indicate that the carrier protein(s) for the molecule under study are normal, but that there is increased availability, either through synthesis of new transport proteins or through increased exposure of existing ones. Alternatively, there may be enhanced carrier mobility through the membrane because an unchanged number of carriers have increased transport capability (99).

Growth and transformation do not affect the uptake of all amino acids. However, as a generalization, amino acids transported primarily by the Na^+ dependent A system (e.g. alanine, glycine, serine, proline, α-amino isobutyric acid) are more subject to growth control than those transported primarily by other systems (21, 99). For example, a pure preparation of the insulin-like growth factor Multiplication-Stimulating Activity (MSA) added to quiescent cultures of chick embryo fibroblasts caused enhanced transport of A system amino acids that preceded the onset of DNA synthesis by several hours, but did not affect the uptake of amino acids transported by the L (Na^+-independent; leucine, isoleucine, phenylalanine) system, or by the ASC (alanine, serine, cysteine-preferring) or Ly^+ (lysine-preferring) systems. A similar effect on A system transport was observed when cells infected with a temperature-sensitive transforming virus moved from a nonpermissive to a permissive temperature. MSA was unable to stimulate transport above that associated with transformation (31). Clearly, however, there is no one transport system alteration unique to malignant cells (8, 99).

The fate of amino acids, once transported into the cell, may also differ in quiescent, proliferating and transformed cells. For example, when the enzymes of the metabolic pathways for the utilization of L-ornithine were examined in hepatomas of varying growth rates and compared to those of normal liver, it was found that the activities of L-ornithine carbamyl transferase (130), the enzyme that channels ornithine into the urea cycle, and ornithine transaminase (123), which directs ornithine into the synthesis of glutamic-γ-semialdehyde and L-glutamate, were decreased, with the amount of the decrease showing a rough inverse correlation with the growth rate of the tumor. In contrast, the activity of ornithine decarboxylase, which directs ornithine into polyamine biosynthesis, is increased in these neoplasms, with the activity of the enzyme roughly paralleling the growth rate of the tumor (133). The requirement of many malignant cell lines for glutamine has been theoretically explained (73) as secondary to the abnormal synthesis of cholesterol and fatty acids, with shunting of substrate away from the Krebs cycle and resultant entry of increased amounts of glutamine distal to the shunt. Abnormally high requirements of the Walker 256 carcinoma cell line for methionine have been suggested (120).

Thus malignant cells may use disproportionately large amounts of certain amino acids; this could impact on the metabolism of the host. A possible regulatory role for some amino acids in cell division remains a possibility.

B. Altered Metabolism of Host Cells: The Divergent Behavior of Liver and Muscle

1. ALTERATIONS IN THE LIVER   Either protein deprivation or starvation produces a marked loss in weight and content of protein (1) and glycogen (46) in the liver. This represents an actual decrease in size of the liver cells due to actual loss of cytoplasm (46). In contrast, liver dry weight frequently increases in rodents bearing either spontaneous or transplanted tumors (88, 119). There is also evidence that transplanted tumors induce proliferation of both the hepatocytes and reticuloendothelial cells of the liver (7, 89), with the majority of mitoses occurring in the reticuloendothelial cells.

Hepatic protein synthesis in tumor-bearing animals has been evaluated both in vivo and in vitro by uptake of labeled amino acid into protein. In both mice and men, the rate of uptake is consistently increased (78, 79, 97, 98) when compared to that found in ad lib fed controls. This was not due to an alteration in the precursor pool (79). Quantitatively, the increased label is found primarily in high molecular weight proteins. The low molecular weight peptides and proteins, however, show the greatest relative increase in incorporation when compared to controls. Some molecular weight regions actually show a decrease in incorporation (79). Lysosomal enzyme activity is also increased in the livers of tumor-bearing animals, suggesting that the rate of protein breakdown may also be increased (80). Similar increases in activity are seen in starved mice; however, the V_{max} and K_m of the cathepsin D activity differ in these two groups, suggesting that undernutrition is not the sole cause of the change in the cancer subjects.

There are also marked changes in the activities of many liver enzymes, with prominent reexpression of fetal isozymes (48, 49, 50). In some respects the hepatic enzyme composition resembles that of the fetal liver, and in other respects the composition resembles that of the tumor itself. Certainly this is not unique to cancer (61). Nevertheless, it is important to note that the liver now resembles, to some extent, the tumor itself, in that enzymes important in carbohydrate and amino acid metabolism are altered such that increased glycolysis and disproportionate metabolism of amino acids may occur here, too. Thus the liver, and possibly other organs, may contribute to the disordered metabolism of cancer patients in some of the same ways as the tumor cells.

2. ALTERED METABOLISM OF HOST CELLS: SKELETAL MUSCLE   The mass of skeletal muscle tends to decline during the course of progressive tumor growth. White or phasic muscle tends to atrophy more rapidly than red or tonic muscle, and contractile proteins are more extensively depleted than the sarcoplasmic proteins (22).

Intraperitoneal injection of either radioactive leucine (78) or valine (22) prior to sacrifice results in decreased incorporation of label into muscle protein in tumor-bearing animals compared to either pair-fed (22) or ad lib fed (78) controls. This depression is more marked in the phasic gastrocneimus than in the tonic soleus, and more severe for contractile than for sarcoplasmic proteins (22). A similarly decreased uptake of labeled amino acid has been recorded for skeletal (rectus abdominis) muscle of undernourished cancer patients with well-nourished noncancer cases as controls (78).

The cause of the decreased incorporation of amino acids into muscle protein and its specificity to neoplasia are in dispute. Clark & Goodlad have proposed, on the basis of in vitro studies, that there is a defect in the 40S ribosomal subunit that causes defective translation at a post-initiation stage (23). Since the decrease in skeletal muscle protein synthesis associated with starvation is believed to occur at the level of peptide-chain initiation (103), this suggests a tumor- (or stress-) specific defect in protein synthesis. However, this has been questioned by Lundholm and co-workers (82), who have found many of the changes in amino acid incorporation into skeletal muscle protein to be similar in starvation and the tumor-bearing state. Thus the relative contributions of hypophagia and some tumor- (or stress-) specific anomalies to muscle wasting remain unclear.

An increased fractional rate of degradation may also contribute to the loss of muscle protein. Proteases in muscle of tumor-bearing rats and cancer patients are more active than those in ad lib fed controls (78, 80). The possible quantitative importance of this may be estimated from the fact that in one study the dry weight of tumor-influenced muscle decreased by $48 \pm 11\%$ (S.E., $p<0.025$), while the dry weight of muscle from pair-fed controls decreased only $4 \pm 7\%$ (not significant) despite similar protein synthetic rates (82).

Glucose metabolism is also impeded in muscle of tumor-bearing patients in that rates of uptake and subsequent conversion of glucose to CO_2, glycogen, or lactate are slowed (76), and the levels of several enzymes involved in the oxidative and glycolytic degradation of glucose are reduced (78). Again, the contribution of semi-starvation to these findings is unclear.

C. Altered Metabolism of Host at the Whole Organism Level

1. ALTERED METABOLISM OF HOST AT THE WHOLE ORGANISM LEVEL: CARBOHYDRATE   The rate of endogenous glucose production and turnover is accelerated in undernourished as compared to normally nourished cancer patients by an average of 80%, although the range is wide (55). In uncomplicated starvation, the rate of glucose production declines; however, it increases in calorie deprivation complicated by sepsis or trauma (43, 83). Endogenous gluconeogenesis arises by two main pathways: the recycling of lactate-pyruvate (Cori cycle), and de novo production from glucogenic amino acids, largely mobilized from skeletal muscle proteins.

In normally nourished cancer patients, the Cori cycle accounts for about 20% of glucose turnover. In the undernourished cancer patients of Holroyde, whose glucose turnover averaged 180% of normal, the Cori cycle activity averaged 90 mg/kg/hr (range, 22–193), compared to 18 mg/kg/hr (range, 13–24) in non–weight losing cancer patients (55), and accounted for about 50% of total glucose turnover. Mean lactate production is increased in patients with metastatic cancer, although again the range of values is wide (54). Although there was only a modest increase in the rate of lactate oxidation in these patients, this mechanism still accounted for the disposal of about 60% of the lactate produced. The excessive lactate recycling in cancer patients cannot be attributed to starvation, because it rises even further during the parenteral hyperalimentation of these subjects (56). The extent to which the excess lactate production occurs in tumor tissue, as opposed to host tissues, is unknown.

The rate of gluconeogenesis from plasma ^{14}C alanine in cachectic cancer and noncancer patients was found to be similar (127), and alanine contributed only 4–5% of total glucose production. Furthermore, the alanine

→ glucose conversion was promptly suppressed by exogenous glucose, as it is in normals. Thus glucose production from lactate probably accounts for most of the increase in glucose turnover in cancer patients.

2. ALTERED METABOLISM OF HOST AT THE WHOLE-ORGANISM LEVEL: FAT   In the progressive weight loss of cancer, loss of adipose mass constitutes the major proportion and exceeds that seen in simple starvation (9, 37). Cancer patients oxidize normal amounts of fatty acid to CO_2 after an overnight fast (128). Entry of free fatty acids into the circulation is also similar in fasting cancer patients and normals. However, free fatty acid oxidation showed a much less than normal decrease in response to a glucose load in cancer patients than in controls, suggesting a continued drain on fat stores for oxidative purposes even in the presence of exogenous glucose. Lipogenesis is decreased in tumor-bearing animals, with decreased food intake (102), but the rate of lipogenesis in animals with normal food intake has been reported in different series to be decreased (27) or normal (102).

The marked hyperlipidemia observed in some animal systems has prompted several studies of plasma lipids in man. Fasting levels of free fatty acids tend to be normal (112, 128) or even low (81), and they show a normal decrease after a glucose load (112). More detailed analyses in humans with breast cancer (4, 5) and in rodents (12) suggest that α-lipoprotein levels may be depressed and at least some fraction of the very low density lipoproteins may be elevated, although no consistent abnormalities have been identified.

3. ALTERED METABOLISM OF HOST AT THE WHOLE-ORGANISM LEVEL: PROTEIN   Protein deficiency may result in inequality of the specific activity of the plasma and intracellular pools of protein. This severely limits the reliability of estimates of protein synthesis rate based on infusion or injection of labeled amino acids (117). Using these techniques, measured whole body protein synthesis rates in undernourished cancer subjects are significantly elevated compared to healthy controls (116, 117), with much of the increase in whole body protein turnover apparently in host tissue (116).

Many studies of the concentration of individual amino acids in the plasma and urine have revealed differences between cancer patients and various controls. To date, however, these measurements have not revealed a consistent profile of abnormalities in any neoplastic disease. In patients with acute leukemia, elevated plasma levels of glutamine, phenylalanine, tyrosine, and leucine plus isoleucine, with decreased levels of asparagine and threonine were reported (67). In contrast, Rudman et al found that 60% of their leukemic patients had subnormal fasting plasma levels of total α-amino nitrogen at some point during their disease, with decreases in alanine, glutamine, histidine, proline, threonine, and methionine (108). In solid tumors, no abnormalities in plasma aminograms were noted in some studies (109), while others have reported that plasma aminograms did not become abnormal until the tumors were 30% of host weight (134). In one study (135) of patients with advanced malignant melanoma, although no abnormalities were noted in the plasma aminograms, urinary aminograms revealed decreased excretion of phosphoserine, alanine, isoleucine, ornithine, ethanolamine, and histidine. Others have confirmed the decreased excretion of histidine and also noted decreased glycine excretion (35). Clarke and co-workers (24) compared plasma aminograms in well-nourished cancer patients with normals; they noted increased plasma alanine, isoleucine, and lysine concentrations in the cancer group. When cancer patients who had anorexia and weight loss were compared wih undernourished controls, several differences were noted. Of the gluconeogenic amino acids, glycine concentrations were elevated in the malnourished noncancer patients compared to the malnourished cancer patients, and proline and aspartate/asparagine values were decreased. Of the branched-chain amino acids, both valine and leucine were lower in the malnourished noncancer patients than in the undernourished cancer patients. In addition, methionine levels were lower in the noncancer malnourished patients. All these discrepancies represent instances in which the malnourished patients' values have changed, but the cancer patients' values have failed to show adaptation to semistarvation.

4. BASAL METABOLIC RATE   Several clinical studies have found generally higher metabolic rate in cancer patients than in subjects with primary undernutrition (who are hypometabolic in comparison to normal subjects) (11, 125). Nevertheless, in none of these studies is it possible to eliminate the possible influence of fever, anemia, recent surgery, infection, or the presence of necrotic tissue, all of which are common in cancer patients. Thus the effect of tumor-bearing per se on basal metabolic rate is unclear.

5. MEDIATORS   Although some of the metabolic abnormalities of the tumor-bearing host are due to characteristics of the cancer cells themselves, others are clearly secondary to alterations in host tissues. These effects are almost certainly mediated by circulating factors, as originally demonstrated by Lucké et al (75) in parabiotic rats, one tumor-bearing and one free of tumor. These factors may be altered levels of normal hormones, either

produced in response to the tumor or by the tumor cells themselves, or other products of either host or tumor cells.

Insulin resistance and increased cortisol secretion are the two most frequently discussed hormonal changes in malignant disease. Other hormones (especially catecholamines and growth hormone/somatomedin) deserve further study. Glucose tolerance tests have revealed "diabetic" responses in both cachectic (112) and noncachectic (84) cancer patients. Baseline plasma glucose concentrations were not significantly different in two studies (81, 112) but were increased in another (77). The amount of insulin released in response to a glucose challenge has been reported to be normal (112) and decreased (77, 81); the disappearance rate of this hormone is normal (81). The disappearance rate of plasma glucose has been reported to be normal (77, 81) and decreased (10). The steady-state concentration of glucose during infusion of a known amount of glucose plus insulin was higher in cancer patients than in controls (112).

Although most of the results above are compatible with a degree of insulin resistance, the finding of a normal disappearance rate of glucose in association with lower than normal plasma insulin concentrations is more compatible with insulin sensitivity (77, 81), a discrepancy that has not been explained. The possible contribution of enhanced gluconeogenesis to this picture has not been completely evaluated (81, 84).

The mechanism of "insulin resistance" is also unclear. Binding of ^{125}I-labeled insulin to insulin receptors on circulating monocytes is normal (112). The incorporation rate of glucose carbon into glycogen and CO_2 and the ability of insulin to stimulate this effect were both less than control in isolated skeletal muscle fibers of cancer patients; however, the incorporation of palmitic acid and leucine into CO_2 was not different from control (81). These results are compatible with a cellular defect in carbohydrate metabolism beyond the receptor level (i.e. abnormal enzyme activity, as previously discussed), but clearly more work is needed in this area. There are also changes in cortisol metabolism associated with cancer. In animals with transplanted tumors there is marked adrenal hypertrophy that is not prevented by force-feeding (9). Hypophysectomy does prevent the hypertrophy (3), indicating at least a permissive role for pituitary-derived or pituitary-dependent factors. The mean fasting plasma cortisol is elevated in patients and animals with various cancers when compared to normal controls (110, 111), but this is not a universal finding (105). Some of the apparent discrepancies in these studies may be due to the inclusion of patients at different points in their natural histories. In the early stages of tumor growth the adrenals have been shown to be hyporesponsive to ACTH (66). As tumor growth progresses, the cortex becomes hyperresponsive for a time; however, as the animal or patient enters the final stages of his disease, the adrenals become markedly hyporesponsive again.

There is increasing evidence that tumor cells, often specifically the neoplastic cell rather than a host cell, produce a host of hormones and hormone-like products that exert powerful effects on host metabolism. Humorally mediated paraneoplastic "syndromes" range from identification of a product without detectable clinical manifestations to well-defined clinical findings without a known causative humoral factor (e.g. neuropathies, myopathies, hypercalcemia without detectable bone disease). Odell and co-workers have demonstrated that most cancer patients have increased plasma levels of materials that cross-react immunologically with a variety of hormones (96), and have hypothesized that virtually all cancers synthesize ectopic proteins. Many of these are biologically inactive as determined by lack of binding in radioreceptor assays (e.g. high molecular weight ACTH), but others produce clinically recognizable syndromes. The extent to which these peptide hormones or hormone-associated tumor products exert subclinical, but deleterious, effects, is unknown.

Recently, a new group of growth-promoting substances called growth factors have been extracted from a variety of malignant and nonmalignant cell lines (42). Elevated levels of nonsuppressible insulin-like activity have been detected in the serum of patients with tumor-associated hypoglycemia (63), and elevated levels of immunoreactive nerve growth factor have been detected in patients with neurofibromatosis (36); thus these peptides may represent a new class of mediators of paraneoplastic syndromes. In addition, tumor cells have been shown to release mitogenic peptides related to several of these growth factors into culture medium (70, 121, 122); similar activities are extractable from tumor cells (104). Several features of these tumor-derived growth factors suggest that they may account for some of the systemic effects of tumors. First, they are mitogenic for some normal cells (70, 121, 122); although not yet directly tested, this ability could account for some of the increased mitoses seen in liver cells of tumor-bearing hosts and for tumor-associated fibrosis. Second, some of them have the ability to confer transformed characteristics (ability to grow in soft agar) on nontransformed cells (121, 122). This capacity could account for the reexpression of fetal isozymes in host livers in patterns somewhat similar to those seen in tumors. Third, growth factors in general are metabolically active, with the ability to stimulate uptake of some, but not all, amino acids (31, 52) and to stimulate glycolysis, apparently by a direct effect on phosphofructokinase (34). Such effects could contribute to the abnormal plasma aminograms and increased lactate production seen in cancer patients. Finally, some of these tumor-derived growth factors have been shown to bind to receptors for normal growth factors (121, 122). Thus a tumor-derived growth factor could conceivably compete with normal growth factors and hormones, induce down-regulation of receptors, and, by inducing an incomplete or abnormal metabolic response in the target cell, have the effect of altering the pattern of nutrient utilization in some host cells.

Several other tumor-associated factors with possible significance in the cancer cachexia syndrome have been reported. Nakahara & Fukuoka described an activity (called toxohormone) extractable from all the tumors they studied which, when injected into normal animals, caused many of the host changes associated with neoplastic disease (91, 93). The possibility that this activity actually reflects bacterial contamination has been raised (64) and denied (92). It is likely that several components are responsible for all the effects attributed to toxohormone (38). Lipid-mobilizing substances in tumor extracts and body fluids of patients and animals with tumors have been reported. One of the better characterized is a 75,000 dalton protein isolated from cell-free ascitic fluid of mice inoculated intraperitoneally with sarcoma 180 cells (85) and from ascitic fluid of humans with hepatoma and carcinoma of the kidney, but not from ascites caused by peritonitis or cirrhosis. Tumor production of prostaglandins is well documented; there is some evidence that these factors may be mediators of tumor-associated hypercalcemia (65). Many tumor cells secrete active proteinases (29, 107) that may have systemic effects we well as contribute to tissue destruction. Finally, Theologides (118) has postulated that tumors produce a host of small, metabolically active peptides and other factors that interfere nonspecifically with the metabolism of the host.

In addition to metabolically active factors produced by tumor cells themselves, the presence of a cancer in the body elicits a host response, with prominent involvement of macrophages and other cells. These cells have been shown to release proteinases, complement components, plasmin inhibitors, reactive metabolites of oxygen, prostaglandins, factors capable of affecting protein synthesis in hepatocytes and other cells, and other products with potentially significant effects upon the host (94).

Clearly, then, there are many possible humoral mediators of the cancer cachexia syndrome. What remains is to determine the biological significance of these factors.

III. CONCLUSIONS

1. Wasting of skeletal muscle and adipose tissue is a general feature of advanced cancer; however, the liver, spleen, and adrenals tend to enlarge. Protein synthesis and carbohydrate utilization are suppressed in skeletal

muscle. In the liver, enzymes of glucose metabolism and amino acid catabolism are altered, with increased activity and reexpression of isozymes
normally suppressed during adult life.

2. Cancer cachexia is usually associated with decreased food intake,
which results from mechanical effects of the tumor, treatment effects, associated infection, and incompletely understood biochemical disturbances in
the tumor-bearing subject.

3. Like patients with cachexia caused by prolonged infections or inflammatory diseases, the cancer subject manifests both semi-starvation and
stress. Undernutrition, with associated abnormalities in insulin metabolism,
probably accounts for most of the wasting of muscle and fat, while hepatic
enlargement and enzymatic alterations may be the liver's response to the
release of bioactive products from the tumor. Hypercorticoidism further
contributes to the changes in both organs.

4. The truly unique feature of cancer is the cancer cells themselves. In
addition to the mechanical effects of tumors, these cells affect host metabolism in two ways: (a) their own uptake and metabolism of nutrients; and
(b) hormones and hormone-like factors they secrete. Accelerated glucose
utilization and lactate production are the most widely discussed of these;
the possibility of a "disordered" pattern of amino acid utilization also
deserves consideration. The possible effects of tumor-secreted metabolically
active products on host metabolism are also potentially fruitful areas of
investigation. The presence of large amounts of growing tissue is not sufficient to account for cachexia, as is demonstrated by uncomplicated pregnancy.

5. Tumors are composed of not only neoplastic cells but also host cells
(macrophages, lymphocytes, neutrophils); the host cells are also capable of
releasing biologically active factors. In addition, the tumors are often super-
infected, and low grade infection may be present in other organs (e.g. GI
tract, bronchial tree). Furthermore, there are zones of necrosis in most, but
not all, tumors. Each of these features may contribute to the cachexia
associated with malignant disease and may account for some of the similarities between cancer cachexia and the wasting associated with infectious
diseases.

6. Almost all studies comparing tumor growth rates with and without
nutritional supplementation show an acceleration in tumor growth rate
when nutrient intake is increased in anorexic animals (17, 18, 30). While
this may make little difference in the rat with a nonmetastasizing tumor
implanted on the hip, even a slight stimulation of tumor growth may hasten
death or debility in the patient with brain or spinal cord metastases, tumor
threatening to obstruct bronchi or bowel, or tumors infiltrating vital organs

such as lung or liver. Clearly these patients represent a majority of individuals with advanced cancer. This may account for the failure of vigorous nutritional support to prolong the life of patients with advanced cancer (13). 7. The challenge of cancer cachexia is thus two-fold. First of all, the characteristics of cancer cells that give them an advantage in the competition for "building block" nutrients must be elucidated and circumvented. Second, the tumor-related causes of anorexia, hypermetabolism, and hepatopathy must be determined and ways found to reverse their effects. Both tasks are formidable, but it is unlikely that truly effective approaches to cancer cachexia will be found that do not deal with these basic questions.

Literature Cited

1. Addis, T., Poo, L. J., Lew, W. 1936. The quantities of protein lost by the various organs and tissues of the body during a fast. *J. Biol. Chem.* 115:111–16
2. Bailey, J. M. 1980. Essential fatty acid requirements and metabolism of cells in tissue culture. *Adv. Prostagl. Thrombox. Res.* 6:549–65
3. Ball, H. A., Samuels, L. T. 1938. Adrenal weights in tumor-bearing rats. *Proc. Soc. Exp. Biol. Med.* 38:441–43
4. Barclay, M., Calathes, D., DiLorenzo, J. C., Helper, A., Kaufman, R. J. 1959. The relation between plasma lipoproteins and breast carcinoma. Effect of degree of breast disease on plasma lipoproteins and the possible role of lipid metabolic aberrations. *Cancer* 12:1163–70
5. Barclay, M., Cogin, G. E., Escher, G. C., Kaufman, R. G., Kidder, E. D., Petermann, M. L. 1955. Human plasma lipoproteins. I. In normal women and in women with advanced carcinoma of the breast. *Cancer* 8:253–60
6. Barsh, G. S., Cunningham, D. D. 1977. Nutrient uptake and control of animal cell proliferation. *J. Supramol. Struct.* 7:61–77
7. Baserga, R., Ksielski, W. E. 1961. Cell proliferation in tumor-bearing mice. *Arch. Pathol.* 72:24–30
8. Bass, R., Hedegaard, H. B., Dillehay, L., Moffett, J., Englesberg, E. 1981. The A, ASC, and L systems for the transport of amino acids in Chinese hamster ovary cells (CHO-K1). *J. Biol. Chem.* 256:10259–66
9. Begg, R. W. 1958. Tumor-host relations. *Adv. Cancer Res.* 5:1–54
10. Bishop, J. S., Marks, P. A. 1959. Studies on carbohydrate metabolism in patients with neoplastic disease. II. Response to insulin administrations. *J. Clin. Invest.* 38:668–72

11. Bozzetti, F., Pagnoni, A., Del Vecchio, M. 1980. Excessive caloric expenditure as a cause of malnutrition in patients with cancer. *Surg. Gynecol. Obstet.* 150:229–34
12. Brennan, D. E., Mathur, S. N., Spector, A. A. 1975. Characterization of the hyperlipidemia in mice bearing the Ehrlich ascites tumor. *Eur. J. Cancer* 11:225–30
13. Brennan, M. F. 1981. Total parenteral nutrition in the management of the cancer patient. *Ann. Rev. Med.* 32:233–43
14. Burke, M., Bryson, E. I., Kark, A. E. 1980. Dietary intakes, resting metabolic rates, and body composition in benign and malignant gastrointestinal disease. *Br. Med. J.* 280:211–15
15. Burns, C. P., Luttenegger, D. G., Dudley, D. T., Buettner, G. R., Spector, A. A. 1979. Effect of modification of plasma membrane fatty acid composition on fluidity and methotrexate transport in L1210 murine leukemia cells. *Cancer Res.* 39:1726–32
16. Burt, M. E., Lowry, S. F., Gorschboth, C., Brennan, M. F. 1981. Metabolic alterations in a noncachectic animal tumor system. *Cancer* 47:2138–46
17. Buzby, G. P., Mullen, J. L., Stein, T. P., Miller, E. E., Hobbs, C. L., Rosato, E. F. 1980. Host-tumor interaction and nutrient supply. *Cancer* 45:2940–48
18. Cameron, I. L., Rogers, W. 1977. Total intravenous hyperalimentation and hydroxyurea chemotherapy in hepatoma-bearing rats. *J. Surg. Res.* 23:279–88
19. Cederbaum, A. I., Rubin, E. 1976. Fatty acid oxidation, substrate shuttles, and activity of the citric acid cycle in hepatocellular carcinomas of varying differentiation. *Cancer Res.* 36:2980–87
20. Chen, H. W., Kandutsch, A. A., Heiniger, H. J. 1978. The role of cholesterol

in malignancy. *Prog. Exp. Tumor Res.* 22:275–316

21. Christensen, H. N. 1975. Recognition sites for material transport and information transfer. *Curr. Top. Membr. Transp.* 6:227–58

22. Clark, C. M., Goodlad, G. A. J. 1971. Depletion of proteins of phasic and tonic muscles in tumor-bearing rats. *Eur. J. Cancer* 7:3–9

23. Clark, C. M., Goodlad, G. A. J. 1975. Muscle protein biosynthesis in the tumor-bearing rat: A defect in a postinitiation stage of translation. *Biochim. Biophys. Acta* 373:230–40

24. Clarke, E. F., Lewis, A. M., Waterhouse, C. 1978. Peripheral amino acid levels in patients with cancer. *Cancer* 42:2909–13

25. Coleman, R. 1973. Membrane bound enzymes and membrane ultrastructure. *Biochim. Biophys. Acta* 300:1–30

26. Costa, G. 1963. Cachexia, the metabolic component of neoplastic diseases. *Prog. Exp. Tumor Res.* 3:321–69

27. Costa, G., Holland, J. F. 1962. Effects of Krebs-2 carcinoma on the lipide metabolism of male Swiss mice. *Cancer Res.* 22:1081–83

28. Costa, G., Lane, W. W., Vincent, R. G., Siebold, J. A., Aragon, M., Bewley, P. T. 1980. Weight loss and cachexia in lung cancer. *Nutr. Cancer* 2:98–103

29. Dabbous, M. K., Roberts, A. N., Brinkley, B. 1977. Collagenase and neutral protease activities in cultures of rabbit VX-2 carcinoma. *Cancer Res.* 37: 3537–44

30. Daly, J. M., Reynolds, H. M., Rowlands, B. J., Dudrick, S. J., Copeland, E. M. 1980. Tumor growth in experimental animals. Nutritional manipulation and chemotherapeutic response in the rat. *Ann. Surg.* 191:316–22

31. Derr, J. T., Smith, G. L. 1980. Regulation of amino acid transport in chicken embryo fibroblasts by purified multiplication-stimulating activity (MSA). *J. Cell. Physiol.* 102:55–62

32. DeWys, W. D. 1979. Anorexia as a general effect of cancer. *Cancer* 43: 2013–19

33. DeWys, W. D., Begg, C., Lavin, P. T., Band, P. R., Bennett, J. M., Bertino, J. R., Cohen, M. H., Douglass, H. D. Jr., Engstrom, P. F., Ezdinli, E. Z., Horton, J., Johnson, G. J., Moertel, C. G., Oken, M. M., Perlia, C., Rosenbaum, C., Silverstein, M. N., Skeel, R. T., Sponzo, R. W., Tormey, D. C. 1980. Prognostic effect of weight loss prior to chemotherapy in cancer patients. *Am. J. Med.* 69:491–97

34. Diamond, I., Legg, A., Schneider, J. A., Rozengurt, E. 1978. Glycolysis in quiescent 3T3 cells. Stimulation by serum, epidermal growth factor and insulin in intact cells and persistence of the stimulation after cell homogenization. *J. Biol. Chem.* 253:866–71

35. Eades, C. H. Jr., Pollack, R. L. 1954. Urinary excretion of fourteen amino acids by normal and cancer subjects. *J. Natl. Cancer Inst.* 15:421–27

36. Fabricant, R. N., Todaro, G. J., Eldridge, R. 1979. Increased levels of a nerve-growth-factor cross-reacting protein in "central" neurofibromatosis. *Lancet* 1:4–7

37. Fenninger, L. D., Mider, G. B. 1954. Energy and nitrogen metabolism in cancer. *Adv. Cancer Res.* 2:229–53

38. Fujii, S., Yuasa, A., Kawachi, T., Okamura, Y., Wakasugi, H., Yamamura, Y. 1964. Purification of toxohormone by carboxymethylcellulose column chromatography. *Gann* 55:67–71

39. Galanti, N., Tsutsui, J., Jonak, G., Kawasaki, S., Soprano, K., Baserga, R. 1982. Nuclear events in normal and malignant cells and the control of cell proliferation. *Proc. 34th Ann. M. D. Anderson Hosp. Tumor Inst. Symp. on Fund. Cancer Res.* Houston, 1982. In press

40. Garattini, S., Bizzi, A., Donelli, M. G., Guaitani, A., Samanin, R., Spreafico, F. 1980. Anorexia and cancer in animals and man. *Cancer Treat. Rev.* 7:115–40

41. Glossmann, H., Presek, P., Eigenbrodt, E. 1981. Association of the src-gene product of Rous Sarcoma Virus with a pyruvate-kinase inactivating factor. *Mol. Cell. Endocrinol.* 23:49–63

42. Gospodarowicz, D., Moran, J. S. 1976. Growth factors in mammalian cell culture. *Ann. Biochem.* 45:531–57

43. Gump, F. E., Long, C. L., Geiger, J. W., Kinney, J. M. 1975. The significance of altered gluconeogenesis in surgical catabolism. *J. Trauma* 15:704–13

44. Harley, C. B., Goldstein, S., Posner, B. I., Guyda, H. J. 1980. Insulin-like peptides stimulate metabolism but not proliferation of human fibroblasts. *Am. J. Physiol.* 239:E125–31

45. Harnett, W. L. 1952. *British Empire Cancer Campaign: A Survey of Cancer in London,* p. 26 London: British Empire Cancer Campaign

46. Harrison, M. F. 1953. Effect of starvation on the composition of the liver cell. *Biochem. J.* 55:204–11

47. Haven, F. L., Bloor, W. R. 1956. Lipids in cancer. *Adv. Cancer Res.* 4:237–314

48. Herzfeld, A., Greengard, O. 1972. The dedifferentiated pattern of enzymes in livers of tumor-bearing rats. *Cancer Res.* 32:1826–32

49. Herzfeld, A., Greengard, O. 1977. The effect of lymphoma and other neoplasms on hepatic and plasma enzymes of the host rat. *Cancer Res.* 37:231–38

50. Herzfeld, A., Greengard, O., McDermott, W. V. 1980. Enzyme pathology of the liver in patients with and without nonhepatic cancer. *Cancer* 45:2383–88

51. Heymsfield, S. B., Horowitz, J., Lawson, D. H. Enteral hyperalimentation. In *Developments in Digestive Diseases,* ed. J. E. Berk, 3:59–83. Philadelphia: Lea and Febiger. 258 pp.

52. Hochstadt, J., Quinlan, D. C., Owen, A. J., Cooper, K. O. 1970. Regulation of transport upon interaction of fibroblast growth factor and epidermal growth factor with quiescent (Go) 3T3 cells and plasma-membrane vesicles isolated from them. In *Hormones and Cell Culture,* ed. G. H. Sato, R. Ross, *Cold Spring Harbor Conf. Cell Prolif.* 6:752–72

53. Holley, R. W. 1972. A unifying hypothesis concerning the nature of malignant growth. *Proc. Natl. Acad. Sci. USA* 69:2840–41

54. Holroyde, C. P., Axelrod, R. S., Skutches, C. L., Haff, A. C., Paul, P., Reichard, G. A. 1979. Lactate metabolism in patients with metastatic colorectal cancer. *Cancer Res.* 39:4900–4

55. Holroyde, C. P., Gabuzda, T. G., Putnam, R. C., Paul, P., Reichard, G. A. 1975. Altered glucose metabolism in metastatic carcinoma. *Cancer Res.* 35:3710–14

56. Holroyde, C. P., Meyers, R. N., Smink, R. D., Putnam, R. C., Reichard, G. A. 1977. Metabolic response to total parenteral nutrition in cancer patients. *Cancer Res.* 37:3109–14

57. Horwitz, A. F., Hatten, M. E., Burger, M. M. 1974. Membrane fatty acid requirements and their effect on growth and lectin-induced agglutinability. *Proc. Natl. Acad. Sci. USA* 71:3115–19

58. Houten, L., Reilley, A. A. 1980. An investigation of the cause of death from cancer. *J. Surg. Oncol.* 13:111–16

59. Hume, D. A., Weidemann, M. J. 1979. Role and regulation of glucose metabolism in proliferating cells. *J. Natl. Cancer Inst.* 62:3–8

60. Ibsen, K. H. 1977. Interrelationships and functions of the pyruvate kinase isozymes and their variant forms: A review. *Cancer Res.* 37:341–53

61. Ibsen, K. H., Fishman, W. H. 1979. Developmental gene expression in cancer. *Biochim. Biophys. Acta* 560:243–80

62. Im, W. B., Deutchler, J. T., Spector, A. A. 1979. Effects of membrane fatty acid composition on sodium-independent phenylalanine transport in Ehrlich cells. *Lipids* 14:1003–8

63. Kahn, C. R. 1980. The riddle of tumour hypoglycaemia revisited. *Clin. Endocrinol. Metab.* 9:335–61

64. Kampschmidt, R. F., Schultz, G. A. 1963. Absence of toxohormone in rat tumors free of bacterial contamination. *Cancer Res.* 23:751–61

65. Karmali, R. A. 1980. Review: Prostaglandins and cancer. *Prostagl. Med.* 5:11–28

66. Kavetsky, R. E., Samundgean, E. M., Butenko, Z. A. 1962. Changes in the functional state of the adrenal cortex during development of tumours. *Acta Unio. Int. Contra Cancrum* 18:115–17

67. Kelley, J. J., Waisman, H. A. 1957. Quantitative plasma amino acid values in leukemic blood. *Blood* 12:635–43

68. Kidwell, W. R., Knazek, R. A., Vonderhaar, B. K., Losonczy, I. 1982. Effects of unsaturated fatty acids on the development and proliferation of normal and neoplastic breast epithelium. See Ref. 39. In press

69. Klock, J. C., Pieprzyk, J. K. 1979. Cholesterol, phospholipids, and fatty acids of normal immature neutrophils: comparison with acute myeloblastic leukemia cells and normal neutrophils. *J. Lipid Res.* 20:908–11

70. Knauer, D. J., Iyer, A. P., Banerjee, M. R., Smith, G. L. 1980. Identification of somatomedin-like polypeptides produced by mammary tumors of BALB/c mice. *Cancer Res.* 40:4368–72

71. Lage-Davila, A., Hofmann-Clerc, F., Torpier, G., Montagnier, L. 1979. Glucose-regulated membrane properties of untransformed and virus-transformed BHK21 cells. *Exp. Cell Res.* 120:181–89

72. Lanks, K. W., Kasambalides, E. J. 1980. Factors that regulate proliferation of normal and transformed cells in culture. *Pathobiol. Annu.* 10:35–50

73. Lavietes, B. B., Coleman, P. S. 1980. The role of lipid metabolism in neoplastic differentiation. *J. Theor. Biol.* 85:523–42

74. Lawrence, W. Jr. 1979. Effects of cancer on nutrition: Impaired organ system effects. *Cancer* 43:2020–29

75. Lucke, B., Berwick, M., Zeckwer, I. 1952/53. Liver catalase activity in

parabiotic rats with one partner tumor-bearing. *J. Natl. Cancer Inst.* 13:681–86

76. Lundholm, K., Bylund, A-C., Holm, J., Schersten, T. 1976. Skeletal muscle metabolism in patients with malignant tumour. *Eur. J. Cancer* 12:465–73

77. Lundholm, K., Bylund, A-C., Schersten, T. 1977. Glucose tolerance in relation to skeletal muscle enzyme activities in cancer patients. *Scand. J. Clin. Lab. Invest.* 37:267–72

78. Lundholm, K., Edström, S., Ekman, L., Karlberg, I., Bylund, A-C., Schersten, T. 1978. A comparative study of the influence of malignant tumor on host metabolism in mice and man: evaluation of an experimental model. *Cancer* 42:453–61

79. Lundholm, K., Ekman, L., Edström, S., Karlberg, I., Jagenburg, R., Schersten, T. 1979. Protein synthesis in liver tissue under the influence of a methylcholanthrene-induced sarcoma in mice. *Cancer Res.* 39:4657–61

80. Lundholm, K., Ekman, L., Karlberg, I., Edström, S., Schersten, T. 1980. Comparison of hepatic cathepsin D activity in response to tumor growth and to caloric restriction in mice. *Cancer Res.* 40:1680–85

81. Lundholm, K., Holm, G., Schersten, T. 1978. Insulin resistance in patients with cancer. *Cancer Res.* 38:4665–70

82. Lundholm, K., Karlberg, I., Ekman, L., Edström, S., Schersten, T. 1981. Evaluation of anorexia as the cause of altered protein synthesis in skeletal muscles from non-growing mice with sarcoma. *Cancer Res.* 41:1989–96

83. Long, C. L., Kinney, J. M., Geiger, J. W. 1976. Nonsuppressibility of gluconeogenesis by glucose in septic patients. *Metabolism* 25:193–201

84. Marks, P. A., Bishop, J. S. 1957. The glucose metabolism of patients with malignant disease and of normal subjects as studied by means of an intravenous glucose tolerance test. *J. Clin. Invest.* 36:254–64

85. Masuno, H., Yamasaki, N., Okuda, H. 1981. Purification and characterization of a lipolytic factor (toxohormone-L) from cell-free fluid of ascites sarcoma 180. *Cancer Res.* 41:284–88

86. McKeehan, W. L., McKeehan, K. A. 1981. Extracellular regulation of fibroblast multiplication: A direct kinetic approach to analysis of role of low molecular weight nutrients and serum growth factors. *J. Supramol. Struct. Cell. Biochem.* 15:83–110

87. McKeehan, W. L., McKeehan, K. A. 1979. Oxocarboxylic acids, pyridine nucleotide-linked oxidoreductases and serum factors in regulation of cell proliferation. *J. Cell. Physiol.* 101:9–16

88. Medigreceanu, F. 1910. On the relative sizes of the organs of rats and mice bearing malignant new growths. *Proc. R. Soc. London, Ser. B* 82:286–92

89. Morgan, W. W., Cameron, I. L. 1973. Effect of fast-growing transplantable hepatoma on cell proliferation in host tissue of the mouse. *Cancer Res.* 33:441–48

90. Morrison, S. D. 1982. Control of food intake in the experimental cancerous host. See Ref. 39. In press

91. Nakahara, W. 1960. A chemical basis for tumor-host relations. *J. Natl. Cancer Inst.* 24:77–86

92. Nakahara, W. 1974. A pilgrim's progress in cancer research, 1918–1974: autobiographical essay. *Cancer Res.* 34:1767–74

93. Nakahara, W., Fukuoka, F. 1958. The newer concept of cancer toxin. *Adv. Cancer Res.* 5:157–77

94. Nathan, C. F., Murray, H. W., Cohn, Z. A. 1980. The macrophage as an effector cell. *N. Engl. J. Med.* 303:622–26

95. Nixon, D. W., Heymsfield, S. B., Cohen, A. E., Kutner, M. H., Ansley, J., Lawson, D. H., Rudman, D. 1980. Protein-calorie undernutrition in hospitalized cancer patients. *Am. J. Med.* 68:683–90

96. Odell, W. D., Wolfsen, A. R. 1980. Hormones from tumors: are they ubiquitous? *Am. J. Med.* 68:317–18

97. Oram-Smith, J. C., Stein, T. P., Wallace, H. W., Mullen, J. L. 1977. Intravenous nutrition and tumor host protein metabolism. *J. Surg. Res.* 22:499–503

98. Pain, V. M., Garlick, P. J. 1980. The effect of an Ehrlich ascites tumour on the rate of protein synthesis in muscle and liver of the host. *Biochem. Soc. Trans.* 8:334

99. Parnes, J. R., Isselbacher, K. J. 1978. Transport alterations in virus-transformed cells. *Prog. Exp. Tumor Res.* 22:79–122

100. Pouyssegur, J., Franchi, A., Salomon, J.-C., Silvestre, P. 1980. Isolation of a Chinese hamster fibroblast mutant defective in hexose transport and aerobic glycolysis: Its use to dissect the malignant phenotype. *Proc. Natl. Acad. Sci. USA* 77:2698–701

101. Quesney-Huneeus, V., Wiley, M. H., Siperstein, M. D. 1979. Essential role for mevalonate synthesis in DNA repli-

cation. *Proc. Natl. Acad. Sci. USA* 76:5056–60

102. Ramaswamy, K., Lyon, I., Baker, N. 1980. Dietary control of lipogenesis in vivo in host tissues and tumours of mice bearing Ehrlich ascites carcinoma. *Cancer Res.* 40:4606–11

103. Rannels, D. E., Pegg, A. E., Rannels, S. R. 1976. Starvation results in descreased initiation factor activity in rat skeletal muscle. *Biochem. Biophys. Res. Commun.* 72:1481–88

104. Roberts, A. B., Lamb, L. C., Newton, D. L., Sporn, M. B., DeLarco, J. E., Todaro, G. J. 1980. Transforming growth factors: Isolation of polypeptides from virally and chemically transformed cells by acid-ethanol extraction. *Proc. Natl. Acad. Sci. USA* 77:3494–98

105. Rose, D. P., Stauber, P., Thiel, A., Crowley, J. J., Milbraths, J. R. 1977. Plasma dehydroepiandrosterone sulfate, androstenedione and cortisol excretion in breast cancer. *Eur. J. Cancer* 13:43–47

106. Rosenfeld, C., Jasmin, C., Mathe, G., Inbar, M. 1979. Dynamic and composition of cellular membranes and serum lipids in malignant disorders. *Rec. Results Cancer Res.* 67:63–77

107. Recklies, A. D., Tiltman, K. J., Stoker, A. M., Poole, A. R. 1980. Secretion of proteinases from malignant and nonmalignant human breast tissue. *Cancer Res.* 40:550–56

108. Rudman, D., Vogler, W. R., Howard, C. H., Gerron, G. G. 1971. Observations on the plasma amino acids of patients with acute leukemia. *Cancer Res.* 31:1159–65

109. Sassenrath, E. N., Greenburg, D. M. 1954. Tumor host relationships. I. Effects on free amino acid concentrations of certain tissues. *Cancer Res.* 14:563–69

110. Schaur, R. J., Fellier, H., Gleispach, H., Fink, E., Kronberger, L. 1979. Tumor host relations. I. Increased plasma cortisol in tumor-bearing humans compared with patients with benign surgical diseases. *J. Cancer Res. Clin. Oncol.* 93:281–85

111. Schaur, R. J., Semmelrock, H-J., Schauenstein, E., Kronberger, L. 1979. Tumor host relations II. Influence of tumor extent and tumor site on plasma cortisol of patients with malignant diseases. *J. Cancer Res. Clin. Oncol.* 93:287–92

112. Schein, P. S., Kisner, D., Haller, D., Blecher, M., Hamosh, M. 1979. Cachexia of malignancy: potential role of insulin in nutritional management. *Cancer* 43:2070–76

113. Sherman, C. D. Jr., Morton, J. J., Mider, G. B. 1950. Potential sources of tumor nitrogen. *Cancer Res.* 10:374–78

114. Shinitzky, M., Rivnay, B. 1977. Degree of exposure of membrane proteins determined by fluorescence quenching. *Biochemistry* 16:982–86

115. Spector, A. A. 1975. Fatty acid metabolism in tumors. *Prog. Biochem. Pharmacol.* 10:42–75

116. Stein, T. P. 1982. Tumor-induced changes in the host's protein metabolism. See Ref. 39. In press

117. Stein, T. P., Buzby, G. P., Rosato, E. F., Mullen, J. L. 1981. Effect of parenteral nutrition on protein synthesis in adult cancer patients. *Am. J. Clin. Nutr.* 34:1484–88

118. Theologides, A. 1972. Pathogenesis of cachexia in cancer. *Cancer* 29:484–88

119. Theologides, A., Pegelow, C. H. 1970. Liver weight changes during distant growth of transplanted tumor. *Proc. Exp. Biol. Med.* 134:1104–8

120. Tisdale, M. J. 1980. Methionine metabolism in Walker carcinosarcoma in vitro. *Eur. J. Cancer* 16:407–14

121. Todaro, G. J., DeLarco, J. E. 1978. Growth factors produced by sarcoma virus-transformed cells. *Cancer Res.* 38:4147–54

122. Todaro, G. J., DeLarco, J. E., Fryling, C., Johnson, P. A., Sporn, M. B. 1981. Transforming growth factors (TGFs): Properties and possible mechanisms of action. *J. Supramol. Struct. Cell. Biochem.* 15:287–301

123. Tomino, I., Katunuma, N., Morris, H. P., Weber, G. 1974. Imbalance in ornithine metabolism in hepatomas of different growth rates as expressed in behavior of L-ornithine: 2-oxoacid aminotransferase (ornithine transaminase, EC 2.6.1.13). *Cancer Res.* 34:627–36

124. Warburg, O. 1956. On the origin of cancer cells. *Science* 123:309–14

125. Warnold, I., Lundholm, K., Schersten, T. 1978. Energy balance and body composition in cancer patients. *Cancer Res.* 38:1801–7

126. Warren, S. 1932. The immediate causes of death in cancer. *Am. J. Med. Sci.* 184:610–15

127. Waterhouse, C., Jeanpretre, N., Keilson, J. 1979. Gluconeogenesis from alanine in patients with progressive malignant disease. *Cancer Res.* 39:1968–72

128. Waterhouse, C., Kemperman, J. H. 1971. Carbohydrate metabolism in sub-

jects with cancer. *Cancer Res.* 31: 1273–78

129. Weber, G. 1982. Differential carbohydrate metabolism in tumor and host. See Ref. 39. In press

130. Weber, G., Queener, S. F., Morris, H. P. 1972. Imbalance in ornithine metabolism in hepatomas of different growth rates as expressed in behavior of L-ornithine carbamyl transferase activity. *Cancer Res.* 32:1933–40

131. Weber, M. J., Salter, D. W., McNair, T. E. 1982. Increased glucose transport in malignant cells: Analysis of its molecular basis. See Ref. 39. In press

132. Weinhouse, S. 1982. Changing perceptions of carbohydrate metabolism in tu-

mors. See Ref. 39. In press

133. Williams-Ashman, H. G., Coppoc, G. L., Weber, G. 1972. Imbalance in ornithine metabolism in hepatomas of different growth rates as expressed in formation of putrescine, spermidine, and spermine. *Cancer Res.* 32:1924–32

134. Wu, C., Bauer, J. M. 1960. A study of free amino acids and of glutamine synthesis in tumor-bearing rats. *Cancer Res.* 20:848–57

135. Young, S. E., Griffin, A. C., Milner, A. N., Stehlin, J. S. Jr. 1967. Free amino acids and related compounds in the blood and urine of patients with malignant melanoma. *Cancer Res.* 27:15–17

Ann. Rev. Nutr. 1982. 2:303–22
Copyright © 1982 by Annual Reviews Inc. All rights reserved

PICA AND NUTRITION

Darla Erhard Danford

Clinical Nutrition Research Center, University of Chicago, Chicago, Illinois
60637 and USDA Human Nutrition Research Center on Aging at Tufts
University, Boston, Massachusetts

CONTENTS

INTRODUCTION

Pica is a pathological craving for normal food constituents or for substances
not commonly regarded as food. It has fascinated the physician and nutrition scientist because it is frequently associated with nutrient deficiency,
notably mineral malabsorption, although it can occasionally result in excessive intakes of substances such as potassium or carotene. To the psychiatrist
or psychologist, it represents a behavioral challenge that is sometimes associated with mental retardation. On a world-wide scale, pica is of anthropo-
logical interest, often being a consequence of cultural patterns ingrained in
the food habits of a region and possibly related to an ancestral food-short-
age. To the veterinarian or zoologist, it is evidence of a nutrient-specific
appetite in wild and/or domestic animals.

303

0199-9885/82/0715-0303$02.00

Against this background I discuss pica as a nutritional aberration that provides opportunities to observe deficiency diseases, to make nutritional interventions, and to reflect on the factors that determine food habits.

The word "pica" was first used to describe a syndrome by the French physician Ambrose Paré in the 16th century (82). Pica is a medieval Latin word meaning magpie, a bird which, according to Cooper (37), was known to early writers for its tendency to pick up a diversity of things to satisfy hunger or curiosity. Other terms that have been applied to this or related syndromes from antiquity to the 19th century include: mal d'estomac[1] (French); erdessen,[2] das Gelusten der Schwangern Frauen,[3] die Schwangern Weiberlust[4] (German); geophagy[5] (Aristotle); allotriophagia[6] (Sophocles); and cachexia Africana.[7] In 1638 Boezo (16) first classified pica systematically. For Boezo the word pica denoted the craving for absurd things; the avid consumption of accustomed foods he termed malacia.

In this review, the term pica will be applied to a pathological craving both for items normally considered food by the population, such as that sometimes reported during pregnancy (e.g. for 10 heads of lettuce daily), and for substances not normally regarded as food (e.g. clay, coal). This definition does not categorize such behaviors as the chewing of gum or tobacco.

Historically the term pica has been vague and its meanings have been confounded owing to culturally based judgments. Certain early writers, for example, declared cravings for foods such as raw cabbage, yeast, and lobster to be pica (56), while in some societies earth is considered food and is used as a seasoning agent (122). In the mid 19th century it was customary for some people in northern Sweden to mix earth with flour when making bread (202). Thus the diagnosis of pica depends upon cultural attitudes as well as amounts ingested and degrees of craving. No sharp demarcation exists between pathological states and normality, nor between the ages at which some form of pica is considered normal.

Descriptions of pica as a syndrome are found in antiquity. Examples are summarized in Table 1. Records from as early as 40 B.C. indicate that Terra Sigillatta, the sacred "Sealed Earth," was used to treat a variety of diseases in Greece. Galen visited the island of Lemnos two centuries later and took back to Rome clay lozenges that for almost 2000 years had been used to treat poisoning. It is related that in Germany in 1581 a condemned prisoner

[1]stomach illness
[2]earth eating
[3]the hunger of pregnant women
[4]the pregnant wives' craving
[5]consumption of soil or clay
[6]indiscriminate craving
[7]wasting away in Africans

Table 1 Historical record of information concerning pica

Year	Event	References
10 B.C.	Clay lozenges ingested to treat illness and poisoning	211
1000 A.D.	Avicenna treated pica with iron	16
1542	Aëtius associated pica with pregnancy	2
1630	Earth eaten in bread dough. 30 Years War: pica associated with superstition	121
1638	Distinction made between pica for food items and pica for nonfood items	16
1668	Stress suggested as cause of pica	124
1698	Hereditary basis for pica proposed	47
1742	Food allergy and idiosyncrasy associated with pica	212
1799–1804	First explorer report of endemic pica in South America	222
1831	Pica associated with lack of nutritious diet	89
1835	Geophagia in Africa—Cachexia Africana described	38
1843	Cachexia Africana disappeared in Dominica secondary to life-style changes	100
1845	Cachexia Africana spreads from West Indies to Southern US with slave trade	24, 38, 169
1846	Animal studies indicate relationship between geophagia and nutrient deficiency	123
1849	Pica reported among insane	215
1851	Infusorial earth mixed with bread flour by choice in Northern Sweden	202
1868	Case report of pica cured by iron	68
1870	Pica associated with anemia	129
1880	Pica associated with worm infestation	37
1900	Pica thought to be a racial phenomenon	150
1900	Pica in India reported among all classes and both sexes	97
1910	Geophagia reported in Egyptian Sudan, pica in pregnant women assumed normal	29
1912	Analysis of soil from 16th century, cation exchange properties noted	211
1924	Lead poisoning associated with pica	182
1960s	Further studies of pica responding to iron therapy	119
1960	Dwarfism, hypogonadism, hepatosplenomegaly and iron deficiency syndrome identified in the Middle East	86
1961	Zinc deficiency described in the syndrome of dwarfism in Middle East	170, 171
1968	Analysis of clay shown to have property of cation exchange	147
1970	Geophagia and amylophagia associated with pregnancy	109
1970s	Pagophagia identified and responds to iron therapy	33, 175
1981	Geophagia and other types of pica in the mentally retarded associated with low plasma iron and zinc	43

asked to be given 6 grams of mercuric chloride (2 grams were considered fatal) if he could eat terra sigillata at the same time. By taking his poison along with "a dram of Terra Sigillata in olde wine" he survived and was freed (211).

In the early 16th century, Aëtius of Amida (2) attributed the pica of pregnancy to pressure on the viscera associated with the growth of the fetus, while in Germany Hubrigkt (98) interpreted the same phenomenon as due to fantasies associated with pregnancy. Avicenna (85), who lived around 1000 A.D., first mentioned beneficial effects of iron therapy in pica. Others recommended the consumption of pigeons along with their bones, thus foreshadowing treatment for the malabsorption of minerals associated with certain types of pica (16). During the remainder of the 17th century, physicians continued to speculate on the origins and nature of pica, prescribing varied and exotic measures, including both dietary treatment (including iron supplementation) and the need for psychological intervention against the mental aberrations supposed to underlie pica.

During the course of expeditions and colonization in various parts of the world in the 18th and 19th centuries, pica was identified under a variety of new circumstances. The Otomac Indians of South America were observed to eat clay colored with iron oxide without ill effects (222). In Java, a reddish baked clay was sold in the public market; its ingestion was supposed to make the individual slender (5, 77). Clay items to be eaten were sold in sections of India, Ghana, Afghanistan, Africa, and other tropical areas (5, 75, 85, 97, 101, 122, 199, 222). In Peru dietary powdered lime was sold in the market place (222). The Chinese, wrote the traveler Medhurst, mixed gypsum into a jelly for consumption (137, 141).

Pica was practiced by the native inhabitants of North America before the arrival of Columbus (131, 219). On plantations of the United States and the Caribbean, slaves sometimes exhibited a craving for clay, a practice probably passed down from their African forebears. When pica is superimposed on the classical pellagragenic diet of salt pork, corn bread, and molasses a variety of deficiency states may appear (169). On the American plantations, symptoms of these deficiencies were known as cachexia Africana, which consisted of weakness, pallor and edema, enlargement of the liver, spleen, and lymph nodes, anorexia, and rapid pulse, with later pre-terminal ulceration of the skin and eventual death (5, 24, 38, 55, 84, 100). It was commonly accepted that nutritional treatment, including administration of iron sulfate was effective in reversing the syndrome (89, 135). In this context, Hancock (89) noted that slaves on Tiger Island, who also practiced clay-eating, did not develop the cachexia, presumably because they used water from an iron cistern. Volpata (221) reported that in 111 males and 115 females with geophagia, 85% developed subsequent gastroenteritis, 91% chlorosis, and

46% pellagra. The role of various B-vitamin deficiencies concurrent with pica remains confusing (156).

INCIDENCE OF PICA

The incidence of pica is difficult to establish, although several surveys of selected groups have been made. Interpretation of survey findings is complicated by inconsistent definitions of pica, reluctance of subjects to admit to the practice, limitations of statistical methods applied, and the impossibility of generalization from a few observed cases. Table 2 provides examples of selected estimates.

The craving for particular food substances during pregnancy is a widely recognized phenomenon (39, 51). In one series of women studied in Bir-

Table 2 Incidence of pica selected reports

Study (Ref.)	Number of subjects	Description and/or age of group	Percentage population with pica
1937, Baltimore (107)	30	retarded children	50
1950, Mississippi (57)	331	pregnant ♀, black	44
1957, Baltimore (37)	386	black, > 6 mo.	27
	398	white, > 6 mo.	17
1962, Washington DC (145)	486	black, 1–6 years	32
	294	white, 1–6 years	10
1963, Washington DC (131)	859	children, low income	55
		children, high income	30
1966, Boston interview (9)	439	children, 1–6 years	15
Mail survey	277	children, 1–6 years	20
1966, England (163)	40	institutionalized, psychotic, 3–13 years	66
1967, Georgia (165)	200	pregnant ♀	55
1968, Chicago (110)	987	pregnant ♀	35
1969, Chicago (112)	500	pregnant ♀	24
1971, California (19)	25	Spanish American, pregnant ♀	38
	10	Spanish American, nonpregnant ♀	15
	21	Spanish American children	32
1979, Mississippi (219)	56	nonpregnant ♀	57
	115	children	16
	33	males	0
	27	adolescents	0
	112	pregnant ♀	28
1981, Boston (41)	991	institutionalized, retarded, 11–89 years	26

mingham, England (91), 51% reported food cravings, with or without aversions and alterations in their sense of taste. The most common cravings were for fruit and other sweet-sour, sour, or sharp-tasting foods. Several positive correlations emerged, including one between pica during pregnancy and a history of pica and food fads in childhood. Similar food preferences were observed in a series of pregnant women studied in New York (96); but in Aberdeen, Taggart (206) did not find pica among 800 pregnant women studied. Pregnant women sometimes also eat nonfood substances. Fifty percent of the pregnant Southern black women in two studies (57, 165) ate clay and starch. In a one-year study, Keith et al (111) noted that 35% of 987 pregnant black and white women exhibited amylophagia (starch eating). Bruhn & Pangborn (19) reported a similar proportion (38%) of pica in pregnant Mexican women. McGanity et al (140) found 28% of 800 pregnant adolescents had a history of pica for clay, soil, starch, and refrigerator frost. Some authors have reported a decline over time in the incidence of pica among similar populations of pregnant women—e.g. of geophagia in rural populations from 55% in 1967 (165) to 18% in 1974 (18), and of amylophagia in urban populations from 35% in 1968 (110) to 20% in 1969 (112). The reasons for these changes are not evident.

Pica in adult men appears to be underreported. Some studies note that the incidence of pica may be decreasing in some male populations as its victims convert to smoking or chewing tobacco (131). In a study of 302 adults in Columbus, Ohio, 25% of the pica cases were male (85). Sayers et al (188) found that 11% of their male outpatient population reported consumption of ash or earth.

Pica is also prevalent among children, being reported especially in black children. Three authors (9, 37, 145) agree that about 30% of black children aged 1–6 years and 10–18% of white children of the same age attending their clinics have pica, mostly for nonfood substances. Among psychotic mentally retarded children, the incidence of pica exceeds 50% (107, 163). In a group of 991 mentally retarded adults the incidence of pica was found to be 26% (41), greater than that of such other eating dysfunctions as anorexia, rumination, or hyperphagia.

In 1974, Klein (115) estimated that 5–10% of all children 1–5 years of age had lead poisoning. More than 30% of children with pica have been found to have lead poisoning (102); conversely, 70–90% of children with lead poisoning give a history of pica (15, 28, 30, 184).

ETIOLOGY AND MECHANISM OF PICA

The causation of pica has been the subject of speculation since ancient times, and several hypotheses from that era have been mentioned above. Hypotheses currently advanced include nutritional, psychological, cultural, phar-macologic, and disease (74, 161).

Nutritional Hypothesis

Pica has been hypothetized to be a craving generated by nutrient deficiency. The "salt lick" of wild animals is widely considered a response to a deficiency (17). Osteophagia in cattle, reported in many countries (71, 123, 209), is associated with phosphorus deficiency (209). Pica has also been described in pellagrous animals (54). Animals deprived of specific nutrients such as potassium (138), thiamin (92, 177, 179), and iron (65, 138, 224) often lick or selectively ingest items high in the depleted nutrient (58, 92, 176). However, this animal model of deficiency-induced pica has not always been confirmed (53, 213).

Davis (44, 45) tried to prove that children will without external guidance select a nutritionally complete diet. However, since the foods provided experimentally to children by Davis were mostly balanced in nutrients, these studies failed to test this hypothesis. On the basis of information from rat studies, Snowdon & Sanderson (197) proposed that a child deficient in calcium may discover that lead ingestion (pica) relieves some of the deficiency symptoms. Specific nutrient deficiencies, such as those of vitamin D (106), phosphorus (104), and vitamin C (79), have been thought to prompt the consumption of nonfood substances. However, pica for nonfood items did not decline in children given supplements of vitamins and minerals (unfortunately not including iron) (81). Hunter (99) hypothesizes that the ingestion of iron and calcium-rich clays by iron- and calcium-deficient individuals in Ghana represents diet supplementation. Similarly, it was postulated that consumption of clay rich in calcium and magnesium was to fulfill a physiologic deficit in Nigerian pregnant women (216).

Attempts to link pica with nutritional states have concentrated on iron (7). Several studies agree that anemia associated with pica for nonfood substances in children (119, 139, 151) and adults (33, 175) can be cured by administering iron. Case reports indicate a similar effect of iron on food pica (32, 39, 40, 166, 183). Unfortunately, no control groups were included in these studies. A special form of pica associated with iron deficiency is pagophagia, in which the pregnant woman consumes large amounts of ice (averaging 700 g daily). Controlled studies by Coltman (33–35) and Rey-nolds et al (175) demonstrated that the subnormal hemoglobin levels and the low concentrations of serum iron in such cases respond to iron therapy, following which the pagophagia disappears. In one series, parenteral admin-istration of iron was effective within 5 days, while oral administration required 11 days to stop the pica (175). Whether the ice induces iron deficiency remains unknown.

Results supporting the hypothesis that iron deficiency causes pica and that such pica can be cured by giving iron have not always been obtained (79, 81, 164, 165). The occurrence of nutrient deficiencies and pica in the same subject does not prove a causal relationship. The disappearance of pica after iron therapy in subjects with very low hemoglobin values suggests that in some cases there may be a causal relationship. However, despite the high incidence of pica associated with anemia (39, 40), only a small percentage of individuals with anemia exhibit pica and vice versa. In cases of food pica (39, 40), the substance craved is rarely a good source of iron, nor does food pica during pregnancy always cease after delivery (2, 131).

Psychological Hypothesis

Pica has been explained as a persistence of the infantile hand-to-mouth behavior pattern (178). Lourie et al (131) determined the psychological status of the mother and child in cases of children with pica. The mother was often found to have personality disturbances and to relate poorly to the child, while the child sometimes had emotional problems, suffered from abnormal dependence and anxiety, and exhibited neurotic and depressive patterns. These authors suggest that pica is an expression of oral fixation (146), and Cooper (37) has noted that pica occurs more frequently in children with feeding problems such as anorexia or refusal of certain foods. Neumann (159) suggested that pica in both children and adults expresses a vestigial instinct related to the need to chew something solid. Others (5, 41, 122, 133) have also reported that texture, color, odor and taste are important components of the craving in pica. Specific neurological changes may be associated with pica results from lead poisoning but evidence indicates that the pica encourages the child to consume sources of lead and not the reverse (14). Several specific brain lesions have been associated with pica. Lesions of the left temporal lobe in monkeys (94) and the analogous Klüver-Bucy syndrome in humans (116) are accompanied by pica, as is damage to the amygdala of the cat (63). Mentally retarded individuals with seizures may have severe pica (13, 41). In instances of pica associated with specific brain lesions, the eating dysfunction seems confined to nonfood substances.

In addition to the individuals with seizures referred to above, the entire population of mentally retarded adults shows a high incidence of pica, which varies with the degree of retardation. In our series (41), the incidence of pica varied from 10% in mild mental deficiency to 33% in severe mental deficiency. However, incidence of pica for food items only was not correlated with severity of mental deficit.

Cultural Hypothesis

Pica has been associated with cultural and familial factors. In antiquity, clay lozenges were prepared on the Greek island of Lemnos, stamped with religious symbols, and exported throughout the Mediterranean area (74). Clay eating was encouraged among the male youths of Greece because it was believed to produce the desirable 'leucophlegmatic' skin and a slender, effeminate body (211). Symbolic geophagy occurs in many cultures (5). Earth-eating, irrespective of cravings, has frequently been associated with religious belief. Clay lozenges bearing Christian symbols are sold today in the Mexican city of Oaxaca (74). It has been noted that when Muslims erase sentences from the Koran by rubbing chalk from the board they sometimes consume the chalk dust out of respect for the book (74).

In parts of Africa it is believed that magical properties of the soil promote well-being. This belief results in the consumption of earth upon entering a territory, to promote fertility in women, and during pregnancy to increase lactation (5, 122, 216, 217). The consumption of earth during the first trimester of pregnancy is believed to suppress nausea, and in some African cultures young girls are taught in childhood that during pregnancy the consumption of earth as desirable (5, 56).

Vermeer & Frate (218, 219) consider the eating of clay to be deeply ingrained in Southern black society. There clay is fed as a pacifier for the infant, a practice also observed in Africa (5). Geophagy occurs among the adults (151), and it may be practiced at group social functions (131). Given the deeply ingrained geophagy of the African cultures that supplied the bulk of slaves to the New World, it is not surprising that the practice persists in the black subculture of the United States (5, 218, 219). On the other hand, geophagy is historically recorded both from Europe and the indigenous Indian population in the New World, individuals in the United States could also have acquired the practice from either.

Other Hypotheses

Pica may sometimes manifest itself in a person's effort to medicate himself. For example, medicinal properties against anemia have been attributed to clay (5, 55, 211). Individuals who consume extraordinarily large amounts of ground coffee (caffeine), cigarette butts (nicotine), oak leaves (tannins), and so forth, may be seeking pharmacological effects (20, 41, 67, 69, 120, 158, 168, 205). It has been reported (41) that 59 individuals who consumed such substances pathologically tended to exhibit behavior characteristic of addiction (83, 130, 148), increasing both the frequency and volume of ingested material. Such obsessive pica has been associated with nocturnal searching for (41), and constant dreams about (125), the craved substance.

Other physiological factors that have been thought to cause pica include gastrointestinal malaise (5, 56, 72, 97, 99, 122, 148, 216), stress and inflammatory processes (13, 21, 117), toxicosis (149), parasitic infestations (56, 66, 156), disease states (122, 172, 190), and hunger (5, 122, 201).

CLINICAL DESCRIPTION OF PICA

Pica is widely thought to be age-related, with the majority of reported cases occurring in children and pregnant women. Recent data [(41) and case reports cited below] indicate that pica is not limited to any age, sex, or racial group; it can occur anywhere.

Geophagia is the most commonly reported and reviewed form (5, 37, 75, 85, 122). However, the substances eaten in pica are almost limitless and their benefits or hazards vary with the amount and type consumed (42).

Metabolic Associations

Most metabolic changes associated with pica have been observed in case studies and interpretation in terms of cause and effect frequently is clouded by the concurrent conditions.

Pica in children has been primarily associated with lead poisoning; as early as 1927 Ruddock (182) described this association. As recently as the early 1950s blood lead levels were not universally available, and the diagnosis of lead poisoning was primarily a clinical one. Despite the continuing controversy over what constitutes lead toxicity, diagnosis is now based on biochemical, gastrointestinal, and neurological parameters. Mahaffey (132) has provided an excellent critique of current knowledge of nutritional factors in lead poisoning.

Symptoms reported in children with pica and lead toxicity include altered hematological values (12, 83, 106, 128, 199), increased serum and urine Δ-aminolevulinic acid (83, 106), elevated protoporphyrin in erythrocytes (106), excretion of coproporphyrin II in the urine (83, 106), high blood lead (13, 14, 31, 127, 152, 163, 192, 199), high dental lead (46), and response to calcium EDTA-lead excretion tests (13, 14, 31, 83). The range of blood lead levels diagnostic for lead toxicity remains debated (36, 76, 127, 128, 199). These changes can occur before the appearance of clinical symptoms such as vague abdominal pain, constipation, anorexia, nonspecific gastroenteritis, and recurrent emesis (83, 106). The most serious manifestations of pediatric plumbism are those involving the central nervous system (drowsiness, coma, grand mal seizures, permanent brain damage) and the renal system (83, 106). Excessive lead ingestion can impose further brain damage and behavioral problems upon the mentally retarded (14, 31, 220, 223). Death rates associated with severe lead toxicity have been as high as 25% (83).

As in adults, pica in childhood has frequently been linked to iron deficiency anemia. Geophagia has been associated with low hemoglobin levels (79, 119, 139, 151), low serum iron (151), hypokalemia (142), low ascorbic acid (30), normal serum protein (119), low albumin (119), high incidence of respiratory infections (79), and normal anthropometric measurements including height and weight (79). Two children thought to have potassium craving secondary to Bartter's syndrome, a potassium wasting disease, consumed over a kilo of potatoes daily (70 mEq potassium/kg body weight) and had persistent hypokalemia (172). Fulton (62) reported a case of pica for beetles, slugs, and invertebrates that stopped suddenly without intervention at the age of 14. In another case (108) a boy who consumed Comet cleanser and had zinc deficiency was cured of his pica following oral zinc sulfate. A patient with pica for metal (88), exhibiting poor growth and appetite and low hair- and serum-zinc levels, improved following zinc therapy.

In many cultures pregnant women are expected to practice pica (5, 118). An extensive list of the varieties of pica in pregnancy emerged from a British Broadcast Corporation program (91) that generated 514 letters from listeners reporting 820 pregnancies (366 cravings for fruits and vegetables, and 187 cravings for nonfood substances such as coal, soap, and paper). In the United States geophagia, amylophagia, and pagophagia are the most commonly reported types of practices in pregnant women. With all three forms association with anemia (33–35, 85, 109–113, 160, 185, 187, 203, 207) has been observed. Bronstein & Dollar (18) observed iron/total-iron binding capacity ratios under 16% in pregnant women with amylophagia. Parotid enlargement has been reported in association with starch-eaters' anemia (144, 191), although it was not found by Roselle (181). Other documented effects of pica during pregnancy include gastric obstruction (4), increased incidence of toxemia (165) [not verified by Keith (113)], delivery complications (78, 95), successive picas (180), and repeated pica during multiple pregnancies (5, 56, 118). One young pregnant woman developed an appetite for blocks of toilet-bowl freshener (para-dichlorobenzene). She presented with anemia and was treated with iron and folic acid. This treatment improved neither her hemoglobin level nor her pica (23).

Pica also occurs in nonpregnant adult females and in adult males. Case reports of nonpregnant adult females include: anemia and olive consumption that ceased upon oral treatment with ferrous sulfate (27); pagophagia in a diabetic who started consuming heads of lettuce when she was prevented from eating ice and whose hematocrit then decreased from 27 to 23% (153); consumption of tomato seeds that ceased following parenteral administration of iron (32); and consumption of burned matches (167, 184). A study of a mentally retarded adolescent who consumed up to two packages of cigarettes a day and had low plasma zinc levels, elevated copper levels, and wounds that would not heal, showed a reversal of all signs after oral administration of zinc sulfate (43). A 74 year-old black woman presenting with severe microcytic hypochromic anemia without blood loss was consuming 60–180 g of magnesium carbonate daily (125). Other cases of pica in nonpregnant women have involved cigarette ash, peanuts (gooberphagia), hair (trichophagia) and lettuce (lectophagia) (49, 134, 157, 164, 195).

The clinical phenomena associated with pica in males has not been well studied. However, in one study of mentally retarded adults the men suffered more severe anemia than did their female counterparts (43). This appeared to be a result of the higher consumption of the craved substance among the males.

In an institutionalized, mentally retarded, primarily adult population, pica was observed in both sexes (41–43). Clinical symptoms varied with the type of pica. Some types of pica (geophagia, cigarette tobacco, coprophagia, paper, string, metal/paint, and twigs) were associated with low hematocrit, low hemoglobin, low plasma iron, elevated total-iron binding saturation, low plasma ferritin, low plasma zinc, elevated plasma copper, normal hair zinc, and some abnormal hair copper and magnesium (43). Other types of pica (cravings for grass, leaves, and insects) were associated with normal plasma values of metals and minerals (43). Five cases of geophagia with hyperkalemia (attributed to the potassium content of the clay) have been reported in male and female individuals with chronic renal failure (67).

Geographic

The combination of a diet high in phytate and fiber and the consumption of clay and soil that can chelate metals has resulted in numerous cases of iron and zinc deficiency in Middle Eastern populations (reviewed in 85). The first descriptions of a syndrome characterized by geophagia, iron deficiency anemia, hepatosplenomegaly, and hypogonadism appeared in the Turkish literature in 1942 (208). Subsequently, the syndrome has been reported in Turkey (26, 162, 186) and Iran (86, 87, 170, 171, 187). Prasad et al (170) first described the same syndrome (nutritional dwarfism) in male Iranians consuming clay and subsequently demonstrated that the dwarfism was due to zinc deficiency (171). This syndrome has been reported more recently in females (180). Many biochemical parameters have been evaluated in populations with pica and zinc-deficient dwarfism, including low hemoglobin (7, 26, 86, 162, 170, 183, 186), pallor (26, 186), low serum iron (7, 26, 73, 86, 87, 170, 180, 186), low hematocrit (26, 86, 180), elevated serum TIBC (7, 26, 86, 186), low transferrin saturation (7), increased erythrocyte fragility (26), no stainable iron in bone marrow (26, 186), reduced hemoglobin A_2 (26); low serum zinc (7, 26, 87, 170), low and elevated serum copper (26, 186), low serum magnesium (26), low serum phosphorus (26), high alkaline phosphatase (86), achlorhydria (86), elevated or normal SGOT, SGPT, BSP, CCF (26, 186); abnormal glucose tolerance (186), decreased vitamin A absorption (26), increased iron absorption test (26), decreased plasma zinc tolerance (7), decreased total protein (26), low albumin (26, 186), elevated globulin (186), low PBI (180, 186), decreased folic acid (186); hepatosplenomegaly (7, 26, 73, 86, 186), liver biopsy changes (86, 186, 187), histological changes with peroral intestinal biopsy (7, 186), retarded bone age (7, 26, 86, 87, 186), growth retardation (26, 73, 87, 170), delayed secondary sex characteristics (7, 73, 86, 170, 186). Essentially normal findings include cholesterol (26), calcium (26), prothrombin time (26), alkaline phosphatase (26), total protein (87, 186), erythrocyte glucose-6-phosphate (26), and d-xylose absorption (186).

Complications

Complications of pica repeatedly encountered include bezoars (22, 42, 107, 195, 214), intestinal perforation (48, 70), dental injury (1), intestinal obstruction (42, 93, 155, 214), achlorhydria (23, 64), parasitic infection (50, 55, 66, 136, 151, 189), and constipation (4, 42, 59, 106). Isolated examples of conditions such as ulcerative colitis (50) and urinary retention (189) are reported. Plain abdominal radiography that can visualize, depending on their mineral content, certain of the substances consumed in pica (42, 64, 114, 119, 133, 142, 219) has been proposed as a diagnostic tool (30).

NUTRITIONAL CONSEQUENCES OF PICA

Because pica is associated with and in some cases may be caused by nutritional deficiencies, the nutrient intakes of individuals with pica have been studied. As mentioned above, Gutelius (80) found that individuals with pica consumed less meat and milk, fewer vitamin C–rich sources, and a smaller variety of foods than normal subjects. Geophagia has been associated with diets low in iron-rich foods (52, 56), calories (56), thiamine (56), and niacin. Sand eating has been encountered in children with excessive milk intake who refuse solid food (25). In the Middle East the diets of individuals with geophagia rarely include animal-protein foods but rather consist of bread, rice, and a few vegetables; however, such diets are not uncommon in the region (170). Danford et al (43) calculated the nutrient intakes of 66 mentally retarded adults (15–71 years old) with and without pica. Dietary intakes of calories, protein, vitamin D, ascorbic acid, thiamin, riboflavin, niacin, calcium, phosphorus, iron, and zinc were within the amounts specified by the Recommended Dietary Allowances. Low intakes of vitamin A, magnesium, and copper were noted in both individuals with and without pica. Thus pica did not appear to interfere with total food intake in this population. Individuals with pica consumed more coffee and water than those without (42, 69, 205).

Dietary factors that may influence a child's susceptibility to lead toxicity are poorly understood. Johnson (103) found an inverse correlation between children's blood-lead levels and their calcium and milk intake. This relationship had previously been shown in an animal model (173). Three-day food records revealed intakes low in calcium, iron, magnesium, pantothenic acid, and zinc in this population (103). Mooty (154) found no dietary intake differences between children with high and low blood lead levels. Several studies in animals have suggested that nutritional inadequacies may potentiate the toxic effects of lead. These relationships have been comprehensively reviewed (106, 126, 128, 132, 198, 204). Sources of lead ingested by children with pica continue to be identified (10, 74, 90, 103, 105, 115, 193, 194, 198, 200).

Nutritional status may be influenced by pica in several ways. First, the consumption of the craved substance can reduce the intake of normal dietary sources of nutrients. For instance, large intakes of laundry starch have been reported to depress intake of regular foods (6, 18, 110, 181, 185, 207). However, amylophagia may not interfere with appetite (43, 56), and can cause obesity (133). Second, pica can reduce the bioavailability of minerals. To geophagia has been attributed reduced absorption of iron (7, 26, 43, 143, 147), zinc (7, 26, 43), and potassium (146), perhaps due to chelation. Others have observed high phytate diets in geophagic populations which could potentially decrease absorption of iron and zinc (174). Starch has been shown to reduce iron absorption (15, 207, 210), and magnesium carbonate was reported to interfere with iron absorption (125). On the other hand, some clays can be a source of such minerals as magnesium (216), potassium (67), iron (99), zinc (196), and calcium (99, 216).

THERAPY FOR PICA

Two major treatment modalities—the nutritional and the behavioral—are recommended in the literature. Many early references advocate the use of iron and "nutritious" food (37). The anemia and low plasma zinc of individuals with pica (especially geophagia) indicate appropriate mineral therapy.

Iron and zinc supplementation may result in improvements in the clinical picture. This is illustrated by cases of Middle Eastern dwarfism, wherein oral zinc administration (26, 58, 87, 170, 180) for pica-induced zinc deficiency resulted in sexual maturation and improved growth rates and iron therapy reversed anemia (7, 26, 86). Many instances of apparent responses to treatment with iron (11, 26, 104, 119, 139, 151) and zinc (88, 108) can be cited. More rapid disappearance of the pica following parenteral iron has been claimed (25, 28, 151, 175). Not all nutrient therapies affect pica. In the series studied by Gutelius et al (81), the oral administration of fat-soluble vitamins, B-vitamins and ascorbic acid supplements raised the plasma ascorbic acid levels of children with pica, but failed to cure the pica. Cure rates have rarely been evaluated over a long period. In a double-blind controlled trial McDonald & Marshall (139) observed a relapse of pica in individuals after 6 months of iron therapy (this was accompanied by a decrease in hemoglobin).

The sporadic success of iron therapy for pica has been postulated to be related to whether the therapy causes critical threshold levels of hemoglobin (139) or serum iron levels (175) to be exceeded. Others hypothesize that the defect behind pica involves iron-dependent tissue enzymes (35, 101, 175). Pica tends to disappear with age. Even double-blind iron therapy studies in young children have not accounted for this (80). Caution must therefore be exercized in evaluating and accepting the results of treatment, notably in the numerous single case reports in the literature.

Pica has in the past been, and is still being, "treated" by physical restraint of its practitioners/sufferers with masks and other devices. However, since individuals with pica persistently seek the specific substances they crave (42, 131, 178)—sometimes, for example, traveling great distances to obtain clay from special areas (5, 218, 219), a behavior also observed in lower animals (60) and primates (B. Marriott, personal communications)—attempts to restrain them are often unsuccessful.

Modern psychotherapy has concentrated on overcorrection techniques in which the pica practitioner is punished with mouth wash-outs (negative reinforcement) for indulgence of the craving and rewarded for the absence of pica with pleasant foods (positive reinforcement). A series of behavioral treatments (8, 20, 59, 61), has resulted in some regression of pica, even in the mentally retarded individuals in whom little spontaneous change was likely. Reviewing the literature on behavioral treatment, Albin (3) notes that experimental conditions are poor, follow-up data inadequate, and thus conclusions difficult.

CONCLUSIONS

The medical and nutritional implications of certain types of pica have been grossly underestimated. Despite extensive investigation, few studies present a comprehensive nutrition picture and none elucidate the etiology of pica. A review of the literature reveals that pica appears to have multiple etiologies. One may not be able to compare the results of one study to another, particularly if the two studies consider different forms of pica. Thus the type of pica should be elucidated, the significant preceding events determined.

Like alcoholism, the consumption of nonfood items is difficult to diagnose by means of an interview. Often the condition is first revealed when the sufferer is X-rayed for other reasons. Identification of individuals at risk is extremely important, especially children and pregnant women who present with anemia and/or other nutrient deficiencies.

In populations habituated to geophagia, amylophagia, and other types of pica associated with iron deficiency, trace element and mineral status should be evaluated. Trace element levels in the body may be subnormal, with consequences that are as yet unknown but perhaps nutritionally significant. Heavy metal toxicity can still be a problem for individuals ingesting substances containing metals such as lead. Treatment modalities vary with the type of pica. Nutritional therapy should be instituted when appropriate and the effects of such intervention systematically documented.

Literature Cited

1. Abbey, L. M., Lombard, J. A. 1973. *J. Am. Dent. Assoc.* 87:885–87
2. Aetius-Aëtios of Amida. 1542. *The Gynecology and Obstetrics of the VIth Century.* (Transl. from the Latin edition of Coronarius by J. V. Ricci). Cited in Ref. 37
3. Albin, J. B. 1977. *Ment. Retard.* 15:14–17
4. Allan, J. D., Woodruff, J. 1963. *N. Engl. J. Med.* 268:776–78
5. Anel, B., Lagercrantz, S. 1958. *Geographical Customs. Stud. Ethnogr. Upsaliensia* 17:1–84
6. Ansell, J. E., Wheby, M. S. 1972. *VA Med. Mon.* 99:951–54
7. Arcasoy, A., Cavdar, A., Babacan, E. 1978. *Acta Haematol.* 60:76–84
8. Ausman, J., Ball, T. S., Alexander, D. 1974. *Ment. Retard.* 12:16–18
9. Barltrop, D. 1966. *Am. J. Dis. Child.* 112:116–23
10. Barltrop, D., Stehlow, C. D., Thorton, I., Webb, J. S. 1974. *Environ. Health Perspect.* 7:75–82
11. Ber, R., Valero, A. 1961. *Harefuah* 61:35–39
12. Betts, P. R., Astley, R., Raine, D. N. 1973. *Br. Med. J.* 1:402–6
13. Bicknell, D. J. 1975. *Pica A Childhood Symptom.* Southampton, England: Camelot Press. pp. 191
14. Bicknell, J., Clayton, B. E., Delves, H. T. 1968. *J. Ment. Defic. Res.* 12:282–93
15. Blum, M., Orton, C. G., Rose, L. 1968. *Ann. Intern. Med.* 68:1165
16. Boezo, M. H. 1638. *De Pica.* Sm. Lipsiae. Cited in Ref. 37
17. Bott, E., Denton, D. A., Goding, J. K., Sabine, J. R. 1964. *Nature* 202:461–63
18. Bronstein, E. S., Dollar, J. 1974. *J. Med. Assoc. Ga.* 63:332–35
19. Bruhn, C. M., Pangborn, R. M. 1971. *J. Am. Diet. Assoc.* 58:417–20
20. Bucher, B., Reykdal, B., Albin, J. B. 1976. *J. Behav. Ther. Exper. Psychol.* 2:137–40
21. Burchfield, S. R., Elich, M. S., Woods, S. C. 1977. *Psychol. Behav.* 19:265–67
22. Butterworth, W. W. 1909. *J. Am. Med. Assoc.* 53:617
23. Campbell, D. M., Davidson, R. J. L. 1970. *J. Obstet. Gynecol. Br. Commonw.* 77:657–59
24. Carpenter, W. M. 1844. *New Orl. Med. Surg. J.* 1:146–68
25. Catzel, P. 1963. *Pediatrics* 31:1056
26. Cavdar, A. O., Arcasoy, A. 1972. *Clin. Pediatr.* 11:215–23
27. Chandra, P., Rosner, F. 1973. *Ann. Intern. Med.* 78:973–74
28. Chisholm, J. J., Kaplan, E. 1968. *J. Pediatr.* 73:942–50
29. Christopherson, J. B. 1910. *J. Trop. Med.* 13:3–7
30. Clayton, R. S., Goodman, P. H. 1955. *Am. J. Roentgenol.* 73:203–7
31. Cohen, D. J., Johnson, W. T. 1976. *Am. J. Dis. Child.* 130:47–48
32. Coleman, D. L., Greenberg, C. S., Ries, C. A. 1981. *N. Engl. J. Med.* 304:848
33. Coltman, C. A. 1969. *J. Am. Med. Assoc.* 207:513–16

34. Coltman, C. A. 1969. *Nutr. Rev.* 27:244
35. Coltman, C. A. 1971. *Arch. Intern. Med.* 128:472–73
36. Committee on Biologic Effects of Atmospheric Pollutants. 1972. Lead. Washington DC: *Nat. Acad. Sci.* 330 pp.
37. Cooper, M. 1957. *Pica.* Springfield, IL: Charles C. Thomas. 109 pp.
38. Craigin, F. W. 1835. *Am. J. Med. Sci.* 17:365–74
39. Crosby, W. H. 1976. *J. Am. Med. Assoc.* 235:2765
40. Crosby, W. H. 1971. *Arch. Intern. Med.* 127:960–61
41. Danford, D. E., Huber, A. M. 1981. *Appetite.* 2:281–92
42. Danford, D. E., Huber, A. M. 1982. *Am. J. Ment. Defic.* In press
43. Danford, D. E., Smith, J. C., Huber, A. M. 1982. *Am. J. Clin. Nutr.* In press
44. Davis, C. M. 1928. *Am. J. Dis. Child.* 36:651–79
45. Davis, C. M. 1939. *Can. Med. Assoc. J.* 41:257–61
46. de la Burdé, B., Shapiro, I. M. 1975. *Arch. Environ. Health* 30:281–84
47. Dehne, T. 1698. *Inauguralis Medica Appetiti Ventriculi Depravato in Pica et Malacia.* Disertatio. Jenae: Literis Christophori Krebsii. Cited in Ref. 37
48. Delaitre, B., Lemaigre, G., Acar, J. F., Atsamena, M., Bouhroum, A. 1976. *Nouv. Presse Med.* 5:1743–46
49. DeSilva, R. A. 1974. *Ann. Intern. Med.* 80:115–16
50. DiCagno, L., Castello, D., Savio, M. T. 1974. *Minerva Pediatr.* 26:1768–77
51. Dickens, G., Trethowan, W. H. 1971. *J. Psychosom. Res.* 15:259–68
52. Dickins, D., Ford, R. N. 1942. *Am. Sociol. Rev.* 7:59–65
53. Donhoffer, S. 1960. *Triangle* 4:233–39
54. Dupont. 1959. *Union Med. Gironde, Bordeaux* 4:400, 498, 545. Cited in Ref. 37
55. Duprey, A. J. B. 1900. *Lancet* 2:1192
56. Edwards, C. H., McDonald, S., Mitchell, D., Jones, S., Mason, L., Kemp, A. M., Laing, D., Trigg, L. 1959. *J. Am. Diet. Assoc.* 35:810–15
57. Ferguson, J. H., Keaton, A. G. 1950. *New Orleans Med. Surg. J.* 102:460–63
58. Foster, J. W. 1927. *E. African Med. J.* 4:63–76
59. Foxx, R. M., Martin, E. D. 1975. *Behav. Res. Ther.* 13:153–62
60. French, M. H. 1945. *E. African Med. J.* 22:103–10
61. Friedin, B. D., Johnson, H. K. 1979. *J. Ment. Defic. Res.* 23:55–61
62. Fulton, J. 1979. *Aust. Med. J. Melbourne* 1:257
63. Ganong, W. F. 1977. *Review of Medical Physiology.* Los Altos, CA: Lange Med. Publ. pp. 178, 362
64. Gardner, J. E., Tevetoglu, F. 1957. *J. Pediatr.* 51:667–71
65. Garretson, F. D., Conrad, M. E. 1967. *Proc. Soc. Exp. Biol. Med.* 126:304–8
66. Gelfand, M. 1945. *E. African Med. J.* 22:98–103
67. Gelfand, M. C., Zarate, A., Knepshield, J. H. 1975. *J. Am. Med. Assoc.* 234:738–40
68. Gould, A. N. 1876. *Boston Med. Surg. J.* 94:417
69. Graham, D. M. 1978. *Nutr. Rev.* 36:97–102
70. Graham, P. W. 1976. *Med. J. Aust.* 2:385–86
71. Green, H. H. 1925. *Physiol. Rev.* 5: 336–48
72. Green, J., Jones, A. 1968. Los Panecitos Benditos: Clay eating in Oaxca. *Ethnic Techn. Notes No. 2.* San Diego, CA: San Diego Museum of Man, Balboa Park
73. Griscelli, C., Raux, M., Attal, C., Barthelemy, C., Mozziconacci, P. 1970. *Ann. Pediatr. (Paris)* 17:214–19
74. Grivetti, L. E. 1978. *BioScience* 28: 172–73
75. Grivetti, L. E. 1981. *Ann. Rev. Nutr.* 1:47–68
76. Guinee, V. F. 1971. *Nutr. Rev.* 29: 267–69
77. Gumilla, J. 1791. *Historia Natural, Civil y Geographica de Rio Orinoco,* Barcelona. Cited in Ref. 37
78. Gusdon, J. P., Tunca, C. 1974. *Obstet. Gynecol.* 43:197–99
79. Gutelius, M. F., Millican, F. K., Layman, E. M., Cohen, G. J., Dublin, C. C. 1962. *Pediatrics* 29:1012–17
80. Gutelius, M. F., Millican, F. K., Layman, E. M., Cohen, G. J., Dublin, C. C. 1962. *Pediatrics* 29:1018–23
81. Gutelius, M. F., Millican, F. K., Layman, E. M., Cohen, G. J., Dublin, C. C. 1963. *Am. J. Nutr.* 12:388–93
82. Hale, M., Lepow, M. L. 1971. *Conn. Med.* 35:492–97
83. Haley, T. J. 1971. *Clin. Toxicol.* 4:11–29
84. Haller, J. S. 1972. *Med. Hist.* 16:238–53
85. Halsted, J. A. 1968. *Am. J. Clin. Nutr.* 21:1384–93
86. Halsted, J. A., Prasad, A. S. 1960. *Trans. Am. Clin. Climatol. Assoc.* 72: 130–49
87. Halsted, J. A., Ronaghy, H. A., Abadi, P., Haghshnass, M., Amirhakemi, G.

H., Barakat, R. M., Reinhold, J. G. 1972. *Am. J. Med.* 53:277–83
88. Hambidge, K. M., Silverman, A. 1973. *Arch. Dis. Child.* 48:567–68
89. Hancock, J. 1831. *Edinburgh Med. Surg. J.* 35:67–73
90. Hankin, L., Heichel, G. H., Botsford, R. A. 1973. *Clin. Pediatr.* 12:654–55
91. Harries, J. M., Hughes, T. F. 1957. *Proc. Nutr. Soc.* 16:20–21
92. Harris, L. J., Clay, J., Hargreaves, J., Ward, A. 1933. *Proc. R. Soc. Lond. Biol. Sci.* 113:161–90
93. Henderson, F. F., Gaston, E. A. 1938. *Arch. Surg.* 36:66–95
94. Holden, C. 1979. *Science* 204:1066–68
95. Holt, W. A., Hendricks, C. H. 1969. *Obstet. Gynecol.* 34:502–4
96. Hook, E. B. 1978. *Am. J. Clin. Nutr.* 31:1355–62
97. Hooper, D., Mann, H. H. 1906. *Mem. Asiatic Soc. Bengal* 1:249–70
98. Hubrigkt, J. F. 1562. *De Appetitu Depravato Pica Dicto,* Altdorff. Cited in Ref. 37
99. Hunter, J. M. 1973. *Geog. Rev.* 63: 170–95
100. Imray, J. 1843. *Edinburg Med. Surg. J.* 59:304–21
101. Jacobs, A. 1961. *Lancet* 2:1331–33
102. Jacobziner, H., Raybin, H. W. 1962. *Arch Pediatr.* 79:72–76
103. Johnson, N. E., Tenuta, K. 1979. *Environ. Res.* 18:369–76
104. Jolly, H. L. 1963. *Practitioner* 191: 417–25
105. Joselow, M. M., Bogden, J. D. 1974. *Am. J. Public Health* 64:238–40
106. Kalisz, K., Ekvall, S., Palmer, S. 1978. *Pediatric Nutrition in Developmental Disorders,* pp. 150–55. Springfield, IL: Charles C. Thomas
107. Kanner, L. 1937. *Child Psychiatry,* pp. 340–53. Springfield, IL: Charles C. Thomas
108. Karayalcin, G., Lanzkowsky, P. 1976. *Lancet* 2:687
109. Keith, L., Brown, E. R., Rosenberg, C. 1970. *Perspect. Biol. Med.* 13:626–32
110. Keith, L., Evenhouse, H., Webster, A. 1968. *Obstet. Gynecol.* 32:415–18
111. Keith, L. G., Rosenberg, C. D., Brown, E. 1969. *J. Am. Med. Assoc.* 208:535
112. Keith, L., Rosenberg, C., Brown, E., Webster, A. 1969. *Chicago Med. Sch. Q.* 28:109–14
113. Keith, L., Rosenberg, C., Brown, E., Webster, A. 1969. *Proc. Soc. Exp. Biol. Med.* 131:1285–87
114. Kennedy, R. S. 1935. *Brit. Med. J.* 1:1262–64

115. Klein, R. 1974. *Pediatr. Clin. North Am.* 21:277–84
116. Klüver, H., Bucy, P. C. 1939. *Arch. Neurol. Psychiatr.* 42:979–1000
117. Koptagel, G., Reimann, F. 1973. *Psychother. Psychosom.* 22:351–58
118. Lackey, C. J. 1978. *The Anthropology of Health,* pp. 121–29. St. Louis: C. V. Mosby
119. Lanzkowsky, P. 1959. *Arch. Dis. Child.* 34:140–48
120. Larson, P. S., Haag, H. B., Silvette, H. 1961. *Tobacco-Experimental and Clinical Studies,* pp. 491–501. Baltimore: Williams and Wilkins
121. Lasch, R. 1898. *Mitt. Anthropol. Gesellsch.* 28:214–22
122. Laufer, B. 1930. *Field Mus. Natl. Hist. Publ. 280, Anthropol. Ser.* 18:99
123. LeConte, J. 1846. *Southern Med. Surg. J.* 1:417–44
124. Ledelius, J. 1668. *De Pica.* Jenae. Cited in Ref. 37
125. Leming, P. D., Reed, D. C., Martelo, O. J. 1981. *Ann. Intern. Med.* 94:660
126. Levander, O. A. 1979. *Environ. Health Perspect.* 29:115–25
127. Lin-Fu, J. S. 1973. *N. Engl. J. Med.* 289:1229–89
128. Lin-Fu, J. S. 1973. *N. Engl. J. Med.* 289:1289–93
129. Livingstone, D. 1870. *Last Journals,* p. 346. Cited in Ref. 37
130. Lourie, R. S., Layman, E. M., Millican, F. K. 1958. *Problems of Addiction and Habituation.* NY: Grune and Stratton
131. Lourie, R. S., Layman, E. M., Millican, F. K. 1963. *Children* 10:143–46
132. Mahaffey, K. R. 1981. *Nutr. Rev.* 39(10):353–62
133. Maravilla, A. M., Berk, R. N. 1978. *Am. J. Gastro.* 70:94–99
134. Marks, J. W. 1973. *Ann. Intern. Med.* 79:612
135. Mason, D. 1833. *Edinburgh Med. Surg. J.* 34:289–96
136. Mathieu, J. 1927. *Arch. de Med. d. Enf.* 30:591–97
137. Maxwell, J. 1835. *Jamaica Phys. J.* 2:416–27
138. McCollum, E. V., Orent-Keiles, E., Gay, H. G. 1939. *The Newer Knowledge of Nutrition.* NY: Macmillan. pp. 577
139. McDonald, R., Marshall, S. R. 1964. *Pediatrics* 34:558–62
140. McGanity, W. J., Little, H. M., Fogelman, A., Jennings, L., Calhoun, E., Dawson, E. B. 1969. *Am. J. Obstet. Gynecol.* 103:773–88
141. Medhurst, W. H. 1838. *China, Its State and Prospects,* p. 38. Cited in Ref. 37

142. Mengel, C. E., Carter, W. A. 1964. *J. Am. Med. Assoc.* 187:955–56
143. Mengel, C., Carter, W. A., Horton, E. S. 1964. *Arch. Intern. Med.* 114:470–74
144. Merkatz, I. R. 1961. *N. Engl. J. Med.* 265:1304–6
145. Millican, F. K., Layman, E. M., Lourie, R. S. Takahashi, L. Y., Dublin, C. C. 1962. *Clin. Proc. Child. Hosp. (Wash.)* 18:207–14
146. Millican, F. K., Layman, E. M., Lourie, R. S., Takahashi, L. Y. 1968. *J. Am. Acad. Child. Psychiatr.* 7:79–107
147. Minnich, V., Okçuoglu, A., Tarcon, Y., Arcasoy, A., Cin, S., Yörükoglu, O., Renda, F., Demirag, B. 1968. *Am. J. Clin. Nutr.* 21:78–86
148. Mitchell, D., Laycock, J. D., Stephens, W. F. 1977. *Am. J. Clin. Nutr.* 30:147–50
149. Mitchell, D., Wells, C., Hoch, N., Lind, K., Woods, S. C., Mitchell, L. K. 1976. *Physiol. Behav.* 17:691–97
150. Mitra, S. C. 1904–7. *J. Anthropol. Soc. Bombay* 7:284–90
151. Mohan, M., Agarwal, K. N., Bhutt, I., Khanduja, P. C. 1968. *J. Indian Med. Assoc.* 51:16–18
152. Moncrieff, A. A., Koumides, O. P., Clayton, B. E., Patrick, A. D., Renwick, A. G. C., Roberts, G. E. 1964. *Arch. Dis. Child.* 39:1–13
153. Moss, J., Nissenblatt, M. J., Inui, T. S. 1974. *Ann. Intern. Med.* 80:425
154. Mooty, J., Ferrand, C. F., Harris, P. 1975. *Pediatrics* 55:636–39
155. Murty, T. V., Rao, N. N., Bopardikar, K. U. 1976. *Indian Pediatr.* 13:575–76
156. Mustacchi, P. 1971. *J. Am. Med. Assoc.* 218:229–32
157. Nawalkha, P. L., Mehta, M. C. 1972. *J. Assoc. Phys. India* 20:339–41
158. Neil, J., Horn, T. L., Himmelhoch, J. M. 1977. *Dis. Nerv. Syst.* 38:724–26
159. Neumann, H. H. 1970. *Pediatrics* 46:441–44
160. Nutrition Foundation. 1969. *Nutr. Rev.* 27:52–54
161. Ohara, T., Shibata, F. 1969. *Iryo* 23:1248–55
162. Okcuoglu, A., Arcasoy, A., Minnich, V., Tarcon, Y., Cin, S., Yörükoglu, O., Bahtiyar, D., Renda, F. 1966. *Am. J. Clin. Nutr.* 19:125–31
163. Oliver, B. E., O'Gorman, G. 1966. *Develop. Med. Child. Neurol.* 8:704–6
164. O'Brien, W., Arkin, R. M. 1969. *Ann. Intern. Med.* 70:232
165. O'Rourke, D. E., Quinn, J. G., Nicholson, J. O., Gibson, H. H. 1967. *Obstet. Gynecol.* 29:581–84
166. Patterson, E. C., Staszak, D. J. 1977. *J. Nutr.* 107:2020–25
167. Perry, M. C. 1977. *N. Engl. J. Med.* 296:824
168. Podboy, J. W., Mallory, W. A. 1977. *Ment. Retard.* 15:40
169. Postell, W. D. 1951. *The Health of Slaves on Southern Plantations.* Baton Rouge: Louisiana State Univ. Press
170. Prasad, A. S., Halsted, J. A., Nadimi, M. 1961. *Am. J. Med.* 31:532–46
171. Prasad, A. S., Miale, A., Farid, Z., Sandstead, H. H., Darby, W. J. 1963. *Arch. Intern. Med.* 11:407–27
172. Pynoos, R. S., Charrow, J., Gribetz, D. 1978. *Am. J. Dis. Child.* 132:420–21
173. Quarterman, J., Morrison, J. N. 1975. *Brit. J. Nutr.* 34:351–62
174. Reinhold, J. G., Nasr, K., Lahimgarzadeh, A., Hedayati, H. 1973. *Lancet* 1:283–88
175. Reynolds, R. D., Binder, H. J., Miller, M. B., Chang, W., Horan, S. 1968. *Ann. Int. Med.* 69:435–40
176. Richter, C. P. 1947. *J. Comp. Physiol. Psychol.* 40:129–41
177. Richter, C. P., Holt, L. E., Barelare, B. 1937. *Science* 86:354
178. Robischon, P. 1971. *Nurs. Res.* 20:4–16
179. Rodgers, W., Rozin, P. 1966. *J. Comp. Physiol. Psychol.* 61:1–4
180. Ronaghy, H. A., Halsted, J. A. 1975. *Am. J. Clin. Nutr.* 28:831–36
181. Roselle, H. A. 1970. *Arch. Intern. Med.* 125:57–61
182. Ruddock, J. C. 1924. *J. Am. Med. Assoc.* 82:1682–84
183. Sachs, H. K., Blanksma, L. A., Murray, E. F. 1970. *Pediatrics* 46:389–96
184. Sacks, S., Tapia, A., Varela, M., Morales, A. 1971. *Rev. Med. De Chile* 99:848–51
185. Sage, J. C. 1962. *The practice, incidence and effect of starch eating in Negro woman at Temple University Medical Center.* PhD thesis. Temple Univ. Med. Sch., Philadelphia
186. Say, B., Özsöylu, S., Berkel, I. 1969. *Clin. Pediatr.* 8:661–68
187. Sayar, S. N., Sarlatti, R., Naficy, M. 1975. *Acta Med. Iran* 18:137–47
188. Sayers, G., Lipschitz, D. A., Sayers, M., Seftel, H. C., Bothwell, T. H., Charlton, R. W. 1974. *S. A. Med. J.* 53:1655–70
189. Shrand, H. 1964. *Lancet* 1:1357–59
190. Shrimali, R., Jain, A. M., Bhandari, B. 1971. *J. Assoc. Physicians India* 19:285–86
191. Silverman, M., Perkins, R. 1966. *Ann. Intern. Med.* 64:842
192. Sinclair, S., Mittal, S. K., Basu, N.,

Ghai, O. P., Bhide, N. K. 1973. *Indian Pediatr.* 10:13–18

193. Six, K. M., Goyer, R. A. 1970. *J. Lab. Clin. Med.* 76:933–42

194. Six, K. M., Goyer, R. A. 1972. *J. Lab. Clin. Med.* 79:128–36

195. Small, A., Muehlbauer, M., Kleinhaus, S. 1968. *Am. J. Gastroenterol.* 50:297–302

196. Smith, J. C., Halsted, J. A. 1970. *N. Nutr.* 100:973–80

197. Snowdon, C. T., Sanderson, B. A. 1974. *Science* 183:92–94

198. Snowdon, C. T. 1977. *Physiol. Behav.* 18:885–93

199. Sobel, R. 1970. *Pediatr. Clin. N. Am.* 17:653–85

200. Sohler, A., Pfeiffer, C. C. 1977. *J. Am. Med. Assoc.* 238:936–42

201. Solien, N. L. 1954. *Fla. Anthropol.* 7:1–9

202. Spengler, O. 1851. *Wochenschr. Ges. Heilk. Berlin* 321–27

203. Speirs, J., Jacobson, R. 1976. *S. A. Med. Tydskrif.* 58:1742

204. Stephens, R., Waldron, H. A. 1975. *Food Cosmet. Toxicol.* 13:555–63

205. Stephenson, P. E. 1977. *J. Am. Diet. Assoc.* 71:240–47

206. Taggart, N. 1961. *Proc. Nutr. Soc.* 20:35–40

207. Talkington, K. M., Gant, N. F., Scott, D. E., Pritchard, J. A. 1970. *Am. J. Obstet. Gynecol.* 108:262–67

208. Tayanc, M. M. 1942. *Tip Dünyasi* 15:175–77

209. Theiler, A., Green, H. H., Dutoit, P. J. 1924. *J. Dept. Agri. So. Africa* 18:1–47

210. Thomas, F. B., Falko, J. M., Zuckerman, K. 1976. *Gastroenterology* 71:1028–32

211. Thompson, G. J. S. 1913. *17th Intern. Med. Congr. Hist. Med.* 23:433. Cited in Ref. 85

212. Trew, C. J. 1742. *Acta Acad. Nat. Curios. Norimb.* 6:458–64

213. Underwood, E. J. 1966. *The Mineral Nutrition of Livestock.* Scotland: The Central Press. pp. 237

214. Uretsky, B. F. 1974. *Arch. Surg.* 109:123

215. Verga, A. 1849. *Gaz. Med. Lombarda* 2:18–20

216. Vermeer, D. E. 1966. *Assoc. Am. Geog. Ann.* 56:197–204

217. Vermeer, D. E. 1971. *Ethnology* 10:56–72

218. Vermeer, D. E., Frate, D. A. 1975. *Assoc. Am. Geog. Ann.* 65:414–24

219. Vermeer, D. E., Frate, D. A. 1979. *Am. J. Clin. Nutr.* 32:2129–35

220. Vessal, K., Ronaghy, H. A., Zarabi, M. 1975. *Am. J. Clin. Nutr.* 28:1095–98

221. Volpato, S. 1848. *Gaz. Med. Lombarda* 2(1):49–52

222. Von Humboldt, A., Bonpland, A. 1821. *Personal Narrative of Travels to the Equinoctial Regions of the New Continent During the Years 1799–1804.* (Transl. H. M. Williams), London, 5:2. Cited in Ref. 37

223. Wiener, G. 1970. *Public Health Rep.* 85:19–24

224. Woods, S. C., Weisinger, R. S. 1970. *Science* 169:1334–36

Ann. Rev. Nutr. 1982. 2:323–41

CAFFEINE

P. B. Dews

Laboratory of Psychobiology, Department of Psychiatry, Harvard Medical
School, Boston, Massachusetts, 02115

CONTENTS

INTRODUCTION

Caffeine is consumed in varying amounts by most people of the world.
Several million kg of caffeine are consumed annually in the United States
alone, and more than 80% of the adult population consumes caffeine in
some form (33). By reason of its ubiquity it is therefore a component of the
diet that merits consideration by students of nutrition. The most important
nutritional aspects of caffeine are its pharmacokinetics and metabolism and
its effects on physiological systems at levels attained by dietary intakes. The
present review primarily concerns the latter. Possible therapeutic uses and
use in over-the-counter proprietary medicines are of little interest in nutri-

323

0199-9885/82/0715-0323$02.00

tion provided they do not interfere with nutriture in other ways. Since such interference does not seem likely and has not been shown to occur in a nutritionally significant manner, the use of caffeine as a drug is not covered here. The effects at high doses of the variety of pharmacologically active components of the diet is not generally considered nutrition.

The chemistry and pharmacology of coffee and caffeine were recently exhaustively reviewed by Eichler et al (20); readers interested primarily in pharmacologic aspects of caffeine are referred to that volume.

SOURCES AND AMOUNTS IN DIET

Dietary caffeine is overwhelmingly derived from beverages. Chocolate and some confectionery, the only other dietary sources of caffeine, contain only a few mg/100 g. The amount in a cup of coffee or tea obviously varies with the strength of the infusion and the size of the cup. A round figure for the caffeine content of a cup of coffee is 80 mg with an extreme range from about one half to twice that amount. Caffeine-containing soft drinks contain about 0.01% caffeine; a 200 ml serving contains about 20 mg of caffeine.

While estimates of caffeine consumption are not well documented in refereed scientific journals, there seems to be little dispute about the general range (23). As one cup of coffee provides about 1 mg of caffeine per kg of body weight for an adult, amounts of up to 3 mg/kg or so can be taken over relatively short periods. The mean consumption of caffeine by people over 18 in the United States was estimated to be about 2.6 mg/kg per day, and the 90th percentile was 5.4 mg/kg per day; that is, 10% of the population consume more than 5.4 mg/kg per day. Both estimates were lower for younger people. These consumption figures come from a Market Research Corporation of America survey (10). Only in recent years have tissue levels of caffeine been measured with any regularity in studies on caffeine, so for most of the work reported on caffeine we know how much was given rather than what tissue levels were produced. Caffeine, however, is a readily absorbed and freely diffusible substance, so dose is a reliable predictor of tissue level under standardized circumstances—e.g. when a dose is taken as a bolus on an empty stomach. When taken in the usual manner in the diet, however—slowly and often with or after food—peak levels following a given intake are much lower and less predictable. There is a dearth of data on the caffeine loads (concentrations and durations of levels of caffeine in body fluids and tissues) that actually occur in the population.

Axelrod & Reichenthal (3) found a plasma level of about 10 mg/l in three subjects one hour after 7 mg/kg caffeine either intravenously or orally. A 250 mg dose of caffeine in 350 ml fluid taken on an empty stomach by 9 young adults produced a mean peak level in plasma of 12 mg/l, falling to

8 mg/l two hours later (59). When Axelrod & Reichenthal (3) had their subjects drink two cups of 80 mg caffeine/cup coffee at 8 A.M., noon, 3 P.M., and 6 P.M., the highest level attained, at 7 P.M., was only about 4 mg/l. The level was close to zero at 8 A.M. next day. From the results just given, it appears that the levels of caffeine attained by high normal consumers might range up to 5–6 mg/l maintained over a few hours per day. Hence, in looking for physiological effects that may be produced regularly by dietary caffeine, one is concerned about effects that occur at plasma caffeine levels of less than 10 mg/l. Such levels will be produced experimentally by single-bolus doses of less than 10 mg/kg.

EFFECTS ON PHYSIOLOGICAL SYSTEMS

Caffeine and other methylxanthines have been studied since the beginning of scientific pharmacology. They are said to "stimulate the central nervous system"; they cause diuresis, relax various smooth muscles; they have positive inotropic effects on the heart muscle and characteristic effects on skeletal muscles. In the following sections we consider how these classical pharmacological effects, obtained usually with large doses and in anesthetized animals or isolated tissues, relate to intakes of caffeine by persons with sane dietary and beverage habits. We then consider studies on the effects of dietary caffeine on health.

It should be emphasized at the outset that the biological effects of reasonable dietary intakes of caffeine are slight and not easy to detect. The most important effects are behavioral, and even these are undramatic and even subtle.

Central Nervous System (CNS)

The injection of doses of 50 mg/kg and greater in animals causes changes in electrical activity of brain. (33). Such doses lead to levels far beyond those achieved in man by dietary intake. When caffeine is described as a CNS "stimulant" it is usually in reference to behavioral effects rather than to directly recorded changes in CNS activity. Behavioral effects are alterations in the interchanges of a subject with the environment. Many authors use the term "behavioral effects" as though it implied direct CNS effects, but such usage is not logically justified. As the techniques and findings in studies of behavioral effects are currently quite different from those of neuropharmacological studies it is convenient to discuss them separately recognizing that, when enough is known, neurological and behavioral phenomena will no doubt be seen to be intimately related.

Directly recorded CNS effects of levels of caffeine achieved by dietary intakes are not well established; they are certainly not conspicuous. Indeed, neuropharmacological effects do not seem to have been detected in experimental animals following oral ingestion of caffeine. In a recent study in humans, Elkins et al (21) found only equivocal changes in an evoked optical potential in 19 children following a dose of 3 or of 10 mg/kg caffeine in 6 oz of soft-drink. The 10 mg/kg dose taken in this manner produced salivary levels of 10.4 mg/l of caffeine one hour after ingestion. The standard deviation was only 1.2 mg/l, indicating little variability among the subjects.

Effects on the Cardiovascular System

There is a vast literature on pharmacologic effects of caffeine on cardiovascular functions, in which are described relaxation of smooth muscle of blood vessels and positive inotropic effects on heart. Most such studies have involved large doses injected into anesthetized animals or added to tissues in vitro. This work is not reviewed here (see 33). Cardiovascular effects such as increases in blood pressure may be produced by the CNS effects of caffeine. Such CNS-mediated effects, rather than direct effects, are traditionally attributed to the levels of caffeine achieved by dietary intake. However, the mechanisms of such effects, if they occur, are not established and the problem has not been studied with modern neurophysiologic techniques.

In humans, a bolus intake of 250 mg caffeine in 9 normal young adults who did not normally consume coffee (and who were abstaining from tea and chocolate if they normally consumed them) produced unmistakable cardiovascular effects (59). The mean systolic blood pressure rose from about 106 mm Hg to a peak of some 120 mm Hg, the diastolic blood pressure from 75 to 85 mm Hg, at 0.5 to 1.5 hr after ingestion. The heart rate first decreased and then increased. Plasma renin activity and norepinephrine concentration rose significantly. The mean plasma level of caffeine at 1 hr after ingestion approximated 12 mg/l. When subjects were given 250 mg caffeine three times per day for seven days, however, the effects just described ceased to occur (60). Similar bolus doses of 250 mg produced no detectable cardiovascular changes in regular coffee drinkers. Interestingly, when the 750 mg/day caffeine was discontinued no withdrawal symptoms were detected.

Effects on Other Systems

Many studies exist of the pharmacologic effects of caffeine on respiratory, renal, and other systems, but few effects have been demonstrated to occur at levels attained from dietary intakes. In the study by Robertson et al (59) described above, both respiratory and renal effects of the 250 mg bolus dose were found. The mean respiratory rate increased from 13.4/min one hour after placebo to 16.1/min one hour after caffeine. This increase was correlated with the plasma caffeine level, being insignificant when the level was less than 5 mg/l. In the same study, 3-hr collections of urine averaged 366 ml after placebo and 469 ml after caffeine. Bolus intubation of 250 mg caffeine into the stomach increased gastric secretion of acid (61), and 150 or 300 mg into the jejunum or by mouth changed the the fluid exchange in a segment of jejunum or ileum from net absorption to net secretion (74).

BEHAVIORAL EFFECTS

Acute Behavioral Effects in Experimental Animals

Behavioral effects of caffeine have been measured in mice, rats, and monkeys after parenteral doses as low as 1–3 mg/kg. In mice, for example, effects on "discrimination learning" in an underwater Y-maze were described by Castellano (11) at doses of 1 and 2 mg/kg. While the effects reported are unlikely to have been changes in "learning" as suggested by author, they were nonetheless effects on behavior. Reports of consequences at lower doses do not carry convinction. There is one claim of a detectable behavioral alteration in mice with a dose of 0.2 mg/kg (68), but scrutiny of the results does not reveal the alleged effect and the same laboratory reported subsequently in comparable tests that 50 mg/kg caffeine were required to induce changes. (69). Castellano (11) found no effects at 0.5 mg/kg. Kallman & Isaac (43) found altered activity in rats to result from 2 mg/kg caffeine, the alterations being consistent in old and young animals studied in the light or dark. No dose lower than 2 mg/kg was studied. Higher doses (up to 32 mg/kg) caused progressively greater effects. Responding under schedule control by either FI or a postponement schedule was increased by 1, 3, and 10 mg/kg of caffeine in squirrel monkeys (14). The consistency in the doses of caffeine in mg/kg causing behavioral effects in the different species is unusual among drugs. It is interesting to note the similarity of acute toxicity of caffeine in a variety of species (see below).

Effects on Performance in Humans

With levels of caffeine achieved by even high dietary intakes it is hard to detect changes in subjects already performing well. Restorative changes in degraded performance can be measured, however. Goldstein et al (29) write:

> Adequately designed experiments have shown unequivocally that caffeine (and also amphetamine) counteracts the decrement in various kinds of performance that is caused by fatigue or sleep deprivation. The evidence is much less convincing (and often contradictory) as to whether or not these drugs are capable of enhancing performance over control levels. Where physical endurance and capacity are required (as in athletic performance), such enhancement has been shown [for amphetamine]. There is also some indication that caffeine can increase the normal threshold frequency at which flicker fusion occurs [(54, 46)] but carefully designed experiments have also yielded negative results [(19)]. In the case of tasks requiring motor coordination, monitoring (alertness), or intellectual activity, the preponderance of data is negative.

In their own experiments on a group of 20 medical students working under competitive conditions, Goldstein et al (29) found that "Caffeine (150 mg or 300 mg) had no demonstrable effect upon either objectively measured performance [alertness or psychomotor coordination] although at the same time it made the subjects feel more alert and physically active."

After a comprehensive and authoritative review of studies in humans, Weiss & Laties (76) concluded that caffeine did not improve intellectual performance "except, perhaps, when normal performance has been degraded by fatigue or boredom." Weiss & Laties addressed the problem of whether caffeine can enhance optimal performance of any kind. They, too, found no convincing evidence that caffeine appreciably enhanced any performance already optimal for the subject. These investigators also asked whether the restoration of degraded performance by caffeine exacts a psychological "price"—for example by leading to impaired judgment, or to a subsequent "letdown" to still more degraded performance—and concluded that no detectable "price" is paid after either acute or chronic use of caffeine.

While the effects of caffeine in restoring human performance toward optimal levels are undoubtedly real and consistent, it must be emphasized again that the effects are small. They are well within the range of effects produced by a variety of everyday arousing and alerting influences: changes of environment, noises, cool draughts, pungent smells, and the like.

Effects on Sleep

The function most sensitive to modification by caffeine in adult humans is that of going to sleep. Sleep postponement in human adults has been detected following bolus intakes of about 100 mg caffeine 0.5 hr before retiring, but not at lower intakes. The results of three published studies are shown in Figure 1.

There is a general presumption that certain individuals are peculiarly sensitive to caffeine, being rendered sleepless or "nervous" by quite small amounts, and there is abundant anecdotal testimony to support the notion. However, there is noticeably little hard quantitative information; indeed, it seems the more careful and objective the study, the less gross the detected variability. The similarity of effective doses in many species would not lead one to expect large differences within a species.

An informative experiment was performed by Goldstein and his colleagues on 20 medical students (30). On 10 occasions each subject before retiring to bed drank decaffeinated coffee to which had been added lactose on 5 occasions and 300 mg caffeine on 5 occasions in random sequence and without the subject knowing which had been added. On all 10 following mornings the subjects estimated how long it had taken them to fall asleep. In every subject, the mean estimated time to fall asleep on the 5 caffeine

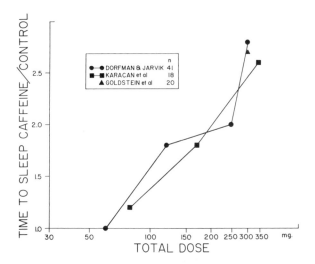

Figure 1 Delay of sleep by caffeine. Caffeine or placebo was taken blindly 0.5 hr before retiring, and the time required to go to sleep was assessed by questionnaire next morning. The delay was expressed as the ratio of mean time to go to sleep after caffeine divided by the mean time on the noncaffeine days. The figure shows the remarkable concordance between the three quite independent studies and also that the effects were slight below 100 mg total dose and undetectable below 80 mg total dose (17, 30, 44).

nights was longer than that on the 5 lactose nights. The mean estimated time that sleep was postponed, however, varied greatly in the 20 subjects from a low of 1.8 min to a high of 53.6 min. But there was also great variability in the estimated time to sleep under the placebo condition, the mean time being 12.2 min with a coefficient of variation of 56%. After caffeine, the mean estimated time was 31.8 min with coefficient of variation of 59%. Thus the caffeine did not appreciably increase the variability in mean estimated time to go to sleep, suggesting a relatively uniform rather than a highly variable response to caffeine.

Yet variability there was. For example, one subject reported a time to sleep of 240 min on one caffeine night, though never reporting more than 45 min on any of the 5 lactose nights; the same subject reported a 15 min time to sleep on another caffeine night. Evidently time to go to sleep was influenced by other factors as much or more than by the presence or absence of caffeine. As has been described, the effect of caffeine on performance is highly dependent on the condition of the subject with respect to fatigue or boredom. While caffeine may consistently establish a tendency, the manifest effect is determined largely by amplification by additional factors. Influences such as slight discomfort, nonoptimal temperature, or noise can postpone sleep and may greatly amplify the effects of caffeine. Even in careful studies, most amplifiers are not identified or controlled, and their

effects are attributed to "innate differences" largely by default. The putatively large individual differences in response to caffeine are probably due
mostly to environmental factors. Such innate differences as do exist may be
exaggerated by strong expectations of large effects of caffeine and by limitations of intake with consequent less tolerance.

Acute Behavioral Effects in Children

Most of the information on effects of caffeine in children concerns subjects
diagnosed as hyperkinetic. Neither the therapeutic effects nor the side
effects of caffeine in such children are impressive, even at doses with clearly
detectable effects in adult humans and animals (21).

Elkins et al (21) studied the effects of 3 mg/kg and 10 mg/kg caffeine
given in a single 6 oz drink to 19 normal prepubertal boys. Salivary levels
(which have been shown to correspond well to plasma levels) were measured in some of the children one hour after ingestion of the caffeine. They
averaged 3.1 mg/l after the 3 mg/kg dose and 10.4 mg/l after the 10 mg/kg
dose. Ratings of mood, side effects, and behavior were made. The children's
activity was assessed by means of an inertial device they wore on their belts.
Visual evoked potentials (EP) in the EEG to 4 light intensities were assessed. Reaction times were measured. Sustained attention (Vigilance Test)
was assessed with a Continuous Performance Test, which permitted recording of errors of both omission and commission and also rapidity of response
to stimuli. A simple memory test was conducted. Finally, blood pressure,
heart rate, and epinephrine and norepinephrine in urine were measured.
The children received mean total doses of 100 mg for the low dose and 369
mg for the high dose. The effects of the 3 mg/kg dose were equivocal. With
the high dose reaction time decreased slightly, omissions decreased on the
Vigilance Test, and activity increased. There were no effects on EPs. No
effects were detected on blood pressure, heart rate, or catecholamine excretion. On some of the tests, scores after 3 mg/kg were between those for
placebo and 10 mg/kg, suggesting a trend and that 3 mg/kg might be
approaching an active dose. Even the high dose caused no significant change
in side effects as a whole. There was a suggestion that a subgroup of 5
children who did not usually consume caffeine showed a slight increase in
side effects. Fidgetiness may have increased. To put these findings in context
of dietary intakes, the 3 mg/kg dose represented an intake of about a quart
of soft drink over the course of a few minutes. The findings of Elkins et al
(21) are of particular interest in view of an oft-quoted comment in a standard textbook of pharmacology (Goodman & Gilman's *The Pharmacological Basis of Therapeutics*) that "Children are more susceptible than adults
to excitation by xanthines" (58). No authority is cited for this opinion,
which was repeated verbatim in the text's first five editions (32, 58). Never-

theless, children appear to be less, and certainly no more, sensitive to measured effects of caffeine than adults, and the clinical reports on hyperkinetic children support such a conclusion (21). Rall (57), writing on methylxanthines in the 6th edition of *The Pharmacological Basis of Therapeutics* makes no claim that children are more susceptible.

Effects of Chronic Intake

Chronic behavioral effects of caffeine have been seen in experimental animals with intakes large enough to cause relatively nonspecific debilitating effects. For example, Estler et al (22) gave mice 150 mg/kg daily caffeine in the drinking water for six weeks. To obtain such high intakes, the concentration in drinking water has to be so high that animals reduce fluid intake, which in turn interferes with food intake. These authors found serious reduction in weight gain of their treated mice as compared to the controls. It is hardly surprising that such debilitated mice performed less well than the controls in swimming performance in cold water. The mice were taking, according to the authors, almost half the acute LD50 of caffeine each day. Even these massive daily doses of caffeine did not have major behavioral effects; the spontaneous motor activity of the treated mice was similar to that of the controls. The lack of information on dose-effect relations in these studies makes extension to lower doses impossible.

In an experiment to see whether dependence on caffeine followed chronic intake, Vitiello & Woods (73) forced rats to drink caffeine solutions at concentrations of 0.17, 0.34, or 0.5 mg/ml for 14 days by making the solutions the only source of drinking water for the experimental groups. Paired controls drank water. The rats were then given for 8 days free choice between the concentration of caffeine they had been drinking, mocha-flavored water (as flavored control for the caffeine), and plain water. If the rats that had been drinking caffeine-solutions were dependent on caffeine it was expected that they would drink more of the caffeine solution to suppress withdrawal symptoms than rats that had not been drinking caffeine-solution. The rats that had been forced to drink caffeine solutions of concentrations of 0.17 or 0.34 mg/ml did not differ, however, in their subsequent choice among the three proffered solutions from rats previously drinking plain water, although the 0.34 mg/ml rats drank more mocha-flavored water. Rats that been drinking 0.5 mg/ml (i.e. intakes of more than 50 mg/kg/day) drank statistically less of the mocha-flavored water than controls. They drank more caffeine solution than their controls, but the difference was not statistically significant. In view of the decrease in intake of mocha-flavored water, the modest increase in intake of caffeine solution could not be attributed to an effect of withdrawal from caffeine. When the control rats for the 0.5 mg/ml group were subsequently forced to drink 0.5

mg/ml caffeine and then given a choice, they too drank significantly less mocha-flavored water. "It is noteworthy" the authors write, "that the rats did not prefer the flavor associated with the caffeine, even on the first day of the free choice period, for there is considerable evidence indicating that the after-effects of drugs are readily associated with flavors." The experiments therefore found no evidence of dependence or withdrawal symptoms from caffeine. It may be noted that the difference between 0.34 mg/ml and 0.5 mg/ml is so small that the increase in consumption of mocha-flavored water in the 0.34 mg/ml group casts serious doubt on the reliability of the decreased consumption by the 0.5 mg/ml group. In any case, the absence of sequelae to intakes of over 50 mg/kg/day is reassuring when the 90th percentile of the distribution of caffeine intakes by humans is about 5.4 mg/kg daily.

HEALTH-RELATED EFFECTS OF CAFFEINE

The previous section concerned measurable effects of dietary caffeine regardless of health consequences. In this section we review studies that have sought to identify any harmful effects of caffeine.

Acute Toxicity

The LD50 of caffeine is fairly consistently approximately 200 mg/kg from species to species (66). It is interesting that it varies little with route of administration; even the intravenous LD50 is only a little lower than the values for oral, subcutaneous, or intraperitoneal administration (66). The consistency is doubtless due to the rapid absorption and distribution of caffeine.

Available evidence suggests that the amount per kg necessary for lethal toxicity in man is not dissimilar from that in experimental animals. Banner & Czajka (4) found case reports in the literature of four adults who had succumbed to caffeine poisoning with post-mortem blood caffeine levels of 1,040, 158, 106, and 79 mg/l. Caffeine has been used in the treatment of apnea in neonates. It was not known at first that neonates metabolize caffeine slowly (1), so the calculated doses of caffeine led to much higher body levels of caffeine than expected. Banner & Czajka (4) report four neonates who received intravenous and intramuscular doses of caffeine of 36–136 mg/kg over a few days. One of the babies developed a plasma caffeine concentration of 80 mg/ml. After a few days there were no detectable sequelae in any of the babies. The authors also report the case of a child who survived a plasma concentration of 190 mg/l caffeine. None of 18 sick infants treated with caffeine for apnea showed detectable sequelae (2). Their plasma levels of caffeine ranged up to 85 mg/l. Only one infant, with a level of 60 mg/l, showed even transient jitteriness attributable to the caffeine (A. H. Neims, personal communication). Such levels are much beyond those that result from ingestion of caffeine in the diet and are sufficient to cause definite effects in experimental animals. There appears to be no acute danger to life from intakes of caffeine attainable from the diet.

At lower levels bolus intakes of caffeine up to 200–400 mg produce such effects as decreased fatigue or decreased ennui resulting in restored performance. With still higher acute doses, the incidence of side effects increases: "Nervousness, feverishness, irritability, headache, and disturbed sleep" are reported (76). These relatively short-lived symptoms are unpleasant rather than indicative of danger and people would probably not tolerate them if they occurred regularly with ordinary intakes. While our information is limited on the levels of plasma caffeine to which people regularly subject themselves through beverage intake, they must rarely attain levels as high as those resulting from bolus doses of 400 mg.

Significant acute toxicity, such as frankly abnormal irritability, requires doses of about 30 mg/kg in rhesus monkeys (P. B. Dews, personal observation); if humans are similarly susceptible, such effects will not be seen with dietary intakes.

Deleterious cardiovascular effects in mice under certain living conditions have been described by Henry and his colleagues (37). When mice were crowded and competed for food and water, blood pressure and blood urea nitrogen were chronically increased, and more mice died than in control cages. Adding caffeine to the drinking water, either as such or as brewed coffee or tea to yield transitory plasma caffeine levels of the order of 6–9 mg/l, exacerbated the deleterious effects of crowding and competition (38). Humans could attain levels of 6–9 mg/l caffeine by dietary intake. The exacerbation by caffeine intake of the increase in blood pressure and blood urea nitrogen was seen only at 3 months in the experimental situation, however, and had disappeared at 5 months even though crowding and caffeine were maintained. The deleterious effects were attributed to the "psychosocial stress" of crowding and competition, which was aggravated by caffeine. Crowding of animals may influence them in many ways besides imposing psychosocial stress, however—for example, by increasing the transmissibility of infections. Chronic interstitial nephritis occurred in the mice, a condition more commonly associated with infection than as a consequence of hypertension. The deleterious effects of crowding and competition on murine cardiovascular function were described as early as 1967 (36).

There have been epidemiological inquiries into the cardiovascular effects of chronic consumption of caffeine. According to the Boston Collaborative Drug Surveillance Program (BCDSP) patients brought into hospital with a myocardial infarction reported higher coffee intakes than did matched controls (42). The surveillance program used hospital records as a means of finding leads to possible associations. A case-control study by Klatsky et al (45) found no such association. In the Framingham study, a prospective longitudinal study of 5209 people that began in 1949, caffeine consumptions of 4492 subjects were assessed by questions of examining physicians, starting 6 years after the beginning of the study. No association between caffeine and any cardiovascular disease was found (15). Another case-control study by Hennekens et al (35) concluded that "the risk, if any, of death from coronary heart disease associated with coffee drinking is small." No relation between coffee intake and blood pressure was found in IBM employees by Bertrand et al (6). The consensus seems to be that the BCDSP finding was a false positive. It appears that the routine proscripion by many physicians of caffeine-containing beverages for patients with cardiovascular diseases, notably myocardial infarction, is based on tradition rather than sound evidence.

Reproductive Effects

In many studies maternal caffeine intakes above (usually much above) 50 mg/kg per day in rodents proved to be deleterious to pregnancy and to the health of the offspring (56). Levels that convincingly affect reproduction approach those that cause maternal toxicity. There is little evidence of selectivity in the lesions in the offspring; that is, no particular deformity seems to result from caffeine administration. Particular deformities—e.g. the phocomelia of thalidomide—are generally regarded as the hallmarks of a true teratogen. Nonspecific interference with reproductive capability is a common consequence of maternal toxicity, and dozens, if not hundreds, of substances are known capable of producing teratogenic effects at high dosage in rats and mice. Most have never been implicated as teratogens in humans (71, 64, 77). Consequently, the demonstration of interference with reproduction by a substance in high dosage in rodents usually means little in terms of human effects at ordinary levels of exposure. One effect of caffeine in pregnant rats that seems to be well established is a delay in calcification of fetal bones during the latter part of pregnancy. This effect has been described as occurring at doses lower than those causing nonspecific effects (56, 55). Ectrodactyly has also been reported in rodents (7).

The possibility has been investigated that caffeine ingestion during pregnancy may produce changes in the behavior of the offspring even though no structural or other functional changes are detectable. Two studies have addressed this problem, one in rats and one in mice (65, 16). In neither was there evidence that caffeine, at doses lower than those causing nonspecific reproductive effects, produced significant deleterious behavioral effects on the offspring.

A number of reports contain information about possible effects of caffeine on human reproduction. A study on 202 malformed babies and 175 normal control babies from a population of 17,979 births suggested that heavy coffee consumption was commoner in the mothers of the malformed babies than in the mothers of normal babies (8). The differences were not impressive. The incidence of malformed babies of women less than 35 years of age who consumed more than 8 cups of coffee per day during pregnancy was 1.07 times the incidence in women who did not drink coffee. No dose-response relationship was established. Further, the information about coffee consumption was obtained after the children were born. Epidemiologists are aware that a mother who has borne a malformed baby is more susceptible to selective recollection of events in pregnancy than is the mother of a normal baby. Finally, the total incidence of severe malformations in the population of 17,970 births was only about one third to one half the incidence reported in other studies (72), so the sampling appears to have been biased.

In a study of babies born in the Kaiser-Permanente hospitals, a crude risk-ratio estimate of 1.3 for all severe congenital anomalies was associated with consumption during pregnancy of 7 or more cups as compared to less than one cup of coffee per day (72). The value 1.3 was not statistically significantly different from 1. The study did find a statistically significant deleterious effect of smoking. A study intended primarily to assess effects of alcohol consumption during pregnancy on outcome found no significant effect of caffeine consumption (67). No association was found between neonate malformations and mother's use of caffeine-containing medications during pregnancy (34).

Only one report has claimed a large effect of caffeine on reproduction (75). The study exhibited many serious defects of sampling and reporting. Its claim that 15 of 16 pregnancies in women who consumed more than 600 mg/day caffeine ended in disaster in one way or another is grossly discrepant from all other studies.

Casual consideration might suggest that the question of whether caffeine consumption has any effect on pregnancy outcome could be settled by a definitive epidemiological study. Unfortunately such may not be the case. Present evidence (e.g. 72) is sufficient to indicate that the association, if present, is slight. Caffeine consumption, however, is associated with a whole variety of influences related to life style, any one or combination of which could affect pregnancy outcome. Mau & Netter (50), who found that women with high coffee consumption more often than nonconsumers had children with small birth weight, concluded "It is nevertheless questionable whether a direct causal relationship exists. Based on other findings, the hypothesis is discussed that the habits of alcohol and coffee consumption are an indicator for a certain constitutional and character type." To the extent that any features of life style with deleterious influences on pregnancy are positively correlated with caffeine consumption, epidemiological studies on caffeine consumption in relation to adverse outcomes of pregnancy would show a positive association, even if caffeine itself in dietary amounts were without effect on pregnancy. Further insight into the effects of caffeine on reproduction is likely to come, not from epidemiological studies, which by nature are not powerful in establishing lack of risk, but from basic research on the physiology of reproduction and embryonic development. When normal mechanisms are known, it is possible to study directly whether additional influences have an effect.

Carcinogenesis

Several studies have been published of long-term administration to rodents of caffeine as such or as coffee in amounts up to the "maximum tolerated level" (79, 78, 56, 70, 5, 49). None of them showed caffeine to be a carcinogen.

In humans, a weak association between coffee consumption and cancer of the lower urinary tract has been reported (13, 9, 62, 51), but further investigations indicate that the association, when it exists, is not due to a causal relation between caffeine and cancer (26, 53, 63) but is due to an association between caffeine consumption and other causal factors.

Of particular interest with respect to caffeine are two recently published case-control studies on pancreatic cancer. One of them identified several factors that were associated with pancreatic cancer, including consumption of decaffeinated coffee but not of untreated coffee (47). The second found an association between pancreatic cancer and coffee drinking but not tea drinking (48). Both studies, therefore, indicate that caffeine itself is not a causative factor.

Fibrocystic Disease of the Breast

Considerable public interest has been generated by a report of effects of methylxanthine consumption on fibrocystic disease of the breast (52). Forty-seven women with clinical fibrocystic disease of the breast were instructed to stop all methylxanthine consumption. Twenty reported that they did stop and 13 of these experienced complete disappearance of all palpable breast nodules and other symptoms within 1–6 months. Only one of the 27 women who said they continued methylxanthine consumption experienced resolution of her disease. Impressive as these figures are as they stand, it must be recognized that they represent no more than clinical impressions. The groups were self-selected, and the assessment was subjective. The results of an uncontrolled clinical study on a disease with a notoriously variable and fluctuating natural history cannot be accepted as scientific evidence (39). Another completely uncontrolled study (8a) to which the same criticisms apply has been published as confirmation of the Minton study. A controlled study published in abstract by Ernster et al (21a) did suggest, however, that reduction in caffeine intake was positively related to reduced fibrocystic breast disease, although the change was "minor and may be of little clinical significance." Part of the concern over fibrocystic disease has arisen from a fear that it may be precancerous. A review by Ernster et al (21b), which suggests that benign breast disease is not a significant predictor of breast cancer, somewhat allays the fear.

Tolerance and Withdrawal

It is generally accepted that regular consumption of caffeine leads to tolerance to its effects. Goldstein (28) reported that caffeine caused distinctly less wakefulness in subjects who habitually drank a great deal of coffee, although even regular coffee drinkers reported sleeping less soundly after 300 mg caffeine than after placebo (29). A comparison of effects of morning caffeine on 18 housewives who were not coffee drinkers with 38 who drank 5 or more cups daily also showed divers differences in the effects on abstainers and consumers (31). Small but significant differences were demonstrated in both frequency and intensity of effects of 150 mg caffeine on pulse rate and sleep between regular caffeine consumers (more than one cup of caffeine-containing beverage per day) and nonconsumers (no more than one cup per day). Caffeine consumers showed a greater tendency to bradycardia and less tendency to disturbed sleep following caffeine. In all these studies abstainers and consumers were self-selected; if more susceptible subjects chose to abstain and less susceptible subjects chose to consume, the observed differences could result without there being a change in susceptibility to caffeine consequent upon consumption. However, the studies of Robertson et al (60) discussed earlier demonstrate unequivocally the development of tolerance in individual subjects.

It is also generally accepted that regular caffeine consumers develop withdrawal headache during the course of a day on which no caffeine is taken. Many years ago, Dreisbach & Pfeiffer (18) gave subjects increasing doses of caffeine in capsules, up to 780 mg; and then one day, without the subjects' knowledge, gave them a capsule containing no caffeine. In 32 out of 38 trials in the 22 subjects, a headache was reported on the placebo day, and in 21 trials the headache was severe. A withdrawal syndrome starting 12–16 hours after the last intake of caffeine was reported by the regularly consuming subjects in the study of Goldstein et al (31). In addition to headache, the consuming subjects complained of being less alert, less active, more sleepy, less content or at ease, more irritable, jittery, nervous, and shaky than abstainers. All these symptoms were promptly relieved by caffeine. The list of statistically significant differences between consumers and abstainers is impressively long, though the syndrome itself was mild and inconstant. No signs of withdrawal were detected by Robertson et al (60) following seven days of 250 mg caffeine three times per day.

ARE THERE BENEFITS OF CAFFEINE CONSUMPTION?

Caffeine is a component of the diet that can produce pharmacologic effects. It is not unique in this regard, as a number of regular dietary components can cause pharmacologic effects (25, 24, 12, 27, 40, 41). Most people of the world elect to imbibe caffeine-containing beverages, thus providing prima facie evidence of perceived benefit. The smooth functioning of industrialized society is associated with people working about eight hours, eating and playing about eight hours, and sleeping about eight hours, with everybody more or less in phase, no matter what their internal rhythms might urge. Perhaps most people appreciate a little help in initiating the work phase; hence the widely accepted practice of consuming a caffeine-containing beverage at or before breakfast as part of the ritual of preparing for work. Some also need help through the work session, so that breaks have been institutionalized when caffeine-containing beverages are often consumed which, along with the alerting effects of change in activity itself, may help restore efficiency. It is surely true that people may harm themselves, their performance, and perhaps in other ways, with excessive intakes of caffeine; but gross overconsumption of any article of diet can be harmful. The deleterious effects of excess intake of caffeine, within some limit, seem to be transient and completely reversible.

ACKNOWLEDGMENT

Preparation of this review was greatly helped by access to a document submitted to the Food and Drug Administration by the International Life Sciences Institute in July, 1981. In particular, I would like to express my indebtedness to the contributions to that document of H. Grice, A. Levitan, and W. Scott. Support of grants from the U.S. Public Health Service (MH02094, MH07658, DA00499, DA02658 and MH14275) is also gratefully noted. I thank my colleague W. H. Morse for his help and Mrs. R. Share for preparation of the manuscript.

CAFFEINE   339

Literature Cited

1. Aldridge, A., Aranda, J. V., Neims, A. H. 1979. Caffeine metabolism in the newborn. *Clin. Pharmacol. Ther.* 25: 447–53
2. Aranda, J. V., Gorman, W., Bergsteinsson, H., Gunn, T. 1977. Efficacy of caffeine in treatment of apnea in the low birth weight infant. *J. Pediatr.* 90:467–72
3. Axelrod, J., Reichenthal, J. 1953. The fate of caffeine in man and a method for its estimation biological material. *J. Pharmacol. Exp. Therap.* 107:519–23
4. Banner, W., Czajka, P. 1980. Acute caffeine overdose in the neonate. *Am. J. Dis. Child.* 134:495–98
5. Bauer, A. R. Jr., Rank, R. K., Kerr, R., Straley, R. L., Mason, J. D. 1977. The effects of prolonged coffee intake on genetically identical mice. *Life Sci.* 21: 63–70
6. Bertrand, C., Pomper, I., Hillman, G., Duffy, J. C., Michell, I., 1978. No relation between coffee and blood pressure. *N. Engl. J. Med.* 299:315–16
7. Bertrand, M., Girod, J., Rigaud, M. F. 1970. Ectrodactyly caused by caffeine in rodents. Effect of genetic and specific factors. *C. R. Soc. Biol.* 159:2199–201
8. Borlee, I., Lechat, M. F., Bouckaert, A., Mission, C. 1978. Coffee, risk factor during pregnancy? *Louvain Med.* 97: 279–84
8a. Brooks, P. G., Gart, S., Heldfond, A. J., Margolin, M. L., Allen, A. S. 1981. Measuring the effect of caffeine restriction on fibrocystic breast disease. *J. Reprod. Med.* 26:279–82
9. Bross, D. J., Tidings, J. 1973. Another look at coffee drinking and cancer of the urinary bladder. *Prev. Med.* 2:445–51
10. Burg, A. W. 1977. Comments on the health aspects of caffeine, especially the contribution of soft drinks, with particular reference to the report of the Select Committee on GRAS Substances. Testimony presented for A.D. Little, Inc. before the Select Committee on GRAS Substances at a public hearing on caffeine, Bethesda, Md.
11. Castellano, C. 1976. Effects of caffeine on discrimination learning, consolidation and learned behavior in mice. *Psychopharmacology* 48:255–60
12. Chiel, H. J., Wurtman, R. J. 1981. Short-term variations in diet composition change the pattern of spontaneous motor activity in rats. *Science* 213: 676–78
13. Cole, P. 1971. Coffee drinking and cancer of the lower urinary tract. *Lancet* 1:1335–37

14. Davis, T. R. A., Kensler, C. J., Dews, P. B. 1973. Comparison of behavioral effects of nicotine, d-amphetamine, caffeine and dimethyheptyl tetrahydrocannabinol in squirrel monkeys. *Pharmacologia* 32:51–65
15. Dawber, T. R., Kannel, W. B., Gordon, T. 1974. Coffee and cardiovascular disease. Observations from the Framingham Study. *N. Engl. J. Med.* 291: 871–74
16. Dews, P. B., Wenger, G. R. 1979. Testing for behavioral effects of agents. In *Test Methods for Definition of Effects of Toxic Substances on Behavior and Neuromotor Function. Neurobehav. Toxicol.* 1: (Suppl. 1) 119–27
17. Dorfman, L. J., Jarvik, M. E. 1970. Comparative stimulant and diuretic actions of caffeine and theobromine in man. *Clin. Pharmacol. Therap.* 11: 869–72
18. Dreisbach, R. H., Pfeiffer, C. 1943. Caffeine-withdrawal headache. *J. Lab. Clin. Med.* 28:1212–19
19. Dureman, E. I. 1962. Differential patterning of behavioral effects from three types of stimulant drugs. *Clin. Pharmacol. Therap.* 3:29–33
20. Eichler, O. 1976. *Kaffee und Coffein.* Berlin: Springer. 491 pp.
21. Elkins, R. N., Rapoport, J. L., Zahn, T. B., Buchsbaum, M. S., Weingartner, H., Kopin, I. J., Langer, D., Johnson, C. 1981. Acute effects of caffeine in normal prepubertal boys. *Am. J. Psychiatry* 138:178–83
21a. Ernster, V. L., Mason, L., Sacks, S., Selvin, S. 1981. Effects of caffeine-free diet on benign breast disease. *Am. J. Epidemiol.* 112:421
21b. Ernster, V. L. 1981. The epidemiology of benign breast disease. *Epidemiologic Reviews* 3:184–202
22. Estler, C. J., Ammon, H.P.T., Herzog, C. 1978. Swimming capacity of mice after prolonged treatment with psychostimulants. *Psychopharmacology* 58: 161–66
23. FASEB. 1978. Select Committee on GRAS Substances. Evaluation of the health aspects of caffeine as a food ingredient. SCOGS-89. Bethesda, MD: Fed. Am. Soc. Exp. Biol.
24. Fernstrom, J. D., Faller, D. V. 1977. Neutral amino acids in the brain: Changes in response to food ingestion of carbohydrate diet. *J. Neurochem.* 30:1531–3823
25. Fernstrom, J. D., Wurtman, R. J. 1971. Brain serotonin content: Increase fol-

lowing ingestion of carbohydrate diet. *Science* 174:1023–25

26. Fraumeni, J. F., Scotto, J., Dunham, L. J. 1971. Coffee-drinking and bladder cancer. *Lancet* 2:1204

27. Gibson, C. J., Wurtman, R. J. 1978. Physiological control of brain norepinephrine synthesis by brain tyrosine concentration. *Life Sci.* 22:1399–406

28. Goldstein, A. 1964. Wakefulness caused by caffeine. *Naunyn-Schmiedebergs Arch. Exp. Pathol. Pharmakol.* 248:269–78

29. Goldstein, A., Kaizer, S., Warren, R. 1965a. Psychotropic effects of caffeine in man. II. Alertness, psychomotor coordination and mood. *J. Pharmacol. Exp. Therap.* 150:146–51

30. Goldstein, A., Warren, R., Kaizer, S. 1965b. Psychotropic effects of caffeine in man. I. Individual differences in sensitivity to caffeine-induced wakefulness. *J. Pharmacol. Exp. Therap.* 149:156–59

31. Goldstein, A., Kaizer, S., Whitby, O. 1969. Psychotropic effects of caffeine in man. IV. Quantitative and qualitative differences associated with habituation to coffee. *Clin. Pharmacol. Therap.* 10:489–97

32. Goodman, L. S., Gilman, A. 1941. *The Pharmacological Basis of Therapeutics.* NY: MacMillan

33. Graham, D. M. 1978. Caffeine: Its identity, dietary sources, intake and biological effects. *Nutr. Rev.* 36:97–102

34. Heinonen, O. P., Slone, D., Shapiro, S. 1977. *Birth Defects and Drugs in Pregnancy.* Littleton, MA: PSG Publ.

35. Hennekens, C. H., Drolette, M. E., Jesse, M. J., Davies, J. E., Hutchison, G. B. 1976. *N. Engl. J. Med.* 294:633–36

36. Henry, J. P., Meehan, J. P., Stephens, P. M. 1967. The use of psychosocial stimuli to induce prolonged systolic hypertension in mice. *Psychosom. Med.* 29:408–32

37. Henry, J. P., Stephens, P. M. 1977. Stress, health and the social environment. NY: Springer. 282 pp.

38. Henry, J. P., Stephens, P. M. 1980. Caffeine as an intensifier of stress-induced hormonal pathophysiologic changes in mice. *Pharmacol. Biochem. Behav.* 13:719–27

39. Heyden, S. 1980. Coffee and fibrocystic breast disease. *Surgery* 88:741–42

40. Hirsch, M. J., Growdon, J. H., Wurtman, R. J. 1978. Relations between dietary choline or lecithin intake, serum choline levels, and various metabolic indices. *Metabolism* 27:953–60

41. Hirsch, M. J., Wurtman, R. J. 1978. Lecithin consumption increases acetylcholine concentrations in rat brain and adrenal gland. *Science* 202:223–25

42. Jick, H., Miettinen, O. S., Neff, R. K., Shapiro, S., Heinonen, O. P., Slone, D. 1973. Coffee and myocardial infarction. *N. Engl. J. Med.* 289:63–67

43. Kallman, W. M., Isaac, W. 1975. The effects of age and illumination on the dose-response curves for three stimulants. *Psychopharmacologia* 40:313–18

44. Karacan, I., Thornby, J. I., Anch, A. M., Booth, G., Williams, R. L. 1976. Dose-related sleep disturbances induced by coffee and caffeine. *J. Clin. Pharmacol. Therap.* 20:682–89

45. Klatsky, A. L., Friedman, G. D., Siegelaub, A. B. 1973. Coffee drinking prior to acute myocardial infarction. *J. Am. Med. Assoc.* 226:540–43

46. Landgrebe, B. 1960. Vergleichende Untersuchungen mit dem Fleinmertest nach coffeinhaltigem und coffeinfreien Kaffee. *Med. Welt,* 27/28:1486–90

47. Lin, R. S., Irving, P. H., Kessler, I. I. 1981. A multifactorial model for pancreatic cancer in man. *J. Am. Med. Assoc.* 245:147–52

48. MacMahon, B., Yen, S., Trichopoulos, D., Warren, K., Nardi, G. 1981. Coffee and cancer of the pancreas. *N. Engl. J. Med.* 304:630–33

49. Macklin, A. W., Szot, R. J. 1980. Eighteen month oral study of aspirin, phenacetin and caffeine in C57Bl/6 mice. *Drug Chem. Toxicol.* 3:135–63

50. Mau, G., Netter, P. 1974. Kaffee- und Alkoholkonsum—Risikofaktoren in der Schwangerschaft? *Geburtsh. Frauenheilk,* 34:1018–22

51. Mettlin, C., Graham, S. 1979. Dietary risk factors in human bladder cancer. *Am. J. Epidemiol.* 110:255–63

52. Minton, J. P., Abou-Issa, H., Reiches, N., Roseman, J. M. 1979. Clinical and biochemical studies on methylxanthine-related fibrocystic breast disease. *Surgery* 86:105

53. Morgan, R. W., Jain, M. G. 1974. Bladder cancer: smoking, beverages and artificial sweeteners. *Can. Med. Assoc. J.* 111:1067–70

54. Mucher, H., Wendt, H. W. 1951. Gruppenversuch zur Bestimmung der kritischen Verschmelzungsfrequenz beim binokulären Sehen: Änderungen unter Koffeine und nach normaler Tagesarbeit. *Naunyn-Schmiedebergs Arch. Exp. Pathol. Pharmakol.* 214:29

55. Nolen, G. A. 1981. The effect of brewed and instant coffee on reproduction and

teratogenesis in the rat. *Toxicol. Appl. Pharmacol.* 58:171–83

56. Palm, P. E., Arnold, E. P., Rachwall, P. C., Leyczek, J. C., Teague, K. W., Kensler, C. J. 1978. Evaluation of the teratogenic potential of fresh-brewed coffee and caffeine in the rat. *Toxicol. Appl. Pharmacol.* 44:1–16

57. Rall, T. W. 1980. In *Pharmacological Basis of Therapeutics,* ed. A. G. Gilman, L. S. Goodman, A. Gilman. NY: Macmillan. 6th ed.

58. Ritchie, J. M. 1975. In *Pharmacological Basis of Therapeutics,* ed. L. S. Goodman, A. Gilman, NY: Macmillan. 1704 pp. 5th ed.

59. Robertson, D., Frolich, J. C., Carr, R. K., Watson, J. T., Hollifield, J. W., Shand, D. G., Oates, J. A. 1978. Effects of caffeine on plasma renin activity, catecholamines and blood pressure. *N. Engl. J. Med.* 298:181–86

60. Robertson, D., Wade, D., Workman, R., Woosley, R. I. 1981. Tolerance to the humoral and hemodynamic effects of caffeine in man. *J. Clin. Invest.* 67:1111–17

61. Roth, J. A., Ivy, A. C. 1944. The effect of caffeine upon gastric secretion in dog, cat and man. *Am. J. Physiol.* 141:1431–61

62. Schmauz, R., Cole, P. 1974. Epidemiology of cancer of the renal pelvis and ureter. *J. Natl. Cancer Inst.* 52:1431–34

63. Simon, D., Yen, S., Cole, P. 1975. Coffee-drinking and cancer of the lower urinary tract. *J. Natl. Cancer Inst.* 54:587

64. Schardein, J. L. 1976. *Drugs as Teratogens.* Cleveland: CRC Press

65. Sobotka, T. J., Spaid, S. L., Brodie, R. E. 1979. Neurobehavioral teratology of caffeine exposure in rats. *Neurotoxicology* 1:403–16

66. Spector, W. S., ed. 1956. Caffeine. In *Handbook of Toxicology. Vol. 1. Acute Toxicities.* Philadelphia: W. B. Saunders

67. Streissguth, A. P., Barr, H. M., Martin, D. C., Herman, C. S. 1980. Effects of maternal alcohol, nicotine, and caffeine use during pregnancy on infant mental

and motor development at eight months. *Alcoholism: Clin. Exp. Res.* 4:152–64

68. Takagi, K., Watanabe, M., Saito, H. 1971. Studies of the spontaneous movement of animals by the hole cross test; Effect of 2-dimethyl-aminoethanol and its acyl esters on the central nervous system. *Jpn. J. Pharmacol.* 21:797–810

69. Takagi, K., Saito, H., Lee, C., Hayashi, T. 1972. Pharmacological studies on fatigue I. *Jpn. J. Pharmacol.* 22:17–26

70. Thayer, P. S., Kensler, C. J. 1973. Exposure of four generations of mice to caffeine in drinking water. *Toxicol. Appl. Pharmacol.* 25:169–79

71. Tuchmann-Duplessis, H. 1975. Screening methods for dysmorphogens. In *Drug Effects on the Fetus.* NY/London: Adis Press. pp. 79–86

72. van den Berg, B. J. 1977. Epidemiologic observations of prematurity: effects of tobacco, coffee and alcohol. In *The Epidemiology of Prematurity,* ed. D. M. Reed, F. J. Stanley. Baltimore/Munich: Urban and Schwarzenberg

73. Vitiello, M. V., Woods, S. C. 1975. Caffeine: preferential consumption by rats. *Pharmacol. Biochem. Behav.* 3:147–49

74. Wald, A., Back, C., Bayless, T. M. 1976. Effect of caffeine on human small intestine. *Gastroenterology* 71:738–42

75. Weathersbee, M. S., Olsen, L. K., Lodge, J. R. 1977. Caffeine and pregnancy: a retrospective survey. *Postgrad. Med.* 62:64–69

76. Weiss, B., Laties, V. G. 1962. Enhancement of human human performance by caffeine and the amphetamines. *Pharmacol. Rev.* 14:1–36

77. Wilson, J. G. 1977. Embryotoxicity of drugs in man. In *Handbook of Teratology,* ed. J. G. Wilson, F. C. Fraser, 1:309–55. NY: Plenum

78. Wurzner, H. P., Lindstrom, E., Vuataz, L. 1977. A 2-year feeding study of instant coffees in rats. II. Incidence and types of neoplasms. *Food Cosmet. Toxicol.* 15:289–96

79. Zeitlin, B. R. 1972. Coffee and bladder cancer. *Lancet* 1:1066

Ann. Rev. Nutr. 1982. 2:343–69

ABSORPTION AND TRANSPORT OF COBALAMIN (VITAMIN B$_{12}$)

Bellur Seetharam and David H. Alpers

Division of Gastroenterology, Washington University School of Medicine, St. Louis, Missouri 63110

CONTENTS

I. PERSPECTIVES AND SUMMARY

This review apprises the reader of recent advances in cobalamin absorption and transport since 1970. This field has been of interest to gastroenterologists, hematologists, and biochemists as well as nutritionists. Clinical condi-

343

0199-9885/82/0715-0343$02.00

tions leading to cobalamin deficiency present especially to the first two of these specialties. Many recent advances involve biochemical definition of the specific transport proteins themselves. Full understanding of the multiple clinical conditions associated with cobalamin deficiency requires some knowledge of these proteins. We do not discuss every paper in the field, especially the early literature (see 47, 61, 150).

Despite rapid strides in understanding the mechanism of absorption and transport of cobalamin both in prokaryotic and eukaryotic cells, the complete sequence of events during cellular absorption at the plasma membrane level and events in the cells that mediate intracellular movement of cobalamin have not been elucidated completely. Here we emphasize the current state of knowledge about cobalamin absorption and transport in man and other mammalian systems, particularly the physiological role and biochemical nature of proteins involved (intrinsic factor, intrinsic factor-cobalamin receptor, transcobalamins).

II. INTRODUCTION

A. Historical Background

The saga of vitamin B_{12} began more than 150 years ago. Between 1824 and 1900 Combe (32) and Addison (1) described "idiopathic anemia," later characterized by Fenwick (52) as the inability (caused by infection or toxins) of acidified scrapings of diseased mucosa to digest hard-boiled eggs. Studies in the early 1900s by Howard Whipple (167), Minot (112), Whipple & Robscheit-Robbins (168), Cohn et al (31) and others lead to the concept that pernicious anemia was due to a nutritional deficiency resulting in decreased red blood cells. Cohn and his associates later prepared a liver extract, administration of which elevated levels of reticulocytes in anemic patients.

In the late 1920s Castle (27) and his associates demonstrated the presence in normal human gastric juice of an "intrinsic factor" that readily combined with an "extrinsic factor" contained in animal protein and resulted in the absorption of an "antipernicious principle." Further identification and isolation of the "antipernicious principle" from liver extracts was a slow process until 1948, when Randolph West (166) proved the clinical activity of crystalline cobalamin isolated by Rickes et al (130a). The discovery by Shorb (147) and Hutner et al (88) that *Lactobacillus lactis* and *Euglena gracilis* required cobalamin for their growth helped to establish a reliable microbial assay for cobalamin, which tool greatly facilitated the purification and isolation of cobalamin.

B. Types of Vitamin B_{12} (Cobalamin, cbl)

Cobalamin is a complex water-soluble molecule (mol wt 1357) essential to the health of all higher animals and some microorganisms. Its structure contains four reduced pyrrol rings linked together and designated "corrin" because they are the core of the molecule. All compounds containing this ring are called corrinoids. The prefix "cob" designates the presence of a cobalt atom. The term cobalamin now denotes those cobamides that play a role in human and mammalian metabolism, the name vitamin B_{12} those corrinoids demonstrating activity in microorganisms and/or mammals. The chemist sometimes uses the term vitamin B_{12} to refer only to cobalamin (Figure 1) where the x group is cyano, or cyanocobalamin. Above the corrin in the cobalamin structure other axial ligands coordinating the central cobalt can be found, such as OH (hydroxy cobalamin), H_2O (aquacobalamin), CH_3 (methylcobalamin), or 5'-deoxyadenosyl (adenosyl cobalamin). The planar tetrapyrrol corrin ring is substituted with acetamide (CH_2CONH_2) and propionamide ($CH_2CH_2CONH_2$) residues at the R and R' positions, respectively. Below the corrin, 1-α-D ribofuranosyl-5-6 dimethyl benzimidazoyl-3-phosphate is present and is linked to the rest of the

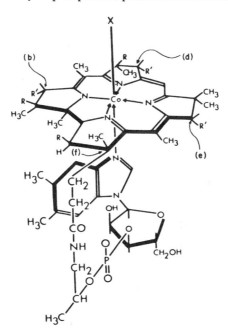

Figure 1   Cobalamin structure. X denotes the beta substituent. R and R' refer to acetamide and proprionamide side chains located on the periphery of the corrin ring.

molecule at two points: (*a*) a phosphodiester linkage to a 1 amino-2 propanol substituent on the propionamide (f), and (*b*) through a coordination linkage to the central cobalt via one of its nitrogens.

The naturally occurring vitamins in man are methyl and adenosyl cobalamins. Since the most stable form chemically is cyanocobalamin, it is the one available for medical use. It must be converted in the body to one of the naturally occurring forms. Compounds lacking the nucleotide moiety are called cobinamides. So far all cobinamides found to be active in human metabolism (cobalamins) have included the nucleotide moiety. Analogs of cobalamins (designated vitamin B_{12} analogs) that are used by bacteria may lack either the ribosyl or amino propanol groups or may have substitutions in these structures. Details of the chemistry, structure, and synthesis of all forms of vitamin B_{12} have been reviewed elsewhere (84, 150).

C. Biological Reactions Involving Cobalamin

In all eukaryotic cells intracellular cobalamin exists mainly in two forms: (*a*) methyl cobalamin found principally in the cytoplasm, and *(b)* adenosyl cobalamin found mainly in mitochondria. These two are cofactors for enzymatic reactions.

The only known reaction mediated by methyl cobalamin in mammalian systems involves the biosynthesis of methionine. In this reaction a methyl group is transferred from a donor N^5-methyl tetrahydrofolate to an acceptor homocysteine, giving rise to methionine. The enzyme concerned is 5-methyl tetrahydrofolate homocysteine methyl transferase. Anaerobic bacteria and acetate-producing bacteria can utilize methyl cobalamin to produce methane and acetate.

Adenosyl cobalamin on the other hand is responsible for two types of reactions: (*a*) intramolecular rearrangements mediated by mutases, and (*b*) formation of aldehydes catalyzed by dehydrases. In mammalian systems methylmalonyl coenzyme A mutase converts methylmalonyl coenzyme A to succinyl coenzyme A, and leucine 2,3-amino mutase converts leucine to beta-leucine (126a). In anaerobic bacteria glutamate mutase converts L glutamate to beta-methyl aspartate. The dehydrases on the other hand, are mostly present in aerobic bacteria and utilize adenosyl cobalamin to convert ethyleneglycol and glycerol to acetaldehyde and glyceraldehyde.

Another reaction in bacteria (e.g. lactobacilli) utilizing adenosyl cobalamin involves the conversion of ribonucleotides to 2' deoxyribonucleotides. This reaction is mediated by the enzyme ribonucleotide reductase and is important in the formation of deoxyribonucleotides.

The interrelationship between cobalamin coenzymes and 5-methyltetrahydrofolate in the formation of methionine is of vital importance. During the formation of methionine from homocysteine, 5-methyltetrahydrofolate is converted to tetrahydrofolate. In the absence of cobalamin the rate of that reaction falls, accompanied by an accumulation of 5-methyltetrahydrofolate. This leads to the inability to form other folic acid vitamers, such as 10-formyl- and 5,10-methylene-tetrahydrofolate, which are required for purine and pyrimidine synthesis. Lack of these vitamers leads to megaloblastic anemia. This hypothesis, known as the methyl folate trap (118), has been the subject of much debate and experimentation; and no clear-cut evidence is available to prove that trapping of 5-methyltetrahydrofolate actually occurs as a result of failure to convert homocysteine to methionine by the cobalamin-dependent methyl transferase.

Indirect evidence has been offered by Scott et al (141a) who have shown in monkeys exposed to nitrous oxide that subacute combined degeneration of the spinal cord develops, and that this lesion can be minimized by maintaining the methionine pool with supplemental dietary methionine. Scott & Weir (141b) have further discussed the hypothesis that kwashoirkor as well as subacute combined degeneration might be related to a deficiency of available methyl groups.

D. Dietary Sources

Cobalamin is made only by microorganisms in nature. Feces are a rich source since colonic microorganisms make large amounts of the vitamin. The usual dietary sources of cobalamin are meat and meat products and to a lesser extent milk and milk products. Fruits and vegetables have very little or no cobalamins, and hence vegans and other strict vegetarians probably derive their limited intake from foods or water contaminated with microorganisms contained in manure. Cobalamin biosynthesized in the colon is not absorbed there. All strict vegetarians slowly develop cobalamin deficiency.

Cobalamin present in foods is stable to high temperatures encountered during cooking but becomes labile if ascorbic acid is also present in the heated diet. The dominant forms present in foodstuffs are the enzymatically active forms—i.e. adenosyl and methyl cobalamins, generally linked to polypeptides.

E. Nutritional Requirements

The recommended dietary allowance (RDA) for cobalamin for an adult is 3 μg (56). However, the requirements in patients may vary due to changes in the gastrointestinal tract, since damage either by a gastrectomy or ileal resection would eliminate normal absorption. Scott & Weir (141), Sullivan & Herbert (155), and others (13, 93) have confirmed the earlier studies of the Vanderbilt group (17a, 40a) that 0.5–1 μg of the vitamin given parenterally daily provides maximum hematologic response. Using radioactive cobalamin, the daily turnover has been shown to be about 0.02% of the body stores (1 μg lost from 5000 μg stores), and hence deficiency of cobalamin in an adult takes months to occur. However, an enterohepatic circulation of cobalamin is present and accounts for delivery of approximately 5–10 μg/day into the intestinal lumen. The cobalamin in bile is thought to be bound to R protein (see below). Therefore, when malabsorption is present, daily losses may exceed 5 μg/day, and deficiency occurs more rapidly. Normal serum and liver levels of cobalamin are over 200 pg/ml and over 0.28 mg/gm liver.

The joint FAO/WHO expert group (50) recommends daily intakes of 2 μg, 0.9 μg, and 3–4 μg for adults, children (1–3 years), and pregnant women, respectively. These compare with the RDAs of 3.0 μg, 2.0 μg, and 4.0 μg for these physiologic categories, respectively.

F. Deficiency Manifestations in Humans

The initial symptoms that follow prolonged deficiency of cobalamin are pallor, weakness, fatigue, dyspnea on exertion, paraesthesias, and a sore tongue. Deficiency also causes patchy or diffuse and progressive demyelinization, producing neuropathy. In most patients one or more of these symptoms predominate. Severely anemic patients may evidence cardiac failure. Loss of appetite, diarrhea, skin disorders, and loss of hair may occur in more depleted patients.

The occurrence of macrocytic anemia is typical in cobalamin deficiency; macrocytosis appears early, the erythrocytes being larger than normal, varying in size, but with normal hemoglobin saturation. The bone marrow is megaloblastic as opposed to the usual normoblast pattern. Because of decreased conversion of ribonucleotides to deoxyribonucleotides the cells have a higher RNA/DNA ratio.

Neuropathy usually leads to symmetrical paresthesias in feet and fingers and is due to a generalized demyelinization of nervous tissue. The process begins in peripheral nerves and progresses centrally to involve posterior and lateral columns of the spinal cord and the brain. Loss of memory, irritability, and abnormalities of smell and taste are observed. Even though cobalamin deficiency commonly causes structural damage in two major organ systems the two groups of symptoms are not always manifested together (164).

III. ABSORPTION OF COBALAMIN (cbl) IN HUMANS AND OTHER ANIMALS

A series of complex events takes place before the dietary cobalamins can be delivered for intracellular utilization. Three phases of this process are now well described: (a) the gastric phase involves release of dietary cobalamin and complexing of the released cobalamin with R protein, a glyco-protein secreted by stomach and salivary glands. (*b*) In the intestinal luminal phase, cobalamin is transferred from R protein to intrinsic factor. This transfer is mediated by pancreatic proteases. (*c*) In the mucosal phase, the intrinsic factor-cobalamin complex attaches to ileal mucosal receptors, a necessary step before the cobalamin can be absorbed.

A. Gastric Phase

1. GASTRIC RELEASE OF DIETARY COBALAMIN   Cooper & Castle (34) demonstrated that the low pH of the stomach and peptic digestion release most of the protein-bound cobalamin in food. The acid peptic digestion of food protein–bound cobalamin appears to be a necessary step for the release of cobalamin in some circumstances, since patients with hypo or achlor-hydria, or partially gastrectomized patients, fail to absorb egg [^{57}Co]-cyanocobalamin (44). However, most patients with cobalamin deficiency after gastric surgery also have insufficient intrinsic factor (135). The absence of gastric proteolysis alone probably rarely causes deficiency, because the cobalamin bound to proteins in food can also be released by the pancreatic proteases.

2. COBALAMIN BINDING TO R PROTEIN AND INTRINSIC FACTOR (IF)
    R proteins are a family of cobalamin binding proteins that move more rapidly than intrinsic factor on electrophoresis (63, 65). These R proteins are present in gastric juice (64) and in saliva (15), from which they have been purified (6, 19) and shown to bind cobalamin at both acidic and neutral pH (7). Allen et al (7) further showed that human salivary R protein–bound cobalamin with an affinity that was 50- and 3-fold higher than those of human intrinsic factor (IF) at pH 2 and pH 8.0, respectively. Even coba-lamin bound to IF was transferred to an equal amount of R protein with $T_{1/2}$'s of 2 and 90 minutes at pH 2 and pH 8.0, respectively, whereas the reverse reaction did not occur. Digestion of R protein and R protein-cobalamin complex with pancreatic proteases led to a 150-fold decrease in the affinity of R protein for cobalamin and a complete transfer of cobalamin to intrinsic factor in 10 minutes. These observations are of considerable physiological importance and are discussed in Section III B.
    In the absence of R proteins, binding of cobalamin (cbl) to IF is rapid (78) and occurs over a range of pH values from 3 to 9 (7, 131). The binding is stable; the complex can be broken only with 5 M guanidine hydrochloride and alkaline buffers (66). Binding of cbl induces conformational changes resulting in the formation of IF dimers and oligomers (5, 6). Affinity of binding for cbl is independent of the nature of the axial ligand X (Figure

1). Change in the structure of either corrin ring side chains or the nucleotide portion to produce analogs of cobalamin results in a decrease in affinity for IF, but does not alter the affinity for R proteins. Unlike R protein, pure hog IF or IF-cbl is stable to proteolysis.

3. PROPERTIES, SYNTHESIS AND SECRETION OF R PROTEINS   Immunologically identical proteins that bind cbl have been identified in leukocytes and in plasma and other biological fluids. Various R-type proteins have different electrophoretic mobilities because of the different number of sialic acid residues.

The R proteins of gastric mucosa and salivary glands appear to be synthesized in mucosal cells of each organ and probably are not derived from granulocytes (87). In leukocytes the R protein is mainly associated with secretory granules (95, 148). In vitro release is inhibited by the sulfhydryl inhibitor N-ethylmaleimide (36) and by sodium fluoride (140) and activated by lithium (140) and the calcium ionophore A23187 (149). The R proteins of normal human plasma are of two types: transcobalamin I (TC I) and transcobalamin III (TC III). The former binds to anion exchange resins tightly and the latter weakly (20). TC I contains more sialic acid residues and fewer fucose residues than TC III (20). TC I is 70–100% saturated with cobalamin and accounts for 80–90% of the total endogenous vitamin content in normal plasma (72, 85). Both TC I and TC III are immunologically identical, exhibit heterogeneity, and have been thought to be released from granulocytes. It has not been conclusively proven that TC III and granulocyte R protein are identical, though they appear to have similar elution profiles on DEAE cellulose, carbohydrate composition, and other properties (26). Moreover, using isoelectric focusing Hall (73) has shown that the R protein released from granulocytes was not TCI but TC III.

R proteins have been purified from saliva, milk, normal granulocytes, and human hepatomas. Based on their amino acid compositions all these proteins have a molecular weight of around $60–66 \times 10^3$. A review comparing the various R proteins has recently been published (92).

4. PROPERTIES OF INTRINSIC FACTOR   Using the technique of affinity chromatography (3) Allen & Mehlman have obtained a very pure intrinsic factor from human gastric juice (5). It has a molecular weight of $42–45 \times 10^3$ and 15% carbohydrate per milligram of protein. It has a single cobalamin binding site with an association constant of 1.5×10^{10} M^{-1}. Intrinsic factor found in the gastric mucosa of several other animal species (46) appears to have similar physical properties. Hog intrinsic factor purified by Allen & Mehlman (6) has a molecular weight of $52–57 \times 10^3$ with 17% carbohydrate. IF from both human and hog can bind about 30 μg of cbl per mg protein.

Human IF has serine as its N terminal amino acid. The N terminal 27 amino acids have been identified (121, 159). Cyanogen bromide cleavage of human IF (116) resulted in four fragments only one of which contained a tyrosine residue. This paucity of tyrosine residues could be the reason for the difficulties observed in the radioiodination of IF.

5. SYNTHESIS AND SECRETION OF INTRINSIC FACTOR   Using the technique of immunofluorescence (90, 91) and autoradiography with [^{57}Co]cbl (83) IF has been localized in the parietal cells of the cardiac and fundic regions. Donaldson and his coworkers (146) have shown that radiolabelled IF can be isolated from cultures of rabbit gastric mucosal biopsies incubated with [^{3}H]leucine or [^{35}S]methionine. Using electron microscopic immunocytochemistry Levine et al (106) suggested that in human and guinea pig, IF was associated with the rough endoplasmic reticulum of parietal cells. IF was not located in the contents of secretory granules. IF is presumably transported to the tubulo-vesicular system before secretion into the lumen.

The presence of food in the stomach stimulates the secretion of IF (40, 55). This secretory response is attributed in part to vagal and in part to hormonal stimulation. Atropine (163) blocks the basal IF secretion, and insulin stimulation of vagal activity increases IF secretion (11). Vagotomy decreases both basal and stimulated secretion of IF (111, 162). Atropine abolishes the increase in acetylcholine-induced output of IF in organ cultures of rabbit gastric mucosa (96). Histamine and pentagastrin administered either intramuscularly or intravenously stimulate IF secretion (89, 104), but this increase may be due either to an actual increase of newly synthesized IF or to a "washout" effect of IF already present in parietal cells. Peak IF secretion usually precedes peak acid secretion in tissue (23, 94). Histamine H2-receptor antagonists reduce both basal and stimulated levels of IF (16, 53). However, it is unlikely that such treatment would lead to cobalamin deficiency, since the reduction of IF is only partial. An interesting possibility is that IF may be synthesized as a high molecular weight precursor that is then converted to mature IF in the cell by protease treatment. Such a preprotein has been described for many other secretory proteins.

B. Intestinal Luminal Phase

Cobalamin bound to R proteins in the stomach must be made available to IF before it can be absorbed because R protein does not mediate cobalamin absorption. Okuda (120), Vonderlippe (165), and Toskes (161) suggested that pancreatic proteases might inactivate an endogenous inhibitor allowing cbl to be bound to IF. Allen et al (7) extended this concept and showed that pancreatic proteases such as trypsin and chymotrypsin can partially degrade both free R protein and R protein-cbl complexes. This process releases cbl that will eventually be bound to IF. Both [^{125}I]-R protein and R protein-[^{58}Co]cbl complex with an apparent molecular weight of 150,000 are converted to proteins of lower molecular weight (7). This partial degradation releases cbl. Based on these in vitro observations it was suggested that cbl malabsorption in pancreatic insufficiency (7) was due to a failure to partially degrade R protein to which cbl binds with much greater affinity, especially at acid pH. Allen et al (8) further extended their in vitro studies on patients with pancreatic insufficiency. They showed that cobinamide, an analog of cobalamin that binds to R protein with an affinity much greater than for IF, could correct cbl malabsorption in these patients without the addition of proteases. In such a situation most of the R proteins would preferentially bind cobinamide, and cbl would be free to bind to IF. The Schilling tests carried out on these patients using [^{57}Co]cbl either with the cbl analog or trypsin gave normal results. It was concluded that the transfer of cbl from R protein to IF was a normal physiological event. Thus both in vitro and in vivo experiments demonstrate the role of pancreatic proteases in the release of cbl bound to R proteins.

Based on these observations Burgge et al (22) have developed an absorption test for diagnosing pancreatic insufficiency. In this test equal amounts of either [^{57}Co]- or [^{58}Co]cbl are bound to IF and to R proteins. Normal subjects absorb and excrete in the urine equal amounts of both isotopes. In pancreatic insufficiency the isotope bound to R protein is unavailable since it is not transferred to IF. Thus the ratio of excreted isotopes will vary. Although this test is no more complex to perform than a regular Schilling test, it is not yet commercially available.

Marcoullis et al (110) have extended the observations of Allen et al (7, 8) and showed that ingested ^{57}[Co]cbl assayed in jejunal aspirates is bound to IF in normal healthy volunteers and largely to R protein in patients with pancreatic insufficiency. Nicolas et al (117) proposed the "inhibited cobalamin absorption theory" to explain the observations of Allen et al (7, 8). They further demonstrated that IF-cbl complex traverses the human intestinal tract without any structural alterations. Anderson & Von der Lippe have provided further evidence for the protease sensitivity of R proteins (9).

However, some preliminary reports (152, 153) have raised questions about the hypothesis of Allen et al, since incomplete correlations were observed between cobalamin malabsorption and levels of trypsin or chymotrypsin activity or gastric acidity. In addition, cobinamide was not always effective in correcting cbl malabsorption in all patients. In our opinion these reports do not invalidate the overall scheme outlined above for transfer of cbl from R proteins to IF. It is possible, however, that pancreatic proteases are not the only intraluminal factor that affects the binding of cobalamin to intrinsic factor. Some evidence exists that bile acids may be one of these factors.

A role for bile in the absorption of cbl was suggested by Teo et al (157) when they observed that some patients with obstructive jaundice and T-tube bile duct drainage malabsorbed cbl. The malabsorption was corrected by replacing bile in the T-tube. However, in vitro studies (158) carried out by the same group showed that there was a time- and concentration-dependent inhibition of cbl binding to IF rather than the enhancement predicted by the in vivo studies. Inhibition was a function of dihydroxy bile salts and not trihydroxy bile salts. In order to explain these conflicting results Teo et al proposed the hypothesis that bile salts may bind to the excess free IF present in the intestinal lumen. They argue that such binding might prevent the excess free IF from competing with the IF-cbl for attachment to ileal receptors.

This hypothesis appears to be incorrect since free IF does not bind to the receptor even when present in 100-fold excess (86). Moreover, for their in vitro experiments Teo et al used crude gastric juice as a source of IF. Coronato & Glass (37) have shown an effect of bile salts on the receptor molecule present in the ileal mucosa but not on IF itself. The physiological role, if any, of bile acids in the sequence of events leading to absorption of cbl is still unclear.

C. Mucosal Phase

1. IN VITRO STUDIES   Cobalamin is absorbed in the ileum (17, 30), and Herbert (77) suggested that the absorption of cbl was by means of specialized receptors for IF-cbl complex in the ileum. The presence of ileal binding and presumed receptors has been confirmed from various animal species (38, 39, 70, 108). In humans, binding is present over the entire ileum or second half of the small intestine. In fact the terminal ileum does not contain the most active binding (70). Partially purified receptor fractions have been obtained from various animal species (38, 39, 108).

Kouvonen & Grasbeck (102, 103) have obtained relatively pure receptor for IF-cbl from guinea-pig homogenates and have shown that it has a molecular weight of 200×10^3. However, the purity of receptor was not ascertained by protein stains on electrophoresis. Seetharam et al (142) obtained highly purified homogeneous receptor from canine ileal mucosa in large enough quantities to define the protein. They showed that the receptor has a molecular weight of 220×10^3 and is comprised of two subunits of molecular weight 62×10^3 and 48×10^3. They further showed that free cbl, free IF, and abnormal IF-cbl R-cbl does not bind to the receptor. The canine receptor had little or no carbohydrate and the receptor did not cross-react with anti-IF antibody. In both of these properties it appears that the canine receptor is different from the partially purified porcine and human receptors (103). However, it is possible that these latter preparations contain other proteins, including possibly IF. Using an artificial bilayer (143) the receptor has been shown to be oriented in such a way that greater than 70% of the protein mass and all of the IF-cbl binding sites were on the outside surface. The receptor thus is probably anchored to the membrane by a relatively small hydrophobic anchor piece. Using papain, Seetharam et al (144) have purified the water-soluble IF-cbl binding unit of the receptor from canine mucosa and have shown that this fraction of the receptor has a molecular weight of $180–190 \times 10^3$. The remaining fragment of molecular weight about 36×10^3 probably represents the anchoring structure of the receptor. The topology of the canine receptors as proposed by Seetharam et al (144) is at variance with that proposed by Kouvonen & Grasbeck (103) for porcine and human receptor. The main differences between the studies is the molecular weight of the functional unit (IF-cbl binding) and anchoring units of the receptor. The canine receptor has a functional unit of molecular weight around 180,000 whereas the molecular weight of the proposed functional unit in porcine and human receptor is 70,000. However, this proposed functional unit of 70,000 molecular weight has not yet been directly shown to bind IF-cbl.

2. IN VIVO STUDIES   Even though the nature and structure of IF and its receptor are now well documented, the sequence of events that follow the binding of IF-cbl to receptor is largely unknown. After the attachment of IF-cbl to the receptor there is a delay of up to 3–4 hours before cbl enters the circulation (29, 34, 80). One of the early studies by Rosenthal et al (133) showed that in guinea pigs peak radioactivity was associated with microsomes and mitochondria 1.5 hr after an oral dose of [^{57}Co]CNcbl. Cytosolic radioactivity peaked only after 4 hr. The role of mitochondria in transintestinal transport was confirmed by the work of Peters et al (123) and Peters & Hoffbrand (122). These workers concluded that cobalamin was not absorbed by pinocytosis since no significant amount of radioactivity was detected in the lysosomal fraction. Using everted sacs Hines et al (80) showed that after the attachment of IF-cbl to the receptor only cbl enters the enterocyte, leaving free IF on the cell surface that could accept additional cobalamin. Since free IF does not bind to the receptor, these data suggest the interesting possibility that after discharging its cbl from the IF-cbl complex, the remaining IF is in some way modified to remain bound to the receptor. Using the technique of immune electron microscopy Levine et al (105) concluded that IF is not internalized during absorption. Supporting this concept is the observation of Cooper & White (35), who failed to demonstrate IF in the portal circulation. On the other hand, Kapadia et al

(97) have shown that labelled rabbit IF does penetrate the enterocytes and is present in the cytosol. Using ileal loops Kapadia et al (98) have demonstrated that IF-cbl is absorbed by the enterocytes. After 4.5 hr cbl bound to IF accounted for as much as 40% of cytosolic cbl, while 40% of the radioactivity was found as free cbl. However, Marcoullis & Rothenberg (110a) failed to detect any free cobalamin in canine ileal mucosa 3–5 hr after instilling ^{57}[Co]cbl into the stomach. The question regarding the fate of IF is still not fully answered, and much more biochemical and morphological work is needed before all the details of the transepithelial movement of cobalamin are known. However, we interpret the available data as suggesting that IF is not absorbed into the enterocytes along with cobalamin. Figure 2 demonstrates an overall scheme for the absorption of cobalamin, including all three phases—gastric, luminal, and mucosal.

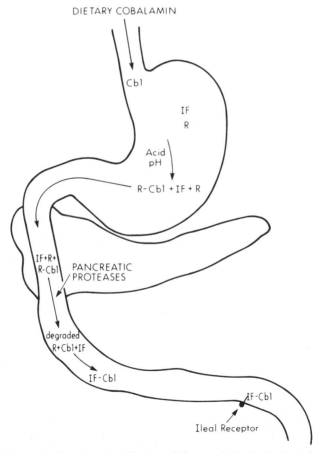

Figure 2 Proposed scheme for the utilization of dietary cobalamin. (Each of the reactions is further discussed in the text.)

IV. TRANSPORT OF COBALAMIN IN THE BODY

After the attachment of IF-cbl to ileal mucosal receptors, cobalamin enters the enterocyte by a mechanism yet to be elucidated. Most of the absorbed cobalamin is found in the mitochondria, and studies using [^{57}Co]CNcbl show that part of this absorbed CNcbl is converted to ado-cbl (122, 123). Cobalamin that exits from the enterocyte is usually not found in free state. In human plasma there are at least three cbl binders—transcobalamins I, II, and III. Most of the circulating levels of cobalamin (200–300 pg/ml plasma) are bound to the R protein, transcobalamin I. Transcobalamin II accounts for most of the unsaturated cbl binding activity found in human plasma (138).

A. Synthesis and Properties of Transcobalamin II (TC II)

TC II is the transport protein that delivers cobalamin to the tissues. Consequently, much work has been carried out on this protein in recent years. Tan & Hansen (156) showed that TC II accumulated in the perfusate of an isolated liver system. Moreover, in an intact animal removal of kidney, stomach, or spleen did not result in any decreased synthesis. De novo synthesis of TC II has been shown in liver perfusates and in cultured rat liver parenchymal cells (33, 49, 136). Extrahepatic synthesis of TC II has been found in dogs (151). TC II production has been demonstrated in macrophages (128) and in fibroblasts (67).

A highly purified TC II has been obtained by Allen and by Puutula & Grasbeck (4, 127). TC II has a molecular weight of 38,000, is not a glycoprotein, and is immunologically different from all other cbl binding proteins. The association constant (Ka) for cbl binding to TC II is $10^{11}M^{-1}$, indicating high affinity (81). The binding is tight, but cbl can be removed by 7.5 M guanidine HCl. TC II has 347 amino acids (2) and a Stokes radius of 2.66 nm (109). One molecule of TC II binds one molecule of cbl and, unlike IF, will bind a wide range of cobamides and other corrinoids at equally high affinity. Molecular microheterogeneity for TC II has been reported by some workers (41, 57) suggesting possible autosomally inherited polymorphism. This observation was based primarily on the different bands obtained on gel electrophoresis. On the other hand, other workers (115, 127) have obtained single bands. The differences between the homogeneity and the heterogeneity of TC II obtained by different workers could also be due to alterations that occur during purification procedures.

B. Function and Metabolism of TC II

The main function of TC II is to transport cobalamin from the intestine after it is absorbed (75) and to deliver the vitamin to other tissues (129). It has been shown by various workers that the TC II mediated uptake of vitamin takes place in a variety of tissues— e. g. Hela cells and human kidney cells and human liver (54), reticulocytes (130), human placental membrane (58), human fibroblasts (132), Erhlich ascites cells (124), and canine spleen and heart (76).

Seligman & Allen (145) have obtained a receptor for TC II in pure form from human placenta, and suggested that TC II and its receptor might have evolved from a common gene. They suggest that TC II might have evolved as a nonglycosylated protein and the latter as a glycoprotein receptor suitable for membrane insertion. The purified receptor had an association constant of $5.6 \times 10^{10} M^{-1}$ for holo TC II, which was twice that for apo TC II ($2.3 \times 10^{10} M^{-1}$). The higher affinity for the TC II-cbl complex confirms the role of the receptor in mediating transmembrane movement of cbl. This high affinity of the plasma membrane receptor for TC II-cbl is probably the explanation for the reduction in TC II levels in plasma after an injection of cbl either intravenously (43) or intramuscularly (14). The TC II level returns to preinjection levels after several hours. However, the in vivo experiments of Schneider et al (138) suggested that there was a 30% faster rate of plasma clearance of [^{125}I]TC II compared to that of [^{125}I]TC II-[^{57}Co]CNcbl. This observation is hard to reconcile with other studies (14, 43, 145) indicating preferential affinity for the receptor for holo TC II compared to apo TC II.

The uptake of TC II-cbl by endocytosis and the involvement of lysosomes in the degradation of TC II appear to be well recognized. Involvement of lysosomes in accumulating administered [^{58}Co]cbl was shown in earlier studies using rat kidney (114). Using partially purified lysosomes from rat liver and kidney, Pletch & Coffey (125, 126) showed that one hour following an intracardiac injection of [^{57}Co]cbl the radioactivity was transiently associated with a protein fraction with a size similar to that of TC II.

The internalization of TC II-cbl and subsequent degradation of TC II by lysosomes have been demonstrated more conclusively using cultured fibroblasts (169, 170). Decreased sensitivity to trypsin of [^{125}I]TC II bound to cell surfaces with an increase in temperature provides evidence for internalization. Decreased release of acid soluble radioactivity into the medium after the addition of 50 μM chloroquine strongly suggests the involvement of lysosomes in the degradation of TC II (126).

The exact mechanism of internalization of TC II-cbl is not known, and more morphological work is needed to ascertain whether cell surface redistribution occurs after binding and results in the formation of specialized structures such as coated pits. Such a mechanism has been demonstrated morphologically for the internalization of low-density lipoproteins (10).

C. Function of R Proteins

The R proteins from saliva or gastric secretion do not appear to have any role in the intestinal absorption of cobalamin, nor do the plasma R proteins TC I and TC III facilitate cellular transport of cobalamin. First, the R-protein-[^{57}Co]cbl complex does not bind to the ileal receptors. Second, two brothers who had deficiencies of all R proteins were hematologically normal (74). Some evidence suggests that binding of cbl by R proteins protects cobalamin from bacterial utilization. Lactoferrin, an iron binding protein with a well-described antibacterial action, has a tissue distribution very similar to that of R proteins. Furthermore, high concentrations of R proteins are present in granulocytes. Gilbert (60) and Gullberg (68, 69) have suggested that the R proteins may play a role in host defense against bacteria. Allen (2) has suggested a role in clearing the cbl analogs found in the intestinal lumen and in the tissues (101).

D. Binding and Uptake of TC I-cbl and TC III-cbl by Hepatic Asialoglycoprotein Receptor

Ashwell & Morell (12) have shown that liver plasma membranes bind a wide variety of plasma glycoproteins as the initial step in their removal from plasma. These glycoproteins bind to this plasma receptor only if the terminal galactose is intact and no sialic acid is present on the glycoprotein. The asialoglycoproteins are internalized and degraded by the lysosomes within 90 minutes. Some R proteins seem to be cleared by the receptor-mediated system. Using the rabbit, Burger et al (21) have shown that [^{125}I]human granulocyte R-[^{57}Co]cbl and [^{125}I]human TC III[^{57}Co]cbl are cleared rapidly ($T_{\frac{1}{2}}$=5 min) from plasma, whereas [^{125}I] human TC I-[^{57}Co]cbl and [^{131}I] bovine serum albumin have prolonged plasma survival. The faster rate of clearance of R-cbl and TC III-cbl can be prolonged by saturating the liver plasma membrane receptor by a prior injection of desialated fetuin. Moreover, the TC I-cbl complex can be cleared more rapidly by desialating it before injection. The physiological significance of asialoglycoprotein receptor in clearing R-cbl from plasma is not fully known. Allen (2) indicates that this mechanism may help in the clearance of cbl analogs that might be formed by bacteria, especially since R proteins are known to bind tightly a wide variety of cbl analogs (8, 62). Analogs will then be secreted into bile after removal by the liver. Reabsorption of the analogs will be poor since IF binds analogs of cobalamin with a lower affinity than cobalamin itself (18). It is interesting to note that in studies involving two brothers (25) who had congenital R protein deficiency, one had neurological illness. However, no harmful effects of noncobalamin analogs of vitamin B_{12} have yet been documented.

Patients deficient in TC II develop pernicious anemia (71, 82) but do not have elevated levels of methylmalonic acid and homocysteine (139) in their urine. It is possible that in these deficient patients cbl is delivered to the liver (but not other tissues) not by TC II internalization but via TC III and the asialoglycoprotein receptor. In one day the amount of TC III produced is so large that it can bind 100–150 μg of cbl.

E. Role of Lysosomes and Mitochondria in Cobalamin Metabolism

The role of lysosomes in the receptor-mediated absorptive endocytosis and the role of mitochondria in further metabolic reactions are not well documented in the intestinal mucosa. Furthermore, it is unclear whether these organelles in other tissues and cells play an important role in the metabolism of cbl bound to TC II. The work of Ryel et al (134) using mouse leukemic lymphoblasts and Pierce et al (124) using Ehrlich ascites carcinoma cells showed that TC III-cbl is not taken up by the classical endocytosis mechanism and TC II was not broken down by lysosomal enzymes. Using rat liver mitochondria Gams et al (59) showed that TC II-cbl was taken up by mitochondria at a rate of 10–30-fold higher than free cbl, and that the uptake was Ca^{2+}-dependent and not affected by 2,4-dinitrophenol. These studies using cyanocobalamin are in sharp contrast to the studies of Fenton et al (51) using hydroxycobalamin. These authors have shown in vitro that swollen mitochondria takes up only free cobalamin by an energy-independent process. In the mitochondria the vitamin was found to be associated with a protein of mol wt 120 X 10^3.

These studies suggesting noninvolvement of lysosomes in the degradation of TC II-cbl are in conflict with the studies using rat kidney (114), rat liver (126), and human fibroblasts (169, 170). The dynamics of cbl movement out of the lysosomes is poorly understood. Lysosomal membranes are fully permeable to molecules of mol wt 400 or less, and hence it is hard to understand fully a mechanism whereby TC II-cbl would enter lysosomes to be degraded with release of free cbl without involving endocytosis. It is also possible that TC II may not penetrate lysosomes but may be degraded on lysosomal membranes or by cytoplasmic proteases. These conflicting results may also be due in part to varied integrity and purity of the isolated organelles.

V. CAUSES OF COBALAMIN DEFICIENCY IN HUMANS

Our current knowledge of normal cobalamin absorption has come from patients with malabsorption of the vitamin and to some extent from in vivo studies on animal models. Deficiency of cobalamin arises with dietary lack, gastric, intestinal, or pancreatic disease, or due to various genetic abnormalities. In many instances the symptoms are insidious and develop over two to three years. Table 1 summarizes causes leading to the deficiency of the vitamin and relates them to the corresponding physiological defect.

VI. DIAGNOSIS OF COBALAMIN DEFICIENCY

A. Tests Determining Intake and Absorption

No reliable method assesses intake of cobalamin, but the Schilling test accurately reflects absorption. This test utilizes the fact that free cobalamin does not occur in the plasma or elsewhere until all binding proteins are saturated. Then the free cobalamin is filtered through the glomerulus. A parenteral injection of 1000 μg of nonlabelled cyanocobalamin is given to saturate tissue and serum binding proteins. Any serum to be drawn for assessment of body stores (see below) must be obtained beforehand. [^{57}Co]- and [^{58}Co]cbl linked to intrinsic factor (IF) are then given by mouth. Excretion of the labeled cobalamin in urine for 24 hr should exceed 10% of the administered dose if absorption is normal. In cases of possible bacterial overgrowth, absorption can be tested after administration of tetracycline, 1 g per day. The use of simultaneous isotope administration allows the test to be performed in one 24 hr period. The problems with the test involve the collection of urine and the intertest variability. When urine

Table 1 Physiological causes of malabsorption of dietary cobalamin

Physiological step	Disorder
1) Impaired food digestion	Gastrectomy, achlorhydria (45)
2) Decreased IF secretion	Pernicious anemia (28)
	Gastrectomy (79)
3) Impaired transfer to IF	Pancreatic insufficiency (7, 160)
	Zollinger-Ellison syndrome (137)
4) Abnormal IF	Decreased ileal binding (99)
5) Competition for uptake	Bacterial overgrowth (42)
	Fish tapeworm infestation (119)
6) Impaired attachment to ileal receptor	Ileal disease or resection (42)
7) Impaired passage through ileal cell	Familial cbl malabsorption (107)
8) Impaired uptake into blood	Transcobalamin II deficiency (24)

collection is incomplete or renal disease is present, a low cobalamin excretion is an unreliable index of absorption. Intertest variability can be as much as 30–50%, though the use of ratios with two isotopes diminishes this somewhat. Thus excretion of less than 7% is clearly low, and over 10% is clearly normal. When excretion is 7–10% interpretation must be cautious. It is a mistake to attach too much importance to precisely 10% excretion as an arbitrary normal limit. Stimulation of urinary excretion by two-fold or more upon addition of intrinsic factor is suggestive of intrinsic factor deficiency, even if the excretion without IF is in the 7–10% range.

Absorption of cobalamin in food requires breakdown by gastric proteases to liberate free cobalamin. Therefore, the Schilling test may not correlate always with physiological alterations in cobalamin absorption, especially when gastric physiology is altered. However, the tests utilizing food sources of labelled cobalamin are not practical. It is unlikely that cobalamin deficiency develops without at least a partial defect in intrinsic factor production.

When absorption of cobalamin with intrinsic factor is low and intestinal disease is not suspected, the following factors should be considered: The preparation of intrinsic factor may not be active and the patient have pernicious anemia; urine collection may be inadequate; or the mild intestinal dysfunction of cobalamin deficiency may have produced the low excretion.

B. Tests Determining Body Stores

Serum cobalamin usually correlates with body stores. Cobalamin concentration in blood cells is not higher than in serum. Thus hemolysis is not a major factor in producing false results. TC II, the serum carrier protein that delivers cobalamin to tissues, is responsible for only 10–30% of total serum cobalamin. Most of the rest is bound to an R protein, transcobalamin I. Therefore, with TC II deficiency serum cobalamin can be normal, but the vitamin is not delivered to tissues and body stores are low. Furthermore, the normal range for serum B_{12} assumes that 2.5% of patients with normal stores will have low levels. Low levels have been found in normal persons, especially the elderly, with no harmful effects. Therefore serum cobalamin does not always correlate with cobalamin body stores.

The assay for vitamin B_{12} used to be microbiological, using *Euglena gracilis* or *Lactobacillus leichmanii.* Although these assays detected a metabolically active vitamin, they required sterile technique, were time-consuming to perform, and were not sensitive below 100 pg/ml. Radioisotopic dilution assays are now generally available and are based on the principle that endogenous serum cobalamin competes with radioactive cobalamin for binding to a limited amount of cobalamin binding protein (113). However, cobalamin analogs bind to cobalamin protein binders and can interfere with the serum assay. This is especially true since the commercially prepared binding proteins contain some R protein rather than 100% intrinsic factor. Cobalamin analogs bind more avidly to R proteins than to intrinsic factor. Therefore cobalamin deficiency can be masked by the presence of analogs in the serum resulting in a falsely normal serum value (100). As many as 20% of cobalamin deficient patients might be mistaken in this way. If suspicion still exists that deficiency is present, the microbiological assay should be used to confirm this diagnosis.

Further problems with the serum vitamin B_{12} assay have been noted (48). These levels can be low when the patient has normal body stores. Thirty percent of patients with folate deficiency have low serum vitamin B_{12} levels, though the reason is not clear. Protein deficiency will lower the amount of total serum vitamin B_{12} without having much effect on delivery of cobalamin to tissues, because most of the vitamin B_{12} binding activity in serum is due to transcobalamin I. Up to 75% of strict vegetarians have low serum cobalamin levels without evidence of deficiency (28). It is likely that these patients would develop some signs of anemia with continued inadequate intake. Finally, in pregnancy serum vitamin B_{12} level is low due to dilution and redistribution of the binding proteins. Less than 120 pg/ml of vitamin B_{12} is associated with low body stores if the above factors are not present.

High levels of vitamin B_{12} ($>$ 1000 pg/ml) are seen with acute liver disease due to release from the hepatocytes, and with increased white cells, since they produce an R protein that increases the total serum vitamin B_{12} binding capacity.

ACKNOWLEDGMENTS

We sincerely thank Mrs. Catherine Camp for superb secretarial help in preparation of the manuscript. We also thank Ms. Marlene Jimenez for her assistance in proofreading and other help. Part of the work by the authors contained in this review was supported by grants AM14038 and AM26638, both from the National Institutes of Health.

Literature Cited

1. Addison, T. 1855. *On the Constitutional and Local Effects of Disease of the Suprarenal Capsules.* London: S. Highley. pp. 2–4
2. Allen, R. H. 1975. Human vitamin B_{12} transport proteins. *Prog. Hematol.* 9: 57–84
3. Allen, R. H., Majerus, P. W. 1972. Isolation of vitamin B_{12} binding proteins using affinity chromatography. I. Preparation and properties of vita-min B_{12}-sepharose. *J. Biol. Chem.* 247:7695–701
4. Allen, R. H., Majerus, P. W. 1972. Isolation of vitamin B_{12} binding proteins using affinity chromatography. III. Purification and properties of human plasma transcobalamin II. *J. Biol. Chem.* 247:7709–17
5. Allen, R. H., Mehlman, C. S. 1973. Isolation of gastric vitamin B_{12}-binding proteins using affinity chromatography. I. Purification and properties of human

intrinsic factor. *J. Biol. Chem.* 248: 3660–69
6. Allen, R. H., Mehlman, C. S. 1973. Isolation and properties of hog intrinsic factor and hog nonintrinsic factor. *J. Biol. Chem.* 248:3670–80
7. Allen, R. H., Seetharam, B., Podell, E., Alpers, D. H. 1978. Effect of proteolytic enzymes on the binding of cobalamin to R protein and intrinsic factor. *J. Clin. Invest.* 61:47–53
8. Allen, R. H., Seetharam, B., Allen, N. C., Podell, E., Alpers, D. H. 1978. Correction of cobalamin malabsorption in pancreatic insufficiency with a cobalamin analogue that binds with high affinity R protein but not to intrinsic factor. *J. Clin. Invest.* 61:1628–34
9. Andersen, K. J., Von der Lippe, G. 1979. The effect of proteolytic enzymes on the vitamin B_{12}-binding proteins of human gastric juice and saliva. *Scand. J. Gastroent.* 14:833–38
10. Anderson, R. G. W., Goldstein, J. L., Brown, M. S. 1977. A mutation that impairs the ability of lipoprotein receptors to localize in coated pits on the cell surface of human fibroblasts. *Nature* 270:695–99
11. Ardeman, S., Chanarin, I. 1965. Stimulation of gastric intrinsic factor secretion. *Br. Med. J.* 1:1417–18
12. Ashwell, G., Morell, A. G. 1974. The role of surface carbohydrates in the hepatic recognition and transport of circulating glycoproteins. *Adv. Enzymol.* 41:99–128
13. Baker, S. J. 1967. Human vitamin B_{12} deficiency. *World Rev. Nutr. Diet.* 8:62–126
14. Begley, J. A., Morelli, T. A., Hall, C. A. 1977. B_{12} binding proteins after injection of cyanocobalamin. *N. Engl. J. Med.* 297:614–15.
15. Bertcher, R. W., Meyer, L. M., Miller, I. F. 1958. Co^{60} vitamin B_{12} binding capacity of normal human saliva. *Proc. Soc. Exp. Biol. Med.* 99:513–15
16. Binder, H. J., Donaldson, R. M. 1978. Effect of cimetidine on intrinsic factor and pepsin secretion in man. *Gastroenterology* 74:371–75
17. Booth, C. C., Mollin, D. L. 1957. Importance of the ileum in the absorption of vitamin B_{12}. *Lancet* 2:1007
17a. Bozian, R. C., Ferguson, J. L., Heyssel, R. M., Meneely, G. R., Darby, W. J. 1963. Evidence concerning the human requirement for vitamin B_{12}. *Am. J. Clin. Nutr.* 12:117–29
18. Bunge, M. M., Schilling, R. F. 1957. Intrinsic factor studies. VI. Competition for vitamin B_{12} binding site offered by analogues of the vitamin. *Proc. Soc. Exp. Biol. Med.* 96:587–92
19. Burger, R. L., Allen, R. H. 1974. Characterization of vitamin B_{12} binding proteins isolated from human milk and saliva by affinity chromatography. *J. Biol. Chem.* 249:7220–27
20. Burger, R. L., Mehlman, C. S., Allen, R. H. 1975. Human plasma R-type vitamin B_{12} binding proteins. I. Isolation and characterization of transcobalamin I, transcobalamin III and the normal granulocyte vitamin B_{12} binding protein. *J. Biol. Chem.* 250:7700–6
21. Burger, R. L., Schneider, R. J., Mehlman, C. S., Allen, R. H. 1975. Human plasma R-type vitamin B_{12} binding proteins. II. The role of TC I, TC III and normal granulocyte vitamin B_{12}-binding protein in plasma transport of vitamin B_{12}. *J. Biol. Chem.* 250:7707–13
22. Burgge, W. R., Goff, J. S., Allen, N. C., Podell, E. R., Allen, R. H. 1980. Development of dual label Schilling test for pancreatic exocrine function based on differential absorption of cobalamin bound to intrinsic factor and R protein. *Gastroenterology* 78:937–49
23. Burland, W. L., Mills, J. G., Sharpe, P. C., Horton, M. A., Mollin, D. L. 1977. The effect of cimetidine on intrinsic factor secretion. In *Cimetidine. Proc. Second Int. Symp. Histamine H2 Receptor Antagonist.* Amsterdam: Excerpta Med. p. 177–83.
24. Burman, J. F., Molin, D. L., Sladden, R. A., Sourial, M., Greany, M. 1977. Inherited deficiency of transcobalamin II causing megaloblastic anemia. *Brit. J. Hematol.* 35:676–77
25. Carmel, R., Herbert, V. 1969. Deficiency of vitamin B_{12} binding alpha globulin in two brothers. *Blood* 33:1–12
26. Carmel, R., Herbert, V. 1972. Vitamin B_{12} binding proteins of leukocytes as a possible major source of the third vitamin B_{12}-binding protein of serum. *Blood* 40:542–49
27. Castle, W. B., Townsend, W. C. 1929. Observation on the etiologic relationship of achylia gastrica to pernicious anaemia. II. The effect of the administration to patients with pernicious anaemia of beef muscle after incubation with normal human gastric juice. *Am. J. Med. Sci.* 178:764–77
28. Chanarin, I. 1969. *The Megaloblastic Anemias.* Oxford: Blackwell
29. Chanarin, I., Muir, M., Hughes, A., Hoffbrand, A. V. 1978. Evidence for intestinal origin of transcobalamin II dur-

ing vitamin B_{12} absorption. *Br. Med. J.* 1:1453–55

30. Citrin, Y., Derosa, C., Halsted, J. A. 1957. Sites of absorption of vitamin B_{12}. *J. Lab. Clin. Med.* 50:667–72

31. Cohn, E. J., Minot, G. R., Alles, G. A., Salter, W. T. 1928. The nature of the material in liver effective in pernicious anemia. *J. Biol. Chem.* 77:325–58

32. Combe, J. S. 1824. History of a case of anemia. *Trans. Med. Chirurg. Soc. Edinburg* 1:194–203

33. Cooksley, W. G. E., England, J. M., Louis, L., Down, M. C., Tavill, A. S. 1974. Hepatic vitamin B_{12} release and transcobalamin II synthesis in the rat. *Clin. Sci. Mol. Med.* 47:531–45

34. Cooper, B. A., Castle, W. B. 1960. Sequential mechanisms in the enhanced absorption of vitamin B_{12} by intrinsic factor in the rat. *J. Clin. Invest.* 39:199–214

35. Cooper, B. A., White, J. J. 1968. Absence of intrinsic factor from human portal plasma during ^{57}Co B_{12} absorption in man. *Br. J. Haematol.* 14:73–78

36. Corcino, J., Krauss, S., Waxman, S., Herbert, V. 1970. Release of vitamin B_{12}-binding proteins by human leukocytes in vitro. *J. Clin. Invest.* 49:2250–55

37. Coronato, A., Glass, G. B. J. 1973. The effect of deconjugated and conjugated bile salts on the intestinal uptake of radio-vitamin B_{12} in vitro and in vivo. *Proc. Soc. Exp. Biol. Med.* 142:1345–48

38. Cotter, R., Rothenberg, S. P. 1976. Solubilization, partial purification and radioassay for the intrinsic factor receptor from ileal mucosa. *Br. J. Haematol.* 34:477–87

39. Cotter, R., Rothenberg, S. P., Weiss, J. P. 1977. Purification of the intestinal receptor for intrinsic factor by affinity chromatography. *Biochim. Biophys. Acta* 490:19–26

40. Deller, D. J., Germar, H., Witts, L. J. 1961. Effect of food on absorption of radioactive vitamin B_{12}. *Lancet* 1:574–77

40a. Darby, W. J., Bridgforth, E. B., Le Brocquy, J., Clark, S. L. Jr., Dutra De Oliveira, J., Kevany, J., McGanity, W. J., Perez, C. 1958. Vitamin B_{12} requirement of adult man. *Am. J. Med.* 25:726

41. Diager, S. P., Labowe, M. L., Parsons, M., Wang, L., Vacalli-Sforza, L. L. 1978. Detection of genetic variation with radioactive ligands III genetic polymorphism of transcobalamin II in human plasma. *Am. J. Hum. Genet.* 30:202–14

42. Donaldson, R. H. 1975. Mechanism of malabsorption of cobalamin. In *Cobalamins*, ed. B. M. Babior, p. 335. NY: Wiley

43. Donaldson, R. M., Brand, M., Serfilippi, D. 1977. Changes in circulating transcobalamin II after injection of cyanocobalamin. *N. Engl. J. Med.* 296:1427–30

44. Doscherholmen, A., Swaim, W. R. 1973. Impaired assimilation of egg ^{57}Co vitamin B_{12} in patients with hypochlorhydria and achlorhydria and after gastric resection. *Gastroenterology* 64:912–19

45. Doscherholmen, A., McMahon, J., Ripley, D. 1968. Vitamin B_{12} assimilation from chicken meat. *Am. J. Clin. Nutr.* 31:825–30

46. Ellenbogen, L. 1975. Absorption and transport of cobalamin. In *Cobalamin: Biochemistry and Pathophysiology*, ed. B. M. Babior, p. 223. NY: Wiley

47. Ellenbogen, L. 1979. Uptake and transport of cobalamins. *Int Rev. Biochem. Biochem. Nutr.* 1A. 27:45–96

48. England, J. H., Linnell, J. C. 1980. Problems with the serum vitamin B_{12} assay. *Lancet* 2:1072–74

49. England, J. M., Clarke, H. G. M., Down, M. C., Chanarin, I. 1973. Studies on transcobalamins. *Br. J. Haematol.* 25:737–49

50. FAO-WHO Expert Group. 1976. Requirements of ascorbic acid, vitamin D, vitamin B_{12}, folate and iron. *WHO Tech. Rep. Ser.* #452

51. Fenton, W. A., Ambani, L. A., Rosenberg, L. E. 1976. Uptake of hydroxycobalamin by rat liver mitochondria, binding to a mitochondrial protein. *J. Biol. Chem.* 251:6616–23

52. Fenwick, S. 1870. On atrophy of the stomach. *Lancet* 2:78–80

53. Fielding, L. P., Chalmers, D. M., Chanarin, I., Levi, A. J. 1978. Inhibitor of intrinsic factor secretion by cimetidine. *Br. Med. J.* 1:818–19

54. Finkler, A. E., Hall, C. A. 1967. Nature of the relationship between vitamin B_{12} binding and cell uptake. *Arch. Biochem. Biophys.* 120:79–85

55. Finlayson, N. D. C., Simpson, J. D., Tothill, P., Samson, R. R., Girdwood, R. H., Sherman, J. D. C. 1969. Application of whole body counting to the measurement of vitamin B_{12} absorption with reference to achlorhydria. *Scand. J. Gastroenterol.* 4:397–405

56. Food and Nutrition Board. 1980. *National Research Council. Recommended*

Daily Allowances. Washington DC: Nat. Acad. Sci. 9th ed.
57. Frater-Schroder, M., Hitzig, W. H., Butler, R. 1979. Studies on transcobalamin. I. Detection of TC II isoproteins in human serum. *Blood* 53:193–203
58. Friedman, P. A., Shia, M. A., Wallace, J. K. 1977. A saturable high affinity binding site for transcobalamin II-vitamin B_{12} complexes in human placental membrane preparations. *J. Clin. Invest.* 59:51–58
59. Gams, R. A., Ryel, E. M., Ostroy, F. 1976. Protein mediated uptake of vitamin B_{12} by isolated mitochondria. *Blood* 47:923–30
60. Gilbert, H. S. 1974. Proposal of a possible function for granulocyte vitamin B_{12} binding proteins in host defense against bacteria. *Blood* 44:926
61. Glass, G. B. J. 1974. *Gastric Intrinsic Factor and Other Vitamin B_{12} Binders.* Biochemistry, physiology, pathology and relation to vitamin B_{12} metabolism. Stuttgart: Thieme. p. 1–165
62. Gottlieb, C., Retief, F. P., Herbert, V. 1967. Blockade of vitamin B_{12}-binding sites in the gastric juice, serum and saliva by analogues and derivatives of vitamin B_{12} and by antibody to intrinsic factor. *Biochim. Biophys. Acta* 131:560–62
63. Grasbeck, R. 1969. Intrinsic factor and other vitamin B_{12} binding proteins. *Prog. Hematol.* 6:233–60
64. Grasbeck, R., Marcoullis, G. 1975. Studies on a fraction of human gastric mucosa containing intrinsic factor isoproteins typical of mucosa. *Scand. J. Clin. Lab. Invest.* 35:13–18
65. Grasbeck, R., Simons, K., Sinkkonen, I. 1966. Isolation of intrinsic factor and its probable degradation product, as their vitamin B_{12} complexes, from human gastric juice. *Biochim. Biophys. Acta* 127:47–58
66. Grasbeck, R., Stenman, U. H., Puutula, L., Visuri, K. 1968. A procedure for detaching bound vitamin B_{12} from its transport protein. *Biochim. Biophys. Acta* 158:292–95
67. Green, P. D., Savage, C. R., Hall, C. A. 1976. Mouse transcobalamin II biosynthesis and uptake by L 929 cells. *Arch. Biochem. Biophys.* 176:683–89
68. Gullberg, R. 1974. Possible antimicrobial function of the large molecular size vitamin B_{12} binding protein. *Scand. J. Gastroenterol.* 9: (Suppl. 29) 19–21
69. Gullberg, R. 1974. Possible influence of vitamin B_{12} binding proteins in milk on

the intestinal flora in breast fed infants. *Scand. J. Gastroenterol.* 9:287–92
70. Hagedorn, C. H., Alpers, D. H. 1977. Distribution of intrinsic factor-vitamin B_{12} receptors in human intestine. *Gastroenterology* 73:1019–22
71. Hakami, N., Neiman, R. P., Canellos, G. P., Lazerson, J. 1971. Neonatal megaloblastic anemia due to inherited transcobalamin II deficiency in two siblings. *N. Engl. J. Med.* 285:1163–70
72. Hall, C. A. 1975. Transcobalamin I and III as natural transport proteins of vitamin B_{12}. *J. Clin. Invest.* 56:1125–31
73. Hall, C. A. 1976. The failure of granulocytes to produce transobalamin I (TC I). *Scand. J. Haematol.* 16:176–82
74. Hall, C. A., Begley, J. A. 1977. Congenital deficiency of human R-type binding proteins of cobalamin. *Am. J. Hum. Genet.* 29:619–26
75. Hall, C. A., Finkler, A. E. 1965. The dynamics of transcobalamin II. A vitamin B_{12} binding substance in plasma. *J. Lab. Clin. Med.* 65:459–69
76. Hall, C. A., Rappazzo, M. E. 1974. Uptake of protein bound vitamin B_{12} by canine organs. *Proc. Soc. Exp. Biol. Med.* 146:898–900
77. Herbert, V. 1959. Mechanism of intrinsic factor action in everted sacs of rat small intestine. *J. Clin. Invest.* 38:102–9
78. Highley, D. R., Davies, M. C., Ellenbogen, L. 1967. Hog intrinsic factor II. Some physicochemical properties of vitamin B_{12} binding fractions from hog pylorus. *J. Biol. Chem.* 242:1010–15
79. Hines, J. D., Hoffbrand, A. V., Mollin, D. L. 1967. The hematologic complications following gastrectomy. *Am. J. Med.* 43:555–69
80. Hines, J. D., Rosenberg, A., Harris, J. W. 1968. Intrinsic factor-mediated radio B_{12} uptake in sequential incubation studies using everted sacs of guinea pig small intestine. Evidence that IF is not absorbed into the intestinal cell. *Proc. Soc. Exp. Biol. Med.* 129:653–58
81. Hippe, E., Olesen, H. 1971. Nature of vitamin B_{12} binding. III. Thermodynamics of binding to human intrinsic factor and transcobalamins. *Biochim. Biophys. Acta* 243:83–89
82. Hitzig, W. H., Dohmann, V., Pluss, H. J., Vischer, D. 1974. Hereditary transcobalamin II deficiency. Clinical findings in a new family. *J. Pediat.* 85:622–28
83. Hoedemaeker, P. J., Abels, J., Watchers, J. J., Arends, A. H., Niewig, H. O. 1964. Investigation about the site of

production of Castle's gastric intrinsic factor. *Lab. Invest.* 13:394–99

84. Hogenkamp, H. P. C. 1975. See Ref. 46, pp. 21–73

85. Hom, B. L. 1967. Plasma turnover of ⁵⁷Cobalt-vitamin B_{12} bound to transcobalamin I and II. *Scand. J. Haematol.* 4:321–32

86. Hooper, D. C., Alpers, D. H., Burger, R. L., Mehlman, C. S., Allen, R. H. 1973. Characterization of ileal vitamin B_{12} binding using homogeneous human and hog intrinsic factors. *J. Clin. Invest.* 13:3074–83

87. Hurlimann, J., Zuber, C. 1969. Vitamin B_{12} binders in human body fluids. II. Synthesis in vitro. *Clin. Exp. Immunol.* 4:141–48

88. Hutner, S. H., Provasoli, L., Stokstad, E. L. R., Hoffmann, C. E., Belt, M., Franklin, A. L., Jukes, T. H. 1949. Assay of anti-pernicious anemia factor with euglena. *Proc. Soc. Exp. Biol. Med.* 70:118–20

89. Irvine, W. J. 1965. Effect of gastrin I and II on the secretion of intrinsic factor. *Lancet* 1:736–37

90. Jacob, E., Glass, G. B. J. 1971. Localization of intrinsic factor and complement fixing intrinsic factor antibody complex in parietal cells of man. *Clin. Exp. Immunol.* 8:517–27

91. Jacob, E., Glass, G. B. J. 1971. Separation of intrinsic factor antibodies from parietal cell antibodies in pernicious anemia serum by gel filtration. *Proc. Soc. Exp. Biol. Med.* 137:243–47

92. Jacob, E., Baker, S. J., Herbert, V. 1980. Vitamin B_{12}-binding proteins. *Physiol. Rev.* 60:918–60

93. Jadhav, M., Webb, J. K. G., Vaishnava, S., Baker, S. J. 1962. Vitamin B_{12} deficiency in Indian infants. A clinical syndrom. *Lancet* 2:903–7

94. Jeffries, G. H., Sleisenger, M. H. 1965. The pharmacology of intrinsic factor secretion in man. *Gastroenterology* 48:444–48

95. Kane, S. P., Peters, T. J. 1975. Analytical subcellular fractionation of human granulocytes with reference to localization of vitamin B_{12}-binding proteins. *Clin. Sci. Mol. Med.* 49:171–82

96. Kapadia, C. R., Donaldson, R. M. 1978. Macromolecular secretion by isolated gastric mucosa. Fundamental differences in pepsinogen and intrinsic factor secretion. *Gastroenterology* 74:535–39

97. Kapadia, C. R., Serfilippi, D., Donaldson, R. M. 1979. Uptake of biosynthetically labelled intrinsic factor by isolated ileal cells. *Clin. Res.* 27:455 (Abstr.)

98. Kapadia, C. R., Voloshin, K., Donaldson, R. M. 1981. Fate of intrinsic factor–cobalamin complex within ileal enterocytes. *Gastroenterology* 80:1187 (Abstr.)

99. Katz, M., Lee, S. K., Copper, B. A. 1972. Vitamin B_{12} absorption due to a biologically inert intrinsic factor. *N. Engl. J. Med.* 287:425–29

100. Kolhouse, J. F., Kondo, H., Allen, N. C., Podell, E., Allen, R. H. 1978. Cobalamin analogues are present in human plasma and can mask cobalamin deficiency because current radioisotope dilution assays are not specific for true cobalamin. *N. Engl. J. Med.* 299:785–92

101. Kondo, H., Kolhouse, J. F., Allen, R. H. 1980. Presence of cobalamin analogues in animal tissues. *Proc. Natl. Acad. Sci.* 77:817–21

102. Kouvonen, I., Grasbeck, R. 1979. A simplified technique to isolate the porcine and human ileal receptor and studies on their subunit structure. *Biochim. Biophys. Res. Comm.* 86:358–64

103. Kouvonen, I., Grasbeck, R. 1981. Topology of the hog intrinsic factor receptor in the intestine. *J. Biol. Chem.* 256:154–58

104. Lawrie, J. H., Anderson, N. M. 1967. Secretion of gastric intrinsic factor. *Lancet* 1:68–71

105. Levine, J. S., Nakane, P. K., Allen, R. H. 1982. Immunocytochemical localization of intrinsic factor-cobalamin bound to guinea pig ileum in vivo. *Gastroenterology* 82:284–90

106. Levine, J. S., Nakane, P. K., Allen, R. 1981. Phylogenic differences in the site of synthesis of intrinsic factor. *Gastroenterology* 80:P1210 (Abstr.)

107. Mackenzie, J. L., Donaldson, R. M., Trier, J. S., Mathan, V. I. 1972. Ileal mucosa in familial selective vitamin B_{12} malabsorption. *N. Engl. J. Med.* 286:1021–25

108. Marcoullis, G., Grasbeck, R. 1977. Solubilized intrinsic factor receptor from pig ileum and its characteristics. *Biochim. Biophys. Acta* 496:36–51

109. Marcoullis, G., Salonen, E., Grasbeck, R. 1977. Isolation of vitamin B_{12}-binding proteins by combined immuno and affinity chromatography. *Biochim. Biophys. Acta* 495:336–48

110. Marcoullis, G., Parmentier, Y., Nicolas, J. P., Jimenez, M., Gerard, P. 1980. Cobalamin malabsoption due to nondegradable R protein in the human intes-

tine. Inhibited cobalamin absorption in exocrine pancreatic dysfunction. *J. Clin. Invest.* 66:430–40

110a. Marcoullis, G., Rothenberg, S. P. 1981. Intrinsic factor–mediated intestinal absorption of cobalamin in the dog. *Am. J. Physiol.* 241:294–99

111. Meikle, D. D., Bull, J., Callender, S. T., Truelove, S. C. 1977. Intrinsic factor secretion after vagotomy. *Br. J. Surg.* 96:795–97

112. Minot, G. R. 1935. The development of liver therapy in pernicious anaemia. *Lancet* 1:361–64

113. Mollin, D. L., Anderson, B. B., Burman, J. F. 1976. The serum vitamin B_{12} level: Its assay and significance. *Clin. Hematol.* 5:521–46

114. Newmark, P., Newman, G. E., O'Brien, J. R. P. 1970. Vitamin B_{12} in the rat kidney. Evidence for an association with lysosomes. *Arch. Biochem. Biophys.* 141:121–30

115. Nexo, E., Olesen, H., Bucher, D., Thomson, J. 1977. Purification and characterization of rabbit transcobalamin II. *Biochim. Biophys. Acta* 494: 395–402

116. Nexo, E., Olesen, H., Hansen, M. R., Bucher, D., Thomsen, J. 1978. Primary structure of human intrinsic factor. Progress report on cyanogen bromide fragmentation. *Scand. J. Clin. Lab. Invest.* 38:649–53

117. Nicolas, J. P., Jimenez, M., Marcoullis, G., Parmentier, Y. 1981. In vivo evidence that intrinsic factor-cobalamin complex transverses human intestine intact. *Biochim. Biophys. Acta* 675: 328–33

118. Noronha, J. M., Silverman, M. 1961. On folic acid, vitamin B_{12}, methionine, and formiminoglutamic acid metabolism. Vitamin B_{12} and intrinsic factor 2. *Europaisches Symp. Hamburg,* ed. H. C. Heinrich. Stuttgart: Enke. p. 728

119. Nyberg, W., Saarni, M. 1964. Calculations on the dynamics of vitamin B_{12} in fish tape worm carriers spontaneously recovering from vitamin B_{12} deficiency. *Acta Med. Scand. Suppl.* 412:65

120. Okuda, K., Kitazaki, T., Takamatsu, M. 1971. Inactivation of vitamin B_{12} by a binder in rat intestine and the role of intrinsic factor. *Digestion* 4:35–48

121. Olesen, H., Nexo, E., Lous, P., Thomsen, J., Bucher, D. 1976. Aminoterminal sequence of human intrinsic factor. *Scand. J. Clin. Lab. Invest.* 36:527–29

122. Peters, T. J., Hoffbrand, A. V. 1970. Absorption of vitamin B_{12} by the guinea

pig. I. Subcellular localization of vitamin B_{12} in the ileal enterocyte during absorption. *Br. J. Haematol.* 19:369–82

123. Peters, T. J., Linnell, J. C., Matthews, D. M., Hoffbrand, A. V. 1971. Absorption of vitamin B_{12} in the guinea pig. III. The forms of vitamin B_{12} in ileal mucosa and portal plasma in the fasting state and during absorption of cyanocobalamin. *Br. J. Haematol.* 20:299–305

124. Pierce, K., Abe, J., Cooper, B. A. 1975. Incorporation and metabolic conversion of cyanocobalamin by ehrlich ascites carcinoma cells in vitro and in vivo. *Biochim. Biophys. Acta* 381: 348–58

125. Pletsch, Q. A., Coffey, J. W. 1971. Intracellular distribution of radioactive vitamin B_{12} in human serum. *J. Biol. Chem.* 246:4619–29

126. Pletsch, Q. A., Coffey, J. W. 1972. Properties of the proteins that bind vitamin B_{12} in subcellular fractions of rat liver. *Arch. Biochem. Biophys.* 151: 157–67

126a. Poston, M. J. 1980. Cobalamin dependent formation of leucine and β-leucine by rat and human tissue. *J. Biol. Chem.* 255:10067–72

127. Puutula, L., Grasbeck, R. 1972. One million fold purification of transcobalamin II from human plasma. *Biochim. Biophys. Acta* 263:734–46

128. Rachmilewitz, B., Rachmilewitz, M., Chaouat, M., Schlesinger, M. 1977. The synthesis of transcobalamin II, a vitamin B_{12} transport protein by stimulated mouse peritoneal macrophages. *Biomedicine* 27:213–14

129. Rappazzo, M. E., Hall, C. A. 1972. Transport function of transcobalamin II. *J. Clin. Invest.* 51:1915–18

130. Retief, F. P., Gottlieb, C. W., Herbert, V. 1966. Mechanism of vitamin B_{12} uptake by erythrocytes. *J. Clin. Invest.* 45:1907–15

130a. Rickes, E. L., Brink, N. G., Koniusey, F. R., Wood, T. R., Folkers, K. 1948. Crystalline vitamin B_{12}. *Science* 107–396

131. Rose, M. S., Chanarin, I. 1969. Dissociation of intrinsic factor from its antibody: Application to study of pernicious anemia gastric juice specimens. *Br. Med. J.* 1:468–70

132. Rosenberg, L. E., Lilljeqvist, A., Allen, R. H. 1973. Transcobalamin II facilitated uptake of vitamin B_{12} by cultured fibroblasts studies in methylmalonicaciduria. *J. Clin. Invest.* 52: 69–70 (Abstr.)

133. Rosenthal, H. L., Cutler, L., Sobiesz-czanski, W. 1970. Uptake and transport of vitamin B_{12} in subcellular fractions of intestinal mucosa. *Am. J. Physiol.* 218:358–62

134. Ryel, E. M., Meyer, L. M., Gams, R. A. 1974. Uptake and subcellular distribution of vitamin B_{12} in mouse L 1210 leukemic lymphoblasts. *Blood* 44: 427–33

135. Ryvgold, O. 1974. Hypovitaminosis B_{12} following partial gastrectomy by the Billroth II method. *Scand. J. Gastroent.* 9: (Suppl. 27) 57–64

136. Savage, C. R., Green, P. D. 1976. Biosynthesis of transcobalamin II by adult rat liver parenchymal cells in culture. *Arch. Biochem. Biophys.* 173:691–702

137. Schimode, S., Saunders, D. R., Rubin, C. E. 1968. The Zollinger-Ellison Syndrome with steatorrhea. II. The mechanism of fat and vitamin B_{12} malabsorption. *Gastroenterology* 55:705–23

138. Schneider, R. J., Burger, R. L., Mehlman, C. S., Allen, R. H. 1976. The role and fate of rabbit and human transcobalamin II in the plasma transport of vitamin B_{12} in the rabbit. *J. Clin. Invest.* 57:27–38

139. Scott, C. R., Hakami, N., Teng, C. C., Sagerson, R. M. 1972. Hereditary transcobalamin II deficiency. The role transcobalamin II in vitamin B_{12} mediated reactions. *J. Pediat.* 81:1106–11

140. Scott, J. M., Bloomfield, S. J., Stebbins, R., Herbert, V. 1974. Studies on derivation of transcobalamin III from granulocytes by lithium and elimination by fluoride of in vitro increments in vitamin B_{12} binding capacity. *J. Clin. Invest.* 53:228–39

141. Scott, J. M., Weir, D. G. 1976. Folate composition, synthesis and function in natural materials. *Clin. Haematol.* 5: 547–68

141a. Scott, J. M., Wilson, P., Dinn, J. J., Weir, D. G. 1981. Pathogenesis of subacute combined degeneration: a result of methyl group deficiency. *Lancet ii*: 334–37

141b. Scott, J. M., Weir, D. G. 1981. The methyl folate trap hypothesis. *Lancet ii* :337–40

142. Seetharam, B., Alpers, D. H., Allen, R. H. 1981. Isolation and characterization of the ileal receptor for intrinsic factor-cobalamin. *J. Biol. Chem.* 256:3785–90

143. Seetharam, B., Bagur, S. S., Alpers, D. H. 1981. Interaction of ileal receptor for intrinsic factor cobalamin with synthetic and brush border lipids. *J. Biol. Chem.* 256:9813–15

144. Seetharam, B., Bagur, S. S., Alpers, D. H. 1981. Isolation and characterization of proteolytically derived ileal receptor for intrinsic factor-cobalamin. *J. Biol. Chem.* 257:183–89

145. Seligman, P. A., Allen, R. H. 1978. Characterization of receptor for transcobalamin II isolated from human placenta. *J. Biol. Chem.* 253:1766–72

146. Serfilippi, D., Donaldson, R. M. 1979. Biosynthesis of radiolabeled intrinsic factor by isolated gastric mucosa. *Gastoenterology* 76:1241 (Abstr.)

147. Shorab, M. S. 1947. Unidentified growth factors for Lactobacillus lactis in refined liver extracts. *J. Biol. Chem.* 169:455–56

148. Simons, K., Weber, T. 1966. The vitamin B_{12} binding protein in human leukocytes. *Biochim. Biophys. Acta* 117:201–8

149. Simon, J. D., Houck, W. E., Albala, M. M. 1976. Release of unsaturated vitamin B_{12} binding capacity from human granulocytes by the calcium ionophore A23187. *Biochim. Biophys. Res. Commun.* 73:444–50

150. Smith, E. L. 1955. In *The Biochemistry of Vitamin B_{12}*, ed. R. J. Williams, pp. 1–14. London: Cambridge Univ. Press

151. Sonnerborn, D. W., Abouna, G., Mendezpicon, G. 1972. Synthesis of transcobalamin II in totally hepatectomized dogs. *Biochim. Biophys. Acta* 273: 283–86

152. Steinberg, W., Curington, C., Toskes, P. 1978. Evidence that a failure to degrade nonintrinsic factor B_{12} binding proteins is not responsible for B_{12} malabsorption in patients with chronic pancreatitis. *Clin. Res.* 26:749 (Abstr.)

153. Steinberg, W., Toskes, P., Curington, C., Shah, R. 1980. Further studies which cast doubt upon a role for R proteins in the cobalamin malabsorption in chronic pancreatitis. *Gastroenterology* 78:1270 (Abstr.)

154. Deleted in proof

155. Sullivan, L. W., Herbert, V. 1965. Studies on the minimum daily requirement for vitamin B_{12}. Hematopoietic responses to 0.1 microgm. of cyanocobalamin or coenzyme B_{12}, and comparison of their relative potency. *N. Engl. J. Med.* 282:340–46

156. Tan, C. H., Hansen, H. J. 1968. Studies on the site of synthesis of transcobalamin II. *Proc. Soc. Exp. Biol. Med.* 127:740–44

157. Teo, N. H., Scott, J. M., Neale, G., Weir, D. G. 1980. Effect of bile on vita-

min B$_{12}$ absorption. *Br. Med. J.* 281:831–33

158. Teo, N. H., Scott, J. M., Neale, G., Weir, D. G. 1981. Bile acid and inhibition of vitamin B$_{12}$ binding by intrinsic factor in vitro. *Gut* 22:270–76

159. Thomsen, J., Bucher, D., Brunfeldt, R., Nexo, E., Olesen, H. 1976. An improved procedure for automated Edman degradation used for determing N terminal amino acid sequence of human transcobalamin I and human intrinsic factor. *Eur. J. Biochem.* 69:87–96

160. Toskes, P. P., Hansell, J., Cerda, J., Deren, J. J. 1971. Vitamin B$_{12}$ malabsorption in chronic pancreatic insufficiency. *N. Engl. J. Med.* 284:627–32

161. Toskes, P. P., Smith, G. M., Francis, G. M., Sander, E. G. 1977. Evidence that pancreatic proteases enhance vitamin B$_{12}$ absorption by acting on crude preparations of hog gastric intrinsic factor and human gastric juice. *Gastroenterology* 72:31–36

162. Twomey, J. J., Laughter, A. H., Jordan, P. H. 1971. Studies into human IF secretion. *Am. J. Dig. Dis.* 16:1075–81

163. Vatn, M. H., Semb, L. S., Schrumpf, E. 1975. The effect of atropine and vagotomy on the secretion of gastric intrinsic factor (IF) in man. *Scand. J. Gastroenterol.* 10:59–64

164. Victor, M., Lear, A. A. 1956. Subacute combined degeneration of the spinal cord. Current concepts of the disease process. Value of serum vitamin B$_{12}$ determinations in clarifying some of the common clinical problems. *Am. J. Med.* 20:896–911

165. Von der Lippe, G., Andersen, K., Schjonby, H. 1977. Pancreatic extract and the intestinal uptake of vitamin B$_{12}$. III. Stimulatory effect in the presence of a nonintrinsic factor vitamin B$_{12}$ binder. *Scand. J. Gastroenterol.* 12:183–87

166. West, R. 1948. Activity of vitamin B$_{12}$ in Addisonian pernicious anemia. *Science* 107:398

167. Whipple, G. H. 1922. Pigment metabolism and regeneration of hemoglobin in the body. *Arch. Int. Med.* 29:711–31

168. Whipple, G. H., Robscheit-Robbins, F. S. 1925. Blood regeneration in severe anemia. II. Favorable influence of liver, heart and skeletal muscle in diet. *Am. J. Physiol.* 72:408–18

169. Youngdahl-Turner, P., Rosenberg, L. E., Allen, R. H. 1978. Binding and uptake of transcobalamin II by human fibroblasts. *J. Clin. Invest.* 61:133–41

170. Youngdahl-Turner, P., Mellman, I. S., Allen, R. H., Rosenberg, L. E. 1979. Protein mediated vitamin uptake. Absorptive endocytosis of transcobalamin II-cobalamin complex by cultured human fibroblasts. *Exp. Cell. Res.* 118:127–34

Ann. Rev. Nutr. 1982. 2:371–418
Copyright © 1982 by Annual Reviews Inc. All rights reserved

PHYSIOLOGY OF THE CONTROL OF FOOD INTAKE

Harry R. Kissileff and Theodore B. Van Itallie[1]

Departments of Medicine and Psychiatry, St. Luke's-Roosevelt Hospital and
Columbia University, New York, NY 10025

CONTENTS

INTRODUCTION AND SCOPE

Purpose and Extent

First we introduce the novice to the field by briefly describing the major phenomena and theories, with reference to other reviews for further discussion. This part of the review will also remind specialists of the diversity of behavioral, physiological, and ecological functions served by ingestion. Next we review in depth the many experiments that bear on the origin and function of neural or humoral signals arising from the acts and consequences of ingestion. The roles of these signals have been evaluated mainly by administering nutrients, neurotransmitters, or inert substances and observing their effects on food intake or food-motivated behavior—e.g. for rats, running in an alley or pressing a lever to obtain food. Finally we point

[1]Supported by Obesity Core Center Grant AM-26867. We thank Joseph R. Vasselli for
constructive comments.

0199-9885/82/0715-0371$02.00

out that our present knowledge does not allow definitive tests of current hypotheses, in large part because the conduct of experiments and presentation of data are not uniform. The diversity of data presentation forms makes it difficult and sometimes impossible to compare results of similar manipulations from different laboratories or even to compare results of the same investigator over several years. We suggest certain basic criteria that would ease the burden for reviewers in the future.

Methods of Study and Types of Control

Food intake is commonly measured by providing an animal or human subject with a mixed diet and measuring the amount consumed in fixed units of time, usually minutes, hours or days. However, in order to understand the physiological controls that lead to cumulative intakes at these time periods, it is necessary to divide the controls into phasic elements (those that initiate or terminate feeding or food-motivated behavior) and tonic elements (those that sustain a state of eating or a state of suppression of eating).

As a result of the operation of tonic and phasic controls (or perhaps it would be more accurate to state that these controls are inferred from the fact that) feeding behavior is episodic in most animals. All animals spend some portion of their time in quiescence (sleep for some), so that even grazing animals like cattle do not eat constantly (169). We shall refer to the times when feeding is the predominant activity of the animal as *meals,* and to those times when feeding is not occurring as *intermeal intervals.* While it may not be logically necessary to have both tonic and phasic elements controlling eating in order for meal patterns to occur, the limited evidence suggests that the controls operate as though such elements existed. The main evidence for this argument is differential effectiveness of physiological and neurological manipulations on the sizes of meals and intermeal intervals (15, 140, 165, 220, 259, 295).

Some types of control apparently act for only brief periods (hours) and are referred to as short-term, while others act for much longer periods (days or months) and are referred to as long-term controls. Signals for short-term controls include the osmolarity of gut contents, fullness of the gut, and fluctuations of hormone or nutrient levels in the blood. Signals for long-term controls could include body fat content (295) or cerebroventricular insulin level (213). Little is known about how these factors influence the tonic and phasic elements although some progress has been made (151).

Direction of Theories

Food intake is largely self-controlled. The absence of food promotes search and ingestion, while ingestion is self-limiting. Theories about food intake have concentrated on specifying sites where nutrients act to modulate ingestion. In addition, theories of food intake control have sought to determine what properties of nutrients are responsible for modulation of the sites.

Theories have also developed along neurobehavioral lines and have utilized psychological constructs to account for the variety of situations in which eating occurs. The concepts of hunger, satiety, palatability, and malaise, to name a few, have been commonly used to relate feeding behavior to a variety of circumstances that presumably end in a final common path in the nervous system. Although it is possible to review the controls of food intake without regard to these constructs, their pervasiveness in the thought of experimenters and use in the literature make them difficult to ignore. However, caution must be urged in attributing a final common behavior like eating to a unitary controlling center in the brain. It is now well-established that a variety of procedures induce eating by diverse neural pathways. This statement is based mainly on the differential effectiveness of brain manipulations on eating in response to food deprivation, body cooling, glucoprivation (reduction in availability of glucose for metabolism) and stress (8, 23, 80, 170, 186).

DEFINITIONS AND CRITERIA FOR THEIR APPLICATION

We here define such common words as hunger, appetite, and satiety in technical terms. Most investigators would agree with these definitions unless stated otherwise.

Hunger

Hunger refers to the internal state or level that disposes an animal or person to eat. It is manifest in verbal reports of desire to eat in man and inferred from human and animal behavior that increases in intensity when followed by the opportunity to obtain food and eat. Hunger is more than the sensation of an empty stomach as proposed by Cannon & Washburn (49), although stomach emptiness can be part of the mechanism by which hunger is induced. Furthermore, hunger is not a simple all-or-none state but may be graded in magnitude; it therefore has motivational properties that can be measured by amount and rate (135) of consumption (75) or rate of performance of an arbitrary behavior to obtain food (180, 255, 282).

Appetite

Appetite (246) refers to the state of willingness to accept food primarily for its pleasurable or rewarding properties. While reward undoubtedly plays a role in behavior driven by hunger, in appetite the urgency or need to replace nutrient is believed to be absent. Hunger is a necessity while appetite is a luxury. When food is eaten with no obvious internal need to be satisfied, appetite is inferred as the intervening variable. The distinction between appetite and hunger therefore rests on determining the neediness of the subject, which is practically impossible to measure. Much attention has been devoted to what may be an artificial distinction.

It may be unnecessary to retain concepts (like appetite and hunger) whose study is unlikely to yield new mechanisms of operation for the control of food intake. Rather, it should be recognized that reinforcement (pleasure) and some degree of deficit always contribute to ingestive behavior. The components of "need" should be expanded to include psychological deficits from constant feeding with the same food and internal depletion at specific loci (221) rather than in the animal as a whole. Only an animal whose gastrointestinal tract is full and which has been fed on a variety of foods can be considered completely without deficits with regard to controls of food intake. When such animals can be induced to eat, we can infer the existence of appetite. It should be noted that not all authors distinguish appetite from hunger, and it has been suggested that the original definition, "desire to satisfy natural needs of the body," is still the most appropriate definition of appetite (25).

Food Intake

Food intake refers to the amount of nourishing substance consumed by a subject. Usually it is stated in terms of weight, calories, or volume of a mixed quantity of macro- and micro-nutrients, although intakes of separate sources of macro-nutrients such as fat, carbohydrate, and protein have been studied as well (201).

Satiety

Satiety (258, 296) refers to an internal state that leads to termination of eating. It is manifest by verbal reports of comfort, pleasantness, and satisfaction in humans, and by rest (9) in animals. It is also characterized by willingness to repeat the behavior that produced the state when it wears off. Like hunger, satiety is graded in intensity; its continuously changing value (280), in conjunction with other variables during a meal, leads to meal termination. That satiety is only one determinant of meal termination is shown by experiments in which rats are fed on quinine (bitter-tasting) food. Feeding stops but rest, which characterizes normal satiety, does not follow (9). We have found that human volunteers stop eating sooner, eat less, and give lower satiety ratings when they are fed a diet they like less than a control diet (24). If satiety were the sole determinant of the termination of eating, we would have obtained the same satiety rating even though less was eaten. Furthermore, subjects reported they would be unlikely to eat the diet again in another setting, therefore not meeting our criterion that satiety be an experience an organism seeks to repeat.

Malaise

Malaise is a state of discomfort manifested by verbal report in man and avoidance of stimuli associated with it in animals. An active debate currently flourishes in the literature over whether certain experimental treatments decrease food intake by inducing satiety or malaise (71, 93). Resolution of the issue by use of conditioned taste aversion was proposed by Deutsch (70, 71). According to this hypothesis, if illness is produced by an experimental procedure and a flavor is paired with that procedure, the animal will develop an aversion for the flavor and consume less of a food in which the flavor is placed. Smith & Gibbs (258), however, pointed out that conditioned taste aversions can be formed by association of flavors with intravenous injection of isotonic saline. They therefore questioned the assertion that illness is indicated whenever a taste aversion is formed.

Booth (27) has also pointed out that association of flavors with foods that produce earlier satiety or lower intakes, such as concentrated starch compared with dilute starch, will also produce conditioned reduction of intake for flavors paired with their ingestion. This reduction, however, occurs late in the meal, and is called conditioned satiety. It differs from conditioned aversion, which reduces intake from the very outset of the meal. Early and late are arbitrary designations. Booth (27) also based his conclusions in part on slowing of the rate of intake, which parallels the overall reduction. However, he used curves averaged from individual animals that stop at different times. Kissileff et al (136) have proposed that the question could be resolved more accurately by fitting equations to the cumulative intake curves to determine whether the rate of consumption at the beginning of the meal or rate of deceleration is affected by various conditioning procedures. To make matters even more complicated, it is not clear whether satiety and malaise are separable states, or degrees on a continuum of inhibition, or whether incipient malaise is a component of satiety in accord with the dictionary definition of being filled beyond need (37, 258, 296).

PHENOMENA TO BE EXPLAINED

Consistency of Food Intake

Theories of food intake control must explain the relative consistency in daily or weekly food intake of animals maintained on a diet of homogeneous composition under constant ambient temperature. Such consistency has been reported in most species of homeotherms—e.g. dogs (59), rabbits (89), rats (3), monkeys (105), quail (294), pigeons (314), and pigs (87). Adolph (3), for example, reported that food intake over 94 days in 7 rats averaged 5.5% of body weight per day with a coefficient of variation (standard deviation divided by mean times 100) of 10.7%. Hamilton (105) reported that a group of six monkeys had mean daily food intakes for a 4-week period ranging from 88 g/day in the monkey whose overall average intake was lowest, to 347 g/day in the monkey whose overall average intake was highest. Within individual monkeys the coefficients of variation ranged from 19.9% to 28.5%. More noteworthy however was the stability in these measures over a year. The coefficient of variation for 13 4-week periods ranged from only 12.6 to 30.3. This consistency, which has been observed in other species as well, suggested that a control system for food intake corrects errors in daily energy balance to maintain a long-term constancy (172). This idea has been explored by the classic means of varying nutritive density of the diet and observing compensatory changes in food intake.

Response to Nutrient Dilution and Concentration

When the nutritive density of a diet is decreased by adding nonnutritive substances, food intake (measured in units of weight or volume) increases; when fat is added, thereby increasing nutritive density, food intake decreases (159, 277). However, the accuracy of adjustment in calories (i.e. compensation) is perfect only when the change in caloric density is small or when water is used as the diluent (see Table 1); the accuracy is not uniform across species. The literature on response to dietary dilution is large [see (107) and (108) for summaries]. We describe below the results from reports whose data are readily comparable in order to extract the most general statements, which in any case are limited by at least the following seven factors: (a) type of diluent, (b) duration of maintenance on the diet, (c) level of dilution, (d) fat content of the diluted diet, (e) time allowed for eating the diet, (f) body composition of the animal, and (g) species.

First, response to dilution is better when water is used as the diluent than when solids are used. Compare the results of Snowdon (266) with those of Kanarek (122) on Table 1 for rats, and the results of Porikos et al (212) with those of Campbell et al (48) for man. Because the Campbell et al (48) study was longer than that of Porikos et al (212), the second factor, time on the diluted diet, should be considered. The longer a subject is on the diet, the more likely it is that compensation will be completed [(26, 265, 279); see also Table 1]. The same conclusion applies to man [see data of Spiegel (269) in Table 1] and to monkeys (107). The third factor contributing to response magnitude is the degree of dilution or concentration. Adolph (3) showed that, with liquids, intake was within 10% of normal intake when the diet was diluted to 8% solids in water. When solids were used as diluents, full caloric compensation occurred in response to dilutions up to 50% with kaolin but only to 25% with cellulose. Beyond these levels of dilution, compensation was incomplete.

Addition of nutritive fat is the fourth factor that influences response to caloric dilution. High-fat diets result in excessive caloric intake (50, 179,

Table 1 Effect of nutrient concentration on food intake

Type of food	Caloric density	Species	Intake/day g or ml[a]	Intake/day kcal	Meal size g or ml	Meal size kcal	Number of meals	Access time hr/day	Access time days	Avg. wt. (kg)	Reference numbers
Powdered chow	3.6	rat	23.85	85.86	3.0	10.8	8.86	24	15	.371	122
Above + 25% cellulose	2.7	rat	26.42	71.33	3.0	8.1	6.70	24	10	.371	122
Chow + oil	4.5	rat	20.4	91.8	3.1	13.95	9.38	24	10	.371	122
Liquid	1.8	rat	41.2	74.16	3.01	5.4	14.55	24	2–4	.348	266
Liquid ½ strength	0.9	rat	89.6	80.64	5.06	4.5	18.16	24	2–4	.348	266
Liquid ¼ strength	0.45	rat	144.4	64.98	7.57	3.4	19.73	24	2–4	.348	266
Powdered chow	3.5	rat	14.3	50	i			2	7	.271	265
Above + cellulose	2.1	rat	12.5	26.2				2	7	.234	265
Chow + fat	6.0	rat	12.9	77.9				2	7[b]		265
Chow + fat + cellulose	4.75	rat	16.1	76.3				2	7[b]		265
Chow + fat + kaolin	3.5	rat	22.0	77.1				2	5[c]		265
Pellets	3.6	rat	22.7	79.4				24	3[d]		265
Pellets + cellulose	2.1	rat	34	71.4				24	3[d]		265
Ensure	1.35	monkey	453	612.5				24	15–60	5.7–8.8	107
Ensure	1.0	monkey	583	583				24	60	5.7–8.8	107
Ensure	0.5	monkey	1126	563				24	15–60	5.7–8.8	107

Table 1 (Continued)

Type of food	Caloric density	Species	Intake/day g or ml[a]	Intake/day kcal	Meal size g or ml	Meal size kcal	Number of meals	Access time hr/day	Access time days[d]	Avg. wt. (kg)	Reference numbers
Metracal	1.0	human (gp A)[h]	1902	1902	5.86	5.86	3.3	24	4–7		269
Metracal	0.5	human (gp A)	2009	1004.5	1164	582	3.45	24	4–8		269
Metracal	1.0	human	2463	2463	1118	1118	2.2	24	7–9		269
Metracal	0.5	human (gp B)	4288	2144	3232	1616	2.6	24	12–14		269
Mixed		human		3400				24	3[e]	103	211, 212
Mixed + 25% dilution		human		2516				24	3[e]	104	211
Mixed + 25% dilution		human		2822				24	3[f]	104	211
Mixed		human		3600				24	6		211
Mixed + 25% dilution		human		3000				24	12		211
Liquid formula	1.0	human[g]	1795	1795				24	5–8	59	48
Liquid formula		human	2692	1777				24	5–7	59	48

a Units are grams for solids, ml for liquids.
b Second week on diet.
c Last 5 days on diet.
d Last 3 days of 1 week period.
e First 3 days on diluted diet.
f Second 3 days on diluted diet.
g Based on 3 subjects who received both 1.0 and .66 kcal/ml concentrations.
h Group A and group B were treated differently in the experiment. A received meals both inside and out of the laboratory, while S's in B had to come to laboratory to eat all meals.
i Blank spaces in the table indicate that data were not presented for that variable.

277), but compensation for their dilution is better than it is with low-fat diets (265). The fifth factor is time of access, in hours per day, to food. When access is limited, the response to dilution is blunted and/or requires more days to reach equilibrium (26, 265). The sixth factor is body fat stores. Obese animals respond more poorly to dilution than lean ones (42, 127, 279), although this effect can be minimized by using liquid diets (60, 284). These results are consistent with observations that some obese rats are hyperreactive to the sensory qualities of the diet (60, 127, 281). When a pelleted rather than a powdered diet was diluted with 25 or 50% kaolin, obese rats with ventromedial hypothalamic lesions increased their food intakes as much as did control rats (265a).

Finally, the factor of species difference in response to dilution must be considered. In order to make a comparison among species, all other factors should be held constant. Since most studies have not utilized the comparative approach, an accurate assessment cannot be made. However, based on the closest approximations, it appears that dogs, cats, and guinea pigs respond poorly to dilution, while rats, monkeys, and humans respond better. For further information, consult the references listed by species in Table 2.

Response to Changes in Energy Expenditure

Although relative long-term consistency in food intake is circumstantial evidence for existence of a regulation, it is not conclusive. Dilution experiments suggested that within limits nutrient intake is preserved. Evidence that the energy in the food is the quality controlled was provided by experiments that showed compensation in food intake when energy expenditure was varied. These experiments thus shifted emphasis to regulation of the energy balance of the body rather than of nutrient intake (42a, 172). Energy expenditure can be varied by changing the activity level of the animal by

Table 2 Studies using dietary dilution

Species	References
Rat	3, 50, 265, 265a, 266
Dog	59
Cat	121
Guinea pig	110
Hamster	253
Gerbil	126
Quail	294
Ruminants	183
Human	48, 211, 212, 269, 309

enforced exercise or restraint, as well as by changing the environmental temperature.

Hamilton (103) has reviewed experiments on the effects of ambient temperature changes on food intake. Since that review appeared, investigators have concentrated on the pattern of eating by which changes in food intake are mediated. Food intake is inversely proportional to ambient temperature, and the major effect of temperature is on the frequency of meals (132, 138, 139, 295). However, the time course of adaptation to a given ambient temperature suggests that energy requirements are not the only determinant of food intake of a mixed diet. Within a few days after a change in ambient temperature the food intake of rats returns toward normal (102, 295).

An early demonstration of the effect of exercise on food intake is that of Mayer et al (173). They showed a slight decrease in intake as energy expenditure increased from sedentary levels and then a linear increase, proportional to the time the female rats spent on a treadmill, up to 5 hr per day. Beyond 5 hr per day of exercise, food intake decreased. Nikoletseas (193) has recently pointed out that the generality of this effect can be obscured by other factors: sex of the animal, time allowed for feeding, spacing of exercise bouts, and duration of the experiment. The following examples illustrate these limitations to the generality. Food intake of female, but not male, rats increased with exercise (199), although intake of male rats increased if a variety of foods was available (7). Food intake was depressed immediately after exercise, even up to 24 hr, but overshot after a day without exercise both in men (76) and rats (274). Regularly spaced bouts of exercise decreased food intake less than irregularly spaced bouts, and after adaptation the decrease was reduced (274). Limiting the time allowed for eating after exercise resulted in failure to increase food intake, and the imbalance in expenditure led to mortality (233), which could be offset by prior adaptation to the feeding schedule (232). The decrease in food intake following exercise was also not observed in 23-hr fasted male rats that had been trained to run prior to introduction of the deprivation schedule (192). Increases in food intake were seen during weeks when energy expenditure was increased in lean (207) but not obese (304) women.

Effects of Changes in Body Nutrient Content

Excesses or deficiencies in body weight, which reflect body nutrient content when transient changes in body water are controlled, lead to changes in food intake in almost all studies of this phenomenon. Adolph (3) did not observe increased food intake upon restoration of food supply to young rats (150–300 g males) deprived of food (but not of water) for either 1 or 6 days; he did observe such increases upon restoration when both food and water had been removed. However, in older rats weighing 350 g or more, deprivation of food for 24 or 48 hr increased food intake from about 22 to about 28 g on the first day of restoration (11, 104, 157, 158, 159, 209). This increase gradually declined over 3–4 days to the pre-deprivation level. Deprivation for longer than 48 hr decreased the initial day's intake to 26 g in 3-day-fasted, 24 g in 4-day-fasted, and 20 g in 6-day-fasted rats (104). However, following fasts of greater than 2 days, food intake gradually increased after the first day of restoration and remained elevated for a number of days proportional to the length of the fast. However, in no case did the total excess intake exceed the amount taken in a single 24-hr period prior to deprivation (160).

Increases in food intake also occurred when body energy was depleted by limiting caloric intake, either by means of providing less food (209), adding quinine to the food (158), or reducing availability of water (158). Slightly larger food intakes were seen intially upon restoration of ad libitum food following partial restriction of food (209) or following feeding of a nonnutritive diet of vaseline and cellulose (104), than following complete food deprivation, even when animals were reduced to the same body weights. It has been suggested that either gastrointestinal factors (104) or starvation diabetes (209) accounts for the reduced intake of the completely starved, in comparison with the food restricted rats. However, body weight is not a perfect index of body fat mass. We suggest that hypometabolism (61) in the completely starved animals may preserve more fat in them than in the restricted rats, and that the metabolic contribution of this hypothetically larger fat mass may reduce hyperphagia. Hypometabolism could also be responsible for the fact that starved rats recovered to the same body composition as unstarved rats with an increased food efficiency (22) [ratio of weight gain to food intake].

Not all species respond as the rat does to deprivation, and not all studies on the rat find uniform effects, particularly when only limited periods were available for eating [see (14, 158) for further discussion of the rat]. Dogs (2, p. 324) and monkeys (176) made up deficits well even in a limited time. Rabbits made up deficits partially by increasing food intake, (164) as did guinea pigs (110). Hamsters did not make up deficits by increased food intake unless on a high fat diet (39) consisting of sunflower seeds; otherwise they lost weight that was not completely recovered (253).

Weight gain induces reduction of food intake. The magnitude of this reduction depends on several factors: the means by which weight gain was induced, amount of weight gain, age of the animal, and diet. Food intake was reduced after the following weight-gain-inducing procedures were terminated: (a) forced intubation of excess food (52, 230) and (b) overeating induced by either electrical stimulation of the brain (272) or injection of long-acting insulin (114). Food intake declines only gradually during weight gain induced by adding fat to the diet (81) or offering concentrated sugar solutions (124). The precise effect on food intake of terminating these procedures has not been studied. However, a precipitous drop would be predicted, because switching rats from highly palatable "snack food" diets to chow after they have gained weight results in food intake reduction (88, 230, 250), although this effect is not uniformly seen (227). It is not clear whether strain differences are responsible for these different results; but this possibility is likely because rat strains are differentially susceptible to the fattening effects of high-fat diets (244) and varied cafeteria diets (231), possibly as a result of the ability of brown fat to burn off the excess intake (231).

It has been reported (see 151) that after weight-gain inducing procedures are terminated rats are hypophagic until they return to their initial body weight, but the actual functional relationship between food intake and body weight has not been precisely specified. Such a relationship is important to know, because it would suggest the type of mechanism (e.g. constant input vs trigger at a certain level) by which body weight could influence food intake. Furthermore, it is important to separate the effects of the various treatments that induce weight gain from the weight gain itself in order to determine what factors are responsible for the apparent effects of changes in body nutrient stores. Obviously, much more work is needed in this important area of investigation.

Microstructure of Eating: Periodicity and Rate

Another basic phenomenon requiring explanation by theories of food intake control is the intermittent occurrence of feeding and its change in rate throughout the meal. Richter (217) was the first to record feeding patterns in the rat. He found meals regularly spaced at about 4-hr intervals. Subsequent investigators have found that the temporal pattern, like total daily food intake, varies quantitatively with a variety of conditions [see (295) for details].

One of the most interesting meal pattern phenomena is the Le Magnen [(267), p. 74] postprandial correlation, a high and significant correlation between the size of a meal and the interval that follows it. Le Magnen and colleagues (152, 155, 156) also noted absence of correlation between the size of a meal and the interval that precedes it during spontaneous feeding in nondeprived rats. This finding was surprising because previous studies had suggested that the interval of deprivation increases the size of subsequent meals (14). Apparently different rules apply to nondeprived animals. This finding has been found in most species [see (151) for details], including man (20). The Le Magnen correlation refocused attention from a search for an increase in depletion factors that control feeding to a search for satiety factors whose decrease releases feeding from inhibition (30).

Many factors influence the meal pattern. These include species, sex, nutritional status, and type and nutrient density of food, as well as phase of the light-dark cycle and effort required to obtain food. The complex effects of these various factors have been reviewed (55, 295). An excellent discussion of the role of metabolic depletion and repletion in relation to meal patterns has recently been completed (151). In the rat, meals vary in size from 3–10 kcal depending on the density and palatability of the diet, and intermeal intervals range from 20 min to 6 hr depending on meal size and effort expended to obtain food. Intake during the dark phase of a 12–12 light-dark cycle is generally twice as large as during the light. Finally, rats tend to be hyperphagic (eating more than the energy they expend) in the dark and hypophagic (eating less than the energy they expend) in the light (154).

Rate is another microstructural characteristic of eating that has received attention, recently. Most observers agree that the rate of eating gradually drops during a meal (120, 254), although this phenomenon is more apparent in deprived than nondeprived subjects (see Figure 1). Mathematical models (64) and equations (136, 174) have been proposed to describe and explain the shape of curves of cumulative intake during a meal under a variety of conditions. Deprivation and palatability increase the initial rate of eating, while gastrointestinal overfilling induced by ingestion of hyperosmotic fluids slows the rate of eating more quickly during the course of a meal (64, 135). An important clinical issue, still controversial, is the idea that rapid eating results in greater intake. This hypothesis is suggested by Jordan & Spiegel (119), who found increased intake when they increased the rate of delivery of food via a pump or simultaneously delivered diet into the stomach while subjects were taking food from the pump by mouth. It is disputed by the mathematical model of Booth & Mather (38), which suggests that an increased rate of eating will activate post-absorptive satiety systems faster than normal and will therefore hasten satiety. The influence of body weight on rate of eating has also been studied. Some studies report higher rates of eating in obese people, whereas others report no differences [see (270) for review], although most of these studies are confounded by interactions with the type of food and sex of the subject (136). In rats the rate of eating declines after deprivation-induced weight loss (158). The rate of eating after overfeeding has not been reported, although after obesity induced by ventromedial hypothalamic lesion it was found unchanged (284).

Nutrient Selection

Another important basic phenomenon in the control of food intake is the ability of animals to select the proper balance of the three major macronutrients, protein, fat, and carbohydrates, from an array of foods with mixed macronutrient content or from a selection of relatively pure macronutrients themselves (78, 201, 218, 235). The amounts of the three macronutrients

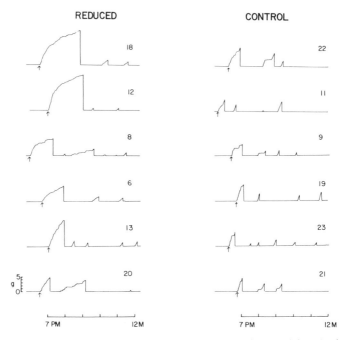

Figure 1   Meal pattern profiles of rats following either a period of 20% weight reduction (left side) as a result of being fed five small (1.5 g) meals per day every 2 hr during the light phase, or no restricted feeding (right side). Both groups were fasted the night before these records were taken and given the same 5 small meals. The last meal was 2 hr before these records were collected. Food was 45 mg Noyes pellets taken from a pellet detecting eatometer (132a). The meal pattern profiles were generated by computer analysis adapted for solid food intake, collected by printout counters (15). (H. R. Kissileff, A. Schmader, unpublished data, 1976).

selected vary with the condition of the animal [e.g. exercised vs sedentary (7, 56), diabetic vs normal (84, 219)], the selections available (78), and the experimental treatments [e.g. insulin administration (125) or ventromedial hypothalamic lesions (123, 131)]. However, under nonintervention conditions, the ratios among spontaneous macronutrient intakes tend to be remarkably constant in humans (percentages of total calories were 11–15% from proteins, 50–58% from carbohydrate, and 26–37% from fat), and somewhat more variable in the rat (see Table 3). Successful survival on self-selection diets also depends on acceptable orosensory qualities of the diet, and Epstein has wisely stated: "The wisdom of the body is not an infallible guide to nutrition" [(78), p. 201].

Availability and Palatability

Availability refers to the ease with which the animal obtains food [procurement cost (53)] and palatability refers to the orosensory qualities that determine acceptance (134). The latter definition may not be accepted by

Table 3 Percentages of macronutrients chosen on self selection diets

Species	Daily intake (kcal)	Fat	Protein	Carbohydrate	Age[a]	Weight[b]	Sex[c]	Source
Rat	46.3	64.0	16.0	20.0	59	130	F	218
Rat[g]	130.0	34.4	9.0	56.6	—	387	M	248
Rat	62.4	26.4	27.5	46.1	49	128–172	F[d]	123
Rat	86.5	18.0	35.0	47.0	—	202–271	F	125
Human	3432.0	33.3	11.8	53.3	19	70	M	76
Human	3296.0	26.1	15.3	58.6	44	103	M & F	212
Human	2460.0[e]	35.0	11.0	54.0	16	55	F	207
Human	2900.0[f]	37.0	13.0	50.0	16	55	F	207
Human	2233.0[e]	31.6	15.8	52.6	42	92	F	303a
Human	2345.0[f]	32.7	15.8	51.5	42	92	F	303a

[a] Years for man, days for rat
[b] g for rat, kg for man
[c] M = male, F = female
[d] Sham group, preoperative
[e] Nonexercising
[f] Exercising
[g] Experiment 2, con-sham

all, as some authors (149, 312) consider the palatability to be a joint function of the animal and the food. However, we believe that in order to delineate the controls of food intake, it makes more sense to consider palatability a quality of the diet and to attribute changes within the animal to changes in its response to the same diet under different experimental conditions (e.g. after fasting, overfeeding, or conditioning).

When food becomes more scarce or more costly to obtain, intake gradually declines (122). When the palatability of the food changes, intake changes with it (224); foods whose acceptance or preferability in short-term tests is high will be overconsumed (281), and foods not preferred in short-term tests will be underconsumed. These changes in intake are not constant over time, however. Rats compensate for changes in diet palatability over time and can maintain almost normal growth on diets that were initially almost totally unacceptable (144, 208). Because units of palatability and availability (or effort) have not been scaled in a standarized way, intake as a function of palatability or effort has not been precisely described. On the theoretical plane, at least two possible relations could be seen. Palatability could yield a graded response in intake if its effects summed with other controls, or it could yield a dichotomous (either high or low) response in food intake if it simply served as a trigger to prevent or prolong eating.

Food variety is also an important factor in intake control. When people were fed three courses, each of a different-flavored yogurt, they consumed more than when the same flavor was given at each course (226). The variety effect has also been observed in rats (150).

Patterns of intake as well as total intake are affected by both palatability and availability of food. As the diet becomes less palatable, meals become smaller and more frequent (249), but they become larger and less frequent as the effort to obtain them is increased (122). For example, on a sweetened condensed milk diet rats took 18 meals per day of 3 ml. When the diet was adulterated with quinine, meal size dropped to 1.7 ml and meal frequency rose to 20 meals per day (249). Meal frequency dropped from 8.8 per day with no effort to .62 per day when 640 lever presses were required to obtain access to the food. Meal size increased from 3 g per meal to 12 g per meal under these conditions. The average rate of eating was unaffected by the increased effort (122).

Summary of Phenomena

When experimenters manipulate the composition of the diet and the time of access to it or when the nutrient content of the animal is altered experimentally, compensatory responses are made in such a way as to restore the prior state of intake of the animal or its body composition. Such responses suggest the existence of detectors that monitor either the intake or its consequent effects on body composition or distribution of nutrients within the body. They also suggest that some response system exists that brings about appropriate changes in intake or energy expenditure. However, responses to some changes in diet composition, such as to those that affect primarily sensory rather than nutritional quality, contradict the idea that intake is determined solely by compensatory changes in response to perturbations in body constituents (283). Not all phenomena can be explained by any simple account of the control of food intake, such as the contraction of an empty stomach (49) or depletion or reduction in utilization of a critical metabolite (172) or even metabolites in general (86, 128).

THEORIES

The theories advanced to explain the results described above are either homeostatic (i.e. they posit attempts to preserve constancy in a variable) or nonhomeostatic. The homeostatic hypotheses often suppose the existence of a reference value or set point (302, 303) against which current values in the regulated variable are compared. Such theories suggest that the discrepancy between this set point and the current value is then used to drive or inhibit a response such as eating. Since no direct evidence for set points has ever been found, it has also been proposed that the sensitivity of detectors and their connections to a response system could restore imbalances and therefore act as a regulatory system (45, 302). Several homeostatic theories of feeding have been advanced over the last 30 years. For those that have been repeatedly reviewed we provide only brief descriptions here and refer the reader to other reviews (4, 40, 203) for details of evidence in their support.

Nonhomeostatic theories do not posit mechanisms that preserve constancies. Instead, such theories assert that the primary control of food intake originates in the configuration of the environment and the genetic adaptations built into the animal to cope with that environment, or to psychological constructs such as drives or incentives that induce the animal to engage in feeding behavior not for the purpose of restoring some deficiency but in order to obtain pleasure or reward. While a single unifying theory would be preferable to the present dichotomy, no such theory exists; the mathematical model of Booth & Mather (38) is an attempt to unify both types of theories in a rigorous way.

Homeostatic Theories

The homeostatic theories propose that a variable is regulated [i.e. maintained constant by means of detectors for its value or some function of it (44)] and that controls (management of rates of functioning) are set in motion to accomplish these regulations. Two kinds of homeostatic theories can be distinguished: those proposing that specific chemicals in the body are regulated [e.g. fats, carbohydrates (mainly glucose), or proteins (i.e. specific amino acids)], and those that propose regulation of energy or some function of it such as body temperature. The lipostatic theory, for example, proposed that depot fat was the regulated variable and that rates of food intake and energy expenditure were its controls (128, 295). The glucostatic theory proposed that utilization of glucose by privileged cells was maintained constant by initiating eating when utilization was low and inhibiting eating when utilization was high (79, 172). The aminostatic theory (178) likewise proposes that excesses and deficiencies of plasma amino acids are responsible for initiating or inhibiting food intake.

Another now-classical theory that attempted to link all these changes was the thermostatic theory (43, 45), which proposed that the heat generated by metabolic fuels either stimulated or inhibited feeding in accordance with the body's need to maintain a constant temperature. Recent adaptations of this theory propose that the energy produced by the metabolism of absorbed nutrients is monitored (28). However, neither the location of the detectors that perform this function nor the nature of the energy being monitored (i.e. electrical, chemical, or thermal) has been determined. The detectors could be in the brain, since it has been established that thermal detectors exist in the hypothalamus (106). There are, however, a number of difficulties with a strict thermal theory (see 86). Chemoreceptors have likewise been discovered in the brain (5, 198), but their relation to chemical energy remains a mystery. Evidence has been advanced for the liver as the organ that monitors the state of the body's energy stores. It has been proposed that "hunger arises in the liver when fuel delivery from the intestines and adipose tissue is inadequate for the maintenance of body functions without significant hepatic contributions" [(86), p. 423].

The problem of the location of detectors and effectors for homeostatic response has been central to discussions of ingestive behavior for decades and merits more consideration than our brief review can provide. We (295) recently reviewed the status of the "dual center" theory originally proposed by Brobeck (42a). In brief this theory stated that feeding was elicited by a lateral hypothalamic center that was inhibited by a ventromedial hypothalamic center as a result of certain (unspecified) post-feeding changes in the body. When the food eaten was disposed of, the lateral hypothalamic center became active again, and the cycle was renewed. Although the concept of diffuse excitatory and inhibitory systems has replaced that of discrete centers (273), the notion of dual controls, one that excites and one that inhibits feeding, is still very much a part of most thinking about the neural control of intake. Evidence for the theory comes from the incontestable facts that (a) lesions (46) or anesthetization (77) of the ventromedial hypothalamus induce hyperphagia, while stimulation of it inhibits eating (143); and (b) lesions of the lateral hypothalamus induce aphagia (6) or hypophagia, while stimulation of it induces eating (181). The theory was also tied to chemostatic theories by locating detectors in the ventromedial hypothalamus (128, 172). This part of the theory initially ran into difficulty when anatomically direct stimulation by injection of putatively monitored metabolites failed to suppress food intake (77, 298) in acute experiments. However, it now appears that chronically administered nutrients do suppress food intake when injected intracranially in both the ventromedial hypothalamus (203, 205) and ventricles (66, 67, 306). Booth (30) seriously questions the interpretation of the lesion/stimulation approach, and his cautious critique should be read by any serious student of food intake.

The other suggested major site for homeostatic control of food intake is the liver. Russek (236) first proposed that hepatic glucoreceptors were involved in feeding because intraperitoneal glucose depressed intake more than equal doses injected into the jugular vein. According to current versions of the theory (237, 238), hunger is the result of decrease in the carbohydrate reserves signaled to the brain by discharges from the hepatocytes in the liver. The pathway for these discharges is in dispute (17, 162, 238). The system operates as follows: "Some metabolite of the glycolytic chain (i.e. pyruvate), related both to liver glycogen content and glucose input of the hepatocytes, has an hyperpolarizing effect on their membranes, perhaps through an increase in the sodium pump. Thus, hunger would normally appear when intestinal absorption and liver glycogen (and liver pyruvate) decrease to a certain critical level" [(237), pp. 137–38]. Note that the wording is almost identical to that of Friedman & Stricker (86). Hyperpolarization and disappearance of the hunger discharges would occur as soon as absorption of glucose and/or amino acids from the intestine increased liver pyruvate, thereby inducing satiety. "Preabsorptive satiation is hypothesized to be caused by a reflex secretion of intrahepatic adrenaline from hepatic chromaffin cells located in the portal spaces [(171, 216)], elicited by information originating in the oropharyngeal, gastric and duodenal receptors [(63, 189, 190, 197, 252, 292)]. Duodenal (and possibly gastric) glucose and amino acid receptors might be the unconditional afferentation of this reflex, while oropharyngeal receptors and gastric distension receptors might produce a conditional effect which can be adapted to the changes in caloric content of food" [(237), p. 138]. Russek goes on to conclude that hepatic receptors might be the most important receptors determining hunger and satiety because "all the numerous factors that have been shown to influence food intake may act as modulators of this mechanism" [237), p. 141]. This is probably the most comprehensive theory proposed since the dual center theory and its chemostatic associates. It is heuristic, like the old glucostatic theory, because the major metabolic fluxes of the body converge on the liver. It is supported by the facts that intraportal injection of adrenaline and/or infusion of glucose inhibit feeding while equivalent doses elsewhere are less effective (36, 194, 196, 240). Electrophysiological studies support the existence of receptors (239). The theory has not gone unscathed, however; its critics point out that vagotomy fails to affect food intake patterns (162) and that glycogen levels gradually rise during the night and fall during the day (153), following, rather than leading, accumulation in food intake. Russek has responded to these and other criticisms (238), and the theory certainly merits further testing.

Two other organs, the stomach and intestine, have been considered as primary foci for homeostatic theories of food intake. McHugh & Moran (177) consider them as a unit, such that the intestine controls the rate of stomach emptying according to caloric homeostasis of emptying rate. Smith & Gibbs (258) and Deutsch (70) view them as units providing independent contributions. According to each of these authors, neural and/or humoral signals arise in these organs that inhibit food intake. When the signals are absent, intake will occur again. This theory is appealing because of its simplicity and because it makes easily tested predictions about the effects on food intake of manipulating the stomach and intestine by means of loading or emptying them, by stimulating or ablating their neural connections, or by simulating actions of their hormones. More of this evidence is detailed in the section on nutrient administration, below. Here we outline only the most compelling evidence and indicate the theory's limitations.

McHugh (175) has shown that caloric intake could be controlled by distension of the stomach, which is in turn controlled by an intestinal mechanism that operates as though calories delivered to the intestine were the key signal controlling emptying of the stomach. Accordingly, preloads of the three macronutrients in equicaloric amounts suppressed subsequent food intake by the same amount (176) and emptied from the stomach at the same caloric rate (177). These results suggested the possibility that the "regulation of caloric delivery by the stomach could have a direct role in the control of food intake" [(177), p. R259]. The stomach and intestine could play a role in the phenomena of feeding we have described above only if emptying were controlled by some function of previously eaten food that had released its calories in a detectable way (i.e. by generating heat or being converted to detectable nutrient store). The theory predicts that stomach emptying will be slower and feeding inhibited after caloric intake exceeds energy expenditure. Doubts about such a mechanism, expressed by Van Itallie et al (295), now seem to be receiving confirmation in more recent studies by Moran & McHugh (185). Two predictions from the theory failed. First, glucose and xylose (a poorly metabolized pentose) leave the stomach at the same rate, yet only glucose contains potentially detectable calories. Nevertheless, each preload results in equal suppression of intake in a 4-hr test. The caloric deficit incurred after the xylose preload is made up the following day. Second, fructose leaves the stomach twice as rapidly as glucose, yet both hexoses inhibit food intake equally in a 4-hr test. Nevertheless, glucose inhibits food intake more than fructose during the first 80 min.

Thus although the gastrointestinal theory of homeostatic control of food intake cannot always account for the phenomena of regulation of energy balance, it can provide an explanation for satiety, whose putative link with energy expenditure must still be provided.

Nonhomeostatic Theories

Three major types of nonhomeostatic theory have been proposed: ecological, psychological, and computable. They differ from the homeostatic theory in that they do not posit the maintenance of a constancy in some body constituent. They do not deny the existence of regulation but propose that it is handled by physiological rather than behavioral processes. The ecological theories propose that feeding behavior is simply one of several alternative behaviors an animal can perform at any given time, and that the selection of a behavior is determined not so much by internal state of the animal as by ecological variables such as cost, abundance, and value (53). According to the theory, animals use an optimizing strategy for controlling meal patterns. An optimal feeding strategy maximizes energy intake relative to the time and/or energy spent feeding. This theory predicts that animals will reduce meal frequency and increase meal size as the effort required to obtain food is increased, a prediction borne out in several species (54, 111, 121, 122). Obviously, the theory is a viable alternative to homeostatic theories for explaining meal patterns; but it certainly is not as general, since it does not attempt to explain the many other phenomena, such as nutrient selection or the variety of meal pattern responses to caloric density, deprivation, or palatability.

The second nonhomeostatic theory, reinforcement or incentive theory [see (288) for discussion], proposes that feeding, once initiated (by an unspecified mechanism), is maintained by certain sensory qualities of food that activate "reward" neurons. These neurons can only be activated by the food when the animal is hungry (228). These neurons are in turn modulated by the internal states of the animal, such as levels of hormones or metabolites. This proposal differs from homeostatic theories in positing no detection of departure from a set point to which the system must return after a disturbance is removed. Reinforcement theory suggests that food intake is controlled by cycles of depletion that permit reward neurons to be activated, and of repletion that block their activation. Behavioral evidence in support of this theory comes from studies showing that brain stimulation at certain sites both reinforces operant behavior (i.e. causes animals to sustain responses that result in further stimulation) and elicits feeding (113, 168). Furthermore, modulation of the reward effects of brain stimulation is obtained by body weight manipulations (112), and body weight manipulations also influence the ingestion of palatable solutions (47, 99, 184, 204).

The third type of nonhomeostatic theory is computable theory (i.e. food intake quantitatively predicted from physiological variables such as rates of stomach emptying, absorption, and metabolism), developed most fully by Booth and his colleagues (30, 33, 38). This theory accounts for meal patterns, adjustments to changes in energy balance, and rewarding effects of sensory quality in combination with energy flows, gastroduodenal control of absorption rate, and learning. It is predicated on the idea that feeding is initiated when net energy flow from lean body mass is detected and stops when there is a net energy flow to lean body mass, provided that orogastrointestinal cues are present, which have been associated with previous energy flows to lean body mass (31). The accuracy of computable theory exceeds that of nonmathematical theories and permits the inclusion of a greater number of variables. Since the components of the model can be manipulated mathematically, the theory permits accurate prediction of the effects of a particular treatment on all variables. The advantages and disadvantages of such a theory have been discussed (30, 38, 182). The theory has yet to incorporate the effects of neurotransmitters and hormones but is presently the most comprehensive of all theories and has the potential to surpass all other theories in accuracy of prediction.

TESTS OF THE THEORIES BY NUTRIENT ADMINISTRATION

Dependent Variables

The predominant theory is that control of food intake is energostatic (see the section above on Homeostatic Theories). The major evidence for this theory is the reduction in feeding activity when nutrients are administered and the lack of effect of administering nonnutritive substances. These reductions have been measured in terms of consumatory (amount eaten) and appetitive (performance of arbitrary responses to obtain food) behaviors. The major dependent variables used to assess consumatory behavior are (a) total daily food intake, expressed in units of weight, volume, or energy or (b) intake at a single session lasting either for a fixed time (e.g. 1–12 hr) or until the subject stops eating for a fixed interval of time. Within each of these measures some finer-grain analyses have been attempted. Meal patterns have been analyzed to determine whether administration of nutrients affects an onset or termination (95, 215, 285) mechanism for control of daily intake, and rate of eating during the course of a meal has been analyzed in the single-meal situation (65, 136).

Appetitive behavior has also been used to assess the effects of nutrient administration when the amount of consumatory (133) activity is limited. Animals are trained to press a lever to obtain food; the rate of pressing on a low-density reinforcement schedule (i.e. several presses are required to obtain a single aliquot of 40–100 mg) is the measure of feeding activity (137, 262a). These details are emphasized at the outset because inconsistent results could be explained by differences in both dependent and independent variables.

Independent Variables

Various manipulations have been shown to influence the outcome of nutrient administration experiments, including type of substance, rate and frequency of administration, interval from administration to testing, nutritional status (hours of deprivation, prior feeding history, body weight), species and surgical preparation, route of administration, and test diet for determining the effect of the experimental treatment. With such an array of factors it is little wonder that it is difficult to make sweeping generalizations. Nevertheless, there is universal agreement that prior administration of nutrients reduces both appetitive and consumatory behavior. This generalization is in accord with predictions of the energostatic theory. On the other hand, quantitative details differ across the range of independent variables.

Type of Substance

In this section we consider the effects of administering different substances when species, route, rate, and other variables are held constant; in subsequent sections we consider the effects of other variables when substance injected is held constant. We deal with interactions (i.e. effects of one independent variable that are not uniform in combination with other independent variables) along the way rather than in a separate discussion at the end. The effects of route of administration are discussed in the section on mechanisms, below, in relation to the issue of sites where nutrients and nutrient derived signals act to influence food intake.

This section addresses three questions: (a) How well does a subject (animal or person) compensate for administration of a nutritionally adequate mixture of nutrients to its body? We evaluate this response by means of an index known as the "suppression efficiency" (215), which is the amount of reduction in voluntary intake expressed as a percentage of the administered load. (b) How much of such reduction is attributable to bulk in the gastrointestinal tract? This question is answered by comparing the effects of administering nonnutritive, poorly absorbed, or poorly metabolized substances with those of administering nothing at all. (c) Do nutrients have specific chemical effects, or do they reduce food intake by some common property such as energy release (28), its time derivative, power (191), or osmolarity (65, 262, 264, 287)?

Loads of Nutritionally Adequate Mixtures

The hypothesis that food intake is controlled by a homeostatic mechanism predicts that disturbing the system by overloading the body with nutrients should be precisely compensated for by reduction in intake equal to the magnitude of the load. If this homeostatic hypothesis were substantiated, it would be logical to determine next what aspect of nutrient loads (including their bulk, which theoretically could be regulated) is detected. In two early tests of this hypothesis, deprived animals were offered food [a solid food for dogs (116) and milk for rats (18)] in two sessions separated by a short interval. Intake was almost the same as it was in the control condition, which was a single session (see Table 4). However, if the food was placed directly in the stomach first, intake in the second session was not reduced as much as it was by food actually eaten in the first session. This difference between second session intakes following eaten vs administered food was smaller in the rat feeding on chow (263), than on milk (compare lines 3 and 4 on Table 4). In monkeys (177a), compensation was almost perfect (lines 8–10, Table 4). In human subjects (269), who were only 3–4 hr deprived, when oral intake in the first session was rapid there was a failure to compensate by adequately reducing intake in the second, so that two sessions of intake, one after the other, resulted in greater intake than a single session. Results of these types of studies depend on the choice of foods and cognitive state of the subject [see (270) for an exhaustive treatment of this paradigm]. Even though compensation was incomplete, reduction in intake was proportional to the size of the load, when loads of different amounts were given [(300); lines 5–7, Table 4].

Some of the trends in these acute studies suggest that better compensation might be seen with animals on ad libitum access to food and with liquid rather than solid foods. It was therefore surprising that Thomas & Mayer (285) did not find any better compensation obtained by use of chronic intragastric infusion of liquid diet than the earlier studies had found using acute injections (compare lines 11 & 12 with line 3 in Table 4). In another study (215) in which intragastric infusions were programmed to correspond to periods during which the animals normally ate, compensation rose from 75 to 87%. Finally, in the most recent study of this type, Rothwell & Stock (229) found that when rats were loaded with from one to three widely spaced meals, their daily intake was reduced in almost perfect compensation (see lines 14–16, Table 4). Similar results were also seen when dogs were chronically given a large fraction of the daily requirement intragastrically (117). However, the rats, unlike the dogs gained from .9 to 2.3 g/day more than controls over 21–30 days (229), and approximately 80% of the gain was fat. Results similar in magnitude to these were also obtained with intravenous nutrient infusions [(1); see line 17, Table 4].

Some of the results above appear to be at variance with a homeostatic theory of food intake control. However, homeostatic theories have been vague about the period over which equilibrium should be achieved. These results need not be considered violations of homeostatic principles if absorption and metabolism of the loaded and ingested food are not completed in the time permitted for response. This time is simply the reciprocal of the subject's energy expenditure. It would be about 20 min for each kcal eaten or loaded in the rat and 1 hr for each 100 kcal consumed by man. Furthermore, in animals subject to only a few hours of feeding (263), lack of perfect compensation could be attributed to the constant stimulus to eat (or removal of satiating effects, whatever these may be) resulting from the sustained energy deficit (in comparison to ad libitum fed animals) that such schedules induce. On the other hand homeostatic theory cannot obviously account for the 18% difference in suppression efficiency between orally and intragastrically loaded food in the experiments of Berkun et al (18) or the failure to see 100% suppression efficiency in other studies. It may be that

Table 4 Effects of nutrient administration on food intake

Line	Species	Units	Oral loads Load size	Oral Intake w/o load	Oral Intake w. load	Oral Intake Diff.[a]	Oral Percentage comp.[b]	Intragastric loads Load size	Intragastric Intake w/o load	Intragastric Intake w. load	Intragastric Intake Diff.[a]	Intragastric Percentage comp.	Reference number
1	Dog	g	200[d]	932	694	238	119	200	1251.0	1308.0	-57	-28	116
2	Dog	g						450	999.5	515.5	484.5	107	116
3	Rat	ml	14.0[d]	19.7	7.1	12.6	90	14.0	19.7	9.6	10.1	72	18
4	Rat	g	4.2[d]	15.0	12.9	2.1	50	4.2	15.0	13.4	1.6	38	263
5	Human	ml	190.0[d]	635.0	476.0	159.0	83						300
6	Human	ml	317.0[d]	635.0	372.0	262.0	83						300
7	Human	ml	698.0[d]	635.0	152.0	483.0	69						300
8	Monkey	kcal	150.0[d]	437.0	273.0	164.0	109	150.0[d]	437.0	273.0	164.0	109	177a
9	Monkey	kcal						300.0[d]	442.0	134.0	306.0	102	177a
10	Monkey	kcal						450.0[d]	446.0	38.0	408.0	91	177a
11	Rat	ml						44.0[e]	72.0	40.0	32.0	72	285
12	Rat	ml						56.0[f]	63.0	21.0	42.0	75	285
13	Rat	ml						36.0	34.8	3.8	31.0	86	215c
14	Rat	kcal						31.0[g]	90.7	61.2	29.5	92	229
15	Rat	kcal						45.6[h]	97.2	50.4	46.8	102	229
16	Rat	kcal						59.9[i]	92.4	27.9	64.5	107	229
17	Rat	kcal						49.5[j]	74.5	28.8	45.7	92	1

[a] Difference in intake (without load − with load).
[b] Percentage compensation = difference in intake/load size.
[c] Based on mean data and report that intake was reduced .86 ml for each ml loaded in a meal paired paradigm.
[d] Single preload.
[e] Continuous load via chronically implanted nasogastric tube, 24 hr.
[f] Load with each meal via chronically implanted nasogastric tube, 24 hr.
[g] One load per day via gavage.
[h] Two loads per day via gavage.
[i] Three loads per day via gavage.
[j] Continuous intravenous load, 24 hr.

about one fifth of the satiation that results from eating is contributed by the oropharyngeal stimulation. This percentage approximately matches the 20% reduction in intake seen when rats, and 30% reduction when humans, feed themselves intragastrically (118).

Bulk

As a result of Cannon's (49) influential theory of hunger it has been commonly assumed that a major determinant of satiety and hence the amount of food consumed at a meal is a full stomach. Many observations have been consistent with this view. For example, Janowitz & Grossman (116) found that placing food or bulk in the stomach of a dog 20 min before its normal daily meal inhibited food intake by the same amount. In the rat, Smith & Duffy concluded that "food in the stomach inhibits further eating, but the immediate effect seems attributable to the physical properties (bulk) of the food" [(263), p. 608]. They found that preloads of food and of nonnutritive bulk depressed food intake about equally (see Table 5). Other lines of investigation, however, have led to the conclusion that bulk is not very important in the control of food intake. The many dilution studies previously discussed are examples (see the section on Dietary Dilution and Concentration). Other examples include the effects of bulk preloads in monkeys (176), simultaneous loads of water in man (118), and intragastric infusions of sodium and urea solutions with meals in the rat (268) (see Table 5 for details). Can these disparate findings be reconciled, and what can be concluded about the role of bulk in the control of food intake? Examination of Table 5 reveals several striking inadequacies in our knowledge of the effects of nonnutritive loads or mechanical distension (e.g. by balloon). In each report, only a few (sometimes only one) levels of bulk have been used. It is therefore impossible to determine the functional relationship between bulk and intake. The data suggest that the relation is linear, but not one to one—i.e. before the bulk effect begins to operate it must be in excess of 20% of the normal intake. The second major problem is the effect of the time factor. As Booth (29) has shown, it appears that in the nondeprived rat, bulk (induced by an osmotic load) has an inhibiting effect that lasts up to 2 hr and has disappeared after the fourth hour following a load. On the other hand, Smith & Duffy's (263) work in the deprived rat suggests that the effect lasts for two hours without change (compare lines 6–9 with 12–13 on Table 5). The time course of the effect may interact with deprivation.

A recent study by Deutsch, Gonzalez & Young (73) has attempted to evaluate what intragastric factors led to satiety. When rats were injected with an equal volume of saline as they drank a condensed milk diet, it was found that intake was reduced to about half of what would have been

Table 5 Effects of administration of bulk on food intake

Species	Type of bulk	Mode of administration	Deprivation (hr)	Delay[a]	Duration (hr)	Units Load	Units Intake	Load size	Amount eaten w/o load	Amount eaten w. load	Reference number
Dog	gum	gastric fistula	23.25	0	.75	% dry[b]	g	15	841.5	809.0	251
Dog	cellulose	gastric fistula	23.25	0	.75	% dry	g	15	841.5	650.0	251
Dog	balloon	inflation w. water	23.25	0	.75	ml	g	300	892.0	704.5	251
Dog	balloon	inflation w. water	23.25	0	.75	ml	g	500	892.0	578.0	251
Dog	balloon	inflation w. water	23.25	0	.75	ml	g	700[c]	937.0	388.0	251
Rat	kaolin	gavage of 66% slurry	22.00	0	.16	ml	g	10	2.9	2.8	263
Rat	kaolin	gavage of 66% slurry	22.00	0	2.0	ml	g	10	15.0	11.7	263
Rat	kaolin	gavage	22.00	0	.16	ml	g	15	2.9	1.8	263
Rat	kaolin	gavage	22.00	0	2.0	ml	g	15	15.0	9.4	263
Rat	.9% NaCl	nasogastric tube	0.	0	24.0	ml	kcal	47.3	64.4	70.9	268
Rat	1 M urea	nasogastric tube	0.	0	24.0	ml	kcal	46.9	64.8	70.4	268
Rat	1 M urea	gavage	0.	1	1.0	ml	g	5.0	1.7	.2	29
Rat	1 M urea	gavage	0.	1	3.0	ml	g	5.0	1.7	2.0	29
Rat	.9% NaCl	gastric tube	14.0	f	.5	ml	ml	11.7	21.1	11.7	73[d]
Monkey	cellulose	gastric fistula	20.0	0	4.0	ml	kcal	150.0	—	-.8[e]	176
Human	water	gastric tube	3–4	f	.33	ml	ml	370.0	414.0	296.0	118

[a] Interval from load to presentation of food (hr).
[b] % of dry weight of intake without load.
[c] Actually 75% of intake without food for each dog.
[d] Data averaged from all values in experiment 1.
[e] Cellulose suspension (unspecified concentration) was reported to reduce intake by 0.8 kcal.
[f] Load was simultaneous and contingent upon, eating.

expected if volume were the only factor controlling it. Conversely, when 5 ml were removed from the stomach as the rat drank, it overconsumed by almost half as much (7.2) as expected. These findings are consistent with the idea that both nutrient and bulk factors contribute to satiety. Until a quantitative manipulation of the bulk factor alone is made, we will not know exactly how much this factor contributes to the control of food intake. One of the problems in assessing this role is that the volume and contents in the stomach change as the rat eats. In order to circumvent this problem, experimenters have used esophagostomized animals (116), animals with open gastric fistula (258), or animals in which diet is removed as it is drunk (62, 74). In each case, the effects of preloading the stomach with bulk have reduced intake for the duration of sham feeding. However, the data available are insufficient to determine the functional relationship and thereby the mechanism of operation of distension on intake.

Osmotic Effects

Besides filling the gastrointestinal tract, nutrients can exert potential osmotic effects owing to their ability to draw water across semipermeable membranes into the gastrointestinal tract, thus filling it and also inhibiting food intake by temporarily dehydrating the rest of the body (68). Schwartzbaum & Ward (245) showed that food intake was depressed as much by stomach loads of hypertonic sodium chloride solutions as by equiosmotic glucose. Jacobs (115) pointed out that the two substances do not produce equivalent thirst effects and suggested that different inhibitory mechanisms were involved. This suggestion received some confirmation by Yin et al (311), who showed in an 8-hr test that intragastric glucose loads (10 ml, 45%) continued to suppress intake even when the rat was hydrated by the intravenous route, but that the suppression of intake induced by equiosmotic sodium chloride (10 ml, 8.1%) loads was almost totally abolished by intravenous water. This confirmation cannot be considered complete because it does not address the question of osmotic effects within the first few hours. Booth (29) showed that glucose, equiosmotic urea, and 3-o-methyl glucose—all poor inducers of thirst—have equal suppressing effects on food intake for the first two hours after a 1 M load of 5 ml. In the third hour only glucose continues to suppress intake. Booth suggests that inhibition by glucose in the first hour is mediated by a chemoreceptor with which 3-o-methyl glucose has a less effective interaction. It is therefore clear that at best osmotic effects are short-lived, but it is not clear whether the initial suppression by glucose is chemospecific, osmotic, or physical.

Energy vs Specific Nutrients

Since other reviewers (4, 30, 40, 203, 295) have provided evidence for and against the classic homeostatic hypotheses, we proceed directly to the question of whether chemospecific or energy-related properties of nutrients control intake. Because the macronutrients have differing sensory qualities, we consider only studies in which the sensory contributions from the oropharynx have been effectively eliminated (34, 35, 91) either by anesthesia, disguise of taste and flavor, or loading of nutrients directly into the circulation or digestive tract. Because energy regulation requires time for food to be absorbed and metabolized before its energy yield could be sensed directly, as either heat or stored nutrient, experiments bearing on this question must last long enough for these processes to occur. The longer the experiment lasts, the more likely the control of food intake by energy regulation will be confirmed. We therefore consider the longest studies first.

Liu & Yin (161) chronically loaded rats intragastrically with either 45% glucose solution or Crisco™ (fat with a 3:1 ratio of unsaturated to saturated fatty acids) in equicaloric amounts (27 kcal/day) for 5 weeks. Food intake was reduced in proportion to the calories loaded throughout the period, and body composition was no different between loading conditions when determined 1 week after termination of the loading. These results support an energy regulation hypothesis. Rothwell & Stock (229) using a similar procedure for only 30 days, but employing butter (3:5 ratio of unsaturated to saturated fatty acids) instead of Crisco™, reported that compensation was only 48% efficient, although when their animals were loaded with an equicaloric volume of a complete diet, suppression was 92% effective (see Table 4). They suggested that because of imbalances in dietary nutrients induced by the fat loads rats were eating to obtain sufficient amounts of other nutrients. Geliebter (92) reported in a longer study (6 weeks) that daily loads of either butter, corn oil, sucrose, or albumin gave nonsignificant differences in food intake across nutrients, and nonsignificant differences in body weight gain and Lee index. He did, however, note a persistent reduction in intake after protein loads 3.5 hr after the load.

These results suggest that any shorter term studies that showed differences in intake suppression across macronutrients (90, 91, 202) would not necessarily preclude adjustment of intake according to an energy balance regulation mechanism, but could be explained as a result of transient chemospecific effects on satiety. Examples of both energy regulatory and chemospecific effects have been found in short-term experiments. Energy regulation is favored by Booth (28), who found that when allowance was made for absorption and metabolism after a load, before food is presented, small nutrient loads (about the size of a normal meal) in otherwise undeprived rats depressed food intake by amounts almost equal to their metabolizable energy. When preabsorptive effects were examined, Booth (28) found a wide variety of intakes in the first hour of access after a 1 hr delay. Intake was least after glucose (0.9 g), highest after glycerol (2.4 g) and oleate (2.1

g) and intermediate after the amino acids valine (1.6 g) and lactate (1.4 g). Geary (90), however, found that suppression efficiency was greater for protein (1.51 kcal reduction in intake per kcal loaded) than glucose (.87) after 12 hr, but the difference was smaller after 24 hr (1.32 for protein and .81 for glucose). The difference from the results of Booth (28) could be attributed to use of proteins rather than amino acids in Geary's (90) study and to the fact that early effects of proteins were included in the 12 hr measures. The convergence of the suppression ratios at 24 hr suggests that longer times would be needed to adequately refute the hypothesis that enhanced nutrient-specific satiety effects of protein are eventually balanced by an energy regulatory mechanism that restores intake. Similar short-term effects of protein on human appetite have been reported (35).

Other studies suggest that the effects of nutrient administration interact with deprivation and possibly with the time of testing. For example, Panksepp (202) found no differences in the effects of equicaloric fat, carbohydrate, and protein loads, but his animals were 12 hr deprived and only tested for 0.5 hr in the light. The half-hour test probably only picks up gastric filling effects, and the animals may be less sensitive to the nutrient effects because of the deprivation, since Booth & Jarman (36) have shown that intake-suppressing effects of small amounts of glucose disappear after 4 hr of deprivation. Panksepp (202) did, however, find a 3.6 g larger suppression of intake following administration of protein than fat or carbohydrate in the first half hour of access to food after a period of spaced loads of 6 meals over 30 hr without other food available. Over the next 24 hr this difference was completely made up. He also found that fat loads suppressed intake less than did carbohydrate or protein loads after a 1-hr delay but not a 3-hr delay from load to eating in rats that were 3.5 hr deprived and tested in the light phase. These apparently conflicting results will not be resolved until we know more about the interaction of nutrient administration with metabolic effects of deprivation and light-dark cycle [see (151) for discussion of these effects]. Problems of interactions of nutrient administration with other factors abound in the long-term studies as well. Differences between the results of Geliebter (92) and Rothwell & Stock (229) could be attributed to the age of the animals, the schedule of nutrient administration, and/or duration of the experiment. Our answer to the question of whether intake is controlled by a nutrient-specific or an energy-regulatory mechanism must be tentative. It appears that in the short run satiety is under chemospecific control, in which the effectiveness per calorie increases in the order: fats, carbohydrates, and proteins. In the long run, when these nutrients are metabolized they exert their effects on food intake by means of their energy yield.

Nonnutritive Influences on the Outcome of Nutrient-Administration Experiments

In addition to the examples of nonnutritive effects presented above, there are several other important illustrations of the interaction of nutrient administration with other variables. The interaction between administration site and deprivation is a case in point: Isotonic glucose infusion suppressed food intake when injected duodenally into nondeprived rabbits or into the hepatic portal vein of deprived rabbits, but the same infusion had no effect when infused into the duodenum of a deprived rabbit or the hepatic portal vein of a nondeprived rabbit (291). The explanation for these findings, consistent with Russek's hepatostatic theory (236), is that duodenal infusion released more gut glucagon than did hepatic portal infusion, thereby raising the intrahepatic concentration of glucose in the nondeprived rabbit and inhibiting a vagally mediated activating signal (197, 291). In the deprived rabbit, glycogen is depleted and thus glucagon released by the duodenal infusion would have no effect. In the nondeprived rabbit, hepatic-portal infusion does not raise the glucose level in hepatic cells because there is already a high carbohydrate level in them, presumably preventing further uptake of glucose necessary to raise the glucose concentration within the cells. Further evidence for glucagon's role in mediating this effect has been obtained (289–290, 293). The importance of route of administration was also shown by the results of Snowdon (268), who found that meal-contingent duodenal infusion of hyperosmotic substances as well as nutrients reduced spontaneous meal size but did not reduce total nutrient intake, while only nutritive substances reduced meal size when infused into the stomach. These results suggested a duodenal rather than gastric locus for the osmotic inhibition of feeding.

The importance of nutritional status (deprived vs nondeprived) was shown by Baile et al (13), who found that glucose inhibited food intake in monkeys when infused intragastrically along with a meal (thus the animal was not in the deprived state), but not when it was given during a half-hour period preceding the meal, after a 22-hr fast. Suppression by preloaded glucose in deprived monkeys was observed, however, by McHugh & Moran (176). The latter believe that differences in the results are due to differences in the length of time food was available and the restraint imposed in the earlier (13) study. In man, Booth et al (34) have shown that a glucose load 15 min before a meal suppressed intake in proportion to the calories in the load, but did not do so if given just before the meal. On the other hand, intravenous infusion of glucose alone (21, 100) or along with insulin (305) failed to either increase or decrease food intake in man. In the rat, intravenous addition of insulin to glucose infusion did improve the suppression efficiency (191), but this effect could be attributable to the higher basal feeding level against which the results were compared when insulin alone was administered. It is clear that factors other than the kind of nutrients must be considered in the interpretation of the results of nutrient administration.

MECHANISMS

Much of the current work on the physiology of food intake control concerns the mechanisms underlying the phenomena and experimental results described above. Some of these, such as the hepatostatic hypothesis and gastrointestinal controls, have already been described. We now provide an overview of hormonal and vagal mediators of satiety, humoral and neural controls of the chronic effects of body weight on food intake, and the glucoprivic control of hunger. The reader may wish to consult one of the many recent symposium proceedings (51, 145, 195) or books (33, 241, 278) for further information.

Mechanisms of Satiety

We consider first the signals by which nutrient ingestion tells the central nervous system to terminate feeding. Both Kraly & Smith (142) and Deutsch and colleagues (74) have shown, using a pyloric noose to prevent outflow from the stomach to intestine, that the oropharynx and stomach together provide signals sufficient to induce satiety. Distension and nutrients induce satiety by different mechanisms, since vagotomy abolishes the response to distension but not to nutrients (96, 141). The stomach may also contain receptors for fat, since Deutsch & Gonzalez (72) found that intake of a 50% fat emulsion was the same whether the pylorus was occluded by cuff or not; intake of the emulsion increased when some of it was removed as they drank but remained the same when saline was injected as they drank. Unfortunately, a critical alternative condition—infusion of saline while the animals drank the emulsion with the pyloric cuff on—was not studied. Thus fat could have inhibited ingestion by a duodenal mechanism in the cuff-off condition while distension of the stomach inhibited it in the cuff-on condition.

Satiety signals can also arise from the intestine as shown by the effects of nutrient infusions into it. These effects could be mediated by one of several hormones released from the gut, stomach, or pancreas (259, 308). The hormone most thoroughly studied is cholecystokinin (CCK) (261). The target of its activity is probably not the brain but a vagally innervated structure, since vagotomy blocks its effect in the rat (260). Since CCK did reduce food intake when infused (though it did not when injected as a bolus) into the cerebral ventricles of sheep (69), there may be species differences in its mechanisms of action. Rats do not respond to intraventricular CCK (69). If the mechanisms of action are different in the two species, vagotomy should not affect the response to peripherally administered CCK in sheep. Administration of several other peptides found in the gut also led to reduction in food intake [see (259, 308) for reviews].

The neurotransmitters involved in the control of food intake are also being studied [see (147) for an encyclopedic review]. Feeding can be stimulated by norepinephrine injections into the paraventricular nucleus [apparently the target or origin of fibers whose damage leads to hyperphagia (187)] by means of an alpha-adrenergic mechanism (146). Feeding is inhibited by norepinephrine injection into the perifornical area of the hypothalamus [whose damage results in aphagia (6)] by means of a beta-adrenergic mechanism (148). When nutrients were infused into the duodenum, synaptic release of norepinephrine was enhanced at lateral sites where norepinephrine injections did not induce feeding [but suppressed it in other studies (148)], and synaptic norepinephrine release was suppressed at medial sites where norepinephrine injections enhanced feeding (188). Because norepinephrine is an inhibitory transmitter, the simplest hypothesis consistent with earlier lesion and stimulation studies is that norepinephrine elevation in the medial area suppresses "satiety" neurons by means of an alpha-adrenergic mechanism; feeding is then suppressed by a duodenally activated mechanism that increases norepinephrine in the lateral area, thereby inhibiting "feeding" neurons by means of a beta-adrenergic mechanism.

Serotonin is also probably involved in inhibition of food intake [see (299) for recent evidence and a brief review]. This inhibition may be linked to carbohydrate (82, 310), but probably not to protein, ingestion (210).

The latest in the series of neurotransmitters involved with feeding are the endogenous opioids (166, 308). Feeding is enhanced by the administration of beta-endorphin (97, 130) and its agonist, D-ala^2-metenkephalinimide (12) and is decreased by the opiate antagonist naloxone (167). However, it is not clear whether this reduction in appetitive behavior is general or specific to food intake, because naloxone reduces several appetitive behaviors (200, 271). The possibility that the endorphin system is specifically involved in the overeating of palatable foods or in the weight gain ensuing from it was suggested by the finding that naltrexone, another opiate antagonist, reduced food intake in animals that were eating an array of palatable foods but not in rats that were eating laboratory chow (10).

Mechanisms For Detecting Energy Deficits

No one has ever isolated a factor that directly induces appetite. However, food intake can be stimulated by administration of insulin (163), 2-deoxy-D-glucose [2-DG (257, 286)], and 5-thioglucose [5-TG (222)]. All of these substances result in reduction of glucose utilization in the brain, the last two in all glucose utilizing cells. The eating effect can be blocked or attenuated by administering metabolic fuels that can be used by liver or brain in the case of insulin administration (234, 276), or by the brain alone in the case of 2-DG administration (275). Therefore these treatments probably induce eating not by glucoprivation but rather by energy privation. The eating response is probably linked not directly to insufficiency of circulating fuels but rather to depletion of an organ. For example, increased eating persists in insulin- or 2-DG-treated animals even after 6 hr without food, at a time when all circulating parameters have returned to normal (221). One possible locus for this effect is the liver, since its glycogen stores remain depleted (85, 98), although not empty (221), until feeding is allowed and since fructose administration blocks the increased eating only in hepatic-vagally intact animals (98). The other possibility is the brain, since its norepinephrine turnover (which would inhibit "satiety" neurons) remains high unless feeding occurs (16). The site for the action of glucoprivic stimuli may be the caudal hindbrain, since injections of 5-TG into the fourth ventricle increased food intake (223, 256).

Mechanisms of Long-Term Control

On the basis of initial hyperphagia and weight gain after ventromedial hypothalamic (VMH) damage, and subsequent reduction in intake after weight had stabilized, Kennedy (128) proposed that a circulating factor correlated with the size of the fat depots suppressed intake in the obese animal. He further proposed that the ventromedial satiety mechanism was directly or indirectly sensitive to the state of the energy reserves so that after VMH damage a greater stimulus was required to inhibit eating (129). Evidence for a circulating factor came from parabiosis experiments in which two animals were sewn together so that they shared a fraction of a common blood supply. When one member of the pair was overfed, the partner ate less and became emaciated (109, 206).

The identity of the circulating factor remains a mystery, but recent evidence suggests it is either insulin in the cerebrospinal fluid (213) or glycerol (67). Cerebrospinal insulin level has been shown to covary with plasma level (307), but fluctuations are greatly damped in the CSF. Plasma insulin covaries in turn with the state of the fat stores (19). Infusion of insulin into the cerebral ventricles of baboons resulted in a loss in body weight and reduction in food intake (306). Glycerol has been proposed as a signal of fat store size because fat catabolism yields it quantitatively and it is not reutilized by that tissue. Administration of glycerol by various routes inhibits food intake and induces weight loss (94, 101, 301). Other metabolites share this ability to a lesser extent when injected into the brain (66), and the glycerol effect is most pronounced in the vicinity of the third ventricle (67).

Not all investigators agree with the hypothesis that the function of the ventromedial hypothalamic area is to detect the size of body energy stores and control food intake accordingly. The interpretation of the ventromedial lesion syndrome has been controversial since its discovery. Sclafani (247) has recently summarized the evidence favoring a primary hyperphagia, and Bray et al (41) and Powley (214) have summarized evidence for primary endocrine and autonomic disturbances that could lead to hyperphagia by means of increased insulin secretion. It has also been suggested that the two sequelae of the lesion (hyperphagia and hyperinsulinemia) are independent effects of damage to overlapping systems (15), because each can be induced in the absence of the other.

Further evidence for this independence of effects comes from recent work on vagotomy in rats with ventromedial hypothalamic damage (either by lesion or knife cut). Cox & Powley (57) have definitively shown that a doubling of body fat is attained after VMH lesions when food intake is limited, by a special infusion pair-feeding paradigm, to the pattern and amount consumed by a neurologically intact rat. This effect is blocked by vagotomy (58). However, it should be noted that the weight gain of animals with restricted feeding was considerably less (1.3 g/day) than it was on a comparable diet eaten ad libitum [5.4 g/day (15)]. Therefore, although VMH lesions predispose toward obesity, hyperphagia greatly enhances it. The argument over which sequela (hyperphagia or hyperinsulinemia) of VMH damage is "primary" for obesity is a sterile one. This conclusion is further shown by the work of Sawchenko and colleagues (242), who found that the coeliac branch of the vagus must remain intact for increased weight gain to occur after VMH damage only on a chow and not on a high-fat diet (243). On high-fat diets vagotomy is less effective in attenuating weight gain and hyperphagia after VMH damage than it is on high-carbohydrate diets (248). These results are consistent with the hypothesis that vagotomy may reduce obesity by suppressing insulin secretion, which is necessary for carbohydrate, but not fat, utilization; but this hypothesis cannot account for persistence of hyperphagia in VMH-lesioned diabetic rats (83, 297, 313), whose insulin secretion is severely impaired. Such animals, of course, fail to become obese on high carbohydrate diets. It is still a mystery why hyperphagia is attenuated in VMH-damaged animals with coeliac vagotomy (242) on low fat diets while hyperphagia persists in the VMH-damaged diabetic animal, since both animals have impaired insulin secretion.

CONCLUSIONS

Given the array of factors that influence feeding behavior and the variety of theories proposed to account for them, is it possible to effect a synthesis that is both explanatory and predictive? The multiplicity of signals and sites involved in the control of intake makes it difficult, if not impossible, to accept simplistic explanations such as dual centers in the brain or primary control by a single organ such as the stomach or liver. Understanding amid such complexity is best gained by expressing relationships among variables in mathematical terms and testing hypotheses by comparing computed outcomes of alternatives against empirically obtained data. However, since many readers are not familiar with this approach, we attempt here to summarize verbally what has been discovered.

Search for food is initiated when certain portions of the brain are activated by (a) disinhibition of its spontaneous activity as a result of removal of inhibitory input from either the blood stream or cerebrospinal fluid, and/or (b) increased excitation from neural or humoral signals from the liver. These inputs influence the brain cells by means of specific neurotransmitters. The same brain cells are also influenced in their activity by direct or indirect detection of fat stores, possibly through links with circumventricular organs or by combination with the normal changes in metabolism believed to influence feeding. Once food is located, feeding is initiated under the control of cells in overlapping but possibly anatomically distinct regions and is maintained by "reward-sensitive" neurons whose activity is gated as a result of disinhibition (i.e. these cells will only be active when the animal is in a "hunger" state). As feeding proceeds, inhibitory inputs impinge on the "reward" cells and at a certain level of inhibition they will no longer be activated by the sensory qualities of the food. Eating of that particular food would then stop, although other foods could still activate the reward neurons, thereby accounting for sensory-specific satiety (225). Absolute satiety would be evidenced by behavioral quiescence and neural inhibition of the regions responsible for search and initiation of eating. Because learning also contributes to control of food intake (32), we suggest that the response of reward neurons to the stimulus qualities of food is modified by postingestive events, and that this modification contributes to the activity of the reward neurons by either enhancing their activity if the postingestive effect results in reward (satiety), or reducing their activity if it results in punishment (illness). This scheme is no doubt filled with flaws but is proposed as a challenge on which to improve.

Finally, we would like to note that the burden of review would be considerably eased and information would be easier to digest if data from comparable methods were presented in comparable units. It is impossible to compare results from such widely divergent units as percentages of control values, percentages of body weights, difference scores across conditions, and simple weight of food consumed. To improve the situation it is suggested that intake data be reported in the units in which they are collected. An author who wishes to convert these data to some other format could then do so separately. When there is more than one source of variance (e.g. animals and times—i.e. repeated observations on an animal at intervals, or replicate observations), analysis of variance would allow the reader to determine how much variability to expect from each source when experiments are replicated or extended. Enough details of the experimental conditions should be presented to enable replication. At a minimum these should include species, sex, strain, breeder, age, and weight of the animal; conditions of illumination, temperature, housing or restraint; macronutrient content of the diet and its energy density. As our ability to collect data increases, owing to automatic weighing and other instruments, our ability to understand them will decline unless we adopt a strategy to organize them. Quantitative data in comparable units are amenable to computerized storage and retrieval. Perhaps if the data are published in a more quantitatively comparable way than they are at present, the next generation of reviews in this field will be prepared with the aid of computerized data bases.

Literature Cited

1. Adair, E. R., Miller, N. E., Booth, D. A. 1968. Effects of continuous intravenous infusion of nutritive substances on consummatory behavior in rats. *Behav. Biol A* 2:25–37
2. Adolph, E. F. 1943. *Physiological Regulations* Lancaster: Cattell. 502 pp.
3. Adolph, E. F. 1947. Urges to eat and drink in rats. *Am. J. Physiol.* 151:110–25
4. Anand, B. K. 1961. Nervous regulation of food intake. *Physiol. Rev.* 41:677–708
5. Anand, B. K. 1967. Central chemosensitive mechanisms related to feeding. In *Handbook of Physiology,* Section 6, *Alimentary Canal,* Vol. 1. *Food and Water Intake,* ed. C. F. Code, pp. 249–63. Washington DC: Am. Physiol. Soc.
6. Anand, B. K., Brobeck, J. R. 1951. Hypothalamic control of food intake in rats and cats. *Yale J. Biol. Med.* 24:123–40
7. Andik, I., Bank, J., Moring, I., Szegvari, G. Y. 1954. Effects of exercise on the intake and selection of food in the rat. *Acta Physiol. Hung.* 5:457–61
8. Antelman, S. M., Szechman, H. 1975. Tail-pinching induces eating in sated rats which appears to depend on nigrostriatal dopamine. *Science* 189:731–33
9. Antin, J., Gibbs, J., Holt, J., Young, R. C., Smith, G. P. 1975. Cholecystokinin elicits the complete behavioral sequence of satiety in rats. *J. Comp. Physiol. Psychol.* 89:784–90
10. Apfelbaum, M., Mandenoff, A. 1981. Naltrexone suppresses hyperphagia induced in the rat by a highly palatable diet. *Pharmacol. Biochem. Behav.* 15:89–91
11. Armstrong, S., Coleman, G., Singer, G. 1980. Food and water deprivation: Changes in rat feeding, drinking, activity, and body weight. *Neurosci. Biobehav. Rev.* 4:377–402
12. Baile, C. A., Keim, D. A., Della-Fera, M. A., McLaughlin, C. L. 1981. Opiate antagonists and agonists and feeding in sheep. *Physiol. Behav.* 26:1019–23
13. Baile, C. A., Zinn, W., Mayer, J. 1971. Feeding behavior of monkeys: Glucose utilization rate and site of glucose entry. *Physiol. Behav.* 6:537–41
14. Bare, J. K., Cicala, G. A. 1960. Deprivation and time of testing as determinants of food intake. *J. Comp. Physiol. Psychol.* 53:151–54
15. Becker, E. E., Kissileff, H. R. 1974. Inhibitory controls of feeding by the ventromedial hypothalamus. *Am. J. Physiol.* 226:383–96
16. Bellin, S., Ritter, S. 1981. Insulin-induced elevation of hypothalamic norepinephrine turnover persists after glucorestoration unless feeding occurs. *Brain Res.* 217:327–37

17. Bellinger, L. L. 1981. Commentary on the "Current status of the hepatostatic theory of food intake control." *Appetite* 2:144–45

18. Berkun, M. M., Kessen, M. L., Miller, N. E. 1952. Hunger-reducing effects of food by stomach fistula versus food by mouth measured by a consummatory response. *J. Comp. Physiol. Psychol.* 45:550–54

19. Bernstein, I. L., Lotter, E. C., Kulkosky, P. J., Porte, D. Jr, Woods, S. C. 1975. Effect of force-feeding upon basal insulin levels of rats. *Proc. Soc. Exp. Biol. Med.* 150:546–48

20. Bernstein, I. L., Zimmerman, J. C., Czeisler, C. A., Weitzman, E. D. 1981. Meal patterns in free-running humans. *Physiol. Behav.* 27:621–23

21. Bernstein, L. M., Grossman, M. I. 1956. An experimental test of the glucostatic theory of the regulation of food intake. *J. Clin. Invest.* 35:627–33

22. Bjorntorp, P., Yang, M.-U. 1982. Refeeding after fasting in the rat I. Effects on body composition and food efficiency. *Int. J. Obesity.* In press

23. Blass, E. M., Kraly, F. S. 1974. Medial forebrain bundle lesions: specific loss of feeding to decreased glucose utilization in rats. *J. Comp. Physiol. Psychol.* 86:679–92

24. Bobroff, E. 1981. Independent measure of palatability correlates with initial rate of eating in men. Presented at Eastern Psychol. Assoc., 52nd, New York

25. Bolles, R. C. 1980. Historical note on the term "appetite." *Appetite* 1:3–6

26. Booth, D. A. 1972. Caloric compensation in rats with continuous or intermittent access to food. *Physiol. Behav.* 8:891–99

27. Booth, D. A. 1972. Conditioned satiety in the rat. *J. Comp. Physiol. Psychol.* 81:457–71

28. Booth, D. A. 1972. Postabsorptively induced suppression of appetite and the energostatic control of feeding. *Physiol. Behav.* 9:199–202

29. Booth, D. A. 1972. Satiety and behavioral caloric compensation following intragastric glucose loads in the rat. *J. Comp. Physiol. Psychol.* 78:412–32

30. Booth, D. A. 1976. Approaches to feeding control. In *Appetite and Food Intake*, ed. T. Silverstone, pp. 417–78. Berlin: Abakon. 497 pp.

31. Booth, D. A. 1977. Appetite and satiety as metabolic expectancies. In *Food Intake and Chemical Senses*, ed. Y. Katsuki, M. Sato, S. F. Takagi, Y. Oomura,

pp. 317–30. Baltimore: University Park Press. 614 pp.

32. Booth, D. A. 1978. Acquired behavior controlling energy intake and output. In *Psychiatric Clinics of North America*, ed. A. J. Stunkard, 1:545–79. Philadelphia: W. B. Saunders 732 pp.

33. Booth, D. A., ed. 1978. *Hunger Models Computable Theory of Feeding Control.* NY: Academic. 478 pp.

34. Booth, D. A., Campbell, A. T., Chase, A. 1970. Temporal bounds of postingestive glucose-induced satiety in man. *Nature* 228:1104–5

35. Booth, D. A., Chase, A., Campbell, A. T. 1970. Relative effectiveness of protein in the late stages of appetite suppression in man. *Physiol. Behav.* 5:1299–1302

36. Booth, D. A., Jarman, S. P. 1976. Inhibition of food intake in the rat following complete absorption of glucose delivered into the stomach, intestine, or liver. *J. Physiol.* 259:501–22

37. Booth, D. A., Lovett, D., McSherry, G. M. 1972. Postingestive modulation of the sweetness preference gradient in the rat. *J. Comp. Physiol. Psychol.* 78:485–512

38. Booth, D. A., Mather, P. 1978. Prototype model of human feeding, growth, and obesity. See Ref. 33, pp. 279–322

39. Borer, K. T., Rowland, N., Mirow, A., Borer, R. C., Kelch, R. P. 1979. Physiological and behavioral responses to starvation in the golden hamster. *Am. J. Physiol.* 236:E105–12

40. Bray, G. A. 1976. Peripheral metabolic factors in the regulation of feeding. See Ref. 30, pp. 141–76

41. Bray, G. A., Inoue, S., Nishizawa, Y. 1981. Hypothalamic obesity. The autonomic hypothesis and the lateral hypothalamus. *Diabetologia* 20: (Suppl.) 366–77

42. Bray, G. A., York, D. A. 1972. Studies on food intake in genetically obese rats. *Am. J. Physiol.* 223:176–79

42a. Brobeck, J. R. 1955. Neural regulation of food intake. *Ann. NY Acad. Sci. 63* (art 1): 44–55

43. Brobeck, J. R. 1960. Food and temperature. *Rec. Adv. Horm. Res.* 16:439–59

44. Brobeck, J. R. 1965. Exchange, control, and regulation. In *Physiological Controls and Regulations*, ed. W. S. Yamamoto, J. R. Brobeck, pp. 1–13. Philadelphia: W. B. Saunders. 362 pp.

45. Brobeck, J. R. 1981. Models for analyzing energy balance in body weight regulation. In *The Body Weight Regulatory System: Normal and Disturbed Mecha-*

nisms, ed. L. A. Cioffi, W. P. T. James, T. B. Van Itallie, pp. 1–9. NY: Raven Press. 380 pp.

46. Brobeck, J. R., Tepperman, J., Long, C. N. H. 1943. Experimental hypothalamic hyperphagia in the albino rat. *Yale J. Biol. Med.* 15:831–53

47. Cabanac, M., Duclaux, R., Spector, N. H. 1971. Sensory feedback in regulation of body weight: Is there a ponderostat? *Nature* 229:125–27

48. Campbell, R. G., Hashim, S., Van Itallie, T. B. 1971. Studies of food-intake regulation in man, responses to variations in nutritive density in lean and obese subjects. *N. Engl. J. Med.* 285:1402–7

49. Cannon, W. B., Washburn, A. L. 1912. An explanation of hunger. *Am. J. Physiol.* 29:444–54

50. Carlisle, H. J., Stellar, E. 1969. Caloric regulation and food preference in normal, hyperphagic and aphagic rats. *J. Comp. Physiol. Psychol.* 69:107–14

51. Cioffi, L. A., James, W. P. T., Van Itallie, T. B., eds. 1981. See Ref. 45.

52. Cohn, C., Joseph, D. 1962. Influence of body weight and body fat on appetite of "normal" lean and obese rats. *Yale J. Biol. Med.* 34:598–607

53. Collier, G. H. 1981. An ecological analysis of motivation. In *Analysis of Motivational Processes,* ed. F. Toates, T. Halliday, pp. 125–51. NY: Academic

54. Collier, G., Hirsch, E., Hamlin, P. H. 1972. The ecological determinants of reinforcement in the rat. *Physiol. Behav.* 9:705–16

55. Collier, G., Hirsch, E., Kanarek, R. 1978. The operant revisited. In *Handbook of Operant Psychology,* ed. W. K. Honig, J. E. R. Staddon, pp. 28–52. Englewood Cliffs, NJ: Prentice Hall

56. Collier, G., Leshner, A. I., Squibb, R. L. 1969. Dietary self-selection in active and non-active rats. *Physiol. Behav.* 4:79–82

57. Cox, J. E., Powley, T. L. 1981. Intragastric pair feeding fails to prevent VMH obesity or hyperinsulinemia. *Am. J. Physiol.* 240:E566–72

58. Cox, J. E., Powley, T. L. 1981. Prior vagotomy blocks VMH obesity in pairfed rats. *Am. J. Physiol.* 240:E573–83

59. Cowgill, G. R. 1928. The energy factor in relation to food intake: Experiments in the dog. *Am. J. Physiol.* 85:45–64

60. Cruce, J. A. F., Greenwood, M. R. C., Johnson, P. R., Quartermain, D. 1974. Genetic versus hypothalamic obesity: Studies of intake and dietary manipulations in rats. *J. Comp. Physiol. Psychol.* 87:295–301

61. Cumming, M., Morrison, S. D. 1960. The total metabolism of rats during fasting and refeeding. *J. Physiol.* 154:219–43

62. Davis, J. D., Campbell, C. S. 1973. Peripheral control of meal size in the rat: Effect of sham feeding on meal size and drinking rate. *J. Comp. Physiol. Psychol.* 83:379–87

63. Davis, J. D., Collins, B. J., Levine, M. W. 1976. Peripheral control of meal size: interaction of gustatory stimulation and postingestional feedback. In *Hunger: Basic Mechanisms and Clinical Implications,* ed. D. Novin, W. Wyricka, G. A. Bray, pp. 395–408. NY: Raven Press

64. Davis, J. D., Collins, B. J., Levine, M. W. 1978. The interactions between gustatory stimulation and gut feedback in the control of ingestion of liquid diets. See Ref. 33, pp. 109–42

65. Davis, J. D., Levine, M. W. 1977. A model for the control of ingestion. *Psychol. Rev.* 84:379–412

66. Davis, J. D. Wirtshafter, D., Asin, K., Brief, D. 1981. Sustained intracerebroventricular infusion of brain fuels reduces body weight and food intake in rats. *Science.* 212:81–83

67. Davis, J. D., Wirtshafter, D., Asin, K., Brief, D. 1983. Sustained intracerebroventricular infusion of glycerol causes body weight loss in rats. *Am. J. Physiol.* In press

68. Deaux, E., Kakolewski, J. W. 1971. Character of osmotic changes resulting in the initiating of eating. *J. Comp. Physiol. Psychol.* 74:248–53

69. Della-Fera, M. A., Baile, C. A. 1980. Cerebral ventricular injections of CCK-octapeptide and feed intake: The importance of continuous injection. *Physiol. Behav.* 24:1133–38

70. Deutsch, J. A. 1978. The stomach in food satiation and the regulation of appetite. *Prog. Neurobiol.* 10:135–53

71. Deutsch, J. A. 1980. Bombesin—satiety or malaise. *Nature* 285:592

72. Deutsch, J. A., Gonzalez, M. F. 1981. Gastric fat content and satiety. *Physiol. Behav.* 26:673–76

73. Deutsch, J. A., Gonzalez, M. F., Young, W. G. 1980. Two factors control meal size. *Brain Res. Bull.* 5: (Suppl 4) 55–57

74. Deutsch, J. A., Young, W. G., Kalogeris, T. J. 1978. The stomach signals satiety. *Science* 201:165–67

75. Dufort, R. H., Wright, J. H. 1962. Food intake as a function of duration of food deprivation. *J. Psychol.* 53:465–68
76. Edholm, O. G., Fletcher, J. G., Widdowson, E. M., McCance, R. A. 1955. The energy expenditure and food intake of individual men. *Brit. J. Nutr.* 9:286–300
77. Epstein, A. N. 1960. Reciprocal changes in feeding behavior produced by intrahypothalamic chemical injections. *Am. J. Physiol.* 199:969–74
78. Epstein, A. N. 1967. Oropharyngeal factors in feeding and drinking. See Ref. 5, pp. 197–218
79. Epstein, A. N., Nicolaidis, S., Miselis, R. 1975. The glucoprivic control of food intake and the glucostatic theory of feeding behavior. In *Neural Integration of Physiological Mechanisms and Behavior*, ed. G. J. Mogenson, F. R. Calaresu, pp. 148–68. Toronto: Univ. Toronto Press. 442 pp.
80. Epstein, A. N., Teitelbaum, P. 1967. Specific loss of the hypoglycemic control of feeding in recovered lateral rats. *Am. J. Physiol.* 213:1159–67
81. Faust, I. M. 1981. Signals from adipose tissue. See Ref. 45, pp. 39–44
82. Fernstrom, J. D., Wurtman, R. J. 1971. Brain serotonin content: increase following ingestion of a carbohydrate diet. *Science* 174:1023–25
83. Friedman, M. I. 1972. Effects of alloxan diabetes on hypothalamic hyperphagia and obesity. *Am. J. Physiol.* 222:174–78
84. Friedman, M. I. 1978. Hyperphagia in rats with experimental diabetes mellitus: A response to a decreased supply of utilizable fuels. *J. Comp. Physiol. Psychol.* 92:109–17
85. Friedman, M. I., Granneman, J. 1982. Food intake and peripheral metabolic factors after recovery from insulin induced hypoglycemia. *Am. J. Physiol.* In press
86. Friedman, M. I., Stricker, E. M. 1976. The physiological psychology of hunger: a physiological perspective. *Psychol. Rev.* 83:409–31
87. Friend, B. W. 1973. Self-selection of feeds and water by unbred gilts. *J. Animal Sci.* 37:1137–41
88. Gale, S. K., Van Itallie, T. B., Faust, I. M. 1981. Effects of palatable diets on body weight and adipose tissue cellularity in the adult obese female Zucker rat (fa/fa). *Metabolism* 30:105–10
89. Gasnier, A., Mayer, A. 1939. Recherches sur la régulation de la nutrition. III. Mechanisms régulateurs de la nutri-

tion et intensité du métabolisme. *Ann. Physiol. Physiochim. Biol.* 15:186–94
90. Geary, N. 1979. Food intake and behavioral caloric compensation after protein repletion in the rat. *Physiol. Behav.* 23:1089–98
91. Geliebter, A. A. 1979. Effects of equicaloric loads of protein, fat, and carbohydrate on food intake in the rat and man. *Physiol. Behav.* 22:267–73
92. Geliebter, A. A. 1980. Effects of longterm loading of isocaloric macronutrients on food intake. Paper presented at Meet. East. Psychol. Assoc., April, 1980, New York
93. Gibbs, J., Smith, G. P. 1980. Reply to Deutsch. *Nature* 285:592
94. Glick, Z. 1980. Food intake of rats administered with glycerol. *Physiol. Behav.* 25:621–26
95. Glick, Z., Modan, M. 1977. Behavioral compensatory responses to continuous duodenal and upper ileal glucose infusion in rats. *Physiol. Behav.* 19:703–5
96. Gonzalez, M. F., Deutsch, J. A. 1981. Vagotomy abolishes cues of satiety produced by gastric distension. *Science* 212:1283–84
97. Grandison, L., Guidotti, A. 1977. Stimulation of food intake by muscimol and beta endorphin. *Neuropharmacol.* 16:533–36
98. Granneman, J., Friedman, M. I. 1982. Cerebral and peripheral factors in the control of food intake following acute effects of 2-deoxy-D-glucose injection. *Am. J. Physiol.* In press
99. Grinker, J. G. 1978. Obesity and sweet taste. *Am. J. Clin. Nutr.* 31:1078–87
100. Grinker, J., Cohn, C., Hirsch, J. 1971. The effects of intravenous administration of glucose, saline, and mannitol on meal regulation in normal-weight human subjects. *Comm. Behav. Biol.* 6:203–8
101. Grinker, J., Strohmayer, A. J., Horowitz, J., Hirsch, J., Leibel, R. 1980. The effect of the metabolite glycerol on food intake and body weight in rats. *Brain Res. Bull.* 5: (Suppl 4):29–35
102. Hamilton, C. L. 1967. Interaction of food intake and temperature regulation in the rat. *J. Comp. Physiol. Psychol.* 56:476–88
103. Hamilton, C. L. 1967. Food and temperature. See Ref. 5, pp. 303–17
104. Hamilton, C. L. 1969. Problems of refeeding after starvation in the rat. *Ann. NY Acad. Sci.* 157 (art. 2):1004–17
105. Hamilton, C. L. 1972. Long term control of food intake in the monkey. *Physiol. Behav.* 9:1–6

106. Hammel, H. T. 1965. Neurons and temperature regulation. See Ref. 44, pp. 71–97
107. Hansen, B. C., Jen, K-L. C., Kripps, P. 1981. Regulation of food intake in monkeys: Response to caloric dilution. *Physiol. Behav.* 26:479–86
108. Harper, A. E., Boyle, P. C. 1976. Nutrients and food intake. See Ref. 30, pp. 177–206
109. Hervey, G. R. 1959. The effects of lesions in the hypothalamus in parabiotic rats. *J. Physiol.* 145:336–52
110. Hirsch, E. 1973. Some determinants of intake and patterns of feeding in the Guinea pig. *Physiol. Behav.* 11:687–704
111. Hirsch, E., Collier, G. 1974. The ecological determinants of reinforcement in the Guinea pig. *Physiol. Behav.* 12:239–49
112. Hoebel, B. G. 1969. Feeding and self-stimulation. *Ann. NY Acad. Sci.* 157 (art 2):758–78
113. Hoebel, B. G., Teitelbaum, P. 1962. Hypothalamic control of feeding and self stimulation. *Science* 135:375–77
114. Hoebel, B. G., Teitelbaum, P. 1966. Weight regulation in normal and hyperphagic rats. *J. Comp. Physiol. Psychol.* 61:189–93
115. Jacobs, H. L. 1962. Some physical, metabolic, and sensory components in the appetite for glucose. *Am. J. Physiol.* 203:1043–54
116. Janowitz, H., Grossman, M. I. 1949. Some factors affecting food intake of normal dogs and dogs with esophagostomy and gastric fistula. *Am. J. Physiol.* 159:143–48
117. Janowitz, H. D., Hollander, F. 1955. The time factor in the adjustment of food intake to varied caloric requirement in the dog: A study of the precision of appetite regulation. *Ann. New York Acad. Sci.* 63 (art 1):56–67
118. Jordan, H. A. 1969. Voluntary intragastric feeding: Oral and gastric contributions to food intake and hunger in man. *J. Comp. Physiol. Psychol.* 68:498–506
119. Jordan, H. A., Spiegel, T. A. 1978. Effects of simultaneous oral-gastric ingestion on meal patterns and satiety in humans. *J. Comp. Physiol. Psychol.* 92:133–47
120. Jordan, H. A., Wieland, W. F., Zebley, S. P., Stellar, E., Stunkard, A. J. 1966. Direct measurement of food intake in man: A method for objective study of eating behavior. *Psychosom. Med.* 28:836–42
121. Kanarek, R. B. 1975. Availability and caloric density of the diet as determi-

nants of meal patterns in cats. *Physiol. Behav.* 15:611–18
122. Kanarek, R. B. 1976. Energetics of meal patterns in rats. *Physiol. Behav.* 17:395–99
123. Kanarek, R. B., Feldman, P. G., Hanes, C. 1981. Pattern of dietary self-selection in VMH lesioned rats. *Physiol. Behav.* 27:337–43
124. Kanarek, R. B., Hirsch, E. 1977. Dietary-induced overeating in experimental animals. *Fed. Proc.* 36:154–58
125. Kanarek, R. B., Marks-Kaufman, R., Lipeles, B. J. 1980. Increased carbohydrate intake as a function of insulin administration in rats. *Physiol. Behav.* 25:779–82
126. Kanarek, R. B., Ogilby, J. D., Mayer, J. 1977. Effects of dietary caloric density on feeding behavior in Mongolian gerbils. *Physiol. Behav.* 19:497–501
127. Kennedy, G. C. 1950. The hypothalamic control of food intake in rats. *Proc. R. Soc. Lond. Ser. B.* 137:535–49
128. Kennedy, G. C. 1953. The role of depot fat in the hypothalamic control of food intake in the rat. *Proc. R. Soc. Lond. Ser. B.* 140:578–92
129. Kennedy, G. C. 1973. Food intake, growth, and obesity in rats. In *Régulation de l'équilibre énergétique chez l'homme,* ed. M. Apfelbaum, pp. 1–11. Paris: Masson et Cie, Editeurs. 353 pp.
130. Kenney, N. J., McKay, L. D., Woods, S. C., Williams, R. H. 1978. Effects of intraventricular beta-endorphin on food intake of rats. *Soc. Neurosci. Abstr.* 4:176
131. Khairy, M., Morgan, T. B., Yudkin, J. 1963. Choice of diets of differing caloric density by normal and hyperphagic rats. *Brit. J. Nutr.* 17:557–68
132. Kissileff, H. R. 1968. The effects of water loading and ambient temperature changes on temporal patterns of food and water intake in the rat. Paper presented at 3rd Int. Conf. Regulation of Food and Water Intake, Haverford College, Pennsylvania, September 1968
132a. Kissileff, H. R. 1970. Free feeding in normal and recovered lateral rats monitored by a pellet-detecting eatometer. *Physiol. Behav.* 5:163–73
133. Kissileff, H. R. 1976. Consumatory behavior. In *International Encyclopedia of Psychiatry, Psychology, Psychoanalysis, & Neurology,* ed. B. Wolman, III: 352–53. NY: Human Sciences Press
134. Kissileff, H. R. 1976. Palatability. See Ref. 133, X:172
135. Kissileff, H. R., Thornton, J. 1982. Facilitation and inhibition in the cumula-

tive food intake curve in man. In *Changing Concepts of the Nervous System*, ed. A. J. Morrison, P. Strick. NY: Academic. In press

136. Kissileff, H. R., Thornton, J., Becker, E. 1982. A quadratic equation adequately describes the cumulative food intake curve in man. *Appetite* 3. In press

137. Kohn, M. 1951. Satiation of hunger from food injected directly into the stomach versus food ingested by mouth. *J. Comp. Physiol. Psychol.* 44:412–22

138. Kraly, F. S., Blass, E. M. 1976. Increased feeding in rats in a low ambient temperature. See Ref. 63, pp. 77–88

139. Kraly, F. S., Blass, E. M. 1976. Mechanisms for enhanced feeding in the cold in rats. *J. Comp. Physiol. Psychol.* 90:714–26

140. Kraly, F. S., Carty, W. J., Resnick, S., Smith, G. P. 1978. Effect of cholecystokinin on meal size and intermeal interval in the sham feeding rat. *J. Comp. Physiol. Psychol.* 92:697–707

141. Kraly, F. S., Gibbs, J. 1980. Vagotomy fails to block the satiating effect of food in the stomach. *Physiol. Behav.* 24:1007–10

142. Kraly, F. S., Smith, G. P. 1978. Combined pregastric and gastric stimulation by food is sufficient for normal meal size. *Physiol. Behav.* 21:405–8

143. Krasne, F. B. 1962. General disruption resulting from electrical stimulus of the ventromedial hypothalamus. *Science.* 138:822–23

144. Kratz, C. M., Levitsky, D. A., Lustick, S. 1978. Differential effects of quinine and sucrose-octa-acetate on food intake in the rat. *Physiol. Behav.* 20:665–67

145. KROC-Symposium. 1981. The nervous system and metabolism. *Diabetologia* 20 (suppl.)

146. Leibowitz, S. F. 1978. Paraventricular nucleus: A primary site mediating adrenergic stimulation of feeding and drinking. *Pharmacol. Biochem. Behav.* 8:163–75

147. Leibowitz, S. F. 1980. Neurochemical systems of the hypothalamus in control of feeding and drinking behavior and water-electrolyte excretion. In *Handbook of the Hypothalamus*, ed. P. J. Morgane, J. Panksepp, 3A:299–437. NY: Marcel Dekker

148. Leibowitz, S. F., Rossakis, C. 1978. Pharmacological characterization of perifornical hypothalamic β-adrenergic receptors mediating feeding inhibition in the rat. *Neuropharmacology* 17:691–702

149. Le Magnen, J. 1971. Advances in studies on the physiological control and regulation of food intake. In *Progress in Physiological Psychology*, ed. E. Stellar, J. M. Sprague, 4:203–61. NY: Academic. 363 pp.

150. Le Magnen, J. 1977. Hunger and food palatability in the control of feeding behavior. See Ref. 31, pp. 263–79

151. Le Magnen, J. 1981. The metabolic basis of the dual periodicity of feeding in rats. *Behav. Brain Sci.* 4:561–607

152. Le Magnen, J., Devos, M. 1980. Parameters of the meal pattern in rats: Their assignment and physiological significance. *Neurosci. Biobehav. Rev.* 4: (Suppl 1): 1–11

153. Le Magnen, J., Devos, M. 1980. Variations of meal-to-meal liver glycogen in rats. *Neurosci. Biobehav. Rev.* 4: (Suppl. 1) 29–32

154. Le Magnen, J., Devos, M. Gaudillière, J., Louis-Sylvestre, J., Tallon, S. 1973. Role of a lipostatic mechanism in regulation by feeding of energy balance in rats. *J. Comp. Physiol. Psychol.* 84:1–23

155. Le Magnen, J., Tallon, S. 1963. Enregistrement et analyse préliminaire de la "périodicité alimentaire spontanée" chez le rat blanc. *J. Physiol. (Paris)* 55:286–87

156. Le Magnen, J., Tallon, S. 1966. La periodicite spontanee de la prise d'aliments ad libitum du rat blanc. *J. Physiol. (Paris)* 58:323–49

157. Le Magnen, J., Tallon, S. 1968. L'effet du jeûne préalable sur les caractéristiques temporelles de la prise d'aliments chez le rat. *J. Physiol. (Paris)* 60:143–54

158. Levitsky, D. A. 1970. Feeding patterns of rats in response to fasts and changes in environmental conditions. *Physiol. Behav.* 5:291–300

159. Levitsky, D. A., Collier, G. 1968. Effects of diet and deprivation on meal eating behavior in rats. *Physiol. Behav.* 3:137–40

160. Levitsky, D. A., Faust, I. M., Glassman, M. 1976. The ingestion of food and the recovery of body weight following fasting in the naive rat. *Physiol. Behav.* 17:575–80

161. Liu, C. M., Yin, T. H. 1974. Caloric compensation to gastric loads in rats with hypothalamic hyperphagia. *Physiol. Behav.* 13:231–38

162. Louis-Sylvestre, J. 1981. Hepatic glucoreceptors do exist but do not control food intake. *Appetite* 2:146–48

163. Mackay, E. M., Calloway, J. W., Barnes, R. H. 1940. Hyperalimentation

in normal animals produced by prota-mine zinc insulin. *J. Nutr.* 20:59–66
164. MacLagan, N. F. 1937. The role of appetite in the control of body weight. *J. Physiol.* 90:385–94
165. Maddison, S. 1977. Intraperitoneal and intracranial cholecystokinin depress operant responding for food. *Physiol. Behav.* 19:819–24
166. Margules, D. L. 1981. Endorphinergic and endoloxonergic states of the diffuse neuroendocrine system in energy balance. See Ref. 45, pp. 361–68
167. Margules, D. L., Moisset, B., Lewis, M., Shibuya, H., Pert, P. B. 1978. β-Endorphin is associated with overeating in genetically obese mice (ob/ob) and rats (fa/fa). *Science* 202:988–91
168. Margules, D. L., Olds, J. 1962. Identical "feeding" and "rewarding" systems in the lateral hypothalamus of rats. *Science* 135:374–75
169. Marler, P., Hamilton, W. J. III. 1966. *Mechanisms of Animal Behavior.* NY: Wiley
170. Marshall, J. F., Teitelbaum, P. 1973. A comparison of the eating in response to hypothermic and glucoprivic challenges after nigral 6-hydroxydopamine and lateral hypothalamic electrolytic lesions in rats. *Brain Res.* 55:229–33
171. Martinez, I., Racotta, R., Russek, M. 1974. Hepatic chromaffin cells. *Life Sci.* 15:267–71
172. Mayer, J. 1955. Regulation of energy intake and the body weight. The glucostatic theory and the lipostatic hypothesis. *Ann. NY Acad. Sci.* 63 (art. 1): 15–43
173. Mayer, J., Marshall, N. B., Vitale, J. J., Christensen, M. B., Mashayekki, M. B., Stare, F. J. 1954. Exercise, food intake and body weight in normal rats, and genetically obese adult mice. *Am. J. Physiol.* 177:544–48
174. McCleery, R. H. 1977. On satiation curves. *Anim. Behav.* 25:1005–15
175. McHugh, P. R. 1979. Aspects of the control of feeding: Application of quantitation in psychobiology. *Johns Hopkins Med. J.* 144:147–55
176. McHugh, P. R., Moran, T. H. 1978. Accuracy of the regulation of caloric ingestion in the rhesus monkey. *Am. J. Physiol.* 235:R29–34
177. McHugh, P. R., Moran, T. H. 1979. Calories and gastric emptying: a regulatory capacity with implications for feeding. *Am. J. Physiol.* 236: R254–60
177a. McHugh, P. R., Moran, T. H., Barton, G. N. 1975. Satiety: A graded behav-

ioral phenomenon regulating caloric intake. *Science* 190:167–69
178. Mellinkoff, S. M., Frankland, M., Boyle, D., Greipel, M. 1956. Relationship between serum amino acid concentration and fluctuations in appetite. *J. Appl. Physiol.* 8:535–38
179. Mickelsen, O., Takahashi, S., Craig, C. 1955. Experimental obesity I. Production of obesity in rats by feeding high-fat diets. *J. Nutr.* 57:541–54
180. Miller, N. E. 1955. Effects of drugs on motivation: The value of using a variety of measures. *Ann. NY Acad. Sci.* 65:318–33
181. Miller, N. E. 1960. Motivational effects of brain stimulation and drugs. *Fed. Proc.* 19:846–53
182. Mogenson, G. J., Calaresu, F. R. 1978. Food intake considered from the viewpoint of systems analysis. See Ref. 33, pp. 1–24
183. Montgomery, M. J., Baumgardt, B. R. 1965. Regulation of food intake in ruminants 2. Rations varying in energy concentration and physical form. *J. Dairy Sci.* 48:1623–28
184. Mook, D. G., Cseh, C. L. 1981. Release of feeding by the sweet taste in rats: the influence of body weight. *Appetite* 2:15–34
185. Moran, T. H., McHugh, P. R. 1981. Distinctions among three sugars in their effects on gastric emptying and satiety. *Am. J. Physiol.* 241:R25–30
186. Morley, J. E., Levine, A. S. 1980. Stress-induced eating is mediated through endogenous opiates. *Science* 209:1259–60
187. Mufson, E. J., Sclafani, A., Aravich, P. F. 1980. Fiber degeneration associated with hyperphagia-inducing knife cuts in the hypothalamus. *Exp. Neurol.* 67:633–45
188. Myers, R. D., McCaleb, M. L. 1980. Feeding: Satiety signal from intestine triggers brain's noradrenergic mechanism. *Science* 209:1035–37
189. Nicolaidis, S. 1969. Early systemic responses to orogastric stimulation in the regulation of food and water balance: functional and electrophysiological data. *Ann. NY Acad. Sci.* 157:1176–200
190. Nicolaidis, S. 1978. Role des réflexes anticipateurs oro-végétatifs dans la régulation hydrominerale et énergétique. *J. Physiol. (Paris)* 74:1–19
191. Nicolaidis, S., Rowland, N. 1976. Metering of intravenous versus oral nutrients and regulation of energy balance. *Am. J. Physiol.* 231:661–68

192. Nikoletseas, M. M. 1978. Effects of forced exercise on the food intake of rats maintained on a 23-h deprivation schedule. *Physiol. Behav.* 20:735–38
193. Nikoletseas, M. M. 1980. Food intake in the exercising rat: A brief review. *Neurosci. Biobehav. Rev.* 4:265–67
194. Novin, D. 1976. Visceral mechanisms in the control of food intake. See Ref. 63, pp. 357–67
195. Novin, D., Oomura, Y., eds. 1980. Integration of central and peripheral receptors in hunger and energy metabolism. *Brain Res. Bull.* 5 (Suppl. 4).
196. Novin, D., Sanderson, J. D., Vander-Weele, D. A. 1974. The effect of isotonic glucose on eating as a function of feeding condition and infusion site. *Physiol. Behav.* 13:3–7
197. Novin, D., VanderWeele, D. A. 1977. Visceral involvement in feeding: there is more to regulation than the hypothalamus. In *Progress in Psychobiology and Physiological Psychology,* ed. J. M. Sprague, A. N. Epstein, 7:193–241. NY: Academic. 257 pp.
198. Oomura, Y., Kita, H. 1981. Insulin acting as a modulator of feeding through the hypothalamus. *Diabetologia* 20: (Suppl.) 290–98
199. Oscai, L. B., Mole, P. A., Holloszy, J. O. 1971. Effects of exercise on cardiac weight and mitochondria in male and female rats. *Am. J. Physiol.* 220: 1944–48
200. Ostrowski, N. L., Foley, T., Lind, M. D., Reid, L. D. 1980. Naloxone reduces fluid intake: effects of water and food deprivation. *Pharmacol. Biochem. Behav.* 12:431–35
201. Overmann, S. R. 1976. Dietary selfselection by animals. *Psychol. Bull.* 83:218–35
202. Panksepp, J. 1971. Effects of fats, proteins, and carbohydrates on food intake in rats. *Psychonomic Monog. Suppl.* 4:85–95
203. Panksepp, J. 1974. Hypothalamic regulation energy balance and feeding behavior. *Fed. Proc.* 33:1150–65
204. Panksepp, J., Meeker, R. 1977. Effects of insulin and hypothalamic lesions on glucose preference in rats. See Ref. 31, pp. 343–56
205. Panksepp, J., Nance, D. M. 1972. Insulin, glucose, and hypothalamic regulation of feeding. *Physiol. Behav.* 9:447–51
206. Parameswaran, S. V., Steffens, A. B., Hervey, G. R., de Ruiter, L. 1977. Involvent of a humoral factor in the regulation of body weight in parabiotic rats. *Am. J. Physiol.* 232:R150–57
207. Parizkova, J., Pupa, O. 1963. Some metabolic consequences of adaptation to muscular work. *Brit. J. Nutr.* 17: 341–45
208. Peck, J. W. 1978. Rats defend different body weights depending on palatability and accessibility of their food. *J. Comp. Physiol. Psychol.* 92:555–70
209. Penicaud, L., Le Magnen, J. 1980. Recovery of body weight following starvation or food restriction in rats. *Neurosci. Biobehav. Res.* 4:47–52
210. Peters, J. C., Harper, A. E. 1981. Protein and energy consumption, plasma amino acid ratios, and brain neurotransmitter concentrations. *Physio. Behav.* 27:287–98
211. Porikos, K. 1981. Control of food intake in man: Response to covert caloric dilution of a conventional and palatable diet. See Ref. 45, pp. 83–87
212. Porikos, K. P., Booth, G., Van Itallie, T. B. 1977. Effect of covert nutritive dilution on the spontaneous food intake of obese individuals: a pilot study. *Am. J. Clin. Nutr.* 30:1638–44
213. Porte, D., Woods, S. C. 1981. Regulation of food intake and body weight by insulin. *Diabetologia.* 20: (Suppl.) 274–80
214. Powley, T. L. 1977. The ventromedial hypothalamic syndrome, satiety, and a cephalic phase hypothesis. *Psychol. Rev.* 84:89–126
215. Quartermain, D., Kissileff, H. R., Shapiro, R., Miller, N. E. 1971. Suppression of food intake with intragastric loading: Relation to natural feeding cycle. *Science* 173:941–43
216. Racotta, R., Vega, C., Russek, M. 1972. Liver catecholamines and preabsorptive satiation. *Fed. Proc.* 31:309 (Abstr.)
217. Richter, C. P. 1927. Animal behavior and internal drives. *Q. Rev. Biol.* 2:307–43
218. Richter, C. P., Holt, L. E., Barelare, B. 1938. Nutritional requirements for normal growth and reproduction in rats studied by the self-selection method. *Am. J. Physiol.* 122:734–44
219. Richter, C. P., Schmidt, E. C. H. 1941. Increased fat and decreased carbohydrate appetite in pancreatectomized rats. *Endocrinology* 28:179–92
220. Ritter, R. C., Epstein, A. N. 1975. Control of meal size by central noradrenergic action. *Proc. Natl. Acad. Sci.* 72:3740–43
221. Ritter, R. C., Roelke, M., Neville, M. 1978. Glucoprivic feeding behavior in

absence of other signs of glucoprivation. *Am. J. Physiol.* 234:E617–21
222. Ritter, R. C., Slusser, P. 1980. 5-Thio-D-glucose causes increased feeding and hyperglycemia in the rat. *Am. J. Physiol.* E141–44
223. Ritter, R. C., Slusser, P., Stone, S. 1981. Glucoreceptors controlling feeding and blood glucose: Location in the hindbrain. *Science* 213:451–53
224. Rolls, B. J. 1981. Palatability and food preference. See Ref. 45, pp. 271–78
225. Rolls, B. J., Rolls, E. T., Rowe, E. A., Sweeney, K. 1981. Sensory specific satiety in man. *Physiol. Behav.* 27:137–42
226. Rolls, B. J., Rowe, E. A., Rolls, E. T., Kingston, B., Megson, A., Gunary, R. 1981. Variety in a meal enhances food intake in man. *Physiol. Behav.* 26:215–21
227. Rolls, B. J., Rowe, E. A., Turner, R. C. 1980. Persistent obesity in rats following a period of consumption of a mixed high energy diet. *J. Physiol.* 298:415–27
228. Rolls, E. T. 1976. Neurophysiology of feeding. See Ref. 30, pp. 21–42
229. Rothwell, N. J., Stock, M. J. 1978. A paradox in the control of energy intake in the rat. *Nature* 273:146–47
230. Rothwell, N. J., Stock, M. J. 1979. Regulation of energy balance in the rat. *J. Comp. Physiol. Psychol.* 93:1024–34
231. Rothwell, N. J., Stock, M. J. 1979. A role for brown adipose tissue in diet-induced thermogenesis. *Nature* 281:31–35
232. Routtenberg, A. 1968. "Self-starvation" of rats living in activity wheels: adaptation effects. *J. Comp. Physiol. Psychol.* 66:234–38
233. Routtenberg, A., Kuznesof, A. W. 1967. "Self-starvation" of rats living in activity wheels on a restricted feeding schedule. *J. Comp. Physiol. Psychol.* 64:414–21
234. Rowland, N., Stricker, E. M. 1979. Differential effects of glucose and fructose infusions on insulin induced feeding in rats. *Physiol. Behav.* 22:387–89
235. Rozin, P. 1968. Are carbohydrate and protein intakes separately regulated: *J. Comp. Physiol. Psychol.* 65:23–29
236. Russek, M. 1963. An hypothesis on the participation of hepatic glucoreceptors in the control of food intake. *Nature* 197:79–80
237. Russek, M. 1981. Current status of the hepatostatic theory of food intake control. *Appetite* 2:137–43
238. Russek, M. 1981. Reply to commentary on "Current status of the hepatostatic

theory of food intake control." *Appetite* 2:157–62
239. Russek, M., Grinstein, S. 1974. Coding of metabolic information by hepatic glucoreceptors. In *Neurohumoral Coding of Brain Function*, ed. R. D. Myers, R. R. Drucker-Colin, pp. 81–97. NY: Plenum
240. Russek, M., Rodriguez-Zenejas, A. M., Piña, S. 1968. Hypothetical liver receptors and the anorexia caused by adrenaline and glucose. *Physiol. Behav.* 3:249–57
241. Samanin, R., Garattini, S., eds. 1978. *Central Mechanisms of Anorectic Drugs.* NY: Raven Press
242. Sawchenko, P. E., Gold, R. M. 1981. Effects of gastric vs complete subdiaphragmatic vagotomy on hypothalamic hyperphagia and obesity. *Physiol. Behav.* 26:281–92
243. Sawchenko, P. E., Gold, R. M., Alexander, J. 1981. Effects of selective vagotomies on knife cut–induced hypothalamic obesity: differential results on lab chow vs high-fat diets. *Physiol. Behav.* 26:293–300
244. Schemmel, R., Mickelsen, O., Gill, J. L. 1970. Dietary obesity in rats: body weight and body fat accretion in seven strains of rat. *J. Nutr.* 100:1941–48
245. Schwartzbaum, J. S., Ward, H. P. 1958. An osmotic factor in the regulation of food intake in the rat. *J. Comp. Physiol. Psychol.* 51:555–60
246. Sclafani, A. 1976. Appetite and hunger in experimental obesity syndromes. See Ref. 63, pp. 281–95
247. Sclafani, A. 1981. The role of hyperinsulinemia and the vagus nerve in hypothalamic hyperphagia reexamined. *Diabetologia* 20:(Suppl.)402–10
248. Sclafani, A., Aravich, P. F., Landman, M. 1981. Vagotomy blocks hypothalamic hyperphagia in rats on a chow diet and sucrose solution, but not on a palatable mixed diet. *J. Comp. Physiol. Psychol.* 95:720–34
249. Sclafani, A., Berner, C. N. 1976. Influence of diet palatability on meal taking behavior of hypothalamic hyperphagic and normal rats. *Physiol. Behav.* 16:355–63
250. Sclafani, A., Gorman, A. N. 1977. Effects of age, sex, and prior body weight on the development of dietary obesity in adult rats. *Physiol. Behav.* 18:1021–26
251. Share, I., Martyniuk, E., Grossman, M. I. 1952. Effect of prolonged intragastric feeding on oral food intake in dogs. *Am. J. Physiol.* 169:229–35

252. Sharma, K. N., Dua-Sharma, S., Jacobs, H. L. 1975. Electrophysiological monitoring of multilevel signals related to food intake. See Ref. 79, pp. 194–212
253. Silverman, H. J., Zucker, I. 1976. Absence of post-fast food compensation in the golden hamster. *Physiol. Behav.* 17:271–85
254. Skinner, B. F. 1932. Drive and reflex strength. *J. Gen. Psychol.* 6:22–47
255. Skinner, B. F. 1936. Conditioning and extinction and their relation to drive. *J. Gen. Psychol.* 14:296–317
256. Slusser, P. G., Ritter, R. C. 1980. Increased feeding and hyperglycemia elicited by intracerebroventricular 5-thioglucose. *Brain Res.* 202:474–78
257. Smith, G. P., Epstein, A. N. 1969. Increased feeding in response to decreased glucose utilization in the rat and monkey. *Am. J. Physiol.* 217:1083–87
258. Smith, G. P., Gibbs, J. 1979. Postprandial satiety. See Ref. 197, pp. 179–242
259. Smith, G. P., Gibbs, J. 1981. Brain gut peptides and the control of food intake. In *Neurosecretion and Brain Peptides,* ed. J. B. Martin, S. Reichlin, K. L. Bick, pp. 389–95. NY: Raven Press
260. Smith, G. P., Jerome, C., Cushin, G. J., Eterno, R., Simansky, K. J. 1981. Abdominal vagotomy blocks the satiety effects of cholecystokinin in the rat. *Science* 213:1036–37
261. Smith, G. P., Gibbs, J., Jerome, C., Pi-Sunyer, F. X., Kissileff, H. R., Thornton, J. 1982. The satiety effect of cholecystokinin: A progress report. *Pharmacol. Biochem. Behav.* In press
262. Smith, M. H. Jr. 1966. Effect of hypertonic preloads on concurrent eating and drinking. *J. Comp. Physiol. Psychol.* 61:398–401
262a. Smith, M., Duffy, M. 1955. The effects of intragastric inejection of various substances on subsequent bar-pressing. *J. Comp. Physiol. Psychol.* 48:387–91
263. Smith, M., Duffy, M. 1957. Some physiological factors that regulate eating behavior. *J. Comp. Physiol. Psychol.* 50:601–8
264. Smith, M., Pool, R., Weinberg, H. 1959. The effect of peripherally induced shifts in water balance on eating. *J. Comp. Physiol. Psychol.* 52:289–93
265. Smith, M., Pool, R., Weinberg, H. 1962. The role of bulk in the control of eating. *J. Comp. Physiol. Psychol.* 55:115–20
265a. Smutz, E. R., Hirsch, E., Jacobs, H. L. 1975. Caloric compensation in hypothalamic obese rats. *Physiol. Behav.* 14:305–9
266. Snowdon, C. T. 1969. Motivation, regulation and the control of meal patterns with oral and intragastric feeding. *J. Comp. Physiol. Psychol.* 69:91–100
267. Snowdon, C. T. 1970. Gastrointestinal sensory and motor control of food intake. *J. Comp. Physiol. Psychol.* 71:68–76
268. Snowdon, C. T. 1975. Production of satiety with small intraduodenal infusions in the rat. *J. Comp. Physiol. Psychol.* 88:231–38
269. Spiegel, T. A. 1973. Caloric regulation of food intake in man. *J. Comp. Physiol. Psychol.* 84:24–37
270. Spitzer, L., Rodin, J. 1981. Studies of human eating behavior: A critical review of normal weight and overweight individuals. *Appetite* 2:293–330
271. Stapelton, J. M., Merriman, V. J., Coogle, C. L., Gelbard, S. D., Reid, L. D. 1979. Naloxone reduces pressing for intracranial stimulation of sites in the periaqueductal gray area, accumbens nucleus, substantia nigra, and lateral hypothalamus. *Physiol. Psychol.* 7:427–36
272. Steffens, A. B. 1975. Influence of reversible obesity on eating behavior, blood glucose, and insulin in the rat. *Am. J. Physiol.* 228:1738–44
273. Stellar, E. 1960. Drive and motivation. In *Handbook of Physiology, Sect. I, Neurophysiology,* ed. H. W. Magoun, 3:1501–27. Washington DC: Am. Physiol. Soc.
274. Stevenson, J. A. F., Box, B. M., Feleki, U., Beaton, J. R. 1966. Bouts of exercise and food intake in the rat. *J. Appl. Physiol.* 21:118–22
275. Stricker, E. M., Rowland, N. 1978. Hepatic versus cerebral origin of stimulus for feeding induced by 2-Deoxy-d-glucose in rats. *J. Comp. Physiol. Psychol.* 92:126–32
276. Stricker, E. M., Rowland, N., Saller, C. F., Friedman, M. I. 1977. Homeostasis during hypoglycemia: central control of adrenal secretion and peripheral control of feeding. *Science* 196:79–81
277. Strominger, J. L., Brobeck, J. R., Cort, R. L. 1953. Regulation of food intake in normal rats and rats with hypothalamic hyperphagia. *Yale J. Biol. Med.* 26:55–74
278. Stunkard, A. J., ed. 1980. *Obesity.* Philadelphia: W. B. Saunders, Co.
279. Sullivan, A. C., Triscari, J., Conai, K. 1978. Caloric compensatory responses to diets containing either nonabsorbable

carbohydrate or lipid by obese and lean Zucker rats. *Am. J. Clin. Nutr.* 31:S261–66

280. Teghtsoonian, M., Becker, E., Edelman, B. 1981. A psychophysical analysis of perceived satiety: its relation to consummatory behavior and degree of overweight. *Appetite* 2:217–29

281. Teitelbaum, P. 1955. Sensory control of hypothalamic hyperphagia. *J. Comp. Physiol. Psychol.* 48:158–63

282. Teitelbaum, P. 1966. The use of operant methods in the assessment and control of motivational states. In *Operant Behavior: Areas of Research and Application,* ed. W. K. Honig, pp. 565–608. NY: Meredith Publ. Co.

283. Teitelbaum, P. 1967. Motivation and control of food intake. See Ref. 5, pp. 319–35

284. Teitelbaum, P., Campbell, B. A. 1958. Ingestion patterns in normal and hyperphagic rats. *J. Comp. Physiol. Psychol.* 51:135–41

285. Thomas, D. W., Mayer, J. 1968. Meal taking and regulation of food intake by normal and hypothalamic hyperphagic rats. *J. Comp. Physiol. Psychol.* 66:642–53

286. Thompson, D. A., Campbell, R. G. 1977. Hunger in humans induced by 2-Deoxy-D-glucose: Glucoprivic control of taste preference and food intake. *Science.* 198:1065–1067.

287. Toates, F. M. 1978. A physiological control theory of the hunger-thirst interaction. See Ref. 33, pp. 347–73

288. Toates, F. M. 1981. The control of ingestive behavior by internal and external stimuli—a theoretical review. *Appetite* 2:35–50

289. VanderWeele, D. A., Geiselman, P. J., Novin, D. 1979. Pancreatic glucagon, food deprivation and feeding in intact and vagotomized rabbits. *Physiol. Behav.* 23:155–58

290. VanderWeele, D. A., Haraczkiewicz, E., Di Conti, M. 1980. Pancreatic glucagon administration, feeding, glycemia and liver glycogen in rats. *Brain Res. Bull.* 5: (Suppl. 4) 17–21

291. VanderWeele, D. A., Novin, D., Rezek, M., Sanderson, J. D. 1974. Duodenal or hepatic-portal glucose perfusion: Evidence for duodenally-based satiety. *Physiol. Behav.* 12:467–73

292. VanderWeele, D. A., Sanderson, J. D. 1976. Peripheral glucosensitive satiety in the rabbit and the rat. See Ref. 33, pp. 383–93

293. VanderWeele, D. A., Skoog, D. R., Novin, D. 1976. Glycogen levels and peripheral mechanism of glucose-induced suppression of feeding. *Am. J. Physiol.* 231:1655–59

294. Van Hemel, S. B., Myer, J. S. 1969. Feeding patterns and response to caloric dilution in the Japanese quail. *Physiol. Behav.* 4:339–44

295. Van Itallie, T. B., Gale, S. K., Kissileff, H. R. 1978. Control of food intake in the regulation of depot fat: an overview. In *Advances in Modern Nutrition,* vol. 2. *Diabetes, Obesity, and Vascular Disease Metabolic and Molecular Interrelationships,* Part 2, ed. H. M. Katzen, R. J. Mahler, pp. 427–92. Washington DC: Hemisphere Publ. Corp.

296. Van Itallie, T. B., VanderWeele, D. A. 1981. The phenomenon of satiety. In *Recent Advances in Obesity Research: III,* ed. P. Bjorntorp, M. Cairella, A. N. Howard, pp. 278–89. London: John Libbey. 392 pp.

297. Vilberg, T. R., Beatty, W. W. 1975. Behavioral changes following VMH lesions in rats with controlled insulin levels. *Pharmacol. Biochem. Behav.* 3: 377–84

298. Wagner, J. W., De Groot, J. 1963. Changes in feeding behavior after intracerebral injections in the rat. *Am. J. Physiol.* 204:483–87

299. Waldbillig, R. J., Bartness, T. J., Stanley, B. G. 1981. Increased food intake, body weight and adiposity, in rats after regional neurochemical depletion of serotonin. *J. Comp. Physiol. Psychol.* 95:391–405

300. Walike, B. C., Jordan, H. A., Stellar, E. 1969. Preloading and the regulation of food intake in man. *J. Comp. Physiol. Psychol.* 68:327–33

301. Wirtshafter, D., Davis, J. D. 1977. Body weight: Reduction by long-term glycerol treatment. *Science* 198: 1271–74

302. Wirtshafter, D., Davis, J. D. 1977. Set points, settling points, and the control of body weight. *Physiol. Behav.* 19:75–78

303. Wolff, F. W., Bartoshuk, L. M., Booth, D. A., Bray, G. A., Chlouverakis, C. S., Curtis-Prior, P. B., Harper, A. E., Hunt, J. N., Novin, D., Russek, M. B., Schneider, K., Smith, G. P. 1976. Peripheral and hormonal mechanisms—group report 2. See Ref. 30, pp. 219–28

303a. Woo, R. 1981. *Effect of exercise on spontaneous caloric intake in obesity.* PhD thesis, Columbia Univ., New York. 194 pp.

304. Woo, R., Garrow, J., Pi-Sunyer, F. X. 1982. Voluntary food intake during pro-

longed exercise in obese women. *Am. J. Clin. Nutr.* In press

305. Woo, R., Kissileff, H. R., Pi-Sunyer, F. X. 1979. Is insulin a satiety hormone? *Fed Proc.* 38:547 (Abstr.)

306. Woods, S. C., Lotter, E. C., McKay, L. D., Porte, D. 1979. Chronic intracerebroventricular infusion of insulin reduces food intake and body weight of baboons. *Nature* 282:503–5

307. Woods, S. C., Porte, D. Jr. 1977. Relationship between plasma and cerebrospinal fluid insulin levels of dogs. *Am. J. Physiol.* 233:E331–34

308. Woods, S. C., West, D. B., Stein, L. J., McKay, L. D., Lotter, E. C., Porte, S. G., Kenney, N. J., Porte, D. Jr. 1981. Peptides and the control of meal size. *Diabetologia.* 20: (Suppl.) 305–13

309. Wooley, O. W. 1971. Long-term food regulation in the obese and nonobese. *Psychosom. Med.* 33:436–44

310. Wurtman, J. J., Wurtman, R. J. 1979. Drugs that enhance serotonergic transmission diminish elective carbohydrate consumption by rats. *Life Sci.* 24:895–904

311. Yin, T. H., Hamilton, C. L., Brobeck, J. R. 1970. Food intake of rats given hypertonic solutions by gavage and water intravenously. *Proc. Soc. Exp. Biol. Med.* 133:83–85

312. Young, P. T. 1967. Palatability: the hedonic response to foodstuffs. See Ref. 5, pp. 353–66

313. Young, T. K., Liu, A. C. 1965. Hyperphagia, insulin and obesity. *Chin. J. Physiol.* 19:247–53

314. Ziegler, H. P., Green, H. L., Siegel, S. 1972. Food and water intake and weight regulation in the pigeon. *Physiol. Behav.* 8:127–34

Ann. Rev. Nutr. 1982. 2:419–54

AMINO ACID IMBALANCE AND HEPATIC ENCEPHALOPATHY[1]

Plinio Bernardini and Josef E. Fischer

Department of Surgery, University of Cincinnati Medical Center, Cincinnati, Ohio 45267

I. BACKGROUND

A. Introduction

Hepatic encephalopathy is one of the most frequent terminal episodes of primary liver disease. It was already known at the time of Hippocrates, and it was well described by Johanne Baptista Margagni, teacher at the Padua Medical School, in the 18th century.

Hepatic encephalopathy is a neuropsychiatric syndrome seen in the presence of hepatic functional impairment secondary to acute liver failure or chronic parenchymal liver disease with or without spontaneous or surgically induced portalsystemic shunting of portal blood. The neuropsychiatric symptoms of liver failure are varied and range from subtle alterations, including mild personality change and disturbance in sleep rhythm, to confusion, drowsiness, stupor, and finally deep coma. In acute liver failure the progression of events may be extremely rapid, taking place in only a few hours. In chronic encephalopathy, in contrast, consciousness may be slowly altered over months, and may occasionally present as progressive and irreversible neurological symptomatology with dementia, parkinsonism, or other extrapyramidal signs suggesting involvement of the cerebellum or basal ganglia (170). Most often in the chronic situation, however, episodes of mental impairment are episodic, the result of defined stresses, and recovery to the premorbid state is the rule.

Other symptoms of hepatic encephalopathy are not specific for liver disease. Asterixis (flapping tremor of the extremities) is probably the most characteristic neurological sign of hepatic encephalopathy, is more common

[1]Supported in part by USPHS Grant #AM 25347

0199-9885/82/0715-0419$02.00

in uremia, and is also seen in patients with respiratory insufficiency, hypokalemia, congestive heart failure, sedative overdose, and even during hypoglycemia (35). Similar tremors can also be elicited in the feet, tightly closed eyelids, pursed lips, or in the protruded tongue. Conn has suggested that asterixis may be associated with a lesion of crossing corticospinal tracts, as it has been observed on the contralateral side of a developing cerebral thrombosis (36). Other neurological abnormalities, when present, are usually transient and are presumed to be a result of a metabolic disturbance rather than of permanent structural damage. Cerebral function may be assessed by simple tests for contructional apraxia such as the ability to draw a five pointed star, by psychometric methods such as the number connection test of Reitan (50, 173), and by electroencephalogram.

In the absence of preexisting liver disease, hepatic encephalopathy associated with acute fulminant hepatic failure is usually seen in the setting of acute viral hepatitis (125, 179), but is observed also with drug-induced liver damage [e.g. paracetamol, halothane (30, 114) or tetracycline (193)] and with the acute fatty degeneration seen in pregnancy (178). Against the background of chronic liver disease, a variety of clinical events, such as gastrointestinal bleeding, infections, and over-diuresis, may provoke hepatic encephalopathy.

B. Pathology

There are no striking findings in the brain pathology of patients dying in hepatic coma. A fairly consistent finding is hyperplasia of protoplasmic type II astrocytes, most prominent in the cortex but also found in other parts of the brain (215). The pseudopods of these cells, which likely are the cells that synthesize glutamine from ammonia, may contribute to the control of the passage of materials across the blood–brain barrier. In the cerebral edema that complicates acute fulminant hepatic failure, which does not respond to steroids, mannitol, urea, or other usual therapeutic measures (222, 229), it is possible that edema of the pseudopods disrupts the tight junctions normally present in brain capillaries and opens up abnormal passages through which toxic materials may enter the brain.

The meaning of these astroglial changes is not clear. It is increasingly thought that the astroglia are the cells that govern the extracellular environment of the brain; as such, their dysfunction may contribute to disruption in neurological function. As discussed elsewhere, glutamine is probably a glial metabolite (10, 12, 228). Elevation of cerebrospinal fluid glutamine is one of the most reliable biochemical correlates of hepatic encephalopathy (83, 98), and thus an anatomical-biochemical correlation may be implicit. Whether the astrocytic protoplasmic hyperplasia observed is an attempt on the part of the glia to maintain neuronal homeostasis or is a pathological response to toxins and even contributes to the mechanism of hepatic encephalopathy is not known. In hepatocerebral degeneration, irreversible neuronal damage and degeneration as well as demyelination may occur.

C. Clinical Laboratory Investigation

In clinical laboratory investigation, there are no "hepatic function tests" or plasma electrolyte disturbances invariably associated with hepatic encephalopathy. Blood ammonia is elevated in the majority of patients with this syndrome; however, its level does not reflect well the degree of coma, and numerous patients with clinical encephalopathy may have normal blood ammonia levels. While arterial ammonia concentration is better correlated with clinical states, 10% of patients with hepatic coma have normal arterial ammonia levels (205); cerebrospinal fluid ammonia and glutamine are more often elevated than peripheral blood ammonia. Clotting factor deficiencies reflect only the severity of hepatic dysfunction, and are not related to the degree of encephalopathy. Electrolyte and acid-base disturbances are common; respiratory alkalosis, which is secondary to hyperventilation and may depress cerebral blood flow, and hypokalemic metabolic alkalosis may occur. Hypoglycemia generally presages a fatal outcome as it is usually encountered in greatly advanced hepatic failure. It is probably due to impaired gluconeogenesis and glycogen synthesis, but it has been reported in noncomatose patients with severe viral hepatitis (56). Renal failure may ensue, and urea and creatinine will rise, but again are not necessarily part of hepatic encephalopathy. Pathological findings in the cerebrospinal fluid (CSF) are not characteristic. CSF is clear and colorless, except when hyperbilirubinemia is present. No characteristic pattern of cells, glucose, protein and electrolytes has been discerned, while CSF glutamine is usually elevated (83, 98).

D. Pathogenesis of Hepatic Encephalopathy

Current knowledge about the pathogenesis of hepatic encephalopathy derives from studies in patients with this disorder and in animals with experimentally induced hepatic coma. Various theories of hepatic encephalopathy have been entertained for the past several decades. Any theory about the etiology and therapy of hepatic coma must accommodate several clinical observations: (a) Decreased hepatic function and shunting of blood around the liver are usually present in hepatic encephalopathy. (b) The substance(s) involved in the etiology of hepatic encephalopathy arise in the gut. (c) Those substances appear to be of nitrogenous origin, as coma is commonly provoked by increased dietary protein or gastrointestinal bleeding. (d) Gut bacteria play a role, since altering gut bacterial flora ameliorates hepatic encephalopathy. (e) While ammonia may not be the sole etiological agent, serum ammonia generally reflects the presence of hepatic coma although the correlation is not exact.

The four prevalent theories of hepatic encephalopathy are those relating to: Ammonia, short-chain fatty acids, the synergistic hypothesis, and the neurotransmitter amino acid hypotheses.

1.AMMONIA   Hyperammonemia has been implicated as a cause of hepatic coma. While patients with hepatic disease are especially sensitive to the cerebral toxic effects of ammonia (163) this does not necessarily mean that spontaneous encephalopathy is the result of ammonia intoxication. Hyperammonemia is common in patients with hepatic encephalopathy (135) and in laboratory animals with portacaval shunt. The concept that hyperammonemia is closely related to portal system encephalopathy is widely held and provides a rationale for treatment by a variety of agents designed to reduce intestinal ammonia production. Blood ammonia determinations are still the most widely performed biochemical tests for hepatic encephalopathy. The mechanism initially proposed by which ammonia exerts its toxic effect was that ammonia blocked energy production by depletion of the cerebral Krebs cycle of 2-oxoglutarate, utilized in the synthesis of glutamine (13). This hypothesis is no longer tenable, as the depletion of 2-oxoglutarate has not been observed in experimental hepatic coma (14, 195), and brain glutamine is derived from the synthesis of ammonia with a rapidly-turning-over pool of glutamic acid rather than directly from 2-oxoglutarate (12). Other possible toxic effects of ammonia that have been proposed include the accumulation of gamma-amino butyric acid (GABA), an inhibitory neurotransmitter (86). However, GABA measured in the brains of animals with acute ammonia intoxication and experimental hepatic coma is normal (192), although recent studies have again suggested that it may play a role in both chemical and experimental hepatic coma (59, 190).

The second major hypothesis is the disruption in energy production. In studies carried out under carefully controlled experimental circumstances using the recently developed ultrarapid freeze-blow technique, slight decreases in phosphocreatine were found in ammonia-intoxicated animals (90). In a more recent study, after 60 minutes of massive ammonia intoxication in animals with portacaval shunts, ATP content was decreased in all regions of the brain, but the reduction in total high-energy phosphate was most marked in the brain stem. In other experiments the authors concluded that the cerebral dysfunction in chronic relapsing ammonia intoxication is not primarily due to energy failure (94).

In vivo toxicity of ammonia may be disassociated from venous ammonia levels by monoamine oxidase inhibitors in man (47) and by inhibitors of glutamine synthesis in experimental animals (223). Arterial ammonia concentrations, while correlating better with encephalopathy than venous ammonia, may still be normal with grade 4 hepatic encephalopathy (205). More recent physiological evidence localized the site of ammonia toxicity to the cortex and perhaps amygdyla, but the reticular activating system and the arousal response are not generally affected by ammonia and thus cannot explain all the symptoms of hepatic encephalopathy (95).

Acute ammonia intoxication does not reproduce all the cerebral changes seen in hepatic encephalopathy such as increased serotonin and tryptophan levels (7, 44, 63, 116), alterations in brain phenylalanine, tyrosine, and their derivative amines (63, 64), and alterations in metabolites of dopamine and serotonin (115). Furthermore, ammonia given to experimental animals in amounts far in excess of levels found in man failed to change cerebral serotonin, and this again suggests that ammonia intoxication does not completely mimic human hepatic encephalopathy (194, 218). Recent experiments from this laboratory have altered this view however.

According to the "glutamine exchange" hypothesis, prolonged infusion of ammonia in normal animals should reproduce, to some extent, the brain amino acid changes seen in experimental animals with impaired hepatic function. Preliminary experiments carried out in this laboratory show that while changes in serotonin and norepinephrine may be achieved by prolonged ammonia infusion, they are not of the same magnitude as seen in hepatic coma (105).

2. SHORT-CHAIN FATTY ACIDS   Butyrate, valerate, and octanoate are increased in the blood and CSF of patients with hepatic encephalopathy (29, 208, 217). A close relationship has been found in at least one instance between slow-wave electrical activity on the EEG and the concentration of fatty acid in the spinal fluid (211). Muto (145) reported elevation in short-chain fatty acids, particularly C4 to C6, in hepatic coma resulting from nonfulminant disease. Precedent exists in another form of coma: that found with the Jamaican vomiting sickness, which is induced by hypoglycin A and results in isovaleric-acidemia (209).

The correlation of blood and CSF concentrations of short-chain fatty acids and grades of coma is not good (27). Furthermore, while the liver is presumably active in the catabolism of such fatty acids absorbed from the gut, it is not clear how such excesses of fatty acids might be linked to ingestion of protein, over-diuresis, sepsis, or some of the other stimuli known to provoke hepatic encephalopathy. Indeed, short-chain fatty acids of this chain length have been administered to patients with known cirrhosis without provoking encephalopathy (138). It is therefore unlikely that short-chain fatty acids alone are responsible for hepatic encephalopathy.

3. THE SYNERGISTIC HYPOTHESIS   Synergism in coma production has been demonstrated experimentally with combined administration of ammonia, fatty acids, and mercaptans (137, 234). Zieve argues that by acting synergistically, smaller amounts of each of these three toxins might be necessary to produce hepatic encephalopathy than if given alone (234). Normal animals have been rendered comatose by ammonium salts supplemented with short-chain fatty acids. However, the concentrations of ammonia achieved in these experiments range from 590 to 1470 μmol/l (1000–2500 μg/dl), values almost never seen in patients except, occasionally, in Reye's syndrome. Thus the results obtained in support of this hypothesis are somewhat controversial.

4. THE NEUROTRANSMITTER AMINO ACID HYPOTHESIS   The neuropsychiatric symptoms associated with hepatic encephalopathy in both acute and chronic circumstances suggest major disturbances in neurotransmission. The past several decades have seen the discovery of many candidates for neurotransmitter function in the central nervous system, including amines, such as acetylcholine, dopamine, norepinephrine (noradrenaline), serotonin, histamine; excitatory amino acids, such as glutamate and aspartate; inhibitory amino acids, including glycine, serine, and GABA; the prostaglandins; substance P; and more recently the peptide neurotransmitters (8). Progress has been made in the physiology of many central neurotransmitters, particularly the neuropharmacology of the adrenergic neurotransmitters, norepinephrine and dopamine. The structural requirements of the peripheral adrenergic system, the sympathetic nervous system, appeared to be a phenolic ring and a short carbon side chain with a hydroxyl group on the B position in the chain (69, 117).

The concept of "false neurochemical transmitters" evolved from evidence that the peripheral adrenergic neurone would take up, protect from destruction, and release in response to electrical stimulation compounds presumably less active sympathomimetically than the putative transmitter norepinephrine; these then could accumulate under toxic or pharmacologic conditions or in response to accumulation of exogenous precursors (42, 144).

The initial evidence for this hypothesis came from the laboratory. Octopamine is a known false neurochemical transmitter with a sympathomimetic action less than 1/50 that of norepinephrine in the periphery; it greatly increases in the brains and the hearts (representative of the peripheral sympathetic nervous system) of rats in acute hepatic coma (63, 66, 70). Norepinephrine, the putative neurotransmitter, decreases at least by approximately 50% in the brains of comatose animals, and the degree of decrease is proportional to level of coma (49, 53, 213). Serotonin can compete with norepinephrine for storage in adrenergic neurons and is inhibitory (8); it has been implicated in normal regulation of consciousness through brainstem mechanisms (141) and is elevated in acute hepatic coma in rats (43).

II. PERIPHERAL AMINO ACID METABOLISM

The importance of the liver in amino acid metabolism was first noted in 1924, when Bollman, Mann & Magath (17) showed that the hepatectomized dog was unable to form urea from amino acids. The earliest studies of amino acid metabolism in hepatic failure utilized paper chromatographic techniques. In analysis of urine (220), no single pattern of abnormalities in amino acid excretion during hepatic failure was documented, presumably because of the relatively crude techniques available and because of deranged renal function in some patients. Excesses, but not deficiencies, of many plasma amino acids were detected with increased plasma tyrosine and methionine being easily detected (100, 231). Several recent studies with more sophisticated analysis have revealed already a considerable amount of information about plasma amino acid levels in patients and animals with hepatic encephalopathy. In chronic liver disease complicated by acute decompensation a pattern was reported consisting of increased plasma phenylalanine, tyrosine, free but not necessarily total tryptophan, methionine, histidine, glutamate and aspartate, together with decreased or low normal levels of the branched-chain amino acids, leucine, isoleucine, and valine (4, 16, 20, 26, 73, 99, 101, 134, 177, 182, 206, 231). These findings assumed increased significance as it became clear that certain neutral amino acids served as precursors for CNS amine neurotransmitters. This group of large neutral amino acids includes tryptophan, tyrosine, phenylalanine, methionine, and histidine; they and the branched-chain amino acids compete for entry across the blood-brain barrier using a common carrier (151). Subsequent investigations have revealed that in addition to the classical amino acid pattern, another distinct amino acid pattern exists (182). While patients with chronic liver disease with superimposed acute insults—i.e. gastrointestinal bleeding, infection, alcoholic hepatitis—manifest the "usual" pattern of increased plasma phenylalanine, tyrosine and methionine, free tryptophan and decreased branched-chain amino acids that appears to be associated with hepatic encephalopathy (67, 72, 148), other investigators claim that it is associated with severe liver disease but not specifically with encephalopathy (140, 226). Others agree that it indicates the presence but not necessarily the grade of encephalopathy, as initially proposed (185). In acute fulminant hepatitis, a second pattern is present: severe hyperaminoacidemia of all amino acids. Only the branched-chain amino acids leucine, isoleucine, and valine remain normal; plasma levels may even be slightly decreased (171, 182).

Tryptophan is thought to be toxic in liver disease (2). Plasma total tryptophan is either slightly elevated (43) or reduced (155) in hepatic encephalopathy while free tryptophan is markedly increased (43). Absolute levels of plasma tryptophan are probably not as important as the ratio of protein-bound to free plasma tryptophan (61), the influence of plasma nonesterified fatty acids (161), and the distribution of branched-chain amino acids (107). Possibly because of these variables, brain tryptophan in animals with liver disease (107, 7) as well as CSF tryptophan and 5-hydroxy-indoleascetic acid (5-HIAA) in both animals (63, 199) and patients with hepatic encephalopathy (115) are greatly increased, despite the relatively small elevations in the plasma concentration of total tryptophan.

Brain tryptophan is increased both because of the decreased plasma concentrations of the competing branched-chain amino acids (43, 60, 107) and because of increased plasma free tryptophan. Serotonin, an inhibitory neurotransmitter amine (89), is greatly increased in the experimental animal with acute hepatic coma (43, 63) and is thought to play a role in hepatic encephalopathy (43, 44, 45, 46, 107, 111, 115, 116, 120, 155, 158). Indeed, some investigators have proposed that the ratio of free tryptophan to competing neutral amino acids may be the most accurate plasma amino acid ratio describing hepatic encephalopathy, both spontaneously and in response to various forms of therapy such as lactulose and infusions of branched-chain amino acids (26, 185, 186). That tryptophan is an essential component of pathogenesis in hepatic encephalopathy is supported by experiments in which a coma–like state is induced by infusion into normal dogs of phenylalanine and tryptophan in combination but not alone (78).

Methionine had previously been used as a lipotropic factor in liver disease, but subsequently it was shown to be toxic (27). Intolerance to methionine has been correlated with the concentration of ammonia in portal blood collaterals (227). Intracarotid arterial injections of large amounts of methionine into normal dogs failed to produce coma (78). Oral tolerance of methionine may be increased by oral antibiotics (162), suggesting that the toxic factor is not methionine but a metabolic product. Other investigators have suggested that methionine may reduce brain ATP by the formation of S-adenosylmethionine (88). However, normal levels of brain ATP have been found in rats in hepatic coma with elevated blood and brain methionine (14). Exogenously administered methionine is probably of less importance to the brain since the brain synthesizes its own methionine when deprived of other sources (156).

Phenylalanine is the amino acid that has the highest concentration in the brain as well as in the blood of animals in hepatic coma. One factor is the decreased conversion of phenylalanine to tyrosine by hepatic phenylalanine-4-hydroxylase, whose activity is decreased early in hepatic impairment.

A constant finding in both patients and experimental animals is the decreased level of the branched-chain amino acids (BCAA) valine, leucine, and isoleucine, both on a relative basis, as in acute fulminant hepatitis, in which they remain normal despite tremendous increases in other amino acids, and on an absolute basis, as in seen in chronic liver disease with acute exacerbation. They have a unique function in that they are not only incorporated into protein but can be catabolized by brain, muscle, and kidney for energy and be subsequently degraded to acetyl-coenzyme A. The low plasma concentration of BCAA is presumably the result of decreased release from muscle (where they are utilized for energy) as well as of increased oxidation by fat (201, 202). Presumably part of the function of the BCAA is to substitute for energy sources such as glucose and ketone bodies, possibly lacking in animals with severe hepatic parenchymal damage. In addition to the liver, the kidney is the one organ that may catabolize the branched-chain amino acids into glucose; it may be using the BCAA as a primary source of oxidizable substrate in an effort to maintain blood glucose when hepatic gluconeogenesis is deficient. In addition to regulation of effects of other amino acids across the muscle cell membrane (152), recent evidence suggestions that infusions of BCAA will increase not only muscle but hepatic protein synthesis (76, 77, 188).

A. Effects of Hormones

Alterations in the levels of insulin, glucagon, and presumably other hormones influence the plasma amino acid imbalance in cirrhotic patients. In advanced liver cirrhosis a remarkable increase in glucagon levels has been demonstrated (132), particularly when portalsystemic shunting is present (194). In spite of increased insulin levels (32), the insulin/glucagon molar ratio is decreased (131). This ratio may be a marker of a catabolic state characterized by enhanced gluconeogenesis from different sources, mainly amino acids (214). Insulin promotes the catabolism of the BCAA by both muscle and fat, and it has been suggested that the decreased concentrations of BCAA within the circulation are secondary to oxidation of these amino acids by muscle under the influence of insulin (142, 201), although increased oxidation by fat certainly plays a role (85, 202).

In animals, following end-to-side portacaval shunt, both insulin and glucagon increased modestly, with a normal insulin/glucagon ratio. As the animal enters hepatic encephalopathy, there is a dramatic rise in the plasma concentration of glucagon while insulin either remains stable or decreases (142, 202). In a recent study, Marchesini et al (130, 131) found that hyperglucagonemia in cirrhotics closely correlates with encephalopathy grade since the plasma concentration of glucagon progressively increases with the deterioration of the mental state. Infusion of glucagon in conjunction with epinephrine and steroids brings about a state of sustained catabolism and gluconeogenesis; with this, aromatic amino acids are presumably released in increased amounts, accumulating within the circulation owing to decreased hepatic catabolism.

B. Effects of Catabolism

In animals and patients with normal liver function, anabolism and catabolism exert relatively minor influences on plasma and brain amino acid levels. However, in animals with liver disease the effects of positive nitrogen balance and intracellular deposition of amino acids are to decrease plasma and brain aromatic amino acids as well as brain amine neurotransmitter derivatives as rats with end-to-side portacaval shunts go into more markedly positive nitrogen balance (183).

C. Effects of Acute Hepatic Necrosis

Patients during the course of fulminant hepatitis with coma have been shown to have grossly abnormal plasma amino acid profiles, characterized by substantially increased levels of most amino acids, but normal or slightly reduced concentrations of the branched-chain amino acids valine, leucine, and isoleucine (171, 182).

The origin of the raised plasma amino acids in fulminant hepatic failure is not certain, although on the basis of a close relationship between plasma tyrosine and serum glutamic oxaloacetic transaminase levels it has been suspected that hepatic necrosis per se is responsible for high plasma amino acid levels (182). Thus the degree of aromatic amino acid elevations, particularly of tyrosine, may be useful in predicting the extent of hepatic necrosis, and possibly outcome, although others have denied this (197).

The concentrations of phenylalanine, tyrosine, and methionine may be as high as 700–800% of normal, and in a series of 15 patients no patient with a tyrosine level higher than 60 μg/ml (or 600% of normal) survived acute fulminant hepatitis regardless of therapy (182). High plasma tyrosine and phenylalanine levels have been found in association with elevated brain concentrations of these amino acids in patients dying from fulminant hepatic failure (171). Conversion of excess tyrosine and phenylalanine to tyramine, octopamine, phenylethylamine and B-hydroxyphenylethanolamine, respectively, act as weak or false neurotransmitters present in excess. Other laboratories have confirmed the hyper-tyrosinemia seen in decompensated cirrhosis and encephalopathy (54, 55). Increased plasma tyrosine and its amine derivative tyramine have also been documented in hepatic encephalopathy (53, 54, 55). Tyramine is, of course, a precursor of octopamine (β–hydroxytyramine), and at present tyramine is not regarded as unique in the amino–acid–neurotransmitter hypothesis of hepatic encephalopathy but rather merely as a representative of the class of phenylethylamines and phenylethanolamines.

Normal BCAA concentration in acute hepatic necrosis is, perhaps, related to two opposing influences: hepatic necrosis releasing branched-chains into the circulation versus increased fat uptake or branched–chain metabolism by muscle for energy.

III. BRAIN AMINO ACID METABOLISM

A. Blood-Brain Barrier

The capillary circulation in the brain is unique in that capillaries do not have pores but tight junctions. The permeability properties of these vessels resemble those of a cell membrane, and these properties have led to the use of the term blood-brain barrier. The blood-brain barrier is altered in a subtle way in chronic liver disease (104) and completely disrupted in experimental models of the late stages of acute hepatic coma (123), but not after 18 hr in a properly supported anhepatic rate (91a).

Blood-brain transport of various substances has been investigated by determining the brain uptake index (BUI) (151). James and his collaborators (104) found that the BUI of tryptophan, phenylalanine, tyrosine, and leucine was significantly increased after portacaval anastomosis (PCA) in rats. No increase was observed in the BUI of tyramine or for inulin (mol wt 5000–5500), which are normally excluded from the brain. The BUI of glucose, for which a hexose-specific transport system has been demonstrated (159), was also unchanged after PCA. In contrast, the BUI of arginine, which is transported by a separate system specific for basic amino acids, was significantly decreased in rats after PCA (104). A significant positive correlation was found between plasma free tryptophan and brain tryptophan, brain tryptophan, and the BUI of tryptophan, strongly suggesting that experimentally obtained BUI values are a valid index of the physiological activity of the blood-brain amino acid transport system. These data suggest that not only brain tryptophan but also brain methionine, tyrosine, phenylalanine, and histidine may be influenced by the activity of the blood-brain transport system.

These results also strongly support the postulated role of the neutral amino acids in the pathogenesis of hepatic encephalopathy. This increase in blood-brain barrier transport activity has been independently confirmed [(91, 93, 235) and D.B.A. Silk, personal communication].

Another phenomenon that appears to be independent of the competition phenomenon is a direct relationship between CSF and, presumably, brain aromatic amino acids and the plasma concentration, suggesting that in acute fulminant hepatitis, when branched-chain amino acids may be normal, the extremely elevated plasma aromatic amino acids will result in flooding of the brain with, for example, phenylalanine and tyrosine. Whether these CSF data are in keeping with a selective active transport phenomenon or whether this is the result of partial breakdown of the blood-brain barrier is not yet clear, although evidence at present favors the former alternative (91a).

B. Glutamine, Ammonia

According to the hypothesis suggested by James et al (109), peripheral hyperammonemia increases the influx of ammonia into the brain where it is detoxified in astrocytes by its reaction with glutamic acid to yield glutamine, a neutral amino acid whose efflux from the brain is mediated by the large neutral amino acid carrier system (108). Glutamine has a low affinity for the neutral amino acid transport system of the blood-brain barrier, whereas it readily exchanges with tryptophan, tyrosine, and methionine in the plasma to enhance the concentration of these amino acids in the brain. There is an excellent correlation between the concentration of glutamine in the brain and tryptophan in the cerebrospinal fluid (199). According to this hypothesis, hyperammonemia contributes indirectly to the brain accumulation of neutral amino acids. Cangiano et al (24) showed that the presence of physiologically high concentration of ammonia significantly increased the uptake of neutral amino acids by isolated brain capillaries. These studies support the concept that hyperammonemia is able to modify the neutral amino acid L-system by increasing the glutamine intracellular levels and then stimulating the exchange of outside neutral amino acids for inside glutamine. The increased level of these precursors alters the balance of neurotransmitter substances in the brain and causes encephalopathy.

C. Significance of the Unified Neurotransmitter Amino Acid Hypothesis

If the above hypothesis is correct, hepatic encephalopathy is the result of altered plasma amino acid profile, changes in the blood-brain barrier, hyperammonemia, and altered neutral amino acid blood-brain barrier transport in turn at least partially related to hyperammonemia and increased exchange for brain glutamine. No single factor, neither ammonia nor plasma amino acid molar ratios, could be expected to have a clear one-to-one correlation with encephalopathy. The various therapeutic approaches, including decreasing ammonia and altering plasma amino acid ratios, would all work via neurotransmitter alterations.

The ultimate proof of this hypothesis in man would be the demonstration that in patients with hepatic coma, decreasing peripheral blood ammonia would result in alterations (decreases) in CSF concentrations of neutral amino acids despite no changes in plasma amino acid concentrations. This apparently has been observed by measuring serial CSF amino acid concentrations in patients in hepatic coma treated with lactulose (L. Capocaccia, personal communication). In those patients, blood ammonia decreased while plasma amino acid concentrations remained unchanged. Nonetheless, CSF aromatic amino acids decreased markedly.

Hyperammonemic Models

If hyperaminonemia increases brain glutamine and this is at least partially responsible for increased exchange, infusing large quantities of ammonia into normal rats should at least partialy mimic amino acid changes seen in animals with portocaval anastomosis. Ammonia infusions, carefully done to avoid seizures, increase brain aromatic amino acids in parallel with rises in brain glutamine (84). Blocking synthesis of brain glutamine appears to prevent at least partially this rise in brain aromatic amino acids (110).

IV. BRAIN TRANSMITTERS

A. Catecholamines

In practice the term "catecholamine" usually implies dihydroxyphenylethylamine (dopamine) and its metabolic products, norepinephrine and epinephrine. At the present time it is well accepted that norepinephrine acts as a neurotransmitter in the central nervous system. Both in the peripheral adrenergic system and the brain, other variables such as exogenous intake, and particularly the liver and its metabolism of amino acids and amines, can control the entry and the concentration of neurotransmitter material into the neurons. The portal circulation absorbs amino acids and amines derived from gut bacterial action. They are generally inactivated by the liver, and their plasma concentrations are kept within a narrow range despite a wide range of intake by hepatic enzymatic function. The blood-brain barrier contributes to the control of neurotransmitter material by selectively allowing precursor amino acids to penetrate and excluding most circulating amines. Although tyrosine is normally the principal precursor for catecholamines, phenylalanine by hydroxylation to tyrosine similarly serves as a precursor for catecholamine synthesis. In liver failure, the peripheral and the central nervous system can accept and synthesize other precursor amino acids or unphysiologic amounts of those precursors, leading to altered neurotransmitter synthesis and derangements in neurotransmission. The depletion of a normal neurotransmitter (norepinephrine) in the periphery (49, 133) might result in a state of high cardiac output and low vascular resistance often seen in hepatic failure (133, 148). Other laboratories have confirmed depletion of brain norpinephrine in animals in acute hepatic coma (53).

B. Indoles

Serotonin (5-HT) is found in many cells that are not neurons, such as platelets, mast cells, and the enterochromaffin cells of the intestinal mucosa. Only about 1–2% of the serotonin in the whole body is found in the brain (41), and as a 5-HT cannot cross the blood-brain barrier it is clear that brain cells must synthesize their own. Within the central nervous system the first important step is the uptake of the amino acid tryptophan, the primary substrate for the synthesis. An active uptake facilitates the entry of tryptophan into cells, and this entry site can be competed for by certain other amino acids, such as phenylalanine or any of the other neutral amino acids. The next step is hydroxylation of tryptophan to form 5-hydroxytryptophan (5-HTP). This step in the synthesis can be specifically blocked by para-chlorophenylalanine, an inhibitor of tryptophan hydroxylase. In the rat, a single intraperitoneal injection of 10 mg/kg of this inhibitor lowers the brain serotonin content (28). Once synthesized, 5-HTP is almost immediately decarboxylated to yield serotonin. The only effective route of continued metabolism for serotonin is deamination by monoamine oxidase (MAO). The products of this reaction can be further oxidized to 5-hydroxyindoleacetic acid.

Disturbances in serotonin metabolism in liver disease have been widely documented. Serotonin, which may replace norepinephrine or dopamine in the adrenergic system, is markedly increased in both chronic encephalopathy and acute hepatic failure (43, 44, 45, 115, 116). Increased 5-HIAA has long been known to be present in the CSF and brain of animals and CSF of patients with hepatic failure (115, 199). In both dogs and primates, when specific nutritional therapy for hepatic encephalopathy is undertaken 5-HIAA promptly returns to normal as the animal recovers (199).

C. "False," Weak, or Inactive Neurochemical Transmitters

In the peripheral sympathetic nervous system, where norepinephrine is the normal transmitter, it has been amply shown that other β-hydroxylated phenylethylamines can replace norepinephrine and act as false or relatively inactive neurochemical transmitters (31, 69). Similar phenolic amines have been shown capable of being taken up, retained, and released in the central nervous system as well as in the peripheral sympathetic nervous system (69).

The role of the false neurochemical transmitters (FNT) may explain the production of some of the symptoms of hepatic failure as follows: Amines are produced in the gut by the action of bacterial amino acid decarboxylases. They and their amino acid precursors, such as phenylalanine and tyrosine, are absorbed into the portal circulation. In normal circumstances these are largely cleared from the portal blood by the liver. When hepatic function is impaired and blood is shunted around the liver, either spontaneously or surgically, these substances flood the peripheral and central nervous system, releasing and replacing the normal endogenous neurotransmitters.

Such events might explain not only the CNS malfunction but also the cardiovascular changes—e.g. the high cardiac output and low peripheral resistance state—that may be associated with hepatic failure (133, 148). The cardiovascular changes associated with the high output state are therefore viewed as secondary. Normally, vascular beds with high resting peripheral vascular resistance are dependent on the presence of norepinephrine in the nerve terminals to maintain normal vascular tone. When norepinephrine is depleted, such normally high vascular resistance areas as skin, muscle, and the splanchnic bed vasodilate, leading to uneconomical shunting of blood through these areas. "High-preference areas" such as the brain, heart, and kidney normally have a relatively low resting peripheral resistance and cannot markedly vasodilate; their metabolic requirements must be satisfied by an increase in cardiac output. Shunting of blood away from the kidney can then cause internal reflex changes, which are associated with the hepatorenal syndrome. The finding of an accumulation of octopamine, a well known FNT, in the brain and blood of experimental animals and in the blood and urine of patients with hepatic encephalopathy has been confirmed with an excellent correlation between octopamine and the grade of encephalopathy (66, 70, 121, 129, 148, 184, 187). Phenylethanolamine, another amine capable of acting as a false neurochemical transmitter, increases as well (187). Similar results have been seen with tyramine, an octopamine precursor, (53, 54, 55). In a recent experiment in which CSF has been measured simultaneously with blood, CSF levels of these inactive or "false" neurochemical transmitters increase even before the elevation of blood octopamine and phenylethanolamine, reaching maximal levels with grade 3–4 coma and decreasing rapidly when appropriate therapy is undertaken. (199).

D. Other Neurotransmitters

The many candidates for neurotransmitter function in the central nervous system include amines such as acetylcholine, norepinephrine, dopamine, serotonin, and histamine. Many other synaptic transmitters are present in the brain and serve various functions, some stimulatory, some inhibitory. GABA, an inhibitory neurotransmitter, is normal in the brains of rats with liver disease or following ammonia administration (14, 172), but more recent work has suggested elevations in plasma GABA levels in experimental animals and man in hepatic coma (59, 190). Brain levels have thus far not been studied. The excitatory neurotransmitters glutamate and aspartate are significantly decreased in the supratentorial part of the brain obtained from rats in acute hepatic coma (94); other inhibitory amino acid neurotransmitter candidates include taurine, serine, and glycine.

Thus a final pathophysiological mechanism would explain (a) the alterations in plasma and brain aromatic amino acids; (b) the depletion of dopamine and norepinephrine, and increased serotonin and β-hydroxyphenolethanolamines; (c) a widespread derangement in neurotransmission; and (d) the relationship between a, b, and c.

V. FACTORS PRECIPITATING HEPATIC COMA

A. Introduction

Many factors may cause encephalopathy and coma in patients with preexisting liver disease, including infection, over-diuresis, gastrointestinal hemorrhage, sedatives, tranquilizers, electrolyte imbalance, surgical procedures, acute alcoholism, abdominal paracentesis, and also occasionally a large protein meal or severe constipation. The most frequent factors in 100 episodes of hepatic coma were, in order of occurrence: azotemia, either spontaneous or diuretic induced; the use of sedatives, tranquilizers, or analgesics; gastrointestinal hemorrhage; hypokalemia; alkalosis; and protein intoxication (62). The syndrome may appear spontaneously, without a precipitating factor, usually in a deeply jaundiced patient with ascites and in the terminal states.

1. DIURETIC THERAPY   The commonest precipitating factor of coma is a brisk response to a potent diuretic that causes hypokalemia and alkalosis. The kidney is an important source of ammonia, and hypokalemia increases ammonia production in the renal vein (5, 81), although whether this increased output represents increased production or a pH-dependent diversion of ammonia from the urine into the circulation is uncertain (164). With the development of metabolic alkalosis, freely diffusible ammonia rises rapidly, favoring the diffusion of ammonia into the brain, whereas a lower pH will convert it to the NH_4^+ form (25). The same may be true for amines. The passage of amines through the blood-brain barrier if it occurs at all (it does occur, for example, with phenylethylamine) should also be facilitated by alkalosis, since they are also weak bases. The mechanism by which diuretics may cause coma need not depend on the toxicity of ammonia. Apart from the liver, the kidney is the only organ capable of manufacturing glucose from amino acids. With a failing liver, the kidney may augment

production in an attempt to maintain peripheral energy supply, thus resulting in decreased BCAA facilitating the entry of the toxic aromatic amino
acids into the brain (72, 107). In addition, one major source of renal venous
ammonia may be the deamination of branched-chain and other amino acids,
which may increase with hypokalemia and alkalosis (164).

Over-diuresis may also decrease intravascular volume, decreasing hepatic
perfusion, and thus further compromise hepatic function.

2. OVERDOSE OF SEDATIVES   The second most common precipitant is
sedative overdose, and half of the episodes of coma are attributed to the use
of chlordiazepoxide, a sedative-tranquilizer often prescribed for alcoholic
patients, who frequently have liver disease. Clearance of chlordiazepoxide
and diazepam, also frequently used in sedating alcholics, is reduced in
advanced liver disease (143). Chlorpromazine resulted in EEG changes
typical of portal systemic encephalopathy in cirrhotic patients (191). Morphine and other opiate derivatives such as methadone, meperidine, and
codeine are metabolized in part by the liver (18, 103, 119), and the excretion
of some barbiturates, especially the short-acting, is dependent on the liver
(23). Factors besides clearance by the liver contribute to clearance of barbiturates, including protein binding and transport by serum albumin, which
is decreased in most patients with liver disease. If the patient is uncontrollable and some sedation is necessary, half the usual dose of barbitone or
oxazepan is given. An antihistaminic such as phenergan may be useful. It
is not clear whether the coma produced by oversedation is similar to spontaneous coma or merely represents oversedation.

3. GASTROINTESTINAL HEMORRHAGE   Gastrointestinal hemorrhage,
usually from esophageal varices, is another common precipitant, and rapid
detection is essential in the treatment of hepatic encephalopathy. Gastrointestinal bleeding increases the protein load of the gut. Blood is particularly
poorly tolerated because it contains large amounts of aromatic amino acids.
In addition, the hypotension associated with gastrointestinal hemorrhage
decreases perfusion of the already compromised liver.

Peripheral intravenous Pitressin (antidiuretic hormone) infusion appears
to be the preferred treatment as few advantages have been demonstrated
with Pitressin infused into the superior mesenteric artery. The Sengstaken-
Blakemore tube may be used as a temporary measure and only postpones
the decision definitely to arrest a variceal bleeding. Other temporary measures include the embolization of either endogenous clot or gelfoam into
varices. Sclerotherapy, recently gaining popularity (188, 210), may serve
until the patient can tolerate a definitive portal hypertension-relieving procedure. Surgery, poorly tolerated in such patients, may be necessary. Emer-

gency shunts tend to have a high mortality, and trials of end-to-side portacaval shunts have revealed only equivocal evidence of life extension, although the mode of death is altered from gastrointestinal bleeding to hepatic failure (102, 157, 175), perhaps secondary to further impairment of hepatic function due to deprivation of the liver of substrate-rich portal blood (7, 16).

4. INFECTION   Especially with bacteremia and including spontaneous bacterial peritonitis in patients with ascites, infection may be the precipitating factor (38). Presumably patients with severe liver disease are less resistant to infection than normal patients. In addition, alcohol has an adverse affect on leukocyte migration (22) and serum bacteriocidal activity (12), depresses white cell mobilization, and impairs phagocytosis (in mice) (124). An active serum inhibitor has recently been invoked (48, 112). Infection and fever increase metabolic demands, resulting in increased lysis of lean body mass to utilize the BCAA, which decrease even further with infection (75, 221). This protein breakdown in turn results in excessive plasma concentration of aromatic amino acids and toxic metabolites. Thus therapy of infection in patients with hepatic decompensation should include proper nutritional support.

IV. THERAPY OF HEPATIC COMA

A. Effects of Established Treatment In Chronic Liver Disease

1. GENERAL SUPPORT
    a. Identify and treat the precipitating factor—e.g. hemorrhage, infection, alcoholism, electrolyte imbalance, sedation, large protein meal.
    b. Carefully adjust fluid and electrolyte balance, particularly avoiding overhydration and hyponatremia. The administration of "salt-poor" 25% albumin to patients with low concentration of serum albumin maintains intravascular volume and urinary output. The measurement of urinary sodium in these patients gives an excellent guide to the requirement for administered sodium.
    c. Adequate oxygenation may be measured by arterial blood gases.
    d. Vitamins, especially of the B group, and calories are essential. Parenteral nutrition may be necessary in patients whose oral intake is interrupted for more than a day or two. These patients have notoriously poor oral intake, and even during unrestricted oral intake many patients with alcholic liver disease are so anorectic that they eat only a thousand calories daily only with difficulty.

e. Finally, other causes of coma may exist in hepatic failure, particularly since trivial trauma may give rise to subdural hematomas or intracranial hemorrage in patients with deficient clotting mechanisms. Meningitis should be ruled out by lumbar puncture.

2. DIET   Protein restriction in patients capable of oral intake is a cornerstone of therapy and usually includes restriction to 40 g protein/24 hr. Oral intake of fewer than 20 g protein/24 hr is not compatible with prolonged survival. Following portacaval shunt, survival in experimental animals has been related to various diets. Those resulting in the shortest survival were rich in the aromatic amino acids, phenylalanine, tyrosine, and tryptophan (33). Milk and cheese are apparently better tolerated than diets containing equal amounts of protein given as meat (57). Perhaps the reason for this is that casein contains more BCAA and fewer aromatic amino acids than meat. Protein derived from vegetables may be tolerated better than animal protein (87). Vegetable protein is less ammoniagenic and contains smaller amounts of methionine and aromatic amino acids. A defined amino acid diet with these properties for patients with chronic encephalopathy is discussed in the section below on BCAA diet.

3. BOWEL STERILIZATION   Bowel sterilization aims to alter bowel flora by the suppression of urease producing organisms, thereby decreasing the production and absorption of ammonia. This is accomplished by means of socalled nonabsorbable antibiotics, generally aminoglycosides, such as neomycin, kanamycin, or paramomycin. Approximately 1% of oral or rectal neomycin is absorbed, with some risk of chronic nephrotoxic or ototoxic effects (11, 118). In the acute case 6–8 g are given daily in divided doses, an amount subsequently reduced to a maintenance dose of 2–4 g/day. In addition to preventing absorption of ammonia, these antibiotics may also cause selective malabsorption of the aromatic amino acids (52, 71). A similar mechanism has been suggested in germ-free animals treated with oral antibiotics(146).

4. LACTULOSE   Lactulose is a nonabsorbable synthetic disaccharide (β-1, 4-galactoside fructose). When given by mouth the bulk reaches the caecum, where it is hydrolyzed by bacterial action to lactic acid and small amounts of acetic acid, producing acidic diarrhea when amounts of 60–160 g/24 hr are utilized. The mechanism of action of lactulose in hepatic encephalopathy is still uncertain (37). It may be mediated by reduction in colonic pH with resulting decreased ammonia absorption, or it may decrease the absorption of aromatic amino acids, and decrease brain octopamine (80). An alternative explanation is that by decreasing the time in which a stool is in

contact with bacteria lactulose decreases ammonia production (3). Since the original observation (15), lactulose has been shown to be effective in three controlled studies (39, 51, 198). An additional study has demonstrated that it may be as effective as neomycin and that the additive effects of lactulose and neomycin may be superior to those of neomycin or lactulose alone (39). Although lactulose is more expensive than neomycin, it is of potential benefit in patients with renal impairment in whom neomycin may be toxic, or in those who fail to respond to neomycin. Other studies have suggested that patients treated with lactulose, despite no changes in plasma amino acid pattern, resulted in decreases in CSF aromatic amino acids, presumably by decreasing exchange for glutamine (L. Capoccia, personal communication).

5. OTHER FORMS OF THERAPY

Colon bypass   Colon bypass may indeed ameliorate chronic portal systemic encephalopathy (136, 174). The operative morbidity and mortality, however, have made this a rare procedure. Ileostomy appears superior to ileorectal anastomosis as colonization of the small intestine above the ileorectal anastomosis decreases the effectiveness of the procedure with time.

Miscellaneous forms of therapy   Recently, bromocriptine, a specific dopamine receptor agonist, in a dose of up to 15 mg daily, has been shown to be effective in patients with chronic encephalopathy (139). Acetohydroxamic acid has not been totally evaluated. In a few patients it has lowered venous blood ammonia but yielded little clinical improvement (204). Colonic lavage with a double-lumen tube has been utilized (230). It is not clear whether this potentially hazardous technique has anything to offer compared with the usual cleansing enemas, and fluid overload is a hazard. Lactobacillus colonization has not been successful (127). The rationale of feeding pure cultures of non-urease-producing lactobacilli is to alter the bowel flora so as to decrease production of ammonia.

B. Effects of Established Treatments In Acute Liver Disease

The management of encephalopathy due to acute hepatic failure is less well understood and much less rewarding than that for portal-systemic encephalopathy. To survive, the patient needs aggressive therapy, which is best administered in an intensive care unit.

The most frequent cause of this condition is acute virus hepatitis of both A and B types (167), although non-A, non-B can also become fulminant (233). Other causes include sensitivity reactions to halothane, to isoniazid, and to monoamine oxidase inhibitors such as iproniazid. Acetaminophen (paracetamol) has a high mortality from acute hepatic necrosis (30). Mushroom poisoning is commonly associated with acute liver disease in France (9).

Therapy in acute hepatic failure is a holding action, an attempt to support the patient until hepatic recovery and regeneration can take place. Numerous heroic measures have been devised to provide temporary biological support. These include exchange transfusion, plasmapheresis, crosscirculation, and perfusion with isolated porcine, bovine, or baboon livers (1, 19, 34, 122, 157, 169, 176, 180, 212). Perfusion using healthy livers has a theoretical advantage if the liver secretes a substance necessary for brain metabolism. Dramatic awakening from hepatic coma has been reported by several investigators, but increased survival has not resulted. In a recent prospective controlled trial, exchange transfusion did not provide any benefit (172). Two uncontrolled studies have recently reported the use of poly-acrylonitrile-membrane hemodialysis (to remove middle molecules) and have reached opposite conclusions. Nusinovici et al (150) concluded that this procedure transiently improved consciousness but did not alter survival; Silk et al (196) reported that survival was improved.

Although corticosteroids are apparently valuable in the treatment of chronic active hepatitis (203), their benefits in fulminant hepatitis have never been adequately documented. The initial report (113) has never been confirmed either in uncontrolled studies (40, 179) or in controlled trials (191). Thus, because of the questionable benefit and the possibility of serious complications, steroid therapy is no longer advocated in the treatment of hepatic encephalopathy.

Hyperbaric oxygenation has also been employed without convincing effect (82).

Conservative but intensive care remains the most reasonable course of action. It includes the furnishing of clotting factors when necessary and at least some minimal means of nutritional support, such as hypertonic dextrose, because patients with fulminant hepatic failure often have impaired hepatic mobilization of glucose, and prolonged hypoglycemia may lead to irreversible deterioration of cerebral function. The provision of nutrition in the form of amino acids and/or protein to patients with hepatitis should theoretically foster hepatic recovery and enable regeneration and more rapid recovery to take place. In a recent study, patients with alcoholic hepatitis who were supplemented with a commercially available amino acid diet had increased survival as compared with patients treated in standard fashion, without emphasis on nutritional support (147). These patients were only moderately ill and hepatic encephalopathy was not a major problem. In sicker patients, where encephalopathy limits oral protein intake, a branched chain enriched amino acid mixture is better tolerated (97). It is tempting to extend these conclusions to sicker patients, but one must do so with caution, as the liver that is destroyed by fulminant hepatitis may be unable to respond with improved regeneration. Thus it is imperative to measure serum glucose frequently and to treat hypoglycemia promptly and aggressively with intravenous dextrose solutions. Also necessary are meticulous attention to fluid and electrolyte balance, prevention and treatment of infection, and the prevention of further gastrointestinal bleeding. Decreasing intestinal flora by administering neomycin or acidifying the stool by lactulose, which may be given orally or by enema, ameliorate the symptomatology of hepatic coma. This may be secondary to decreased production or absorption of ammonia. It has been previously noted that intestinal sterilization in animals with chronic end-to-side portacaval shunts decreases brain FNT amines to almost normal levels (71). Because most FNT amines are similar to ammonia in their pH dependency of absorption, rendering the bowel lumen more acidic certainly decreases the absorption of tyramine, octopamine, and similar substances.

C. Experimental Treatments

1. L-DOPA IN HEPATIC COMA   L-dopa is the precursor of dopamine and norepinephrine in the normal metabolic synthesis of the catecholamines. Since the first report by Parkes et al (160) on the use of L-dopa in hepatic coma, numerous investigators have confirmed the apparent awakening of patients with acute or chronic hepatic encephalopathy with L-dopa therapy (68, 70, 126, 166, 189). The modes of administration have included oral (nasogastric tube), rectal, and intravenous routes. While most studies have been uncontrolled, in crossover studies L-dopa apparently increases cerebral oxygen consumption and decreases response time (126). However, another randomized prospective trial has failed to confirm the efficacy of L-dopa.

Various explanations have been offered for the effect of L–dopa in hepatic encephalopathy. The mode of action may be secondary to a number of mechanisms including replenishment of such normal transmitters as serotonin (149), release of β-hydroxyphenylethanolamines (21, 106), or the absorption of methyl groups, thus preventing the synthesis of potentially toxic methylated amines (232).

Up to 30% of patients may not absorb L-dopa even when antacid is added to aid absorption in the duodenum (181). Recent evidence suggests that coma may pass from a reversible to an irreversible stage; thus if initiated early in the course of hepatic coma, L-dopa therapy may be of some benefit (68). Side effects exist; gastrointestinal tolerance decreases with time, and the incidence of gastritis, nausea, and anorexia increases.

2. AMINO ACID INFUSION   Although most investigators accept the concept that plasma aminograms are variously deranged in patients with chronic liver disease and hepatic encephalopathy, controversy surrounds the interpretation of such data and their relation to the pathogenesis of hepatic encephalopathy.

Part of the problem lies in the nature of our understanding of the blood-brain barrier and its alteration in hepatic encephalopathy (104, 109). Our laboratory had proposed that the ratio (Val + Leu + Ileu)/ (Phe + Tyr) could accurately predict the concentrations of aromatic amino acids in the brain (67, 72). It has long been clear, however, that this is not so (199) and that alterations in the blood-brain barrier (104, 235), particularly via exchange for glutamine (109), may be more important in determining intracerebral neutral amino acid monoamine precursor concentrations. Thus whether this ratio is (148) or is not (140, 226) an accurate prediction of amino acid concentrations within the brain seems unimportant, as it is now known that many other factors influence such concentrations. Furthermore, there may be other differences between medical and surgical patients as well (74). Thus the controversy may be unimportant. Suffice it to say that in most patients, plasma amino acid patterns will show elevated levels of phenylalanine, tyrosine, methionine, free but not necessarily total tryptophan (which may be decreased), and decreased concentrations of the BCAA.

Based in part on these findings that deranged amino acid concentrations are pathogenically related to hepatic coma, corrective amino acid solutions have been proposed (67, 72). The theoretical purpose of this form of therapy is to provide comparatively large amounts of BCAA (a) to decrease muscle catabolism, (b) to decrease the release of aromatic amino acids from muscle and promote their utilization via skeletal muscle and hepatic protein synthesis (76, 77), and (c) to compete with the aromatic amino acids for blood-brain transport at the blood-brain barrier. Infusion of a branched-chain enriched amino acid solutions, will "normalize" the plasma amino acid pattern, increasing BCAA and reducing plasma aromatic amino acids. Following the initial report of improvement in hepatic encephalopathy in patients with chronic liver disease given large amounts of amino acids in the form of special amino acid formulation (F080, a BCAA-enriched solution) (72) many additional studies, including several randomized prospective trials, have been carried out. BCAA enriched mixtures were originally proposed based on abnormal plasma amino acid patterns which were similar in dogs and man (4, 67, 72, 73). In initial animal experiments a randomized trial of a commercially available amino acid mixture vs a branched-chain enriched amino acid mixture demonstrated the superiority of the BCAA-enriched mixture (67). Neurologic normality and prolonged survival were seen when the branched-chain enriched amino acid mixture was given. In contrast, dogs with commercially available amino acid mixtures died regularly in hepatic encephalopathy (67). When animals maintained in neurological normality on prolonged infusions of BCAA were switched to freamine ® they died within 10 days in hepatic coma (67).

Subsequent studies revealed that in patients with hepatic encephalopathy and/or those with impaired hepatic function who did not tolerate commercially available amino acid mixtures, infusion with BCAA enriched mixture resulted in improvement in encephalopathy and nitrogen balance (72). A host of studies from a variety of institutions have subsequently confirmed such efficacy on an anecdotal basis as well as in three randomized prospective multi-centered trials (186).[2]   In five or six other trials in which the randomization is suspect, efficacy has also been claimed (50, 93, 96, 153, 154, 168).

The mechanism is of such an improvement in hepatic encephalopathy is the result of decreased plasma aromatic amino acid concentrations due to increased hepatic and skeletal protein synthesis. Competition of the BCAA at the blood-brain barrier is also important in normalizing brain monamine precursors.

Two studies have appeared in abstract form in which the efficacy of the BCAA in both acute and chronic patients was not demonstrated (165, 216). It should be noted, however, that the principal caloric source in both of these studies was intravenous fat. There is little evidence that fat is utilized in hepatic failure; it may, in fact, be injurious, as nonesterified fatty acids may compete with tryptophan for binding sides on albumin, thereby displacing bound tryptophan, increasing free tryptophan, and increasing central nervous system indoles. In confirmation of the lack of utilization of aromatic amino acids for protein synthesis, the plasma concentrations of aromatic amino acids were unchanged in the study in which acute patients were treated (165). These findings suggest that fat may be an inappropriate caloric source for such infusions and will not be efficacious; glucose in adequate caloric amounts is required.

Further investigations in (a) experimental animals with chronic indwelling cannulas in the lateral ventricles from which CSF may be collected and (b) animals in which brain and sagittal sinus blood amino acids have measured have revealed the following (199): (a) The changes in brain and/or CSF amino acids, amines, and transmitter metabolites precede those of the plasma. (b) In general it is impossible to predict brain and/or CSF concentrations from plasma concentrations of these various substances. (c) Hepatic coma occurs when phenylalanine, tyrosine, tryptophan, and

---

[2]A multi-centered trial in the United States is approaching its conclusion. A multicentered trial in Brazil has also been completed.

their CNS neurotransmitter metabolites, octopamine, phenylethanolamine, and 5-hydroxy indolacetic acid are at their highest levels. (*d*) Improvement and awakening from hepatic encephalopathy appears to occur simultaneously with or immediately following the normalization of these amino acids and neurotransmitter metabolites. With BCAA infusions, CSF and presumably brain concentrations of the aromatic amino acids and their amine derivatives decrease precipitously, as do the sulfur-containing amino acids in both dogs and monkeys (199, 200).

Subsequent studies appear to confirm that exchange for glutamine may be a mechanism for accumulation of CNS amino acids in patients with hepatic encephalopathy. Thus treatment of patients with hepatic encephalopathy with lactulose, which does not change plasma concentrations of amino acids, nonetheless was accompanied by precipitous decreases in aromatic amino acids within the cerebrospinal fluid. CSF ammonia and glutamine decreased as well.

There is a growing trend toward nutritional support and metabolic modification as a major therapeutic approach to encephalopathy. Theoretically, supplying BCAA enriched mixtures with hypertonic dextrose should have the following beneficial effects: (*a*) It should promote muscle protein synthesis, thereby lowering plasma aromatic amino acids. (*b*) In the presence of overall energy deficiency, BCAA may satisfy a greater percentage of peripheral energy requirements than the estimated 5–6% they provide under normal circumstances. (*c*) At the blood-brain barrier, the BCAA compete with the aromatic amino acids for transport by system-L. (*d*) By decreasing catabolism, decrease ammonia production, brain glutamine, and exchange of glutamine for aromatic amino acids across the blood-brain barrier (109). (*e*) BCAA may improve hepatic protein synthesis and regeneration (76, 77).

Up to 120 g protein equivalent in the form of amino acids have been administered to patients with protein intolerance and hepatic encephalopathy with beneficial effects, including the clearing of encephalopathy, positive nitrogen balance (when 80 g protein equivalent and 32–37 kcal/kg/day are administered), and in some cases apparent improvement in hepatic function. Prospective randomized trials have confirmed efficacy.

3. ALPHA-KETO ANALOGS   Another possible approach is the administration of alpha-keto analogs of amino acids, either orally or intravenously. These keto acids are the derivates of the branched chain amino acids. Since abundant nitrogen is available as urea or glutamine, providing the keto-acid carbon-chain skeletons of amino acids facilitates transamination with available nitrogen to convert these keto acids into amino acids, which become available for protein synthesis. In addition, utilization of alpha-keto acids does not depend on the liver (219, 225). In a small series of patients with

chronic hepatic encephalopathy given alpha-keto acids intravenously, improved nutrition and clearing of hepatic encephalopathy were observed in some patients (128). The nitrogen donor in hepatic failure is glutamine, not urea as in renal failure. One beneficial effect of the alpha-keto analogs appears to be decreased muscle catabolism, as decreased plasma levels of tyrosine and glycine were observed in these patients despite the fact that tyrosine and glycine were not given (64, 128). The keto acids become more soluble when made into sodium or calcium salts, but it is questionable whether many patients with chronic hepatic insufficiency could tolerate amounts of calcium or sodium ions that would be contained in useful doses of water-soluble keto-acid formulations. More recent studies suggest that the ornithine salts of the alpha-keto acids are more efficacious than equimolar amounts of the calcium salts or the BCAA themselves (92). Watanabe has utilized a similar approach using ornithine and the BCAA (Hep-OU) (93, 224). Here again the decrease in blood ammonia may be more efficacious, since less glutamine is synthesized and less is available for exchange across the blood-brain barrier. In addition, glutamine itself appears to be the nitrogen donor.

4. BRANCHED-CHAIN AMINO ACID ENRICHED DIET   Until recently there had been few attempts to explore diet therapy (other than protein restriction) of patients with liver disease. Protein restricted diet may increase catabolism and result in deterioration of liver function and mental state. Patients with hepatic encephalopathy are frequently treated with a 40 g protein diet for prolonged periods of time. This may result in negative nitrogen balance since earlier studies indicated that cirrhotics require a minimum of 35–50 g protein/day (153, 207), and negative nitrogen balance cannot be sustained indefinitely. The parenteral approach appears to be useful in an acute or an in-hospital setting where patients cannot take nourishment orally. A much larger problem exists in patients who, either following portacaval shunt or spontaneously, demonstrate severe protein intolerance and hepatic encephalopathy accompanied by incapability of accepting minimal intakes of protein, even when given nonabsorbable antibiotics and lactulose. Recent studies suggest that a nonprotein diet in a patient with hepatic impairment releases large amounts of aromatic amino acids, resulting in greater plasma amino acid imbalances. Many patients with hepatic impairment can tolerate 50–60 g of protein orally. For those who can not, we have proposed a branched-chain enriched amino acid diet: 35% BCAA (Hepatic Aid) with a composition similar to F080. This amino acid-glucose formulation consists of L-amino acids in similar proportion to the intravenous formulation F080 (67, 72). BCAA make up 35% of the amino acids and aromatic amino acids are decreased as compared with normal commercially available diets. The results, especially in patients with

portacaval shunt, have been interesting (58, 65, 79, 97) and include improvement in encephalopathy as well as liver function. A recent prospective randomized study appears to demonstrate the efficacy of such a BCAA diet as compared with conventional protein (97). Some problems remain, especially because the commercially available diets are wedded to high-dose glucose. In patients who are usually diabetic and hyperglucagonemic, such diets make difficult the control of blood glucose. Under these circumstances, we have used up to 30 g of BCAA alone on a daily basis, in divided doses.

Literature Cited

1. Abouna, G. M. 1972. Improved technique of exchange transfusion for hepatic coma. *Surg. Gynecol. Obstet.* 134:658–62
2. Agihara, K., Mozai, T., Hirai, S. 1966. Tryptophan as a cause of hepatic coma. *N. Engl. J. Med.* 275:1255–56
3. Agostini, L., Down, P. F., Murison, J., Wrong, O. M. 1972. Faecal ammonia with pH during lactulose administration in man: a comparison with other cathartics. *Gut* 13:829–66
4. Aguirre, A., Yoshimura, N., Westman, T., Fischer, J. E. 1974. Plasma amino acids in dogs with two experimental forms of liver damage. *J. Surg. Res.* 16:339–45
5. Baertl, J. M., Sancetta, S. M., Gabuzda, G. J. 1963. Relation of acute potassium depletion to renal ammonium metabolism in patient with cirrhosis. *J. Clin. Invest.* 42:696–707
6. Baldessarini, R. J., Fischer, J. E. 1967. S-adenosylmethionine following portacaval anastomosis. *Surgery* 62:311–18
7. Baldessarini, R. J., Fischer, J. E. 1973. Serotonin metabolism in rat brain after surgical diversion of the portal venous circulation. *Nature New Biol.* 254: 272–75
8. Baldessarini, R. J., Karobath, M. 1973. Biochemical physiology of central synapses. *Ann. Rev. Physiol.* 35:273–304
9. Benhamou, J. P., Rueff, B., Sicot, C. 1972. Severe hepatic failure; a critical study of current therapy. In *Liver and Drugs,* ed. F. Orlandi, A. M. Jezequel, p. 213. NY: Academic
10. Benjamin, A. M., Quastel, J. H. 1972. Location of amino acids in brain slices from the rat. *Biochem. J.* 128:631–46
11. Berk, D. P., Chalmers, T. 1970. Deafness complicating antibiotic therapy of hepatic encephalopathy. *Ann. Intern. Med.* 73:393–96
12. Berl, S., Takajaki, G., Clarke, D. D., Waelsch, H. 1962. Metabolic compartments in vivo: ammonia and glutamine

acid metabolism in brain and liver. *J. Biol. Chem.* 237:2562–69
13. Bessman, S. P., Bessman, A. W. 1955. The cerebral and peripheral uptake of ammonia in liver disease with a hypothesis for the mechanism of hepatic coma. *J. Clin. Invest.* 34:622–28
14. Biebuyck, J., Funovics, J., Dedrick, D. F., Scherer, Y. D., Fischer, J. E. 1975. Neurochemistry of hepatic coma. Alterations in putative neurotransmitter amino acids. In *Artificial Liver Support,* ed. R. Williams, I. M. Murray-Lyon, pp. 51–60. London: Pitman Medical
15. Bircher, J., Muller, J., Guggenheim, P. 1966. Treatment of chronic portal-systemic encephalopathy with lactulose. *Lancet* i:890–92
16. Bollman, J. R., Flock, E. V., Grindlay, J. H., Bickford, R. G., Lichtenheld, F. R. 1957. Coma with increased amino acids of brain in dogs with Eck's fistula. *Arch. Surg.* 75:405–11
17. Bollman, J. L., Mann, F. C., Magath, T. B. 1924. Studies on the physiology of the liver. VIII. Effect of total removal of the liver on the formation of urea. *Am. J. Physiol.* 69:371–92
18. Bonnycastel, D. D., Delia, C. W. 1950. Effect of hepatectomy upon the analgesic action of L-methadone. *Proc. Soc. Exp. Biol. Med.* 74:589–91
19. Bosman, S. C. W., Terblanche, J., Saunders, S. J., Harrison, G. G., Barnard, C. N. 1968. Cross-circulation between man and baboon. *Lancet* ii:583–85
20. Bouletreau, P., Delafosse, B., Auboyer, C., Motin, J., Cotte, J., Creyssel, R. 1980. Role of branched-chain amino acids in the encephalopathy of the patients with cirrhosis of the liver. In *Le Foie En Anesthesie et en Reanimation,* ed. Conseiller et al. Jounees, d'enseignement post-Universitaire d'anesthesie et de reamination, Paris, pp. 239–54
21. Brandau, K., Axelrod, J. 1972. The biosynthesis of octopamine. *Naunyn Schmiedebergs Arch. Pharmacol.* 273: 123–33

22. Brayton, R. G., Stokes, P. E., Schwartz, M. S., Louria, D. B. 1970. Effect of alcohol and various diseases on leukocyte mobilization, phagocytosis and intracellular bacterial killing. *N. Engl. J. Med.* 282:123–28

23. Breen, K. J., Shaw, J., Alvin, J., Henderson, G. I., Hoyumpa, A. M., Schenker, S. 1973. The effect of experimental hepatic injury on the clearance of phenobarbital and paraldehyde. *Gastroenterology* 64:992–1004

24. Cangiano, C., Cardelli-Cangiano, P., James, J., Fischer, J. E. 1980. Ammonia stimulates amino acid uptake by isolated bovine brain microvessels. *Gastroenterology* 78:1302 (Abstr.)

25. Carter, C. C., Lifton, J. F., Welch, M. J. 1973. Organ uptake and blood pH and concentration effects of ammonia in dogs determined with ammonia labelled with 10 minutes half-lived nitrogen 13. *Neurology* 23:204–13

26. Cascino, A, Cangiano, C., Calcaterra, V., Rossi-Fanelli, F., Capocaccia, L. 1978. Plasma amino acids imbalance in patients with liver disease. *Am. J. Dig. Dis.* 23:591–98

27. Challenger, F., Walshe, J. M. 1955. Feator hepaticus. *Lancet i*:1239–41

28. Chance, W. T., Herlin, P. M., Bernardini, A. P., James, J. H., Fischer, J. E. 1981. Behavioral and biochemical changes in rats following portacaval anastomosis: effects of parachloroamphetamine. *Surg. Forum* 32:188–91

29. Chen, S., Mahadevan, V., Zieve, L. 1970. Volatile fatty acids in the breath of patients with cirrhosis of the liver. *J. Lab. Clin. Med.* 75:622–27

30. Clark, R., Borirakchanyavat, V., Davidson, A. R., Thompson, R. P. H., Widdop, B., Goulding, R., Williams, R. 1973. Hepatic damage and death from overdose of paracetamol. *Lancet* i:66–70

31. Cohen, R. A., Kopin, I. J., Creveling, C. R., Musacchio, J. M., Fischer, J. E., Crout, J. R., Gill, J. R. Jr. 1966. Clinical conference: False neurochemical transmitters. *Ann. Intern. Med.* 65:347–62

32. Collins, J. R., Crofford, O. B. 1969. Glucose intolerance and insulin resistance in patients with liver disease. *Arch. Intern. Med.* 124:142–48

33. Condon, R. E. 1971. Effect on dietary protein on symptoms and survival in dogs with an Eck fistula. *Am. J. Surg.* 121:107–14

34. Condon, R. E., Bombeck, D. T., Steigmann, P. 1970. Heterologous bovine liver perfusion therapy of acute hepatic failure. *Am. J. Surg.* 119:147–54

35. Conn, H. O. 1960. Asterixis in nonhepatic disorders. *Am. J. Med.* 29: 647–61

36. Conn, H. O. 1973. Current diagnosis and treatment of hepatic coma. *Hosp. Pract.* 8:65–72

37. Conn, H. O. 1978. Lactulose: a drug in search of a modus operandi. *Gastroenterology* 74:624–30

38. Conn, H. O., Fessel, J. M. 1971. Spontaneous bacterial peritonitis in cirrhosis: variation on a theme. *Medicine* 50:161–97

39. Conn, H. O., Leevy, C. M., Maddrey, W. C., Rodgers, J. B., Seeff, L., Vlahcevic, Z. R. 1974. Lactulose in the treatment of chronic portal systemic encephalopathy. A prospective double-blind cooperative comparison of lactulose with neomycin. *Gastroenterology* 67:784 (Abstr.)

40. Cook, G. C., Sherlock, S. 1965. Jaundice and its relation to therapeutic agent. *Lancet i*:175–79

41. Cooper, J. R., Bloom, F. E., Roth, R. H., eds. 1978. The catecholamines I: General Aspects. In *Biochemical Basis of Neuropharmacology.* NY: Oxford Univ. Press. pp. 102–60. 3rd ed.

42. Crout, J. F., Alpers, H. S., Tatum, E. L., Shore, P. A. 1964. Release of metaraminol (Aramine) from the heart by sympathetic nerve stimulation. *Science* 145:828–29

43. Cummings, M. G., James, J. H., Soeters, P. B., Keane, J. M., Foster, J., Fischer, J. E. 1976. Regional brain study of indoleamine metabolism in the rat in acute hepatic failure. *J. Neurochem.* 27:741–46

44. Cummings, M. G., Soeters, P. B., James, J. H., Keane, J. M., Fischer, J. E. 1976. Regional brain indoleamine metabolism following chronic portacaval anastomosis in the rat. *J. Neurochem.* 27:501–9

45. Curzon, G., Kantamaneni, B. D., Winch, J., Rojas-Bueno, A., Murray Lyon, I. M., Williams, R. J. 1973. Plasma and brain tryptophan changes in experimental acute hepatic failure. *J. Neurochem.* 21:137–45

46. Curzon, G., Knott, P. J., Murray-Lyon, I. M., Record, C. O., Williams, R. 1975. Disturbed brain tryptophan metabolism in hepatic coma. *Lancet* i:1092–93

47. Dawson, A. M., Sherlock, S. 1957. Effect of amine oxidase inhibitor on arterial ammonium levels in liver disease. *Lancet* i:1332–33

48. DeMeo, A. N., Andersen, B. R. 1972. Defective chemotaxis associated with a serum inhibitor in cirrhotic patients. *N. Engl. J. Med.* 286:735–40

49. Dodsworth, J. M., James, J. H., Cummings, M. G., Fischer, J. E. 1974. Depletion of brain norepinephrine in acute hepatic coma. *Surgery* 75:811–20

50. Egberts, E. H., Hamster, W., Jurgens, P., Schumaker, H., Fondalinski, G., Reinhard, V., Schomerus, H. 1981. Effect of branched-chain amino acids on latent portal-systemic encephalopathy. In *Metabolism and Clinical Implications of Branched-Chain Amino and Ketoacids*, ed. M. Walser, R. Williamson, pp. 453–463. NY: Elsevier North Holland

51. Elkington, S. G., Floch, M. H., Conn, H. O. 1969. Lactulose in the treatment of chronic portal-systemic encephalopathy. A double-blind clinical trial. *N. Engl. J. Med.* 281:408–13

52. Faloon, W. W., Pase, I., Woodfolk, C., Nankin, H., Wallace, K., Haro, E. N. 1965. Effect of neomycin and kanamycin upon intestinal absorption. *Ann. N.Y. Acad. Sci.* 132:879–87

53. Faraj, B. A., Camp, V. M., Ansley, J. D., Scott, J., Ali, F. M., Malveaux, E. J. 1981. Evidence of central hypertyraminemia in hepatic encephalopathy. *J. Clin. Invest.* 67:395–402

54. Faraj, B. A., Bowen, P. A., Isaacs, J. W., Rudman, D. 1976. Hypertyraminemia in cirrhotic patients. *N. Engl. J. Med.* 294:1360–64

55. Faraj, B. A., Fulenwider, J. T., Rypins, E. B., Nordlinger, B., Ivey, G. L., Jansen, R. D., Ali, F. M., Camp, V. M., Kutner, M., Schmidt, F., Rudman, D. 1979. Tyramine kinetics and metabolism in cirrhosis. *J. Clin. Invest.* 64:413–20

56. Felig, P., Brown, W. V., Levine, R. A., Klatskin, G. 1970. Glucose homeostasis in viral hepatitis. *N. Engl. J. Med.* 283:1436–40

57. Fenton, J. C. B., Knight, E. J., Humpherson, P. L. 1966. Milk and cheese diet in portal-systemic encephalopathy. *Lancet* i:164–65

58. Ferenci, P., Dragosics, B., Wewazka, F. 1981. Oral administration of branched-chain amino acids (BCAA) and keto acids (BCKA) in patients with liver cirrhosis (LC). See Ref. 50, pp. 507–512

59. Ferenci, P., Schafer, D. F., Shrager, R., Jones, E. A. 1981. Metabolism of the inhibitory neurotransmitter γ-amino butyric acid in the rabbit model of acute

hepatic failure. *Hepatology* 1:509 (Abstr.)

60. Fernstrom, J. D., Wurtman, R. J. 1971. Brain serotonin content: physiological dependence on plasma tryptophan levels. *Science* 173:149–51

61. Fernstrom, J. D., Wurtman, R. J. 1972. Brain serotonin content: Physiological regulation by plasma neutral amino acids. *Science* 178:414–16

62. Fessel, J. M., Conn, H. O. 1972. An analysis of the causes and prevention of hepatic coma. *Gastroenterology* 62:191 (Abstr.)

63. Fischer, J. E. 1974. False neurotransmitter and hepatic coma. *Res. Publ. Assoc. Res. Nerv. Ment. Dis.* 53:53–73

64. Fischer, J. E. 1976. Editorial: Non-amino acids: non-toxic or antitoxic. *Gastroenterology* 71:329

65. Fischer, J. E. 1981. Nutritional intervention in hepatic encephalopathy by the use of branched-chain enriched amino acid mixture. See Ref. 50, pp. 441–46

66. Fischer, J. E., Baldessarini, R. J. 1971. False neurotransmitters and hepatic failure. *Lancet* ii:75–79

67. Fischer, J. E., Funovics, J. M., Aguirre, A., James, J. H., Keane, J. M., Wesdorp, R. I. C., Yoshimura, N., Westman, T. 1975. The role of plasma amino acids in hepatic encephalopathy. *Surgery* 78:276–90

68. Fischer, J. E., Funovics, J. M., Falcao, H. A. 1976. L-dopa in hepatic coma. *Ann. Surg.* 183:386–91

69. Fischer, J. E., Horst, W. D., Kopin, I. J. 1965. β-hydroxylated sympathomimetic amines as false neurotransmitters. *Br. J. Pharmacol.* 24:477–84

70. Fischer, J. E., James, J. H. 1972. Treatment of hepatic coma and hepatorenal syndrome: mechanisms of action of L-Dopa in hepatic coma. *Am. J. Surg.* 133:222–30

71. Fischer, J. E., James, J. H., Keane, J. M., Shuman, L., Dodsworth, J., Funovics, J. M. 1974. An alternative mechanism for beneficial effects of intestinal sterilization in hepatic encephalopathy. *Surg. Forum* 25:369–72

72. Fischer, J. E., Rosen, H. M., Ebeid, A. M., James, J. H., Keane, J. M., Soeters, P. B. 1976. The effect of normalization of plasma amino acids on hepatic encephalopathy in man. *Surgery* 80:77–91

73. Fischer, J. E., Yoshimura, N., James, J. H., Cummings, M. G., Abel, R. M., Deindoerfer, F. 1974. Plasma amino acids in patients with hepatic enceph-

alopathy: effects of amino acid infusions. *Am. J. Surg.* 127:40–47

74. Fischer, J. E. 1982. Amino acids and hepatic encephalopathy. *Dig. Dis. Sci.* In press

75. Freund, H., Ryan, J. A., Fischer, J. E. 1979. Amino acid derangements in patients with overwhelming sepsis: treatment with branched-chain amino acid rich infusion. *Ann. Surg.* 188:423–30

76. Freund, H. R., Hoover, H. C. Jr., Atamian, S., Fischer, J. E. 1979. Infusion of the branched-chain amino acids in postoperative patients. Anti-catabolic properties. *Ann. Surg.* 190:18–23

77. Freund, H. R., James, H. J., Fischer, J. E. 1981. Nitrogen sparing mechanisms of singly administered branched-chain amino acids in the injured rat. *Surgery* 90/2:237

78. Freund, H. R., Krause, R., Rossi-Fanelli, F., Smith, A. R., Fischer, J. E. 1978. Amino acid induced coma in normal animals; prevention by branched-chain amino acids. *Gastroenterology* 74:1167 (Abstr.)

79. Freund, H., Yoshimura, N., Fischer, J. E. 1979. Chronic hepatic encephalopathy. Long-term therapy with a branched-chain-amino-acid-enriched elemental diet. *J. Am. Med. Assoc.* 242:347–49

80. Funovics, J. M., Soeters, P. B. 1976. Unpublished observations.

81. Gabuzda, G. J., Hall, P. W. 1966. Relation of potassium depletion to renal ammonium metabolism and hepatic coma. *Medicine* 45:481–91

82. Gaulon, M., Rapin, M., Barois, A., Got, C., Grobuis, S., Gajdos, P., Azizi, P. P. 1971. Essai de traitement des hepatites virales graves par l'oxygen-hyperbare. *Ann. De Med. Interne* 122:93–98

83. Gilon, E., Szeinberg, A., Tauman, G., Bodonyi, E. 1959. Glutamine estimation in cerebrospinal fluid in cases of liver cirrhosis and hepatic coma. *J. Lab. Clin. Med.* 53:714–19

84. Gimmon, Z., James, J. H., Von Meyenfeldt, M., Fischer, J. E. 1981. Opposing effect of prolonged ammonia and branched-chain amino acid infusion on the accumulation of aromatic amino acids by brain. See Ref. 50, pp. 487–92

85. Goodman, H. M., Frier, G. P. 1981. Metabolism of branched-chain amino acids in adipose tissue. See Ref. 50, pp. 167–80

86. Goetchus, J. S., Webster, L. T. 1965. γ-Aminobutyrate and hepatic coma. *J. Lab. Clin. Med.* 65:257–67

87. Greenberger, N. J., Carley, J., Schenker, S. 1977. Effect of vegetables and animal protein diets in chronic hepatic encephalopathy. *Am. J. Dig. Dis.* 22:845–50

88. Hardwick, D. F., Applegarth, D. A., Cockcroft, D. M., Ross, P. M., Calder, R. J. 1970. Pathogenesis of methionine induced toxicity. *Metabolism* 19:381–91

89. Hartmann, E. 1977. L-tryptophan: a rational hypnotic with clinical potential. *Am. J. Psychiatry* 134:366–70

90. Hawkins, J., Miller, A. L., Nielsen, R. C., Veech, R. L. 1973. The acute action of ammonia on rat brain metabolism in vivo. *Biochem. J.* 134:1001–8

91. Hawkins, R. A., Mans, A. M., Biebuyck, J. E. 1981. Regional blood brain permeability in hepatic encephalopathy. *J. Cerebr. Blood Flow Metab.* 1: (Suppl.) 385–86

91a. Herlin, P., James, H., Nauchbauer, C., Fischer, J. E. 1981. The blood-brain barrier is intact eighteen hours after total hepatectomy. *Hepatology* 5:516

92. Herlong, H. F., Maddrey, W. C., Walser, M. 1980. Ornithine salts of branched chain keto-acids in portal systemic encephalopathy. *Ann. Int. Med.* 93:545–50

93. Higashi, T., Watanabe, A., Hayashi, S., Obata, T., Tanei, N., Nagashima, H. 1981. Effect of branched chain amino acid infusion on alterations in CSF neutral amino acids and their transport across the blood brain barrier in hepatic encephalopathy. See Ref. 50, pp. 465–70

94. Hindfeldt, B., Plum, F., Duffy, T. E. 1977. Effect of acute ammonia intoxication on cerebral metabolism in rats with portacaval shunts. *J. Clin. Invest.* 59:386–96

95. Holm, E. 1975. *Ammoniak und hepatische Enzephalopathie.* Stuttgart: Gustav Fischer

96. Holm, E., Streibel, J. P., Moller, P., Hartman, M. 1981. Amino acid solutions for parenteral nutrition and for adjuvant treatment of encephalopathy in liver cirrhosis, studies concerning 120 patients. See Ref. 50, pp. 513–18

97. Horst, D., Grace, N., Conn, H. O., Schiff, E., Schenker, S., Viteri, A., Law, D., Atterbury, C. E. 1981. A double-blind randomized comparison of dietary protein and an oral branched chain amino acid (BCAA) supplement in cirrhotic patients with chronic portal-systemic encephalopathy (PSE) (ABS). *Hepatology* 5:518

98. Hourani, B. T., Hamlin, E. M., Reynolds, T. B. 1971. Cerebrospinal fluid glutamine as a measure of hepatic encephalopathy. *Arch. Int. Med.* 127: 1033–36

99. Iber, F. L., Rosen, H., Levenson, S. M., Chalmers, T. C. 1957. The plasma amino acids in patients with liver failure. *J. Lab. Clin. Med.* 50:417–25

100. Iob, V., Coon, W. W., Sloan, M. 1966. Altered clearance of free amino acids from plasma of patients with cirrhosis of the liver. *J. Surg. Res.* 6:233–39

101. Iob, V., Mattson, W. J. Jr., Sloan, M., Coon, W. W., Turcotte, J. G., Child, C. G. III. 1970. Alterations in plasma-free amino acids in dogs with hepatic insufficiency. *Surg. Gynecol. Obstet.* 130:794–801

102. Jackson, F. C., Perrin, E. B., Feux, W. R., Smith, A. G. 1971. A clinical investigation of the portacaval shunt. V. Survival analysis of the therapeutic operation. *Ann. Surg.* 174:672–98

103. Jaffe, J. H. 1970. Narcotic analgesics. In *The Pharmacologic Basis of Therapeutics.* ed. L. S. Goodman, A. Gilman, pp. 237–75. NY: Macmillan

104. James, J. H., Escourrou, J., Fischer, J. E. 1978. Portacaval anastomosis increases the activity of blood brain neutral amino acid transport. *Science* 200:1395–97

105. James, J. H. Unpublished observation

106. James, J. H., Gischer, J. E. 1975. Release of octopamine and alpha methyloctopamine by L-dopa. *Biochem. Pharm.* 24:1099–1101

107. James, J. H., Hodgman, J. M., Funovics, J. M., Yoshimura, N., Fischer, J. E. 1976. Brain tryptophan, plasma free tryptophan and distribution of plasma neutral amino acids. *Metabolism* 25: 471–76

108. James, J. H., Fischer, J. E. 1981. The transport of neutral amino acids at the blood-brain barrier. *Pharmacology* 22: 1–7

109. James, J. H., Ziparo, V., Jeppsson, B., Fischer, J. E. 1979. Hyperammonaemia, plasma amino acid imbalance, and blood-brain amino acid transport: A unified theory of portal systemic encephalopathy. *Lancet* ii:772–75

110. James, J. H. Unpublished observation

111. Jellinger, K., Riederer, P. 1977. Brain monamines in metabolic (endotoxic) coma: a preliminary biochemical study in human postmortem material. *J. Neural Transm.* 41:275–86

112. Johnson, W. D., Stokes, P., Kaye, D. 1969. The effect of intravenous ethanol on the bactericidal activity of human serum. *Yale J. Biol. Med.* 42:171–85

113. Katz, R., Velasco, M., Klinger, J., Alessandri, H. 1962. Corticosteroids in the treatment of acute hepatitis in coma. *Gastroenterology* 42:258–66

114. Klion, F. M., Schaffner, R., Popper, H. 1969. Hepatitis after exposure to halothane. *Ann. Intern. Med.* 71:467–77

115. Knell, A. J., Davidson, A. R., Williams, R., Kantamaneni, B. D., Curzon, G. 1974. Dopamine and serotonin metabolism in hepatic encephalopathy. *Br. Med. J.* ii:549–51

116. Knott, P. J., Curzon, G. 1974. Effect of increased rat brain tryptophan on 5-hydroxytryptamine and 5-hydroxyindolyl acetic acid in the hypothalamus and other brain regions. *J. Neurochem.* 22:1065–71

117. Kopin, I. J. 1968. False adrenergic transmitters. *Ann. Rev. Pharmacol.* 8: 377–94

118. Kunin, C. M., Chalmers, T. C., Leevy, C. M., Sebastyen, S. C., Lieber, C. S., Finland, M. 1960. Absorption of orally-administered neomycyn and kanamycin. *N. Engl. J. Med.* 262:380–85

119. Laidlaw, J., Read, A. E., Sherlock, S. 1961. Morphine tolerance with hepatic cirrhosis. *Gastroenterology* 40:389–97

120. Lal, S., Young, S. N., Sourkes, T. L. 1975. 5-Hydroxytryptamine and hepatic coma. *Lancet* ii:979–80

121. Lam, K. C., Tall, A. R., Goldstein, G. B., Mistillis, S. P. 1973. Role of a false neurotransmitter, octopamine, in the pathogenesis of hepatic and renal encephalopathy. *Scand. J. Gastroenterol.* 8:465–72

122. Lepore, M. J., Martel, A. J. 1970. Plasmapheresis with plasma exchange in hepatic coma. *Ann. Intern. Med.* 72: 165–74

123. Livingstone, A. S., Potvin, M., Goresky, C. A., Finlayson, M. K., Hinchey, E. J. 1977. Changes in the blood-brain barrier in hepatic coma after hepatectomy in the rat. *Gastroenterology* 73:697–704

124. Louria, D. B. 1963. Susceptibility to infection during experimental alcohol intoxication. *Trans. Assoc. Am. Physicians* 76:102–12

125. Lucke, B., Mallory, T. 1946. The fulminant form of epidemic hepatitis. *Am. J. Pathol.* 22:867–945

126. Lunzer, M., James, I. M., Weisman, J., Sherlock, S. 1974. Treatment of chronic hepatic encephalopathy with levodopa. *Gut* 15:555–62

127. MacBeth, W. A. A. G., Kass, E. H., McDermott, W. V. 1965. Treatment of hepatic encephalopathy by alterations of intestinal flora with lactobacillus acidophilus. *Lancet* i:339–403

128. Maddrey, W. 1976. Effects of keto-analogues of essential amino acids in portal systemic encephalopathy. *Gastroenterology* 73:598–604

129. Manghani, K. K., Lunzer, M. R., Billing, B. H., Sherlock, S. 1975. Urinary and serum octopamine in patients with portal systemic encephalopathy. *Lancet* ii:943–46

130. Marchesini, G., Forlani, G., Zoli, M., Angioli, A., Scolari, M. P., Bianchi, F. B., Pisi, E. 1979. Insulin and glucagon levels in liver cirrhosis. Relationship with plasma amino acid imbalance of chronic hepatic encephalopathy. *Dig. Dis. Sci.* 24:594–601

131. Marchesini, G., Zoli, M., Forlani, G., Angiolini, A., Bianchi, F. B., Pisi, E. 1978. Glucagon levels and insulin/glucagon molar ratios in hepatic encephalopathy. *Int. J. Gastroenterol.* 10:193 (Abstr.)

132. Marco, J., Diego, J., Villamuera, M. L., Diaz-Fierros, M., Valverde, I., Segovia, J. 1973. Elevated plasma glucagon levels in cirrhosis of the liver. *N. Engl. J. Med.* 289:1107–11

133. Mashford, M. L., Mahon, W. A., Chalmers, T. C. 1962. Studies of the cardiovascular system in the hypotension of liver failure. *N. Engl. J. Med.* 267:1071–74

134. Mattson, W. J. Jr, Iob, V., Sloan, M., Coon, W. W., Turcotte, J. G., Child, C. G. III. 1970. Alterations of individual free amino acids in brain during acute hepatic coma. *Surg. Gynecol. Obstet.* 130:263–66

134a. McCollough, A. J., Czaja, A. J., Jones, J. D., Go, V. L. W. 1981. The nature and prognostic significance of serial amino acid determinations in severe chronic active liver disease. *Gastroenterology* 81:645–52

135. McDermott, W. V., Adams, R. D. 1954. Episodic stupor associated with Eck fistula in the human with particular reference to the metabolism of ammonia. *J. Clin. Invest.* 33:1–9

136. McDermott, W. V. Jr, Victor, M., Point, W. W. 1962. Exclusion of the colon in the treatment of hepatic encephalopathy. *N. Engl. J. Med.* 267:850–54

137. Merino, G. E., Jetzer, T., Doizaki, W. M. 1975. Methionine-induced hepatic coma in dogs. *Am. J. Surg.* 130:41–46

138. Morgan, M. H., Bolton, C. H., Morris, J. S., Read, E. A. 1974. Medium chain triglycerides and hepatic encephalopathy. *Gut* 15:180–84

139. Morgan, M. Y., Jakobovits, A. M., Lennox, R. 1980. Successful use of bromocriptine in the treatment of chronic hepatic encephalopathy. *Gastroenterology* 78:663

140. Morgan, M., Milsom, J. P., Sherlock, S. 1977. Plasma ratio of valine, leucine, and isoleucine to phenylalanine and tyrosine in liver disease. *Gut* 19:1068–73

141. Mountcastle, V. B., Baldessarini, R. J. 1974. Synaptic transmission (section on neuroglia). In *Medical Physiology,* ed. V. B. Mountcastle, Vol. 1:182–223 St Louis: C. V. Mosby

142. Munro, H. N., Fernstrom, T. D., Wurtman, R. T. 1975. Insulin plasma amino acid imbalance and hepatic coma. *Lancet* i:722–24

143. Murray-Lyon, I. M., Yong, J., Parkes, J. D., Knill-Jones, R. P., Williams, R. 1971. Clinical and electroencephalographic assessment of diazepan in liver disease. *Br. Med. J.* iv:265–66

144. Muscholl, E., Maitre, L. 1963. Release by sympathetic stimulation of γ-methylnoradrenaline stored in the heart after administration of γ-methyldopa. *Experientia* 19:658–70

145. Muto, Y. 1966. Clinical study on the relationship of short-chain fatty acids and hepatic encephalopathy. *Jpn. J. Gastroenterol.* 63:19–32

146. Nance, F. C., Baston, R. C., Kline, D. G. 1971. Ammonia production in germ-free Eck fistula dogs. *Surgery* 70:169–74

147. Nashalla, S. M., Galambos, J. T. 1980. Amino acid therapy in alcoholic hepatitis. *Lancet* i:1276–77

148. Nespoli, A., Bevilcqua, G., Staudacher, G., Rossi, N., Salerno, E., Castelli, M. R. 1981. The role of false neurotransmitters in the pathogenesis of hepatic encephalopathy and hyperdynamic syndrome in cirrhosis. *Arch. Surg.* 116:1129–38

149. Ng, K. Y., Chase, T. N., Colburn, R. W., Kopin, I. J. 1970. L-dopa induced release of cerebral monoamines. *Science* 170:76–78

150. Nusinovici, V., Crubille, C., Opolon, P., Touboul, J. P., Dainis, F., Caroli, J. 1977. Hepatites fulminantes avec coma. Revue de 137 cases. I. Complications. *Gastroenterol. Clin. Biol.* 1:861–73

151. Oldendorf, W. K. 1971. Brain uptake of radiolabelled amino acids, amines and

hexoses after arterial injection. *Am. J. Physiol.* 221:1629–39

152. Oddessey, R., Goldberg, A. L. 1972. Oxidation of leucine by rat skeletal muscle *Am. J. Physiol.* 223:1376–83

153. Okada, A., Kamata, S., Kim, C. W., Kawashima, Y. 1981. Treatment of hepatic encephalopathy with BCAA-rich amino acid mixture. See Ref. 50, pp. 447–52

154. Okada, A., Ikeda, Y. I., Fanura, T. et al. 1978. Treatment of hepatic encephalopathy with a new parenteral amino acid mixture. *J. Parent. Ent. Nutr.* 2:218

155. Ono, J., Hutson, D. G., Dombro, R. S., Levi, J. V., Livingstone, A., Zeppa, R. 1978. Tryptophan and hepatic coma. *Gastroenterology* 74:136–200

156. Ordonez, L. A., Wurtman, R. J. 1973. Enzymes catalysing the de novo synthesis of methyl groups in the brain and other tissues of the rat. *J. Neurochem.* 21:1447–55

157. Parbhoo, S. P., Kennedy, J., James, I. M., Chalstrey, L. J., Aydukiewicz, A., Brock, P. J., Zanalatos, C., Sayer, P., Sherlock, S. 1971. Extracorporeal pig liver perfusion in treatment of hepatic coma due to fulminant hepatitis. *Lancet* i:659–65

158. Pardridge, W. M. 1975. Tryptophan and hepatic encephalopathy. *Lancet* ii:1035

159. Pardridge, W. M., Oldendorf, W. 1975. Kinetics of blood-brain barrier transport of hexoses. *Biochem. Biophys. Acta* 382:377–92

160. Parkes, J. D., Sharpstone, P., Williams, R. 1970. Levodopa in hepatic coma. *Lancet* ii: 1341–43

161. Perez Cruet, J., Chase, T. N., Murphy, D. L. 1973. Dietary regulation of brain tryptophan metabolism by plasma ratio of free tryptophan and neutral amino acids in human. *Nature* 248:693–95

162. Phear, E. A., Ruebner, B., Sherlock, S., Summerskill, W. H. J. 1956. Methionine toxicity in liver disease and its prevention by chlortetracycline. *Clin. Sci.* 15:93–117

163. Phillips, G. B., Schwartz, R., Gabuzda, G. J., Davidson, C. S. 1952. The syndrome of impending hepatic coma in patients with cirrhosis of liver given nitrogenous substances. *N. Engl. J. Med.* 247:239–46

164. Pitts, R. F. 1971. The role of ammonia production and excretion in regulation of acid base balance. *N. Engl. J. Med.* 284:32–41

165. Pomier-Layrangues, G., Duhamel, O., Cuilleret, G., Bovics, P., Bellet-Hermann, H., Michel, H. 1982. Treatment of hepatic encephalopathy by infusions of a modified amino acid solution. Results of a controlled study in 33 cirrhotic patients. Submitted for publication.

166. Posado, J. G., Penicha, J. H., Tirado-Arroyara, S. 1972. Effect of 3,4-dihidroxy-phenylalanine (L-dopa) in hepatic coma. *Arch. Invest. Med.* 3:1–8

167. Rakela, J., Redeker, A. G., Edwards, V. M., Decker, V. M., Overby, R., Mosley, J. W. 1978. Hepatitis A virus infection in fulminant hepatitis and chronic active hepatitis. *Gastroenterology* 74: 879–82

168. Rakette, S., Fischer, M., Reimann, H. J., Sommoggy, S. F. 1981. Effects of special amino solutions in patients with liver cirrhosis and hepatic encephalopathy. See Ref. 50, pp. 419–27

169. Ranek, L., Hansen, R. I., Hilden, M., Ramsoe, K., Schmidt, A., Winkler, D., Tygstrup, N. 1971. Pig liver perfusion in the treatment of acute hepatic failure. *Scand. J. Gastroenterol.* 9:161–69

170. Read, A. E., Sherlock, S., Laidlaw, J., Walker, J. G. 1967. The neuropsychiatric syndromes associated with chronic liver disease and an extensive portalsystemic collateral circulation. *Q. J. Med.* 36:135–50

171. Record, C. O., Buxton, B., Chase, R. A. 1976. Plasma and brain amino acids in fulminant hepatic failure and their relationship to hepatic encephalopathy. *Eur. J. Clin. Invest.* 6:387–94

172. Redeker, A. G., Yamahiro, H. S. 1973. Controlled trial of exchange transfusion therapy in fulminant hepatitis. *Lancet* i:3–6

173. Reitan, R. M. 1958. Validity of the trailmaking test as an indicator for organic brain damage. *Percept. Mot. Skills* 8:271

174. Resnick, R. H., Ishihara, A., Chalmers, T. C. 1968. A controlled trial of colon bypass in chronic hepatic encephalopathy. *Gastroenterology* 54:1057–69

175. Resnick, R. H., Iber, F. L., Ishihara, A. M., Chalmers, T. C., Zimmerman, H., The Boston Inter-Hospital Liver Group. 1974. A controlled study of therapeutic portacaval shunt. *Gastroenterology* 67:843–57

176. Reynolds, T. B. 1969. Exchange transfusion in fulminant hepatic failure. *Gastroenterology* 56:170–72

177. Richmond, J., Girdwood, R. H. 1962.

Observations on amino acid absorption. *Clin. Sci.* 22:301–14

178. Riely, C. A. 1980. Acute hepatic failure at term. Diagnostic problems posed by broad clinical spectrum antibiotics. *Postgrad. Med.* 68(3):118–27

179. Ritt, D. J., Whelan, G., Werner, D. J., Eigenbrodt, E. H., Schenker, S., Combes, B. 1969. Acute hepatic necrosis with stupor or coma. *Medicine* 48:151–72

180. Rivera, R. A., Slaughter, R. L., Boyce, H. W. 1970. Exchange transfusion in the treatment of patients with acute hepatitis in coma. *Am. J. Dig. Dis.* 15:580–602

181. Rivera-Calimlim, L., Dujovne, C. A., Morgan, J. P., Lasagne, L., Bianchine, J. R. 1970. L-dopa treatment failure: explanation and correction. *Br. Med. J.* ii:93–94

182. Rosen, H. M., Yoshimura, N., Hodgman, J. M., Fischer, J. E. 1977. Plasma amino acid patterns in hepatic encephalopathy of differing etiology. *Gastroenterology* 72:483–87

183. Rosen, H. M., Soeters, P. B., James, J. H., Hodgman, J., Fischer, J. E. 1978. Influences of exogenous intake and nitrogen balance on plasma and brain aromatic amino acid concentrations. *Metabolism* 27:393–404

184. Rossi-Fanelli, F., Cangiano, C., Attili, A., Angelico, M., Cascino, A., Capocaccia, L., Strom, R., Crifo, C. 1976. Octopamine plasma levels and hepatic encephalopathy: a reappraisal of the problem. *Clin. Chim. Acta* 67:255–61

185. Rossi-Fanelli, F., Cangiano, C., Attili, A., Capocaccia, L. 1978. Amino acids in hepatic encephalopathy. *Am. J. Dig. Dis.* 23:591–98

186. Rossi-Fanelli, F., Riggio, D., Cangiano, C., Cascino, A., Deoncilliis, D., Merli, M., Giunchi, G. 1982. Branched-chain amino acids vs. lactulose in the treatment of hepatic coma, an controlled study. *Dig. Dis. Sci.* In press

187. Rossi-Fanelli, F., Smith, A. R., Cangiano, C., Bozzi, A., James, J. H., Kay, L. A., Perelle, B. A., Capocaccia, L., Fischer, J. E. 1978. Simultaneous determination of phenylethanolamine and octopamine in plasma and cerebro-spinal fluid. In *Biochemistry of Phenylethylamines,* ed. A. Moosmaim. NY: Raven

188. Sakamoto, A., Moldawer, L. L., Bothe, A., Bistrian, B. R., Blackburn, G. L. 1980. Are the nitrogen sparing mechanisms of branched chain amino acid ad-ministration really unique? *Surg. Forum* 31:99–100

189. Sarrazen, A., Emerit, J., Oliver, L., Rebelo, F., Bousquet, O. 1971. Traitement du coma hepatique par la L-dopa, premiers resultats. *Presse Med.* 79:2226–27

190. Schafer, D. F., Ferenci, P., Kleinberger, G., Hoofnagle, J. H., Jones, E. A. 1981. Elevated serum concentrations of the inhibitory neurotransmitter γ-amino butyric acid in patients with hepatic cellular disease. *Hepatology* 1:53 (Abstr.)

191. Schenker, S., Breen, K. J., Hoyumpa, A. A. Jr. 1974. Hepatic encephalopathy: Current status. *Gastroenterology* 66:121–51

192. Schenker, S., McCandless, D. W., Brophy, E., Lewis, M. S. 1967. Studies on the intracerebral toxicity of ammonia. *J. Clin. Invest.* 46:838–48

194. Sherwin, R., Joshi, P., Hendler, R., Felig, P., Conn, H. O. 1974. Hyperglucagonemia in Laennec's cirrhosis. *N. Engl. J. Med.* 290:239–42

195. Shorey, J., McCandless, D. W., Schenker, S. 1967. Cerebral alphaketogluterate in ammonia intoxication. *Gastroenterology* 53:706–11

196. Silk, D. B. A., Hanid, M. A., Trewby, P. N. 1977. Treatment of fulminant hepatic failure by polyacrylonitrite membrane haemodialysis. *Lancet* ii:1–3

197. Silk, D. B. A., Williams, R. 1978. Experiences in the treatment of fulminant hepatic failure by conservative therapy charcoal hemoperfusion, and polyacrylonitrile hemodialysis. *Int. J. Artif. Organs* 1:29–33

198. Simmons, F. J., Goldstein, G., Boyle, J. D. 1970. A controlled clinical trial of lactulose in hepatic encephalopathy. *Gastroenterology* 59:827–32

199. Smith, A. R., Rossi-Fanelli, F., Ziparo, V., James, J. H., Perelle, B. A., Fischer, J. E. 1978. Serial alterations in CSF and plasma metabolites, amino acids and 5-hydroxyindole acetic acid in hepatic coma in the dog. *Ann. Surg.* 187:343–50

200. Smith, A. R., Rossi-Fanelli, F., Freund, H., Fischer, J. E. 1979. Sulfur-containing amino acids in experimental hepatic coma in the dog and the monkey. *Surgery* 85:677–83

201. Soeters, P. B., Fischer, J. E. 1976. Insulin, glucagon, amino acid imbalance and hepatic encephalopathy. *Lancet* ii:880–82

202. Soeters, P. B., Weir, G. C., Ebeid, A. M., Fischer, J. E. 1977. Insulin, glucagon, portasystemic shunting and

hepatic failure in the dog. *J. Surg. Res.* 23:183–88

203. Summerskill, W. H. J., Ammon, H. V., Baggenstoss, A. H. 1974. Treatment of chronic hepatitis. In *The Liver and Its Diseases,* ed. F. Schaffner, S. Sherlock, C. M. Leevy. NY: Intercontinental Medical Book Corporation, pp. 218–26

204. Summerskill, W. H. J., Thorsell, F., Feinberg, J. 1968. Effect of urease inhibition in hyperammonemia: clinical and experimental studies with acetohydroxamic acid. *Gastroenterology* 54:20–26

205. Summerskill, W. H. J., Wolfe, S. J. 1957. The metabolism of ammonia and α-keto acids in liver disease and hepatic coma. *J. Clin. Invest.* 36:361–72

206. Svec, M. H., Freeman, S. 1949. Effect of impaired hepatic circulation on plasma free amino acids of dogs. *Am. J. Physiol.* 159:357–64

207. Swart, G. R., Frenkel, M., Von den Berg, V. W. O. 1981. Minimum protein requirements in advanced liver disease: a metabolic ward study of the effects of oral branched chain amino acids. See Ref. 50, pp. 427–33

208. Takahashi, Y. 1963. Serum lipids in liver disease and the relationship of serum lipids and hepatic coma. *Jpn. J. Gastroenterol.* 60:571–79

209. Tanaka, K., Isselbacher, K. F., Shih, V. 1962. Isovaleric and α-methylbutric acidemias induced by hypoglycin A: mechanism of Jamaican vomiting sickness. *Science* 175:69–71

210. Terblanche, J. 1980. The management of patients with portal hypertension and oesophageal varices. *S. Afr. Med. J.* 57:616–19

211. Teychenne, P. R., Walters, I., Claveria, L. E. 1976. The encephalopathic action of five-carbon-atom fatty acids in the rabbit. *Clin. Sci. Mol.* 50:463–72

212. Trey, C., Burns, D., Saunders, S. 1966. Treatment of hepatic coma by exchange blood transfusions. *N. Engl. J. Med.* 274:473–81

213. Tyce, G. M., Owen, C. A. 1978. Dopamine and norepinephrine in the brains of hepatectomized rats. *Life Sci.* 22: 781–86

214. Unger, R. H. 1971. Glucagon physiology and pathophysiology. *N. Engl. J. Med.* 285:443–49

215. Waggoner, R. W., Malamud, N. 1942. Wilson's disease in the light of cerebral changes following ordinary acquired liver disorders. *J. Nerv. Dis.* 96:410–23

216. Wahren, J. J., Denis, J., Desurmont, P., Ericson, S. et al. 1981. Is i.v. administration of branched-chain amino acids effective in the treatment of hepatic encephalopathy of multicenter study? *Eur. Soc. Parent. Enter. Nutr.* FC47:61

217. Walker, C. O., McCandless, D. W., McCarry, J. D., Schenker, S. 1970. Cerebral metabolism in short chain fatty acid-induced coma. *J. Lab. Clin. Med.* 76:569–83

218. Walker, C. O., Speeg, K. V. Jr., Levinson, J. D., Schenker, S. 1971. Cerebral acetylcholine, serotonin and norepinephrine in acute ammonia intoxication. *Proc. Soc. Exp. Biol. Med.* 136:668–71

219. Walser, M., Lund, P., Ruderman, N. B., Coulter, A. W. 1973. Synthesis of essential amino acids from their α-keto analogues by perfused rat liver and muscle. *J. Clin. Invest.* 52:2856–68

220. Walshe, J. M. 1951. Observations on the symptomatology and pathogenesis of hepatic coma. *Q. J. Med.* 20:421–38

221. Wannemacher, R. W. Jr., Dinterman, R. E. 1977. Total body catabolism in starved and infected rats. *Am. J. Clin. Nutr.* 30:1510–12

222. Ware, A. J., D'Agostino, A. N., Combes, B. 1971. Cerebral adema: a major complication of massive hepatic necrosis. *Gastroenterology* 61:877–84

223. Warren, K. S., Shenker, S. 1964. Effect of an inhibitor of glutamine synthesis (methionine sulfoxamine) on ammonia toxicity and metabolism. *J. Lab. Clin. Med.* 64:442–49

224. Watanabe, A. 1979. Serum amino acids in hepatic encephalopathy–effects of branched-chain amino acid infusion in serum aminograms. *Acta Hepatogastroenterol.* 26:346–57

225. Weber, F. L., Maddrey, W. C., Walser, M. et al. 1975. Intestinal absorption and metabolism of α-keto-α-methylvalerate. *Clin. Res.* 23:260A

226. Weber, F. L. Jr., Reiser, B. A. 1981. Relationship of plasma amino acids to nitrogen balance and portal systemic encephalopathy in liver disease. *Dig. Dis. Sci.* In press

227. Webster, L. T., Gabuzda, G. J. 1957. Effect on portal blood ammonium concentration of administering methionine to patients with hepatic cirrhosis. *J. Lab. Clin. Med.* 50:426–31

228. Williams, A. H., Kyu, Ma Hta, Fenton, J. C. B., Cavanagh, J. B. 1972. The glutamine and glutamine content of rat brain after portacaval anastomosis. *J. Neurochem.* 19:1073–77

229. Williams, R. 1973. Hepatic encephalopathy. *J. R. Coll. Physicians London* 8:63–74

230. Wolpers, E., Phillips, S. F., Summerskill, W. H. J. 1970. Ammonia production in the human colon. Effects of clearing, neomycin, and acetohydroxamic acid. *N. Engl. J. Med.* 283:159–64
231. Wu, C. J., Bollman, G., Butt, H. R. 1955. Changes in free amino acids in the plasma during hepatic coma. *J. Clin. Invest.* 34:845–49
232. Wurtman, R. J., Rose, C. M., Mathysse, S., Stephenson, J., Baldessarini, R. 1970. L-dihydroxyphenylalanine: effect on S-adenosylmethionine in brain. *Science* 169:395–97
233. Wyke, R. J., Thornton, A., Portmann, B., Zuckerman, A. J., Tsiquaye, K. N.,

Williams, R. 1979. Transmission of non-A, non-B, hepatitis to chimpanzees by factor IX concentrates in patients with chronic liver disease. *Lancet* i:520–24
234. Zieve, F. J., Zieve, L., Doizaki, W. M., Gilsdorf, R. B. 1974. Synergism between ammonia and fatty acids in the production of coma: implication for hepatic coma. *J. Pharmacol. Exp. Therap.* 191:10–16
235. Zanchin, G., Rigotti, P., Oussini, N., Vassanell, P., Battistin, L. 1979. Cerebral amino acid levels and uptake in rats after portacaval anastomosis: II. *J. Neurosci. Res.* 4:301–10

AUTHOR INDEX

(Names appearing in capital letters indicate authors of chapters in this volume.)

SUBJECT INDEX

A

Acetaldehyde
  colchicine binding to liver
    tubulin and, 37
  physiologic response to, 56
Acetaminophen
  acute hepatic necrosis and,
    438–39
Acetazolamide
  bone changes and, 214
Acetoacetate
  placental transport of, 94
Acetohydroxamic acid
  hepatic encephalopathy
    therapy and, 438
Acid-base balance
  total parenteral nutrition
    and, 190
Acrodermatitis enteropathica
  immune response in, 167
  zinc deficiency and, 160–61
Actinomyces viscosus
  oral
    xylitol and, 140
Acute myeloblastic leukemia
  lipid composition of blast
    cells in, 285
Adenylic acid
  mouth ulceration and, 12–13
ADH
  water intake and, 73–74
ADH release
  osmotic regulation of, 74–76
  RAS and, 81–83
Adipose tissue
  obesity and, 100–2
Adipsia, 85
Adriamycin
  cardiomyopathy and, 60
Alanine
  excretion of
    malignant melanoma and,
      291
Albumin
  liver disease and, 36–37
  zinc transport and, 161
Alcohol
  aortic atherosclerosis and, 65
  cardiomyopathy and, 57–60
  cardiovascular beriberi and,
    60–61
  cardiovascular diseases and
    public health aspects of,
      66–67
  cardiovascular system and,
    51–67
  coronary atherosclerotic
    disease and, 62–65

coronary circulation and,
    55–56
  heart muscle structure and,
    56–57
  heart pumping action and,
    54–55
  heart rate, blood pressure,
    and blood vessel tone
    and, 53
  hypertension and, 61–62
  myocardial biochemistry and,
    56
  noncoronary atherosclerotic
    disease and, 66
  stroke and, 65
  see also Ethanol
Alcoholic cardiomyopathy,
    57–60
Alcoholic hepatitis
  tyrosine formation and, 29
  urea cycle and, 32
    corticosteroid therapy and,
      33
Alcoholics
  dietary intake and nutritional
    status of, 22–23
Alcoholism
  beriberi and, 1
  digestion and absorption
    disorders and, 24–25
Aldoses
  nutritional importance of,
    119
Aldosterone
  alcohol and, 53
Alkaline phosphatase
  zinc and, 164
Allopurinol
  senses of taste and smell and,
    218
Alpha-keto analogs
  hepatic encephalopathy
    therapy and, 443–44
Aluminum hydroxide
  phosphate depletion and, 216
Amino acid absorption
  ethanol and, 25
Amino acid imbalance
  hepatic encephalopathy and,
    419–45
Amino acid infusion
  hepatic encephalopathy
    therapy and, 441–43
Amino acid metabolism
  brain, 429–31
  cancer cells and, 286–87
  peripheral, 425–29
    acute hepatic necrosis and,
      428–29

catabolism and, 428
  hormones and, 427–28
Amino acids
  branched-chain
    hepatic encephalopathy
      therapy and, 444–45
    nitrogen balance and, 183
  hepatic encephalopathy and,
    34
  hepatic encephalopathy
    therapy and, 35–36
  total parenteral nutrition
    and, 182–83
Aminoglycosides
  hepatic coma therapy and,
    437
Amitriptyline
  carbohydrate craving and,
    218
  riboflavin metabolism and,
    217
Ammonia
  hepatic encephalopathy and,
    422–23
  influx of into the brain
    hyperammonemia and, 430
Amylopectin
  dietary significance of, 121
Amylose
  dietary significance of, 121
Anemias
  see specific type
Anesthesia
  vitamin B_{12} metabolism and,
    217
Angina pectoris
  alcohol and, 63
Angiotensin
  ADH- releasing mechanism
    and, 82–83
Anorexia
  neoplastic disease and, 277
Antacids
  phosphate depletion and, 216
Antiarrhythmic agents
  alcoholic cardiomyopathy
    and, 59
Antibiotics
  hepatic coma therapy and,
    437
  hepatic encephalopathy and,
    35
  renal magnesium wasting
    and, 217
Anticholinergic drugs
  pancreatic secretion and, 259
Anticoagulants
  vitamin K and, 216
Anticonvulsants
  folate deficiency and, 214–15

484

CUMULATIVE INDEXES

CONTRIBUTING AUTHORS, VOLUMES 1,2

CHAPTER TITLES, VOLUMES 1, 2